Functional Neurosurgery and Neuromodulation

Functional Neurosurgery and Neuromodulation

AHMED M. RASLAN, MD, FAANS
Associate Professor in Neurological Surgery
Oregon Health and Science University
Portland, OR, United States

KIM J. BURCHIEL, MD, FACS
John Raaf Professor and Head
Division of Functional Neurosurgery
Department of Neurological Surgery
Oregon Health and Science University
Portland, OR, United States

ELSEVIER

ELSEVIER

3251 Riverport Lane
St. Louis, Missouri 63043

Functional Neurosurgery and Neuromodulation ISBN: 978-0-323-48569-2

Content Strategist: Belinda Kuhn
Content Development Manager: Taylor Ball
Content Development Specialist: Taylor Ball
Publishing Services Manager: Deepthi Unni
Project Manager: Nadhiya Sekar
Designer: Gopalakrishnan Venkatraman

Last digit is the print number: 9 8 7 6 5 4 3 2 1

List of Contributors

Walid A. Abdel Ghany, MD, PhD
Associate Professor
Department of Neurological Surgery
Ain Shams University
Cairo, Egypt

Isaac J. Abecassis, MD
Resident Physician
Department of Neurological Surgery
University of Washington
Seattle, WA, United States

Garrett P. Banks, MD
Department of Neurological Surgery
Columbia University
New York, NY, USA

Erik Brown, MD, PhD
Resident Physician
Department of Neurosurgery
Oregon Health & Science University
Portland, OR, United States

Carli Bullis, MD
Resident Physician
Department of Neurological Surgery
Oregon Health and Science University
Portland, OR, United States

Kim J. Burchiel, MD, FACS
Raaf Professor and Head
Division of Functional Neurosurgery
Department of Neurological Surgery
Oregon Health and Science University
Portland, Oregon USA

Purvee Patel, MD
Resident Physician
Department of Neurosurgery
Rutgers University
New Brunswick, NJ, United States

Nitesh V Patel, MD
Resident Physician
Department of Neurosurgery
Rutgers University
New Brunswick, NJ, United States

Shabbar F. Danish, MD, FAANS
Chief, Neurosurgery, Rutgers Cancer Institute Director
Stereotactic and Functional Neurosurgery Director
RWJ Gamma Knife Center Associate Professor
Rutgers-RWJ Medical School New Brunswick, NJ
United States:
Associate Professor
Robert Wood Johnson Medical School

Lia de Leon Ernst, MD
Assistant Professor
Department of Neurology
Epilepsy Center of Excellence
VA Portland Health Care System
Oregon Health and Science University
Portland, OR, United States

Michael J. Kinsman, MD
Department of Neurosurgery
The University of Kansas Medical Center
Kansas City, KS, United States

Christopher Miller, MD
Department of Neurosurgery
The University of Kansas Medical Center
Kansas City, KS, United States

Steven M. Falowski, MD, FAANS
Director Functional Neurosurgery
St. Luke's University Health Network
Bethlehem, PA, United States

Michael G.Z. Ghali, MD, PhD, MS
Resident Physician
Department of Neurosurgery
Baylor College of Medicine
Houston, TX, United States

Kunal Gupta, MBBChir (Cantab), PhD
Resident Physician
Department of Neurological Surgery
Oregon Health & Science University
Portland, OR, United States

Omaditya Khanna, MD
Resident Physician
Department of Neurological Surgery
Jack and Vickie Farber Institute for Neuroscience at Thomas Jefferson University
Philadelphia, PA, United States

Andrew L. Ko, MD
Assistant Professor
Department of Neurological Surgery
University of Washington
Seattle, WA, United States

Michael J. Lang, MD
Resident Physician
Department of Neurological Surgery
Jack and Vickie Farber Institute for Neuroscience at Thomas Jefferson University
Philadelphia, PA, United States

Paul S. Larson, MD
Professor and Vice Chair
UCSF Department of Neurological Surgery
San Francisco, CA, United States

Albert Lee, MD, MSECE, FACS
Assistant Professor
Department of Neurological Surgery
Indiana University
Indianapolis, Indiana, USA

Kevin Mansfield, MD
Instructor
Division of Functional Neurosurgery
Department of Neurological Surgery
Oregon Health and Science University
Portland, Oregon, USA

Shirley McCartney, PhD
Associate Professor
Department of Neurological Surgery
Oregon Health & Science University
Portland, OR, United States

Jonathan P. Miller, FAANS, FACS
Director
Functional and Restorative Neurosurgery Center
George R. and Constance P. Lincoln Professor and Vice Chair
Neurological Surgery
University Hospitals Cleveland Medical Center/Case Western Reserve University
University Hospitals Case Medical Center
Case Western Reserve University School of Medicine
Cleveland, OH, United States

Erika A. Petersen, MD, FAANS, FACS
Associate Professor
Department of Neurological Surgery
University of Arkansas for Medical Sciences
Little Rock, AR, United States

Julie G. Pilitsis, MD, PhD
Albany Medical Center
Albany, NY, United States

Heather N. Pinckard-Dover, MD
Resident Physician
Department of Neurological Surgery
University of Arkansas for Medical Sciences
Little Rock, AR, United States

Mohamed A. Nada, MD, PhD
Consultant Neurosurgeon
Ministry of Health hospitals
Cairo, Egypt

Abigail J. Rao, MD
Fellow
Stereotactic and Functional Neurosurgery
Department of Neurosurgery
University of California-Los Angeles and VA Greater Los Angeles Healthcare System
Los Angeles, CA, United States

Ahmed M. Raslan, MD, FAANS
Associate Professor in Neurological Surgery
Oregon Health and Science University
Portland, OR, United States

Nataly Raviv, MD
Albany Medical Center
Albany, NY, United States

Colin Roberts, MD
Associate Professor of Pediatrics
Division of Neurology
Oregon Health and Science University
Portland, United States

Nathan R. Selden, MD, PhD (Cantab)
Campagna Professor and Chair
Department of Neurological Surgery
Oregon Health & Science University
Portland, United States

Lauren Simpson, MD, MPH
Department of Neurological Surgery
Oregon Health & Science University
Portland, OR, United States

David C. Spencer, MD
Professor
Department of Neurology
Oregon Health & Science University
Portland, OR, United States

Michael D. Staudt, MD, Msc
Neurosurgery Resident
London Health Sciences Centre
The University of Western Ontario
London, ON, Canada

Geoffrey Stricsek, MD
Resident Physician
Department of Neurological Surgery
Jack and Vickie Farber Institute for Neuroscience at Thomas Jefferson University
Philadelphia, PA, United States

Ashwin Viswanathan, MD
Associate Professor
Department of Neurosurgery
Baylor College of Medicine
Houston, TX, United States

Jonathan Weyhenmeyer, MD, BSEE
Resident Physician
Indiana University/Department of Neurological Surgery
Indianapolis, Indiana, United States

Christopher J. Winfree, MD, FAANS
Department of Neurological Surgery
Columbia University
New York, NY, United States

Chengyuan Wu, MD, MSBmE
Assistant Professor
Department of Neurological Surgery
Jack and Vickie Farber Institute for Neuroscience at Thomas Jefferson University
Philadelphia, PA, United States

Christopher C. Young, MBChB, DPhil
Resident Physician
Department of Neurological Surgery
University of Washington
Seattle, WA, United States

Andrew C. Zacest, MBBS, MS, FRACS, FFPMANZCA
Department of Neurosurgery
Royal Adelaide Hospital and University of Adelaide
Adelaide, SA, Australia

Jennifer Sweet, MD
Assistant Professor, Neurosurgery, CWRU School of Medicine
Division of Functional & Stereotactic Neurosurgery
University Hospitals Cleveland Medical Center
Cleveland, Ohio, United States

Introduction

AHMED M. RASLAN, MD, FAANS • KIM J. BURCHIEL, MD, FACS

"Functional Neurosurgery" as a subspecialty has evolved over the years. Historically, stereotaxic surgery and functional neurosurgery have been linked. However, with the evolution of functional neurosurgery and neurosurgery writ large, stereotaxic surgery now encompasses much of cranial neurosurgery and occasionally, functional neurosurgery may not necessarily use stereoatactic principles.

The birth of the specialty is difficult to determine, but by the late 19th century, there were documented attempts to guide probes precisely into animal brains. A guiding arc device had been developed in Russia to be used in humans. The first well-documented description of a stereotactic device is credited to Horsley, who, along with Clark, developed the first stereotactic frame and applied it to animals.

Since then, the stereotactic and functional neurosurgery specialty has been chiefly characterized by innovation and growth.

Throughout the journey of functional neurosurgery, several impactful technologies have been developed. These technologies, were developed originally for functional neurosurgery. However, their impact and penetration extended to the entire neurosurgical field and occasionally outside neurosurgery. Radiofrequency lesioning was developed for functional neurosurgery and its use now extends to liver tumors. Stereoatactic navigation is used everyday for the vast majority of brain tumor surgery. Radiosurgery, which was developed originally for treating tremors, is mostly used nowadays for treatment of brain tumors. Deep brain stimulation and spinal cord stimulation were both originally developed for specific disease conditions, but their use continues to expand beyond their original intended uses.

The contemporary functional neurosurgeon is expected to be able to use and troubleshoot technologies such as; deep brain stimulation (including all newer permutations such as directional and closed loop systems), spinal cord stimulation (including newer permutations such as high frequency and density stimulation) burst stimulation and dorsal root ganglion (DRG) stimulation and laser ablation systems, robotic guidance systems, intraoperative imaging systems using CT or MRI, and many other technologies.

Functional neurosurgery is unique among other neurosurgical specialties since the disease paradigms treated are constantly changing and evolving. The essential concept is that functional neurosurgery does not necessarily treat a structural disorder, but rather it modifies central nervous system circuits to effect a change within or outside the nervous system. This is a powerful indication of the scope of functional neurosurgery. Diseases such as obesity, dementia, depression, or addiction are potential candidates for treatment, alongside the well-established treatable conditions such as chronic pain, epilepsy, movement disorders, and spasticity.

The contemporary definition of functional neurosurgery, therefore, extends beyond disease paradigms, since diseases and disorders treatable by functional neurosurgeons will continue to expand and be modified with time. Functional neurosurgery also extends beyond an approach of treatment. Approaches such as neuromodulation or neural ablation do not define the specialty, but rather the concept of modification of central nervous circuits to change the disease. While for last few decades, neural modulation with electricity or pharmacology had been the main approach versus neural ablation, advances in technology such as high-frequency ultrasound and laser ablation, lead to the return of ablation as an approach for treatment.

It is an exciting time for functional neurosurgery. Ours is a specialty that has benefitted substantially from technological advances in pulse generators such as the high computational power of newer processors, higher battery capacity, advances in computational neuroscience, advanced bioengineering, and sensor technologies.

Functional neurosurgeons cannot define themselves by a disease, a technique, or approach, lest this approach or disease become unfavorable for surgical treatment. Given the fast pace of advancing technology and the maturing understanding of neurological diseases, the functional neurosurgery specialty will see changes and evolution of technology in a never-before-seen pace. It is expected that functional neurosurgeons acquire and learn new, more advanced surgical and technological skills than what they learned in their training. In fact, current functional neurosurgeons graduating more than 5 years ago have had to learn and adapt to newer technologies such as laser ablation, DRG stimulation, robotic aiming, and responsive neural stimulation.

This book is designed to cover the most pertinent topics for the contemporary functional neurosurgeon. Neuromodulation constitutes a significant and important approach in contemporary functional neurosurgery, hence the title. It also serves to help the occasional physicians who use neuromodulation as part of their therapeutic toolbox, but who are not functional neurosurgeons, such as spine or pain physicians using spinal cord stimulation to treat chronic pain. It is worthwhile to note that the practice of functional neurosurgery across institutions is variable. In most academic institutions, functional neurosurgeons treat conditions such as chronic pain, trigeminal neuralgia, movement disorders, epilepsy, spasticity, and brain tumors requiring functional cortical localization using mapping techniques. Other institutions limit the practice of functional neurosurgery to a more limited spectrum of practice, such as to deep brain stimulation. Our hope is that this book will be versatile enough to be useful in a variety of neurosurgical practices.

The future is both exciting and challenging for functional neurosurgery. There will be ethical challenges in conditions treated such as dementia and post-traumatic stress disorder (PTSD). There will be economic challenges to decide which patients might benefit the most from any given treatment and to determine that the burden of disease is greater than the burden of care.

With great power and impact comes great responsibility. This is true for neurosurgery and even more so for functional neurosurgery. Our endeavor is to educate and mentor future generations to prepare them for these challenges and to honor this responsibility. To this effect, we have edited this volume to bring to the graduating and early career neurosurgeon the most pertinent and contemporary view of functional neurosurgery in a concise and accessible fashion.

Contents

CHAPTER 1

Facial Pain Classification and Outcome Measurement

SHIRLEY MCCARTNEY, PHD • KIM J. BURCHIEL, MD, FACS

INTRODUCTION

The diagnostic term "facial pain" includes an extensive list of clinical conditions such as craniofacial pain of musculoskeletal origin, including headache and migraine syndromes; orofacial pain syndromes such as dental pain, sinusitis, or temporomandibular disorders; and cranial neuralgias such as trigeminal neuralgia (TN).[1−3] The Task Force on Taxonomy of the International Association for the Study of Pain defines TN as "sudden, usually unilateral, severe brief stabbing recurrent pains in the distribution of one or more branches of the Vth cranial nerve" (006.X8a).[4] The International Headache Society uses a somewhat more detailed distinction of "Classical trigeminal neuralgia, purely paroxysmal" (13.1.1.1) and "Classical trigeminal neuralgia, with concomitant persistent facial pain" (13.1.1.2).[5] An important feature of TN is a positive response to anticonvulsants such as carbamazepine, gabapentin, or phenytoin.[6,7] This can be helpful in differentiating TN from other orofacial pain syndromes that typically do not respond. The incidence of TN was reported in 1972 as 4.3 per 100,000 persons per year, with a higher incidence for women (5.9 per 100,000) compared with men (3.4 per 100,000).[8] A 2005 study reported TN with a prevalence of 0.1−0.2 per 1000 persons and an incidence of 4−5 per 100,000 persons per year up to 20 per 100,000 persons per year after the age of 60 years,[9] and a UK study in 2006 reported TN incidence as 27 per 100,000 persons.[10] If left untreated, TN can be debilitating.[1]

In some cases, TN seems to be associated with vascular compression of the trigeminal nerve[11−16]; however, recent analysis has indicated that no clear vascular compression of the nerve can be found in approximately one-third of the cases.[17,18] In 2008, the first evidence-based international guidelines for TN management by two neurological societies were published.[19,20] Despite this, the optimal pharmacological and surgical treatments of TN continue to be debated. However, the little dispute that is fundamental to the treatment of TN is the establishment of an accurate diagnosis.[15] This chapter will focus on the diagnosis of TN and how it directly impacts the prognosis for surgical treatment.

FACIAL PAIN CLASSIFICATION

The taxonomies of pain disorders are challenging, and the classification of facial pain is no exception. Simplistic schemes designating broad categories such as TN, atypical TN, and atypical facial pain (AFP) suffered from having no objective category boundaries or grounding in a patient history. Revisions of the clinical definition of TN[4] and the introduction of classification schemes for trigeminal TN and related facial pain syndromes driven by patient history have emerged[21−24] and promise to bring a fresh perspective to the question of diagnosis.

There are few pain conditions that have as stereotyped a history as does TN. It is a diagnosis that is, in fact, completely based on the patient history. Direct questions related to the patient history such as the nature of the pain onset (sudden and memorable, or gradual), descriptors of the pains (electrical, shocklike, stabbing, radiating, burning, aching), frequency and duration of the pains, location of the pains, triggers of the pains, any pain-free intervals, and any relief of the pains by anticonvulsant medications are invaluable for diagnosis.

Fifteen years ago, we proposed a facial pain classification scheme based solely on the patient history (Table 1.1; diagnostic criteria for each diagnosis).[1,2] A patient-centered history questionnaire, with binomial yes/no responses (Fig. 1.1),[22,23] based on our facial pain classification system consisting of seven diagnoses,[1,2] type 1 (TN1), type 2 (TN2), trigeminal neuropathic pain (TNP), trigeminal deafferentation

TABLE 1.1
Classification Scheme for Trigeminal Neuralgia (TN)—Related Facial Pain Syndrome

TN Type	Description
TN1	Trigeminal neuralgia type 1. Idiopathic, spontaneous facial pain that the patient describes as predominantly (>50% of the pain) **episodic**, lancinating, and "electric."
TN2	Trigeminal neuralgia type 2. Idiopathic, spontaneous facial pain that the patient describes as predominantly (>50% of the pain) **constant** dull, aching, burning.
TNP	Trigeminal neuropathic pain. Patient history attributes to the result of accidental or unintentional injury to the trigeminal system (facial injury, dental/oral surgical procedures, or neurosurgical injury to the trigeminal nerve or one of its branches).
TDP	Trigeminal deafferentation pain. Patient history attributes result of intentional injury to the trigeminal system, such as trigeminal neurectomy or rhizotomy, i.e., "anesthesia dolorosa" or its variants.
STN	Symptomatic trigeminal neuralgia. Result of multiple sclerosis.
PHN	Postherpetic neuralgia. Historical result of painful sequela of herpes zoster (shingles) outbreak in the trigeminal distribution (usually V1-2).
AFP	Atypical facial pain. Suspected psychogenic pain, established only by psychologic interview and testing.

pain (TDP), symptomatic TN (STN), postherpetic neuralgia (PHN), and AFP, was developed and published as an artificial neural network (ANN) in 2006[22] and subsequently updated in 2014.[1,2,23] In neurosurgery, ANNs can be effectively used for diagnosis, prognosis, and outcome prediction.[25] Since its inception, this diagnostic facial pain tool has been implemented as a free, web-based application using an ANN. This web-based application (https://neurosurgery.ohsu.edu/tgn.php; Academic Licence OHSU #2271)[26] allows anyone seeking a diagnosis for their facial pain to anonymously answer questions related to the nature of their facial pain and establish a diagnosis. The ANN described here is powered by patient data (collected under an institutional review board–approved research study with subject consent) for which the predicted diagnosis is correct and included in a secured database for future ANN training. The number of datasets has increased over time, and continuous refinement and improvement of the ANN are ongoing. The classification system and the ANN used have proven to have a high sensitivity (number of true positives/number of true positives + number of false negatives) and specificity (number of true negatives/number of true negatives + number of false positives) for TN1, TN2, TNP, and PHN (Fig. 1.2). Statistical analysis of other diagnoses (TDP, STN) is limited by low numbers of patients in our dataset, and by definition, the diagnosis of AFP cannot be made solely on the basis of a questionnaire. The goal of such a diagnostic patient-driven system is to arm patients, particularly those with TN1, with a diagnosis to allow them to seek out proper clinical care, avoid ineffective or ill-advised medical and or surgical therapy, and increase patient satisfaction.

Recently, Cruccu et al. proposed an additional new TN classification and diagnostic grading for practice and research.[27] Their definition and diagnostic classification requirements for idiopathic, classical, and secondary TN were based on review of clinical and etiologic features of TN. As the authors point out, TN caused by neurovascular compression (NVC) is the most frequent form; however, by their estimate, in approximately 11% of TN patients the etiology remains unclear.[18,28–30] Practice guidelines for diagnosis and treatment of classical TN (French Headache Society and French Neurosurgical Society) are also available.[31]

CLINICAL OUTCOMES

Using the diagnostic facial pain classification scheme described above,[1,2] we have reported that the categorization of TN1 and TN2 has significant implications for the outcome of surgery for these conditions,[32] as well as for separating these two entities in distinct clinical, pathologic, and prognostic entities.[33] Pain relief after microvascular decompression (MVD) was strongly correlated with the lancinating pain component of TN, and therefore the type of TN pain is the best predictor of long-term outcome after MVD.[33] TN1 patients were older than TN2 patients, were more likely to have right-sided symptoms, and reported shorter symptom duration. TN1 was significantly more likely to be associated with arterial compression, whereas venous or no compression was more common in TN2 patients. TN1 patients were also more likely to be pain-free immediately after MVD and less likely to have a recurrence of pain within 2 years.[32]

OHSU

Diagnostic Questions

Here at OHSU's Department of Neurological Surgery we have developed a helpful questionnaire for the diagnosis and treatment of patients suffering from varies types of trigeminal neuralgia.

1	Do you have facial pain?	yes/no
2	Do you remember exactly where you were the moment your facial pain started?	yes/no
3	When you have pain, is it predominantly in your face (i.e., forehead, eye, cheek, nose, upper/lower jaw, teeth, lips, etc)?	yes/no
4	Do you have pain just on one side of your face?	yes/no
5	When you have pain, is it predominantly deep in your ear?	yes/no
6	When you have pain, is it predominantly deep in your throat or tongue, near the area of your tonsil?	yes/no
7	Is your pain either entirely or mostly brief (seconds to minutes) and unpredictable sensations (electrical, shocking, stabbing, shooting)?	yes/no
8	Do you have any constant background facial pain (e.g., aching, burning, throbbing, stinging)?	yes/no
9	Do you have constant background facial pain (aching, burning, throbbing, stinging) for more than half of your waking hours?	yes/no
10	Do you have any constant facual numbness? yesno	
11	Can your pain start by something touching your face (for example, by eating, washing your face, shaving, brushing teeth, wind)?	yes/no
12	Since your pain began have you ever experienced periods of weeks, months, or years, when you were pain-free? (This would not include periods after any pain-relieving surgery or while you were on medications for your pain.)	yes/no
13	Have you ever taken Tegretol® (carbamazepine), Neurontin® (gabapentin), Lioresal® (baclofen), Treleptal® (oxcarbazepine), Topamax® (topiramate), Zonegran® (zonisamide), or any other anticonvulsant medication for your pain?	yes/no
14	Did you ever experience any major reduction in facial pain (partial or complete) from taking any of the medications listed in question 13, or any anticonvulsant medication?	yes/no
15	Have you ever had trigeminal nerve surgery for your pain? (e.g., neurectomy, RF rhizotomy/ gangliolysis, glycerol injection, ballon comperession, rhizotomy, MVD, gamma knife)	yes/no
16	Have you ever experienced any major reduction in facial pain (partial or compleet) from trigeminal nerve surgery for your pain? (e.g., neurectomy, RF rhizotomy/gangliolysis, glycerol injection, balloon compression, rhizotomy, MVD, gamma knife)	yes/no
17	Did your current pain start only after trigeminal nerve surgery (neurectomy, RF rhizotomy/ gangliolysis, glycerol injection, balloon compression, rhizotomy, MVD, gamma knife)? (If this is a recurrence of your original pain after a successful trigeminal nerve surgery, answer "no")	yes/no
18	Did your pain start after facial zoster or "shingles" rash (Herpes zoster - not to be confused with "fever blisters" around the mouth)?	yes/no
19	Do you have multiple sclerosis?	yes/no
20	Did your pain start after a facial injury?	yes/no
21	Did your pain start only after facial surgery (oral surgery, ENT suergery, plastic suergery)?	yes/no

FIG. 1.1 Facial pain patient-centered history questionnaire, with binomial yes/no responses (developed at Oregon Health & Science University—18 questions in 2006[22] and updated to 22 questions in 2014[23]; https://neurosurgery.ohsu.edu/tgn.php; Academic Licence OHSU #2271[26]).

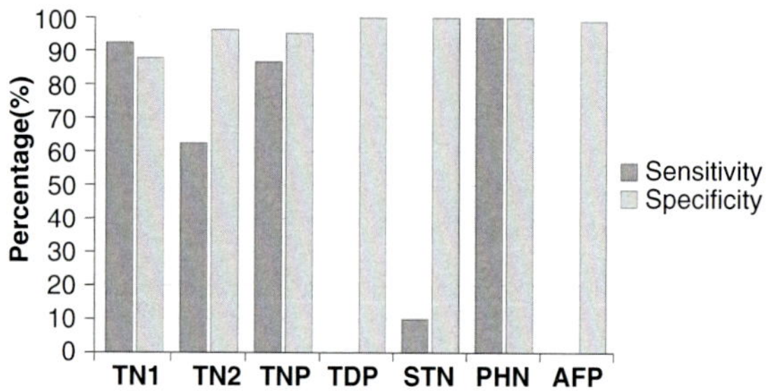

FIG. 1.2 Artificial neural network sensitivity and specificity data for diagnoses TN1, TN2, TNP, TDP, STN, PHN and AFP. *AFP*, atypical facial pain; *TDP*, trigeminal deafferentation pain; *TN1*, trigeminal neuralgia type 1; *TN2*, trigeminal neuralgia type 2; *TNP*, trigeminal neuropathic pain; *PHN*, postherpetic neuralgia.

We have also reported on significant differences in imaging characteristics of TN1 and TN2 patients with regard to the incidence, type, and severity of NVC.[34] With regard to NVC, we reported that NVC is "neither sufficient nor necessary for the development of TN" and patients with TN without NVC may represent a distinct population of younger, predominantly female, patients who may require different surgical interventions such as internal neurolysis.[17,35]

Our facial pain classification scheme has also been used for other outcome assessment for MVD surgery,[36] stereotactic radiosurgery (SRS; γ knife)[37]; an evaluation of reliability and predictive ability of 1.5-T magnetic resonance imaging for diagnosis of symptomatic vascular contact[38]; and a comparison of percutaneous balloon compression (PBC) and percutaneous retrogasserian glycerol rhizotomy (PRGR) as TN treatments.[39] Sekula et al. reported that patients with TN (maxillary nerve; V2) treated by MVD were more likely to be female, tended toward a TN2 classification with venous pathology, and surgical outcomes were similar to TN1.[36] Singh et al. evaluated pain relief using visual analog scale (VAS) scores after SRS in TN1 and TN2 patients. Initial pain relief was similar for TN1 (87.2%) and TN2 (86.8%) patients, a higher initial VAS score was associated with a greater likelihood of treatment success for TN1 patients, and no prognostic factors were found to significantly impact the likelihood of initial pain relief for TN2 patients. Apslund et al. showed that PBC and PRGR were effective as primary surgical treatment for TN1 patients and favored PBC over PRGR as a result of lower incidence of dysesthesia, corneal hypesthesia, and technical failures.[39]

Additionally, the subdivision of TN into TN1 and TN2 has promoted research into the causes and treatment of TN[40] and is now included in the National Institutes of Neurological Disorders and Stroke Trigeminal Neuralgia Fact Sheet, which was published in 2013.[41]

CONCLUSION

If left untreated, TN can be physically and mentally debilitating.[1] TN diagnosis is based primarily on patient history and description of symptoms, along with physical and neurologic examination and imaging results. Accurate diagnosis and timely surgical consultation and intervention are essential to determine future medical and/or surgical course and outcome. With emerging information surrounding presence versus absence of NVC and presentation in a younger age group, careful rethinking of treatment options is warranted.

The use of a patient-centered history-gathering questionnaire directly tied to a facial classification scheme built on an ANN, as described here, has shown success.

REFERENCES

1. Burchiel KJ. A new classification for facial pain. *Neurosurgery*. 2003;53(5):1164–1166.
2. Eller J, Raslan A, Burchiel K. Trigeminal neuralgia: definition and classification. *Neurosurg Focus*. 2005;18(5):E3.
3. Zakrzewska JM, Jensen TS. History of facial pain diagnosis. *Cephalalgia*. 2017. https://doi.org/10.1177/0333102417691045.
4. Merskey H, Bogduk N. *Classification of Chronic Pain: Descriptions of Chronic Pain Syndromes and Definitions of Pain Terms*. 2nd ed. Seattle: IASP Press; 1994.
5. International Headache Society, Headache Classification Committee of the International Headache Society (IHS). The international classification of headache Disorders, 3rd ed. (beta version). *Cephalalgia*; 2013. http://www.ihs-headache.org/binary_data/1437_ichd-iii-beta-cephalalgia-issue-9-2013.pdf.
6. Loeser J. Tic douloureux and atypical facial pain. In: Wall P, Melzack R, eds. *Textbook of Pain*. 3rd ed. London: Churchill Livingstone; 1994:699–710.
7. Wiffen P, Collins S, McQuay H, Carroll D, Jadad A, Moore A. Anticonvulsant drugs for acute and chronic pain. *Cochrane Database Syst Rev*. 2005;(3):CD001133.
8. Yoshimasu F, Kurland LT, Elveback LR. Tic douloureux in Rochester, Minnesota, 1945–1969. *Neurology*. 1972;22(9):952–956.
9. Manzoni GC, Torelli P. Epidemiology of typical and atypical craniofacial neuralgias. *Neurol Sci*. 2005;26(suppl 2):s65–s67.
10. Hall GC, Carroll D, Parry D, McQuay HJ. Epidemiology and treatment of neuropathic pain: the UK primary care perspective. *Pain*. 2006;122(1–2):156–162.

11. Hamlyn PJ. Neurovascular relationships in the posterior cranial fossa, with special reference to trigeminal neuralgia. 1. Review of the literature and development of a new method of vascular injection-filling in cadaveric controls. *Clin Anat*. 1997;10(6):371–379.
12. Hamlyn PJ, King TT. Neurovascular compression in trigeminal neuralgia: a clinical and anatomical study. *J Neurosurg*. 1992;76(6):948–954.
13. Hilton DA, Love S, Gradidge T, Coakham HB. Pathological findings associated with trigeminal neuralgia caused by vascular compression. *Neurosurgery*. 1994;35(2):299–303; discussion 303.
14. Jannetta PJ. Arterial compression of the trigeminal nerve at the pons in patients with trigeminal neuralgia. *J Neurosurg*. 1967;26(suppl 1):159–162.
15. Klun B, Prestor B. Microvascular relations of the trigeminal nerve: an anatomical study. *Neurosurgery*. 1986;19(4): 535–539.
16. Love S, Hilton DA, Coakham HB. Central demyelination of the Vth nerve root in trigeminal neuralgia associated with vascular compression. *Brain Pathol*. 1998;8(1): 1–11; discussion 11–12.
17. Ko AL, Lee A, Raslan AM, Ozpinar A, McCartney S, Burchiel KJ. Trigeminal neuralgia without neurovascular compression presents earlier than trigeminal neuralgia with neurovascular compression. *J Neurosurg*. 2015; 123(6):1519–1527.
18. Lee A, McCartney S, Burbidge C, Raslan AM, Burchiel KJ. Trigeminal neuralgia occurs and recurs in the absence of neurovascular compression. *J Neurosurg*. 2014;120(5): 1048–1054.
19. Gronseth G, Cruccu G, Alksne J, et al. Practice parameter: the diagnostic evaluation and treatment of trigeminal neuralgia (an evidence-based review): report of the Quality Standards Subcommittee of the American Academy of Neurology and the European Federation of Neurological Societies. *Neurology*. 2008;71(15):1183–1190.
20. Cruccu G, Gronseth G, Alksne J, et al. AAN-EFNS guidelines on trigeminal neuralgia management. *Eur J Neurol*. 2008;15(10):1013–1028.
21. Zakrzewska JM. Facial pain: an update. *Curr Opin Support Palliat Care*. 2009;3(2):125–130.
22. Limonadi FM, McCartney S, Burchiel KJ. Design of an artificial neural network for diagnosis of facial pain syndromes. *Stereotact Funct Neurosurg*. 2006;84(5–6): 212–220.
23. McCartney S, Weltin M, Burchiel KJ. Use of an artificial neural network for diagnosis of facial pain syndromes: an update. *Stereotact Funct Neurosurg*. 2014;92(1): 44–52.
24. Siccoli MM, Bassetti CL, Sándor PS. Facial pain: clinical differential diagnosis. *Lancet Neurol*. 2006;5(3):257–267.
25. Azimi P, Mohammadi HR, Benzel EC, Shahzadi S, Azhari S, Montazeri A. Artificial neural networks in neurosurgery. *J Neurol Neurosurg Psychiatry*. 2015;86(3):251–256.
26. Oregon Health & Science University. Academic license for diagnostic classification and questionnaire for facial pain. http://www.ohsu.edu/tech-transfer/portal/agreement_terms.php?agreement_id=42&technology_id=2520309.
27. Cruccu G, Finnerup NB, Jensen TS, et al. Trigeminal neuralgia: new classification and diagnostic grading for practice and research. *Neurology*. 2016;87(2):220–228.
28. Antonini G, Di Pasquale A, Cruccu G, et al. Magnetic resonance imaging contribution for diagnosing symptomatic neurovascular contact in classical trigeminal neuralgia: a blinded case-control study and meta-analysis. *Pain*. 2014;155(8):1464–1471.
29. Miller JP, Acar F, Hamilton BE, Burchiel KJ. Radiographic evaluation of trigeminal neurovascular compression in patients with and without trigeminal neuralgia. *J Neurosurg*. 2009;110(4):627–632.
30. Sindou M, Leston J, Howeidy T, Decullier E, Chapuis F. Micro-vascular decompression for primary trigeminal neuralgia (typical or atypical). Long-term effectiveness on pain; prospective study with survival analysis in a consecutive series of 362 patients. *Acta Neurochir (Wien)*. 2006; 148(12):1235–1245; discussion 1245.
31. Donnet A, Simon E, Cuny E, et al. French guidelines for diagnosis and treatment of classical trigeminal neuralgia (French Headache Society and French Neurosurgical Society). *Rev Neurol (Paris)*. 2017;173(3):131–151. https://doi.org/10.1016/j.neurol.2016.12.033. Epub 2017 Mar 15.
32. Miller JP, Acar F, Burchiel KJ. Classification of trigeminal neuralgia: clinical, therapeutic, and prognostic implications in a series of 144 patients undergoing microvascular decompression. *J Neurosurg*. 2009;111(6):1231–1234.
33. Miller JP, Magill ST, Acar F, Burchiel KJ. Predictors of long-term success after microvascular decompression for trigeminal neuralgia. *J Neurosurg*. 2009;110(4):620–626.
34. Zacest AC, Magill ST, Miller J, Burchiel KJ. Preoperative magnetic resonance imaging in type 2 trigeminal neuralgia. *J Neurosurg*. 2010;113(3):511–515.
35. Ko AL, Ozpinar A, Lee A, Raslan AM, McCartney S, Burchiel KJ. Long-term efficacy and safety of internal neurolysis for trigeminal neuralgia without neurovascular compression. *J Neurosurg*. 2015;122(5):1048–1057.
36. Sekula RF, Frederickson AM, Jannetta PJ, Bhatia S, Quigley MR, Abdel Aziz KM. Microvascular decompression in patients with isolated maxillary division trigeminal neuralgia, with particular attention to venous pathology. *Neurosurg Focus*. 2009;27(5):E10.
37. Singh R, Davis J, Sharma S. Stereotactic radiosurgery for trigeminal neuralgia: a eetrospective multi-institutional examination of treatment outcomes. *Cureus*. 2016;8(4):e554.
38. Panczykowski DM, Frederickson AM, Hughes MA, Oskin JE, Stevens DR, Sekula Jr RF. A blinded, case-control trial assessing the value of steady state free precession magnetic resonance imaging in the diagnosis of trigeminal neuralgia. *World Neurosurg*. 2016;89:427–433.

39. Asplund P, Blomstedt P, Bergenheim AT. Percutaneous balloon compression vs percutaneous retrogasserian glycerol rhizotomy for the primary treatment of trigeminal neuralgia. *Neurosurgery*. 2016;78(3):421–428; discussion 428.
40. Montano N, Conforti G, Di Bonaventura R, Meglio M, Fernandez E, Papacci F. Advances in diagnosis and treatment of trigeminal neuralgia. *Ther Clin Risk Manag*. 2015;11:289–299.
41. National Institutes of Neurological Disorders and Stroke. Trigeminal Neuralgia Fact Sheet. https://www.ninds.nih.gov/Disorders/Patient-Caregiver-Education/Fact-Sheets/Trigeminal-Neuralgia-Fact-Sheet.

CHAPTER 2

Microvascular Decompression

LAUREN SIMPSON, MD, MPH • AHMED M. RASLAN, MD, FAANS

INTRODUCTION

Trigeminal neuralgia (TN) is a syndrome characterized by sudden, usually unilateral, severe brief stabbing recurrent pain in one or more distributions of the trigeminal nerve. The severe lancinating quality of the unilateral facial pain and pattern of paroxysmal episodes separated by pain-free periods are key characteristics that help to distinguish it from other facial pain syndromes. Neurovascular compression of the trigeminal nerve where it enters the brainstem has been pathophysiologically associated with the development of TN in many patients. As such, microvascular decompression via a retrosigmoid approach can be performed to separate the vessel from the trigeminal nerve. Microvascular decompression is the most successful and durable surgical approach for TN. However, care must be taken to wisely choose to operate on the appropriate patient population to provide benefit from microvascular decompression.

HISTORY

Physicians have been studying, evaluating, and treating patients with TN for the past 2.5 millennia. Aretaeus of Cappadocia (AD 150), a celebrated Greek physician, is credited for the first description of TN as a headache in which "spasm and distortion of the countenance take place." Aretaeus documented accounts of hemicranial headaches occurring in paroxysmal attacks accompanied by a facial spasm, followed by a fainting spell, separated by pain-free intervals. Interestingly, as early as the 11th century, Jujani, an Arab physician, suggested that "the proximity of the artery to the nerve" is the cause of a unilateral facial pain syndrome associated with facial spasm and anxiety. Further descriptions throughout the 17th and 18th centuries better characterized TN and helped differentiate it from other facial pain syndromes. In 1671, Fehr spoke about the syndrome in a eulogy. And in 1677, physician John Locke recalled a "fit of such violent and exquisite torment that it forced her to ... cries and shrieks ... which extended itself all over the right side of her face and mouth." André coined the term "tic douloureux" in his description of a convulsive-like condition. In 1756, he described it as "a cruel and obscure illness, which causes ... in the face some violent motions, some hideous grimaces which are an insurmountable obstacle to the reception of food, [and] which put off sleep." John Fothergill gave the first accurate and comprehensive clinical description of TN as in a 1773 writing to the medical society of London about 14 patients with disease.

Early treatment of TN was on the basis of the belief that it was a form of epileptic seizure in the brainstem trigeminal complex. Bergouignan used phenytoin to relieve TN, and patient response to antiepileptic drugs supported this original theory. As such, surgical management aimed to ablate the epileptogenic foci by lesioning of the trigeminal nerve. In 1934, Walter Dandy approached the trigeminal nerve via retrosigmoid craniotomy and wrote, "In many instances the nerve is grooved or bent in an angle by the artery. This I believe is the cause of *tic douloureux*." Although Dandy equated neurovascular compression to the development of TN, he believed that this was an irreversible pathologic process and did not attempt to decompress the trigeminal nerve. In 1959, W. James Gardner performed the first microvascular decompression. He mobilized a vessel from the trigeminal nerve and maintained a barrier by placing a piece of absorbable gelatin sponge (Gelfoam) between them. In the 1970s, Peter Jannetta refined the microvascular decompression technique with the aid of the operating microscope. He performed thousands of microvascular decompressions and popularized surgical management for TN by demonstrating the prospect of lasting pain relief in the appropriately selected population of patients. Microvascular decompression accounts for over 90%

of surgical procedures performed for treatment of neuralgic facial pain. Since the early 1990s, it has remained the most common procedure performed for TN.

PATHOPHYSIOLOGY

Early on, physician scientists determined that the presence of an adjacent vessel, tumor, cyst, arteriovascular malformation, aneurysm, or demyelination plaque in relation to the brainstem trigeminal complex and subsequent development of ipsilateral paroxysmal trigeminal pain leads to formation of the belief that TN is a neuropathic pain state of the central or peripheral nervous system. The popularization of Microvascular Decompression(MVDs) bolstered support for vascular compression and demyelination as the pathophysiologic mechanism of pain production in TN.[1]

The pathophysiology of TN has been associated with vascular compression of the trigeminal nerve at the Obersteiner-Redlich zone, which is the transitional region a few millimeters before the trigeminal nerve enters the brainstem where axons are ensheathed by peripheral myelin produced by Schwann cells and central myelin produced by oligodendrocytes. Specifically, the trigeminal nerve axons ensheathed by central myelin are thought to be particularly susceptible to pathologic changes induced by adjacent dynamic vascular contact. Damage from vascular compression results in demyelination, loss of axons, and altered conduction.[2,3]

The pathology and mechanism of pain production in TN is not fully understood. The theory that sustained or pulsatile vascular compression causes demyelination of sensory axons in trigeminal roots is supported by the high incidence of TN among multiple sclerosis, high incidence of compression in TN, and prolonged relief after microvascular decompression.[4,5] However, activity in myelinated axons is generally associated with vibration sense and touch, not pain. As such, demyelination would be expected to halt impulse propagation and produce patchy numbness rather than pain. Furthermore, several hallmarks of TN symptomatology are conceptually inconsistent with the demyelination theory. The following questions began the case against demyelination: Why is the onset and termination of symptoms abrupt? Why are the symptoms able to be triggered? Why does the pain outlast the trigger? Why do people often have the lesion associated with TN, i.e., compression or demyelinated plaques without having the symptoms? These questions were addressed by the ignition theory.

Histopathologic study of trigeminal nerve biopsy specimens from patients undergoing microvascular decompression and advances in the understanding of abnormal electrical behavior in injured sensory neurons led to the development of the ignition hypothesis. The basis of which are ectopic pacemaker sites, including patches of demyelination, nerve-ending sprouts, and swollen end bulbs. These abnormalities of trigeminal afferent neurons in the trigeminal root or ganglion are plentiful in patients with TN. Axons and axotomized somata are rendered hyperexcitable by these injuries, which give rise to pain paroxysms as a result of synchronized after discharge activity. Ectopic impulse generation with chain reaction formation leads to "ignition" of TN pain. Triggerability with after-discharge phenomena occurs due to neuron acquisition of resonance after axonal injury. The phenomena of resonance, or sinusoidal oscillations in membrane potential, provide the ability to fire in a sustained manner and thus provide the fuel for the pain that outlasts the initial trigger, i.e., autonomous activity. Emphatic contact between denuded axons allows for one-to-one duplication of impulses and neural amplification of impulses. Calcium influx during paroxysms activates calcium-dependent potassium channels which out-flux causing hyperpolarization and refractoriness.[6]

Still, vascular compression plays an important role in patients with TN due to compression. In 2014, Leal et al. sought to prospectively evaluate atrophic changes in trigeminal nerves using measurements of volume and cross-sectional area from high-resolution 3-T MR images obtained in patients with unilateral TN and to correlate these data with patient and neurovascular compression characteristics and with clinical outcomes. They developed the Sindou classification of vascular compression graded I, II, and III whereby Grade I is mere contact between the symptomatic trigeminal nerve and vessel, Grade II is displacement or distortion of root due to vascular compression, and Grade III is marked indentation of the symptomatic trigeminal nerve due to vascular compression. They found that the mean volume and cross-sectional area of the trigeminal nerve on symptomatic side of the face were significantly smaller than those for the asymptomatic side of the face. Patients cured by microvascular decompression had symptomatic trigeminal nerves that were smaller than those in patients with partial pain relief or treatment failure. Thus, trigeminal nerve atrophic changes in patients with TN significantly correlated with the severity of compression and clinical outcomes.[7]

Neurovascular compression in TN can be caused by arteries and veins. The superior cerebellar artery (SCA) is most often the source of compression, and venous structures frequently contribute to compression in 68%. The anterior inferior cerebellar artery is sometimes the offending vessel, and occasionally, veins are the only identified source of compression. The compression vector determines which trigeminal nerve division will be symptomatic based on nerve root fiber lamination pattern.

Cranial compression causes ophthalmic division symptom. As such, it is unusual to have TN only in the first ophthalmic division of the trigeminal nerve. Medial compression causes maxillary division symptoms, and lateral or caudal compression causes mandibular division symptoms. In patients with TN, pathologic changes of the trigeminal nerve may be reversed after microvascular decompression. Investigators performing nerve root and scalp electrode recordings found immediate neurophysiologic improvement once the compressive vessel was separated from the trigeminal nerve (Leandri et al.). Improvement in both sensory thresholds and asymmetric jaw motion has also been demonstrated following microvascular decompression as well.

Vascular compression certainly plays a principal role in root entry zone demyelination and subsequent trigeminal nerve hyperactivity; however, many other factors must contribute to the pathogenesis of TN. Radiographic and anatomic studies have demonstrated that TN occurs and recurs in the absence of neurovascular compression. In addition, vascular contact with the trigeminal nerve is common in asymptomatic individuals. Thus neurovascular compression is neither sufficient nor necessary for the development of TN. Trigeminal and facial nuclei hyperactivity has been implicated in the pathogenesis. Age, gender, and anatomic variation may make contributions as well. Older patients develop artery elongation within the cisternal space, which is thought to increase probability of intimate neurovascular association. Symptomatic patients without neurovascular compression have been shown to be predominantly female and younger than those with neurovascular compression. Volumetric measurements have also been investigated as a possible pathogenic factor and imaging predictor.

ALTERNATIVE TREATMENTS

The first line of treatment for TN is with antiepileptic medications, which provide 100% pain relief in 70% of patients. Carbamazepine is the first drug of choice. Oxcarbazepine is the second drug of choice although it has better tolerability, fewer drug interactions, and similar efficacy as carbamazepine. Baclofen and lamotrigine may be recommended if a patient develops an adverse reaction to carbamazepine and oxcarbazepine. Other medications that may be effective include phenytoin, valproate, gabapentin, pregabalin, baclofen, and clonazepam. Several of these should be trialed before determining that a patient has failed medical management. Most patients achieve adequate pain control initially.

Antiepileptic drugs have a stabilizing effect on trigeminal nerve neurons by decreasing impulse conduction speed. Unfortunately, this action on the central nervous system contributes to poorly tolerated side effects such as drowsiness, dizziness, fatigue, and poor concentration. Furthermore, about half of the patients, who are successfully managed with medications at diagnosis, will be unable to obtain good pain control with pharmacologic therapy after 10 years. This diminished effect is likely linked to the progressive nature of TN pathophysiology. A positive response to neuropathic pain medications often supports the diagnosis of typical TN and potentially predicts a good outcome.

Inadequate pain control in TN has a profound negative impact on quality of life for patients. For this reason, patients suffering with TN should be considered for surgical interventions as soon as they show signs or endorse symptoms of medical intractability. Antiepileptic medications will not provide a meaningful therapeutic response in up to 10% of patients who will qualify for surgical intervention sooner. The surgical intervention options for TN can be categorized as either ablative or nonablative. Ablative procedures intend to deliver a lesion to the trigeminal nerve or ganglion for the purpose of pain control. Most surgical options for trigeminal neuralgia are ablative in nature. MVD, however, is an exception to ablation. These treatments include stereotactic radiosurgery, radiofrequency ablation, glycerol injection, and balloon compression. Stereotactic radiosurgery creates a lesion at the trigeminal nerve by targeting the root entry zone, and as such, it is typically only effective in a delayed fashion on the magnitude of months. Trigeminal nerve access for lesioning is achieved with a needle through the face for radiofrequency ablation, glycerol injection, and balloon compression. These percutaneous procedures are intended to result in more immediate pain control by direct injury to sensory fibers or desensitization. So pain control relies on some degree of facial numbness, and return of facial sensation is inextricably linked to recurrence of painful TN episodes. Patients must be able to tolerate this relationship and accept the greater risk of developing facial dysesthesia and anesthesia dolorosa. Ablative procedure recurrence is sooner than that of nonablative surgery with pain control lasting only a few years.

Each intervention comes with its own set of merits, limitations, and drawbacks. A recent longitudinal prospectively collected study directly compared long-term pain control rates between first-time surgical treatments for idiopathic TN with MVD, stereotactic radiosurgery(SRS), and Radiofrequency ablation(RFA) and found that patients who received MVD had longer pain-free intervals compared with other procedures. Several large series have described MVD efficacy with consistency, showing that 70%–80% of patients remain pain-free at 5–10 years. The literature on stereotactic radiosurgery shows fewer efficacies and more variability. Only 35%–65% of patients are pain-free at 5 years and 20%–45% are pain-free at 10 years. Many potential confounding patient variables make direct comparison between the procedures challenging. Still, some factors prove valuable in guiding management and counseling patients on surgical procedure decision-making. Procedure selection can be guided by the following general considerations. Patients who are poor surgical candidates like older patients with medical comorbidities are better candidates for SRS or RFA. Patients with V1 distribution pain should be counseled against RFA, in general. Postoperative procedure sensory change has been shown to be predictive of favorable outcome for patients who received SRS. Perceived costs and risks of MVD can influence the patient's decision on treatment selection because it is the most invasive and expensive treatment intervention. However, MVD is often recommended for first-time surgical treatment because it treats the primary cause of TN, which is what makes long-term pain relief possible. As the only nonablative surgical option, MVD differs from the other treatments in its primary objective of slowing the progressive nature of the clinical course of TN. Rather than causing intentional damage to the nerve, MVD aims to prevent nerve damage and other pathophysiologic changes from compression and subsequent igniting mechanism. Additionally, patients who have persistent pain after an ablative procedure can still undergo MVD safely with no decrease in effectiveness as long as they do not have trigeminal neuropathy. MVD is associated with the lowest pain recurrence rate and the highest patient satisfaction.

PREOPERATIVE EVALUATION

Obtaining a thorough history is a critical initial step to determine whether a patient is indicated for microvascular decompression. Patients with TN typically have very distinct memory of initial pain onset. The focal point, primary location, and radiation areas of the pain must be described to help differentiate trigeminal distribution pain from migraines, cluster headaches, temporomandibular joint dysfunction, dental disease, orbital disease, temporal arteritis, glossopharyngeal neuralgia, and nervus intermedius neuralgia. TN pain can manifest in any location innervated by the trigeminal nerve, i.e., forehead, eye, cheek, nose, upper/lower jaw, teeth, lips, and is typically unilateral but can be bilateral. Patients describe unpredictable sensations as sharp, severe, sudden, shocking, stabbing, shooting, electrical, buzzing, burning, and lancinating. It is typical for the pain to be either entirely or mostly brief (seconds to minutes). Alternatively, a constant background facial pain characterized by aching, burning, throbbing, and stinging may be the chief complaint. Patients often provide a history of episodic pain with pain-free intervals that become progressively shorter until transition to a constant intractable facial pain. Specific stimuli, such as eating, drinking, face washing, shaving, teeth brushing, light touch, cold temperature, and even wind, can predictably trigger and exacerbate painful episodes. This is often followed by a refractory period, during which time pain cannot be triggered. Trigeminal pain may be short-lived in some patients, and patients below the age of 40 years have a higher risk of recurrence, so the duration of symptoms should be considered before offering MVD.

Burchiel et al. reported a helpful facial pain classification scheme that helps stratify TN from other facial pain syndromes commonly encountered in neurosurgical practice (Table 2.1). The facial pain diagnosis category provides prognostic potential in terms of efficacy of MVD. MVD is more likely to provide relief for lancinating pain. Type 1 TN is predominantly characterized by this type of pain, whereas type 2 TN is predominantly characterized by constant facial pain. Therefore, TN1 is the most responsive to microvascular decompression; however, MVD results in long-term pain control in most patients with both types 1 and 2 TN. Idiopathic TN must be differentiated from trigeminal pain due to certain underlying causes because the latter is unlikely to improve after MVD. Trigeminal neuropathic pain is caused by unintentional injury that may occur in the setting of facial trauma, dental procedures, and interventions by otolaryngologists or oral maxillofacial surgeons. Trigeminal deafferentation pain is caused by intentional injury for therapeutic effect such as rhizotomy, radiation therapy, and radiofrequency lesioning. Trigeminal neuropathic pain and deafferentation pain are characterized by burning and associated

TABLE 2.1
Classification Scheme for Facial Pains Commonly Encountered in Neurosurgical Practice

Diagnosis	History
	Spontaneous onset
Trigeminal neuralgia, type 1	>50% episodic pain
Trigeminal neuralgia, type 2	>50% constant pain
	Trigeminal injury
Trigeminal neuropathic pain	Unintentional, incidental trauma
Trigeminal deafferentation pain	Intentional deafferentation
Symptomatic trigeminal neuralgia	Multiple sclerosis
Postherpetic neuralgia	Trigeminal *Herpes zoster* outbreak
Atypical facial pain[a]	Somatoform pain disorder

[a] Cannot be diagnosed by history alone.
From Burchiel KJ. A new classification for facial pain. *Neurosurgery*. 2003;53:1164–1167.

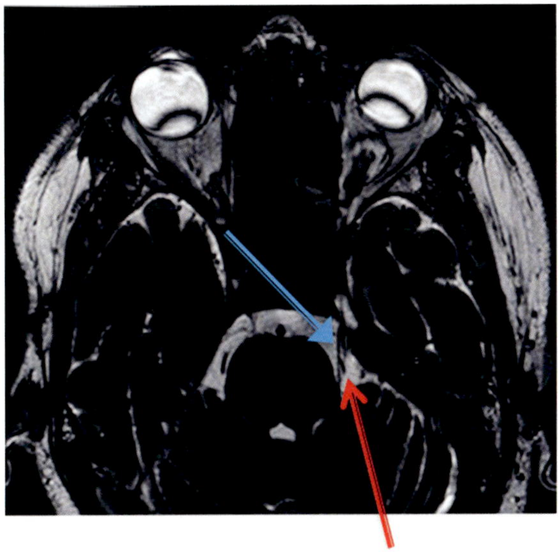

FIG. 2.1 T2 BFFE magnetic resonance imaging demonstrated clear compression of the left trigeminal nerve (*blue arrow*) by the superior cerebellar artery (*red arrow*).

sensory loss, which may be the only demonstrable neurologic deficit on physical examination. Postherpetic neuralgia results from herpes zoster (shingles) infection. Symptomatic TN is present in 2%–4% of patients with multiple sclerosis due to demyelinating plaques within the trigeminal nerve. MVD leads to improvement in some patients with symptomatic TN but is associated with higher rate of recurrence and rare long-lasting relief. Atypical TN has a neuropsychologic component and is unlikely to improve after MVD.

Young, healthy patients with type 1 or type 2 TN suffering with inadequate pain relief are indicated for MVD. Age is an important factor when indicating a patient for MVD if it raises concern that the patient will not tolerate anesthesia and if life expectancy is too short to justify such an invasive procedure. Otherwise there is no difference in complication rate or outcome after MVD in older patients compared with young patients. Interestingly, age-related cerebellar atrophy allows for technically easier MVD owing to less need for retraction. Prohibitive medical comorbidities are the main contraindications for MVD.

Preoperative magnetic resonance imaging (MRI) must be obtained for all patients being considered for MVD. Trigeminal distribution pain can be caused by demyelinating disease, inflammatory changes, and intracranial mass lesions, such as a vestibular schwannoma, epidermoid cyst, cerebellopontine angle(CPA) meningioma, ectopic basilar artery, aneurysm, or arteriovenous malformation. Visualization of neurovascular compression and performance on predicting the symptomatic side are improved by fusion of high-resolution MRI with gadolinium-based contrast enhancement, steady-state sequences, and time-of-flight magnetic resonance angiography. Three-dimensional reconstruction simulates the intraoperative view to aid planning. Failure to identify neurovascular compression on MRI is not a contraindication for posterior fossa exploration for MVD. Prognostic information may also be gleaned from imaging, as atrophy of the symptomatic trigeminal nerve is associated with good prognosis after MVD. In Fig. 2.1, clear compression of the left trigeminal nerve by the SCA is demonstrated on MRI BFFE sequence.

PROCEDURE

Multidisciplinary team discussion should occur before MVD. Anesthesia should apply standard techniques, chemical paralysis, and controlled ventilation to prevent extraneous motion during the case. Anesthesia must be made aware of electrophysiologic intraoperative monitoring of brainstem auditory evoked potentials so that they can plan to adjust anesthesia type and depth accordingly. Therefore total intravenous anesthesia or TIVA is commonly used.

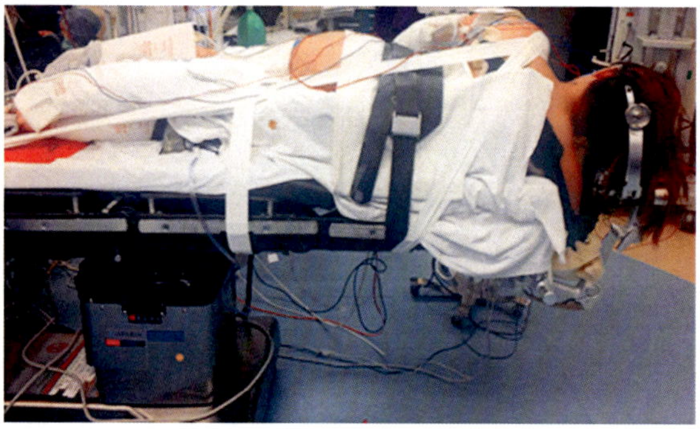

FIG. 2.2 Three-quarter prone position. Some may also place supine with head turned. The ipsilateral shoulder is gently retracted caudally with tape.

After induction and intubation, attention is turned toward positioning, which begins with application of a cranial fixation device. Patients can be positioned supine, lateral decubitus, or three-quarter prone depending on surgeon preference. Supine positioning is simple and offers an unobstructed view. The other positions require flexing the neck and taping the ipsilateral shoulder out of the way. The sitting position can be used as well. Care should be taken to ensure that cranial nerves (CNs) VII and VIII are inferior to the trigeminal nerve by placing the cranial vertex parallel to the floor (Fig. 2.2).

Intraoperative electrodes are placed by neuromonitoring after positioning. Lumbar drain is unnecessary because direct access to the trigeminal cistern via retrosigmoid approach allows for immediate egress of cerebrospinal fluid. Subsequent cerebellar relaxation minimizes the need for retraction, which puts CNs 7 and 8 at increased risk for stretch-induced injury. Brainstem auditory evoked potentials and facial nerve monitoring allow for detection of decreased signal, increased latency, and facial nerve EMG activity. Surgeons loosen cerebellar retraction or other deleterious stimuli until electrophysiologic normalization. Thus, intraoperative monitoring helps prevent injury to the brainstem and CNs (Fig. 2.3).

A longitudinal linear or curvilinear incision should be planned two fingerbreadths behind the ear (Fig. 2.4). The transverse sinus runs along a line from the inion to the external auditory meatus, and only a quarter of the incision should extend beyond this line. The sigmoid sinus runs along a line from the digastric groove posterior to the mastoid eminence. The incision does not need to extend inferior to those landmarks. Superficial and soft-tissue dissection is achieved using monopolar electrocautery until bony exposure of the mastoid eminence and digastric groove is obtained.

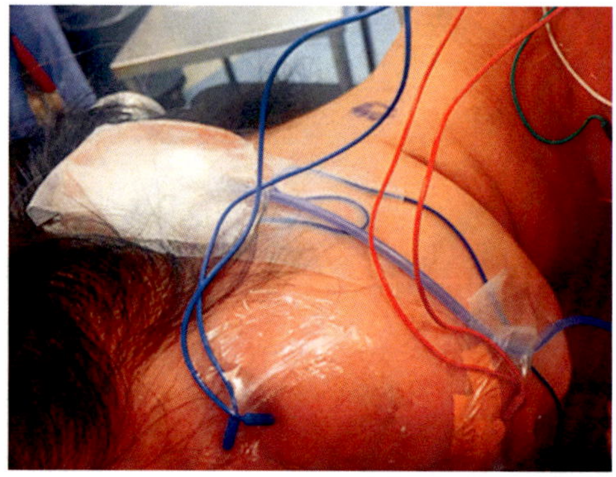

FIG. 2.3 Left facial nerve integrity monitoring used with leads placed in orbicularis oculi *(blue)* and orbicularis oris *(red)*. Brainstem auditory evoked response used.

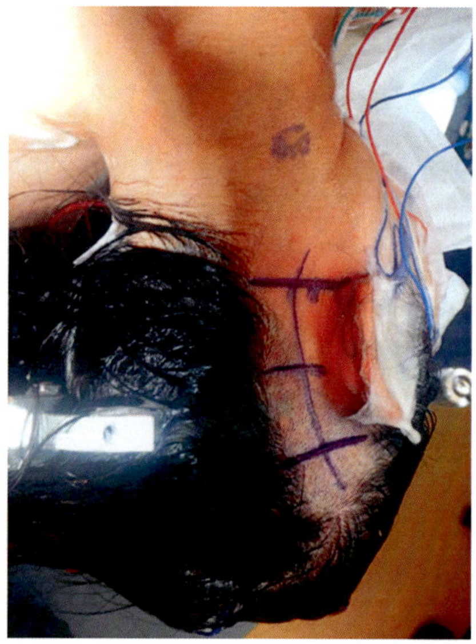

FIG. 2.4 Incision planned by palpating mastoid tip and creating 2 cm posterior to ear extending from mastoid tip to superior aspect of pinna.

Digastric notch palpation demarcates inferior limit. The junction of the transverse and sigmoid sinuses can usually be identified by overlying large mastoid emissary vein. Aterion should be identified as it is junction of lambdoid suture, parietomastoid suture, and occipital-mastoid suture. It approximates the transverse-sigmoid sinus junction (Fig. 2.5).

Next, a small retrosigmoid craniectomy or craniotomy should be performed. Bony removal should start inferiorly and posteriorly to avoid unintentional damage to the sinus (Fig. 2.6). If sinus injury occurs, hemostasis must be achieved without causing venous obstruction. Usually, thrombin-soaked Gelfoam is

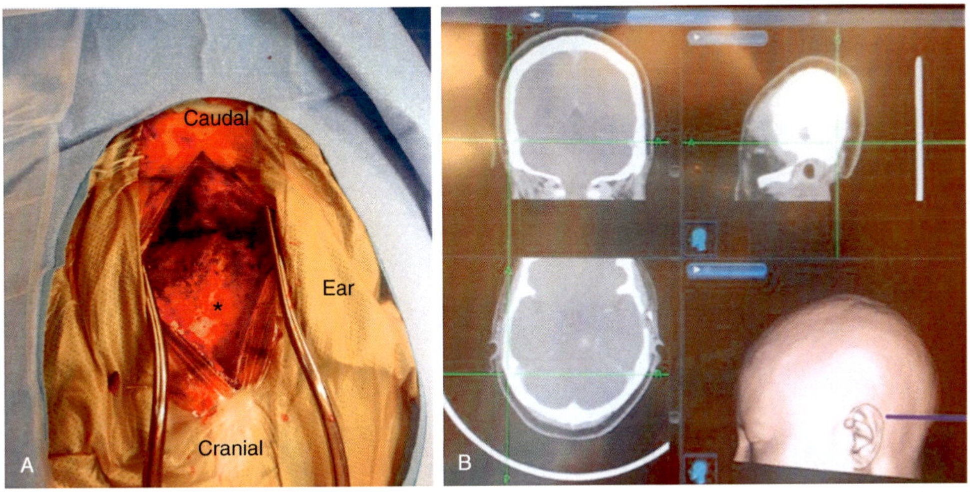

FIG. 2.5 Asterisk marks asterion and correlates to stereotactic navigation demonstrating transverse-sigmoid sinus junction.

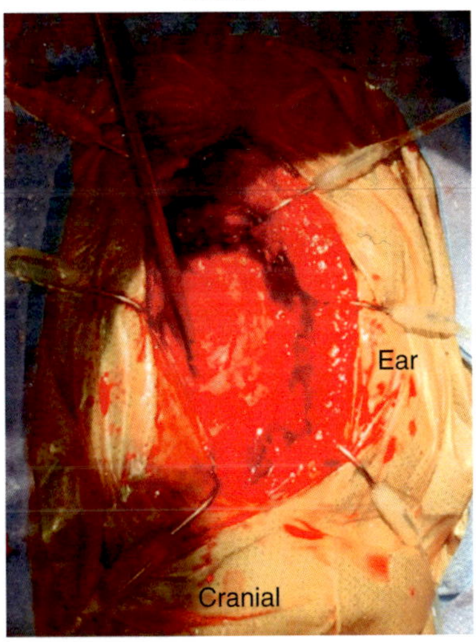

FIG. 2.6 Craniectomy performed with fluted ball bit and kerrison rongeurs. Alternatively, some elect to perform craniotomy. Suction is pointing to transverse-sigmoid junction.

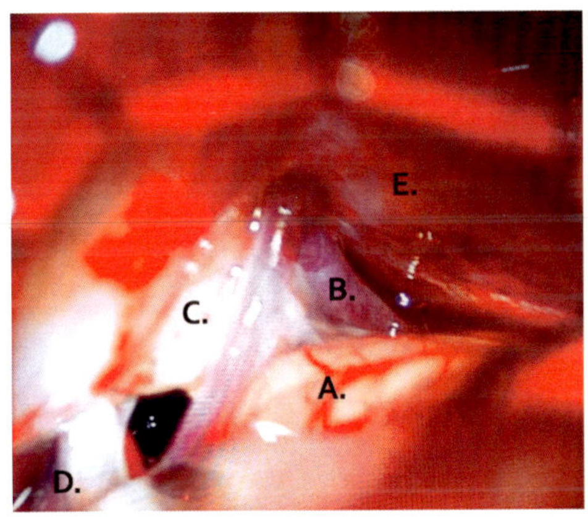

FIG. 2.7 Dura is open in a C-shaped fashion, following a few millimeters from the edge of the sinus. Retractor is placed. (A) Cerebellum. (B) Petrosal vein. (C) Suprameatal tubercle. (D) Cranial nerve VII. (E) Tentorium.

sufficient for management, but occasionally tack-up sutures or dural patch may be necessary. Mastoid air cells should be meticulously waxed during bony exposure and closure to prevent postoperative cerebrospinal fluid leak. Failure to adequately wax creates a pathway for cerebrospinal fluid leakage from the dural opening to the mastoid air cells, through the Eustachian tube and into the nasopharynx causing postoperative rhinorrhea. Cerebrospinal fluid rhinorrhea often necessitates wound exploration for repair of leak with lumbar drain placement to facilitate closure of fistula for definitive management. In addition to mastoid air cell waxing, watertight dural closure can be bolstered with fibrin scaffold, fibrin glue, and patch duraplasty with dural substitute or autograft (e.g., from local muscle, periosteum). Completing these steps with care will help avoidance of this complication.

Adequate exposure is achieved once the transverse and sigmoid sinuses can be seen. Meticulous hemostasis is necessary before dural opening so that subarachnoid hemorrhage does not occur from accumulation of rundown (Fig. 2.7). The dura is opened parallel to the transverse and sigmoid sinuses, a few millimeters away from the edge in the shape of a bow and arrow, and adjacent tack-up sutures are placed. Next, the trigeminal cistern should be penetrated to allow for drainage of cerebrospinal fluid and brain relaxation. This can be achieved by placing a flexible retractor over a cottonoid and gently advancing it.

Using high magnification, typically by use of an operative microscope, but endoscopes have been used as well, arachnoid dissection is performed and the angle of attack is determined by identifying landmarks (Fig. 2.8–2.11). Arterial sacrifice should be avoided as much as possible. Hemorrhagic infarct can occur in the cerebellum if too many veins are sacrificed, so this should be performed judiciously. Upon visualization of the region of interest, neurovascular compression must be identified. The trigeminal nerve must be examined for vascular compression along the root entry zone or its cisternal course. Identification of any

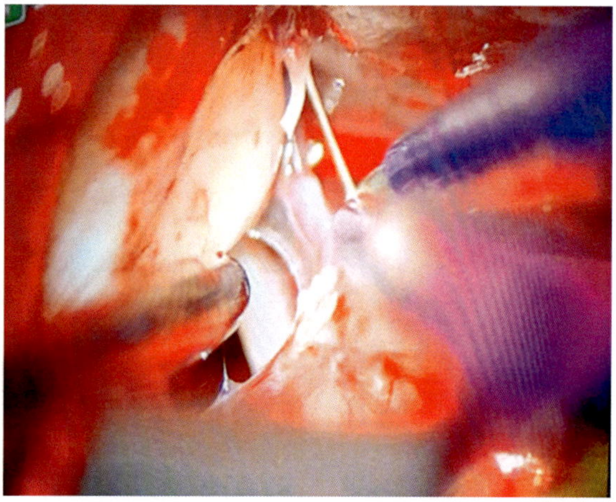

FIG. 2.8 Petrosal vein coagulated and divided, exposing cranial nerve V.

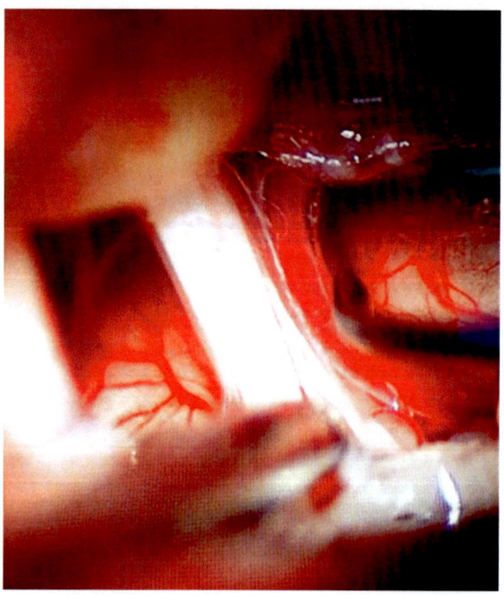

FIG. 2.9 Immediately apparent is the superior cerebellar artery compressing cranial nerve V.

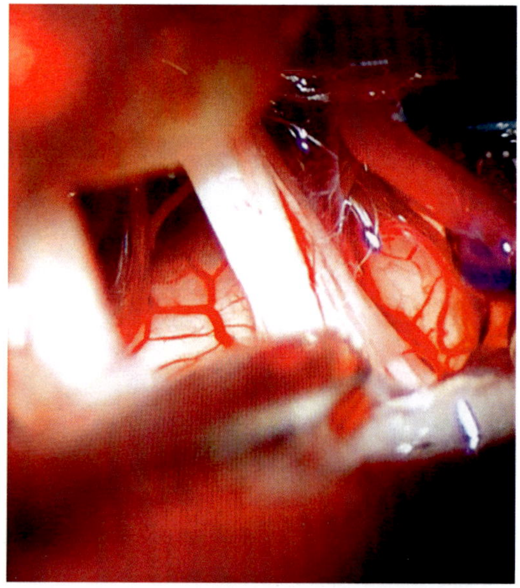

FIG. 2.10 The offending superior cerebellar artery gently retracted off cranial nerve V.

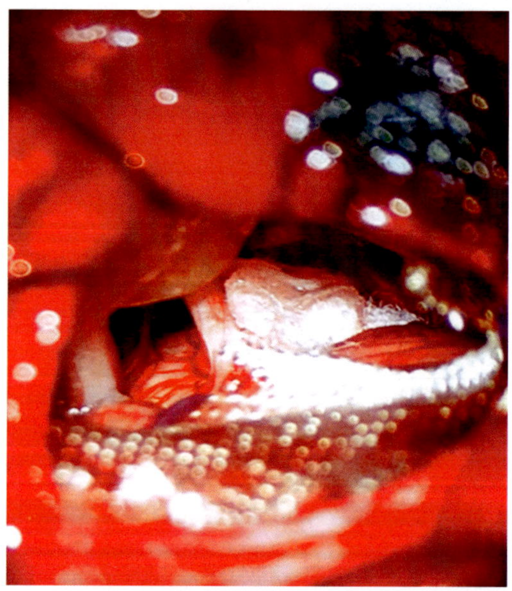

FIG. 2.11 Small thrombin-soaked Teflon balls are placed between superior cerebellar artery and cranial nerve V.

compressive arteries or veins should be followed by careful dissection from the nerve, and placement of small balls of Teflon felt should be used to provide padding. Mobilization of offending vessels is the objective. Sometimes, microvascular decompression by placement of Teflon ball is technically not feasible, in which case transposition of the vessel or interposition can be performed. These procedures are more complex and technically challenging. Biologic adhesive is sometimes used to maintain decompression. It can also be used to keep Teflon in place. Some patients will not have evidence of vascular compression intraoperatively. Patients should be counseled regarding this possibility preoperatively. In these cases, a partial sensory rhizotomy should be performed by gently dividing the nerve along the fascicles to create subtle disruption with a microdissector. The dura is closed in a running or interrupted fashion with Surgilon, covered with dural glue. Ensure watertight closure. Any air cells are copiously sealed with bone wax. The craniectomy defect is covered with titanium mesh and bone cement. The muscle is closed in layers. The skin is closed in a running fashion.

Following microvascular decompression, patients have historically been admitted to the intensive care unit (ICU) for the first night after surgery. As is the case for most craniotomies, close observation, hourly neurologic examinations, and hemodynamic monitoring are important in the immediate postoperative period. Sekula et al., however, recently performed a multiinstitution analysis of ICU utilization during hospital admission for patients undergoing MVD and found that patients who were not admitted to the ICU had shorter length of stay and received less postoperative imaging, both of which led to estimated cost saving of $14,000 per patient. There was no statistically significant difference between complications after surgery related to ICU stay, and the only significant predictor of complications in multivariate analysis was coronary artery disease. Many institutions have moved away from routine postoperative imaging unless there are specific concerns or postoperative neurologic change. Carbamazepine or other neuroleptic medication should be slowly weaned as tolerated.

OUTCOME

CN damage is a rare complication. Trigeminal deafferentation pain is far less common after MVDs compared with ablative procedures. Transient conductive hearing loss can be expected for a few weeks after surgery from mastoid to middle ear fluid. Sensorineural hearing loss has an incidence of less than 1% owing to standardization of brainstem auditory evoked potential monitoring. It tends to be permanent and can be prevented by taking care to avoid retraction and Anterior Inferior Cerebellar Artery(AICA) vasospasm. Postoperative vertigo, tinnitus, and facial weakness tend to improve spontaneously over weeks, whereas trochlear palsy takes months to resolve.

Aseptic meningitis, wound infection, cerebellar injury, and posterior fossa hemorrhage must all be considered in postoperative patients with severe persistent headaches. Cerebrospinal fluid leakage is also a possibility after MVD and could manifest either by obvious fluid leakage from the incision or as rhinorrhea. Cerebellar contusions, edema, and retraction injury can be avoided by being careful, gentle, and minimizing the number of veins sacrificed.

By the 1990s, additional surgical procedures joined MVD as potential treatment options for TN. Jho et al. published a landmark paper in the *New England Journal of Medicine* demonstrating that, of all the available treatments for TN, microvascular decompression is not only safe but also effective with a high rate of long-term success. Approximately 1200 patients who underwent MVD over a 20-year period with a median follow-up with more than 6 years were included in this prospective study. Using Kaplan-Meier analysis, these investigators demonstrated that 70% of these patients were free of pain without analgesic medication 10 years after surgery and additional 4% of these patients had only occasional pain that did not require long-term medication. Furthermore, prior radiofrequency did not prevent these patients from improving after MVD. Patients who had a history of an ablative procedure were no less likely to become pain-free than patients who did not. They did, however, have higher rates of burning and aching facial pain. Annual rate of recurrence was found to be less than 1%. Significant predictors of recurrence were female gender, long duration of symptoms, venous compression, and lack of relief in the immediate postoperative period.[8]

A large body of evidence supports that MVD is an effective treatment for TN. There have been certain characteristics that may be predictive of prognosis. The type of TN is the most significant predictor of TN pain. TN due to venous compression is associated with worse prognosis, likely due to vein regrowth. TN due to arterial versus venous compression may be important for prognostication of postoperative pain relief and recurrence rate. A recent study explored these influences and found that the artery compression group got more early relief and higher recurrence rate than the venous compression group. MVD after an ablative procedure does not portend worse outcome.

REFERENCES

1. Jannetta PJ, Robbins LJ. Trigeminal neuropathy—new observations. *Neurosurgery*. 1980;7(4):347–351.
2. Burchiel KJ. Abnormal impulse generation in focally demyelinated trigeminal roots. *J Neurosurg*. 1980;53(5): 674–683. https://doi.org/10.3171/jns.1980.53.5.0674.
3. Devor M, Govrin-Lippmann R, Rappaport ZH. Mechanism of trigeminal neuralgia: an ultrastructural analysis of trigeminal root specimens obtained during microvascular decompression surgery. *J Neurosurg*. 2002;96(3):532–543. https://doi.org/10.3171/jns.2002.96.3.0532.
4. Gybels J, Kupers R. Deep brain stimulation in the treatment of chronic pain in man: where and why? *Neurophysiol Clin*. 1990;20(5):389–398.
5. Jannetta PJ. Arterial compression of the trigeminal nerve at the pons in patients with trigeminal neuralgia. *J Neurosurg*. 1967;26(suppl 1):159–162. https://doi.org/10.3171/jns.1967.26.1part2.0159.
6. Devor M, Amir R, Rappaport ZH. Pathophysiology of trigeminal neuralgia: the ignition hypothesis. *Clin J Pain*. 2002;18(1):4–13.
7. Leal PR, Barbier C, Hermier M, Souza MA, Cristino-Filho G, Sindou M. Atrophic changes in the trigeminal nerves of patients with trigeminal neuralgia due to neurovascular compression and their association with the severity of compression and clinical outcomes. *J Neurosurg*. 2014;120(6):1484–1495. https://doi.org/10.3171/2014.2.jns131288.
8. Barker 2nd FG, Jannetta PJ, Bissonette DJ, Larkins MV, Jho HD. The long-term outcome of microvascular decompression for trigeminal neuralgia. *N Engl J Med*. 1996; 334(17):1077–1083.

FURTHER READING

1. Anderson VC, Berryhill PC, Sandquist MA, Ciaverella DP, Nesbit GM, Burchiel KJ. High-resolution three-dimensional magnetic resonance angiography and three-dimensional spoiled gradient-recalled imaging in the evaluation of neurovascular compression in patients with trigeminal neuralgia: a double-blind pilot study. *Neurosurgery*. 2006; 58(4):666–673; discussion 666–673. https://doi.org/10.1227/01.neu.0000197117.34888.de.
2. Anichini G, Iqbal M, Rafiq NM, Ironside JW, Kamel M. Sacrificing the superior petrosal vein during microvascular decompression. Is it safe? Learning the hard way. Case report and review of literature. *Surg Neurol Int*. 2016; 7(suppl 14):S415–S420. https://doi.org/10.4103/2152-7806.183520.
3. Ashkan K, Marsh H. Microvascular decompression for trigeminal neuralgia in the elderly: a review of the safety and efficacy. *Neurosurgery*. 2004;55(4):840–850. https://doi.org/10.1227/01.neu.0000137660.06337.c5.
4. Be P, Ka S. Prospective comparison of posterior fossa exploration and stereotactic radiosurgery dorsal root entry zone target as primary surgery for patients with idiopathic trigeminal neuralgia. *Neurosurgery*. 2010;67(3):633–638; discussion 638–639. https://doi.org/10.1227/01.NEU.0000377861.14650.98.
5. Bhangoo SS. Letter to the editor: misuse of the cancer genome atlas? *J Neurosurg*. 2015;123(6):1609–1610. https://doi.org/10.3171/2015.5.JNS151018.
6. Broggi G, Ferroli P, Franzini A, et al. Operative findings and outcomes of microvascular decompression for trigeminal neuralgia in 35 patients affected by multiple sclerosis. *Neurosurgery*. 2004;55(4):830–839. https://doi.org/10.1227/01.neu.0000137656.59536.0e.
7. Burchiel KJ. A new classification for facial pain. *Neurosurgery*. 2003;53(5):1164–1167. https://doi.org/10.1227/01.neu.0000088806.11659.d8.
8. Oesman C, Mooij JJ. Long-term follow-up of microvascular decompression for trigeminal neuralgia. *Skull Base*. 2011;21(5):313–322. https://doi.org/10.1055/s-0031-1284213.
9. Calvin WH, Loeser JD, Howe JF. A neurophysiological theory for the pain mechanism of tic douloureux. *Pain*. 1977; 3(2):147–154.
10. Capel C, Peltier J. Commentary on: trigeminal neuralgia: frequency of occurrence in different nerve branches. *Anesth Pain Med*. 2012;1(3):214–215. https://doi.org/10.5812/kowsar.22287523.3573.
11. Freudenstein D, Wagner A, Gürvit O, Bartz D, Duffner F. Simultaneous virtual representation of both vascular and neural tissue within the subarachnoid space of the basal cistern – technical note. *Med Sci Monit*. 2002;8(9): MT153–158.
12. Dash C, Garg K, Sharma BS. Letter to the editor: reduced incidence of CSF leak following complete calvarial reconstruction of craniectomies. *J Neurosurg*. 2016;125(3):779. https://doi.org/10.3171/2016.3.JNS16514.
13. Daugherty E, Bhavsar S, Hahn SS, Bassano D, Hall W. A successful case of multiple stereotactic radiosurgeries for ipsilateral recurrent trigeminal neuralgia. *J Neurosurg*. 2015;122(6):1324–1329. https://doi.org/10.3171/2014.9.jns13959.
14. Duan Y, Sweet J, Munyon C, Miller J. Degree of distal trigeminal nerve atrophy predicts outcome after microvascular decompression for type 1a trigeminal neuralgia. *J Neurosurg*. 2015;123(6):1512–1518. https://doi.org/10.3171/2014.12.jns142086.
15. Eboli P, Stone JL, Aydin S, Slavin KV. Historical characterization of trigeminal neuralgia. *Neurosurgery*. 2009;64(6): 1183–1186; discussion 1186–1187. https://doi.org/10.1227/01.NEU.0000339412.44397.76.

16. El-Ghandour NM. Microvascular decompression in the treatment of trigeminal neuralgia caused by vertebrobasilar ectasia. *Neurosurgery*. 2010;67(2):330–337. https://doi.org/10.1227/01.NEU.0000371978.86528.60.
17. Eseonu CI, Goodwin CR, Zhou X, et al. Reduced CSF leak in complete calvarial reconstructions of microvascular decompression craniectomies using calcium phosphate cement. *J Neurosurg*. 2015;123(6):1476–1479. https://doi.org/10.3171/2015.1.jns142102.
18. Broggi G, Ferroli P, Franzini A, Servello D, Dones I. Microvascular decompression for trigeminal neuralgia: comments on a series of 250 cases, including 10 patients with multiple sclerosis. *J Neurol Neurosurg Psychiatry*. 2000;68(1):59–64.
19. Report of the Quality Standards Subcommittee of the American Academy of Neurology and the European Federation of Neurological Societies. Neurology, 71, 1183–1190. https://doi.org/10.1212/01.wnl.0000326598.83183.04
20. Ichida MC, de Almeida AN, da Nobrega JC, Teixeira MJ, de Siqueira JT, de Siqueira SR. Sensory abnormalities and masticatory function after microvascular decompression or balloon compression for trigeminal neuralgia compared with carbamazepine and healthy controls. *J Neurosurg*. 2015;122(6):1315–1323. https://doi.org/10.3171/2014.9.jns14346.
21. Jannetta PJ. Preoperative evaluation of neurovascular compression in patients with trigeminal neuralgia by use of three-dimensional reconstruction from two types of high-resolution magnetic resonance imaging. *Neurosurgery*. 2003;52(6):1511. https://doi.org/10.1227/01.neu.0000068352.22859.82Burchiel.
22. Piatt JH, Wilkins RH. Correspondence: microvascular decompression for tic douloureux. *Neurosurgery*. 1984;15(3):456.
23. Kalkanis SN, Eskandar EN, Carter BS, Barker FG. Microvascular decompression surgery in the United States, 1996 to 2000: mortality rates, morbidity rates, and the effects of hospital and surgeon volumes. *Neurosurgery*. 2003;52(6):1251–1262. https://doi.org/10.1227/01.neu.0000065129.25359.ee.
24. Ko AL, Lee A, Raslan AM, Ozpinar A, McCartney S, Burchiel KJ. Trigeminal neuralgia without neurovascular compression presents earlier than trigeminal neuralgia with neurovascular compression. *J Neurosurg*. 2015;123(6):1519–1527. https://doi.org/10.3171/2014.11.jns141741.
25. Ko AL, Ozpinar A, Lee A, Raslan AM, McCartney S, Burchiel KJ. Long-term efficacy and safety of internal neurolysis for trigeminal neuralgia without neurovascular compression. *J Neurosurg*. 2015;122(5):1048–1057. https://doi.org/10.3171/2014.12.jns14469.
26. Lawrence JD, Tuchek C, Cohen-Gadol AA, Sekula Jr RF. Utility of the intensive care unit in patients undergoing microvascular decompression: a multiinstitution comparative analysis. *J Neurosurg*. 2017;126(6):1967–1973. https://doi.org/10.3171/2016.5.jns152118.
27. Leal PR, Hermier M, Souza MA, Cristino-Filho G, Froment JC, Sindou M. Visualization of vascular compression of the trigeminal nerve with high-resolution 3T MRI: a prospective study comparing preoperative imaging analysis to surgical findings in 40 consecutive patients who underwent microvascular decompression for trigeminal neuralgia. *Neurosurgery*. 2011;69(1):15–25; discussion 26. https://doi.org/10.1227/NEU.0b013e318212bafa.
28. Lee A, McCartney S, Burbidge C, Raslan AM, Burchiel KJ. Trigeminal neuralgia occurs and recurs in the absence of neurovascular compression. *J Neurosurg*. 2014;120(5):1048–1054. https://doi.org/10.3171/2014.1.jns131410.
29. Lee JYK, Pierce JT, Sandhu SK, Petrov D, Yang AI. Endoscopic versus microscopic microvascular decompression for trigeminal neuralgia: equivalent pain outcomes with possibly decreased postoperative headache after endoscopic surgery. *J Neurosurg*. 2017;126(5):1676–1684. https://doi.org/10.3171/2016.5.jns1621.
30. Adamczyk M, Bulski T, Sowińska J, Furmanek A, Bekiesińska-Figatowska M. Trigeminal nerve-artery contact in people without trigeminal neuralgia: MR study. *Med Sci Monit*. 2007;13(suppl 1):38–43.
31. Parise M, Acioly MA, Ribeiro CT, Vincent M, Gasparetto EL. The role of the cerebellopontine angle cistern area and trigeminal nerve length in the pathogenesis of trigeminal neuralgia: a prospective case-control study. *Acta Neurochir (Wien)*. 2013;155(5):863–868. https://doi.org/10.1007/s00701-012-1573-0.
32. Matsushima T, Huynh-Le P, Miyazono M. Trigeminal neuralgia caused by venous compression. *Neurosurgery*. 2004;55(2):334–339. https://doi.org/10.1227/01.neu.0000129552.87291.87.
33. McLaughlin N, Upadhyaya P, Buxey F, Martin NA. Value-based neurosurgery: measuring and reducing the cost of microvascular decompression surgery. *J Neurosurg*. 2014;121(3):700–708. https://doi.org/10.3171/2014.5.JNS131996.
34. Miller JP, Acar F, Burchiel KJ. Classification of trigeminal neuralgia: clinical, therapeutic, and prognostic implications in a series of 144 patients undergoing microvascular decompression. *J Neurosurg*. 2009;111(6):1231–1234. https://doi.org/10.3171/2008.6.17604.
35. Miller JP, Acar F, Hamilton BE, Burchiel KJ. Radiographic evaluation of trigeminal neurovascular compression in patients with and without trigeminal neuralgia. *J Neurosurg*. 2009;110(4):627–632. https://doi.org/10.3171/2008.6.17620.
36. Miller JP, Magill ST, Acar F, Burchiel KJ. Predictors of long-term success after microvascular decompression for trigeminal neuralgia. *J Neurosurg*. 2009;110(4):620–626. https://doi.org/10.3171/2008.6.17605.
37. Mortazavi MM, Tubbs RS, Riech S, et al. Anatomy and pathology of the cranial emissary veins: a review with surgical implications. *Neurosurgery*. 2012;70(5):1312–1318; discussion 1318–1319. https://doi.org/10.1227/NEU.0b013e31824388f8.

38. Nurmikko TJ, Eldridge PR. Trigeminal neuralgia—pathophysiology, diagnosis and current treatment. *Br J Anaesth*. 2001;87(1):117–132.
39. Otani N, Toyooka T, Fujii K, et al. "Birdlime" technique using TachoSil tissue sealing sheet soaked with fibrin glue for sutureless vessel transposition in microvascular decompression: operative technique and nuances. *J Neurosurg*. 2017:1–8. https://doi.org/10.3171/2017.1.jns161243.
40. Rampp S, Rensch L, Simmermacher S, Rahne T, Strauss C, Prell J. Intraoperative auditory steady-state monitoring during surgery in the cerebellopontine angle for estimation of postoperative hearing classes. *J Neurosurg*. 2017;127(3):559–568. https://doi.org/10.3171/2016.7.JNS16460.
41. Reinard K, Nerenz DR, Basheer A, et al. Racial disparities in the diagnosis and management of trigeminal neuralgia. *J Neurosurg*. 2017;126(2):368–374. https://doi.org/10.3171/2015.11.jns151177.
42. Rose FC. Trigeminal neuralgia. *Arch Neurol*. 1999;56(9):1163–1164.
43. Love S, Coakham HB. Trigeminal neuralgia pathology and pathogenesis. *Brain*. 2001;124:2347–2360.
44. Satoh T, Onoda K, Date I. Preoperative simulation for microvascular decompression in patients with idiopathic trigeminal neuralgia: visualization with three-dimensional magnetic resonance cisternogram and angiogram fusion imaging. *Neurosurgery*. 2007;60(1):104–113; discussion 113–114. https://doi.org/10.1227/01.neu.0000249213.34838.c9.
45. Microvascular decompression for primary trigeminal neuralgia: long-term effectiveness and prognostic factors in a series of 362 consecutive patients with clear-cut neurovascular conflicts who underwent pure decompression. *J Neurosurg*. 107(6), 1144–1153. https://doi.org/10.3171/jns-07/12/1144.
46. Sivakanthan S, Van Gompel JJ, Alikhani P, van Loveren H, Chen R, Agazzi S. Surgical management of trigeminal neuralgia: use and cost-effectiveness from an analysis of the Medicare claims database. *Neurosurgery*. 2014;75(3):220–226; discussion 225–226. https://doi.org/10.1227/neu.0000000000000430.
47. Suzuki H, Maki H, Maeda M, Shimizu S, Trousset Y, Taki W. Visualization of the intracisternal angioarchitecture at the posterior fossa by use of image fusion. *Neurosurgery*. 2005;56(2):335–342. https://doi.org/10.1227/01.neu.0000148005.29708.1c.
48. Tuleasca C, Carron R, Resseguier N, et al. Decreased probability of initial pain cessation in classic trigeminal neuralgia treated with Gamma Knife surgery in case of previous microvascular decompression: a prospective series of 45 patients with >1 year of follow-up. *Neurosurgery*. 2015;77(1):87–94; discussion 94–85. https://doi.org/10.1227/neu.0000000000000739.
49. Wang DD, Raygor KP, Cage TA, et al. Prospective comparison of long-term pain relief rates after first-time microvascular decompression and stereotactic radiosurgery for trigeminal neuralgia. *J Neurosurg*. 2017:1–10. https://doi.org/10.3171/2016.9.jns16149.
50. Kawano Y, Maehara T, Ohno K. Validation and evaluation of the volumetric measurement of cerebellopontine angle cistern as a prognostic factor of microvascular decompression for primary trigeminal neuralgia. *Acta Neurochir (Wien)*. 2014;156(6):1173–1179. https://doi.org/10.1007/s00701-014-2064-2.
51. Zakrzewska JM, Lopez BC. Quality of reporting in evaluations of surgical treatment of trigeminal neuralgia: recommendations for future reports. *Neurosurgery*. 2003;53(1):110–122. https://doi.org/10.1227/01.neu.0000068862.78930.ee.

CHAPTER 3

Trigeminal Ganglion/Rootlets Ablation for Pain

MICHAEL G.Z. GHALI, MD, PHD, MS • ASHWIN VISWANATHAN, MD • KIM J. BURCHIEL, MD, FACS

INTRODUCTION

Idiopathic trigeminal neuralgia (TN) is a facial pain condition, which involves triggerable, sharp electrical pains in one or more branches of the trigeminal nerve Cranial nerve (CN) V. When choosing a surgical treatment option, idiopathic TN must be differentiated from other facial pain conditions including trigeminal neuropathic pain, symptomatic TN, postherpetic neuralgia, and atypical facial pain.

Many patients with TN will find excellent pain relief with carbamazepine. However, for those patients with persistent pain, or side effects from medication, such as hyponatremia, surgical interventions can provide effective pain relief. Microvascular decompression (MVD) is the surgical intervention for TN, which provides the longest interval of being pain-free off medications.[1] However, for patients who wish to avoid craniotomy, who have recurrent pain after MVD, or who have symptomatic TN, ablative techniques can provide excellent treatment options.[2,3]

Percutaneous radiofrequency trigeminal gangliolysis (PRTG) is an elegant and highly effective procedure in the hands of a skilled surgeon for the treatment of TN.[3] The procedure was first shown to be effective in treating facial pain over four decades ago.[4] Unfortunately, the lack of neurosurgeons trained in radiofrequency techniques, and the perception that PRTG is a more taxing surgical experience for the patient and physician, has led to a decline in the use of this technique. There has been a concomitant rise in the use of techniques such as radiosurgery, balloon compression, and glycerol rhizotomy, which can be performed under general anesthesia without patient cooperation.

Advantages of PRTG when compared with radiosurgery include an immediate benefit, a potentially selective ablation to the trigeminal nerve, and the ability to perform the procedure multiple times with pain recurrence.

PREOPERATIVE CONSIDERATIONS

Counseling patients that the goal of PRTG is to create numbness in the distribution of pain is imperative. Numbness in fact leads to the improvement in pain, and hence numbness should not be viewed as a complication of the procedure, but rather a desired treatment effect.[3] As the third division of CN V innervates the muscles of mastication, patients are also counseled that they may experience weakness of the muscles of mastication, which will likely improve over the course of 2 months following surgery. Although pain relief usually occurs immediately postoperatively, the practice of these authors has been to maintain medication dosage for 1 week postoperatively, to ensure the patient is pain free, before weaning the TN medications.

PRTG is a procedure that requires patient cooperation during surgery to provide feedback to the surgeon regarding two issues. First, during stimulation before lesioning, patients must be able to tell the surgeon in which division of the trigeminal nerve they feel paresthesias. Second, after lesioning, patients must be able to help the surgeon evaluate the degree of hypesthesia that has been created. Hence, for patients who are not able to communicate, or who may not be cooperative during surgery, PRTG may not be the best consideration. For these patients, consideration should be given to radiosurgery, balloon compression, or glycerol injection, which does not require patient cooperation.

SURGICAL CONSIDERATIONS

Anesthesia

A skilled anesthesia team is an essential part of a successful PRTG. The anesthesiologist must be able to deeply sedate the patient during canalization of the foramen ovale. The anesthesiologist also must be able to safely and rapidly wake the patient for intraoperative

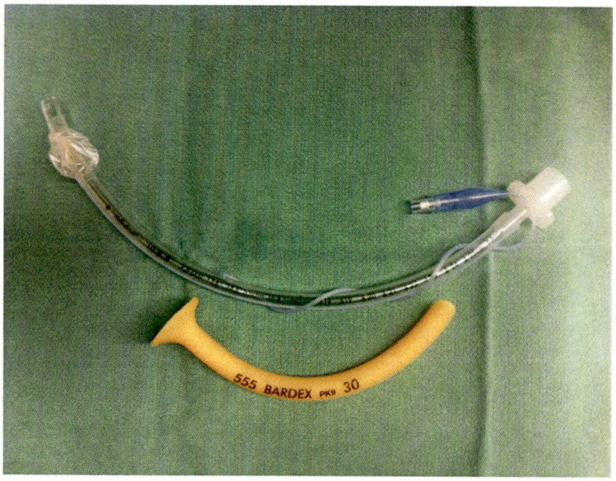

FIG. 3.1 A 30 French nasopharyngeal airway proves a comfortable size for most patients. A 5.5-mm endotracheal tube can be fit snugly into the 30 French aperture.

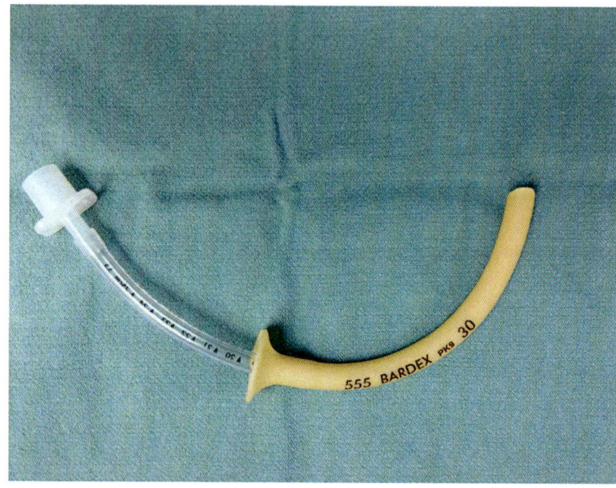

FIG. 3.3 Once inserted, the endotracheal tube should be snug within the nasopharyngeal airway to prevent an air leak.

stimulation and testing. The senior author (KJB) has found the use of a nasopharyngeal airway a safe and effective technique for achieving patient comfort and safety. Here we describe this technique.

The patient is brought to the operating room, and an appropriately sized nasopharyngeal airway is selected based on the patient's nasal passages. For a 30 French airway, a 5.5-mm endotracheal tube proves a snug fit (Fig. 3.1). The endotracheal tube is cut to an appropriate length and inserted into the nasopharyngeal airway (Figs. 3.2 and 3.3). The patient is positioned to obtain an image of the foramen ovale, using submental vertex fluoroscopy projection, and the entry point on the face is sterilely prepared and draped. After an initial amnestic dose of propofol (0.25–0.5 mg/kg) is given, a lubricated nasopharyngeal airway is inserted into the nostril. Once accomplished, a second bolus of propofol (~1 mg/kg) is administered to induce brief general anesthesia. Respiration can be supported through the nasopharyngeal tube, if necessary (Fig. 3.4). If the patient is rendered briefly apneic by the propofol bolus, respirations will promptly resume after a few breaths are administered via the nasopharyngeal tube. A critical aspect of this technique, which can be overlooked, is that the patient's mouth must be closed to allow ventilation to occur. As described, the nostril contralateral to

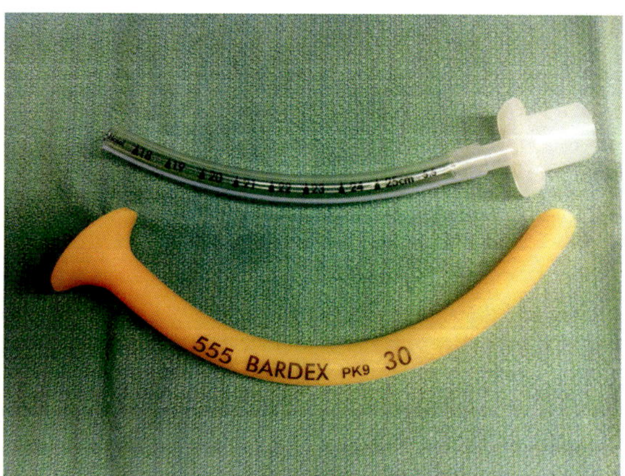

FIG. 3.2 The endotracheal tube has been cut to remove the cuff and allow insertion into the nasopharyngeal airway.

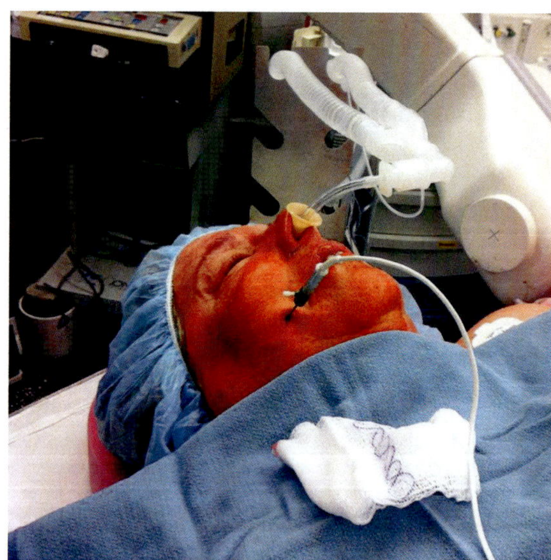

FIG. 3.4 Intraoperative view of an anesthetized patient being ventilated through nasopharyngeal airway connected to the anesthesia circuit.

the nasopharyngeal airway can also be occluded and the jaw thrust anteriorly, if there is a need for brief respiratory support.

Intravenous propofol bolusing provides the advantage of rapid induction of deep anesthesia as well as smooth awakening. Once the effects of the propofol have subsided, patients are awake and cooperative for the procedure and can accurately respond to sensory testing. The technique of a nasopharyngeal airway, fitted with an endotracheal tube, provides easy airway management and deep surgical anesthesia for placement of the cannula. In most cases, patients undergoing the PRTG described above are amnestic for the procedure and thus are not apprehensive to have this repeated in the future, if necessary.

Various other anesthetic strategies for PRTG have been described. Most focus on a combination of methohexital, fentanyl, and a benzodiazepine, commonly either midazolam or diazepam. Kanpolat et al., in their large series of 1600 patients undergoing PRTG, used a combination of alfentanil and midazolam to sedate patients as needed.[5,6] Tew and Grande[6] advocated a rapid infusion of methohexital to anesthetize the patient during cannulation of the foramen ovale and as needed for lesion generation.[7] Regardless of the technique used, the surgeon must develop a technique that allows for patient comfort and for accurate intraoperative testing.

Localization and Targeting of the Foramen Ovale and Gasserian Ganglion

Proper visualization of the foramen ovale is confirmed using intraoperative submental vertex view fluoroscopy. Once the patient is surgically anesthetized, an 11 blade is used to make a stab incision ~2.5 cm lateral to and 1 cm inferior to the labial commissure. The TEW cannula (Cosman Medical, Boston MA) with the stylet is then inserted toward the foramen ovale, with one finger placed within the oral cavity to prevent violation of the oral mucosa. A sequential palpation technique is used to identify the infratemporal fossa and proceed inferiorly until the posteromedial aspect of the foramen ovale is entered (Fig. 3.5). Commonly, entering the foramen ovale is met with a jaw jerk reflex.

Once the foramen ovale is entered, the fluoroscope is moved into the lateral position, and the cannula is advanced until an appropriate depth is reached. For V1 or V2 TN, a curved electrode is often needed. For V1 TN, the radiofrequency electrode may need to be positioned slightly beyond the clival line (Fig. 3.6). For V2 TN, the electrode can usually be positioned at, or just proximal to, the clival line. When treated V3 TN, a straight electrode can be used, and the cannula is positioned well proximal to the clival line.

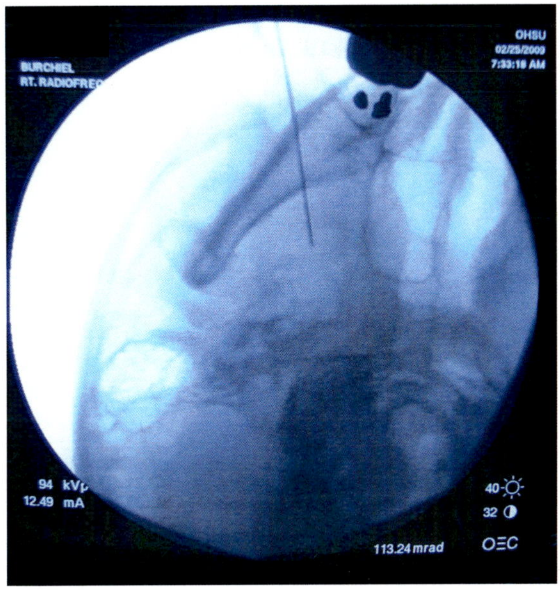

FIG. 3.5 Submental vertex X-ray demonstrating cannula within the foramen ovale. The posterolaterally positioned foramen spinosum is another well-visualized landmark.

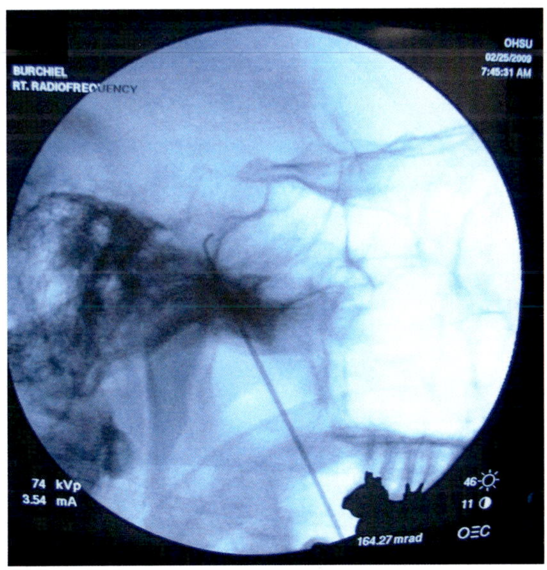

FIG. 3.6 Lateral fluoroscopy with the curved RF electrode positioned just beyond the clival line in the treatment of V1 trigeminal neuralgia.

Prelesional Electrical Stimulation

Once the radiofrequency electrode is in a radiographically satisfactory position, the patient is allowed to awaken. Stimulation testing is then performed (rate of 100 Hz, pulse width 1 ms) with the awake and cooperative patient to ascertain that the desired divisions of the trigeminal nerve are being targeted.[8] Generally, stimulation will be elicited between 0.1 and 0.2 V. However, this sensory threshold can be elevated in patients who have undergone previous PRTG or in multiple sclerosis patients with preexisting deafferentation. If paresthesias are not generated at less than 0.5 V, consideration should be given to ensuring appropriate position of the RF electrode and verifying integrity of the RF system. Once the physiologic location of the electrode has been accomplished, another bolus of propofol is given for sedation and to allow the creation of the first lesion. For V2 and V3 lesions, the first lesion is often made at 70°C for 90 s. For V1 TN, a lesion at 60°C for 60 s may be advisable to minimize the risk of corneal anesthesia.

In lieu of somatotopic mapping of the trigeminal distribution in the awake state,[8] attempts have been made to use antidromic conduction monitoring as an objective correlate of the affected trigeminal distribution to identify target fibers to be lesioned to allow the procedure to be performed under sedation. Antidromic conduction monitoring did indeed correlate in a statistically significant fashion with the patient's subjective description of paresthesias, but correlation proper was weak.[9] Use of trigeminal somatosensory evoked potentials also serves as a potential objective measure for degree of lesioning in PRTG.[10] Although percutaneous trigeminal thermocoagulation has been shown to be 96% and 66% effective immediately and 2 years postintervention, respectively, in nonawake patients,[11] we believe that objective correlates of identification of trigeminal distribution to be lesioned are not sufficiently developed to supplant subjective patient feedback.

Postlesioning

After lesioning, the patient is again awakened and several minutes are allowed to pass such that the patient demonstrates reliable and consistent responses to testing.[12–14] A facial sensory examination is performed, asking the patient to discriminate between pinprick and light touch sensation. A useful adjunct is a safety pin, alternately asking whether the patient can discriminate between the sharp point of the safety pin and the rounded smooth side of the safety pin. The goal of the lesion is the loss of the patient's ability to differentiate sharp and dull sensation. If the desired degree of hypesthesia has not been created with the first lesion, repeat stimulation testing (100 Hz, 1 ms pulse) is again performed to ensure that the RF electrode is targeting the desired division of the trigeminal nerve. Once this is confirmed, the patient is resedated with a bolus of propofol, and further cycles of lesion production can be performed. The additional lesions can be performed at the same temperature as the initial lesion, with the RF electrode in a slightly different position. Alternately, the electrode position can be maintained and the lesion temperature can be increased by 5°C. The process of sensory testing and lesion generation should be repeated until the desired level of hypalgesia is achieved.

DISCUSSION

Treatment of Trigeminal Neuralgia

Carbamazepine is the first-line treatment for TN, and in fact, response to carbamazepine is useful in confirming the diagnosis of TN. For medically refractory patients, several interventions are available, including MVD via retrosigmoid craniectomy, percutaneous trigeminal rhizotomy via radiofrequency (PRTG), glycerol rhizotomy (PGR), or balloon compression (PBC), and stereotactic radiosurgery. Radiofrequency lesioning of the spinal nucleus and tract of V has also been performed via a percutaneous atlantooccipital approach for patients with greater components of neuropathic pain.[15]

MVD has been shown to have excellent initial and long-term results,[16–19] but it does carry the attendant risks of craniotomy including hearing loss, CSF leak, and rare cases of stroke or death. In comparison with MVD, PRTG is an outpatient procedure with minimal recovery time. In addition, it is a very low-risk procedure that can be used even in patients with very poor medical condition.[20–24] However, we continue to encourage MVD as a first-line therapy for appropriate candidates given its nondestructive nature and excellent long-term results.[25]

Outcome of Percutaneous Radiofrequency Trigeminal Gangliolysis

PRTG is associated with >98% of individuals consistently achieving symptom relief immediately following the procedure. In addition, 85%, 68%, and 54% of patients will maintain pain relief at 1, 2, and 3 years postoperatively, respectively.[3,26–28] Sustained efficacy of up to 85% has been reported at 3 years[27]; however, reported rates of recurrence vary widely.[26,29,30] Varying surgeon techniques and varying degrees of hypesthesia created intraoperatively likely account for the variation in outcomes reported in the literature. Our practice is generally to counsel patients that PRTG will last on average 3–4 years and may be repeated multiple times if needed. Patients with multiple sclerosis–related TN may have an earlier recurrence and require higher temperatures used during PRTG.[31–34] The immediacy and lower complication rate of PRTG is attractive, especially in patients who are elderly or deemed to be in poor general medical condition for surgery.[29,35,36]

In comparison with PRTG, pain relief following PBC and PGR lasts between 0.5 and 3.5 years.[31,37–39] PGR and PBC tend to be less division-selective and are thus recommended for multidivision TN. PBC exhibits greater selectivity for injuring large myelinating fibers and is thus recommended for ophthalmic division TN, as it spares the smaller sensory fibers underlying the afferent limb of the corneal reflex.[40]

In patients with imaging evidence of neurovascular conflict (NVC) at the trigeminal root entry zone (REZ), MVD is the most effective treatment.[41] Conversely, PRTG represents a good option for patients without NVC as the initial treatment, as well as in cases of post-MVD recurrence without NVC. PRTG is also effective in treating bilateral TN.[5]

Although ablative techniques provide good immediate relief from TN,[42] all ablative techniques are associated with recurrence. The goal is to have a long-term strategy for managing the patients' pain over the course of their life. Recurrence of TN following PRTG generally occurs within 4 years.[43,44] The largest study evaluating outcomes in patients with TN following PRTG included more than 1500 patients and demonstrated pain relief immediately in ~98%, with sustained pain relief in 58% at 5 years and 42% at 15 years.[3] Those undergoing multiple treatments achieved pain relief rates of greater than 90% at 5–15 years postintervention.

Complications of Percutaneous Radiofrequency Trigeminal Gangliolysis

Complications can occur during PRTG although it is a simple and effective treatment for TN. As an ablative technique, the goal of PRTG is to create hypesthesia for patients, with the degree of sensory loss inversely correlated with the duration of pain relief.[3] In addition, weakness of the muscles of mastication can occur in up to 10% patients, as the trigeminal nerve innervates these muscles. Other complications include dysgeusia, dysesthesias (5%–25%), corneal hypesthesia (~20%) with or without decreased reflex, keratitis (1%–3%), transient oculomotor palsies, and anesthesia dolorosa (1%–4%).[3,8,36,45–47] Reported, but rare, complications have included abducens palsy, extratrigeminal cranial nerve palsies, cardiac asystole, meningitis, intracranial hemorrhage, and death.[3,40,48–52] Foramen ovale puncture can be associated with bradycardia and pressor responses, and prelesional electrical stimulation and radiofrequency thermocoagulation can also be associated with moderate and marked pressor responses, respectively,[53] putatively via invocation of the trigeminocardiac reflex. In contradistinction to balloon compression, the use of atropine and transcutaneous pacing is rarely needed when performing PRTG.

Radiofrequency Thermoablation and Pulsed Radiofrequency

Insufficient thermocoagulation is associated with nonresolution, earlier recurrence, and more frequent recurrence. Conversely, excessive thermocoagulation is associated with higher frequency of facial numbness, thus rendering treatment parameters a critical determinant of procedure safety and efficacy. Neurosurgical experience has shown traditional RF to be the technique of choice for maximizing the long-term pain outcome for the patient. However, pulsed radiofrequency at energies that are nondestructive, alone and in combination with thermoablation, continues to be used as a treatment modality, with the goal of reducing complication rates.[54–56] In treating ophthalmic division TN, PRTG in conjunction with pulsed radiofrequency (PRF) achieved better symptomatic relief at 1, 2, and 3 years, lower recurrence, and lower incidence of corneal hypesthesia compared with PRTG alone.[57] The use of higher voltages can lead to greater efficacy when pulsed radiofrequency is used.[58]

Localization Adjuncts

Intraoperative fluoroscopy remains an excellent modality for safely cannulating the foramen ovale. However, with increasing availability of intraoperative neuronavigation and intraoperative 3D imaging, different methods for localizing the needle to the foramen ovale have been explored. Successful application of these techniques has been reported, with good patient outcomes and low complication rates.[59] Use of neuronavigation guided by CT, MRI and fused MRI, and intraoperative CT images can improve target identification in patients undergoing PRTG.[60–63] C-Arm and CT-guided PRTG ensures correct positioning of the needle in all cases.[64] Such localization modalities may be useful for those without experience in the traditional X-ray approaches or for patients with unusual anatomic variations.[65]

CONCLUSION

PRTG is a unique treatment in that it provides immediate pain relief for patients suffering from TN, has a low morbidity, and is of low cost.[2] It is a skill procedure, however, and consequently, the surgeon must be able to instruct the anesthesiologist on the best anesthetic technique. We believe our technique is easily implemented and provides for optimal patient comfort and cooperation. Although PRTG is a highly effective treatment, counseling patients on the expected duration of pain relief and that the goal of the procedure is to create hypesthesia is important. Further studies of different ablative techniques will enable individualized treatment selection, as well as further refinement of our ability to maintain patient's pain relief and decrease complications.

REFERENCES

1. Barker FG, Jannetta PJ, Bissonette DJ, et al. The long-term outcome of microvascular decompression for trigeminal neuralgia. *N Engl J Med*. 1996;334:1077–1083.
2. Burchiel KJ, Steege TD, Howe JF, et al. Comparison of percutaneous radiofrequency gangliolysis and microvascular decompression for the surgical management of tic douloureux. *Neurosurgery*. 1981;9:111–119.
3. Kanpolat Y, Savas A, Bekar A, et al. Percutaneous controlled radiofrequency trigeminal rhizotomy for the treatment of idiopathic trigeminal neuralgia: 25-year experience with 1,600 patients. *Neurosurgery*. 2001;48:524–532.
4. Sweet WG. Proceedings: analgesia dolorosa after differential retrogasserian thermal or mechanical rhizotomy: tactics employed to decrease its influence. *J Neurol Neurosurg Psychiatry*. 1975;38:407.
5. Bozkurt M, Al-Beyati ES, Ozdemir M, et al. Management of bilateral trigeminal neuralgia with trigeminal radiofrequency rhizotomy: a treatment strategy for the life-long disease. *Acta Neurochir (Wien)*. 2012;154:785–791; discussion 791–782.
6. Tew JM, Grande AW. Percutaneous stereotactic radiofrequency treatment of trigeminal neuralgia. *Cosman Med*. 2008:1–20.
7. Brisman R. Analgesia and sedation during percutaneous radiofrequency electrocoagulation for trigeminal neuralgia. *Neurosurgery*. 1993;32:400–405; discussion 405–406.
8. Cheng JS, Lim DA, Chang EF, et al. A review of percutaneous treatments for trigeminal neuralgia. *Neurosurgery*. 2014;10(suppl 1):25–33; discussion 33.
9. Li X, Yue J, Yang L, et al. Application of antidromic conduction monitoring in ganglion radiofrequency thermocoagulation for locating trigeminal branches in trigeminal neuralgia. *Pain Pract*. 2016;16:305–310.
10. Zhao YX, Miao SH, Tang YZ, et al. Trigeminal somatosensory-evoked potential: a neurophysiological tool to monitor the extent of lesion of ganglion radiofrequency thermocoagulation in idiopathic trigeminal neuralgia: a case-control study. *Medicine (Baltimore)*. 2017;96(3):e5872.
11. Hart MG, Nowell M, Coakham HB. Radiofrequency thermocoagulation for trigeminal neuralgia without intra-operative patient waking. *Br J Neurosurg*. 2012;26:392–396.
12. Vallejo R, Benyamin RM, Aliaga L. Radiofrequency vs. pulse radiofrequency: the end of the controversy [Internet]. *Tech Reg Anesth Pain Manag*. 2010;14:128–132.
13. Sim SE, Kim YH, Kim YC, et al. Pulsed mode radiofrequency lesioning of the mental nerve for the treatment of trigeminal neuralgia [Internet]. *Reg Anesth Pain Med*. 2007;32:69.
14. Kapur D. Radiofrequency lesioning techniques in the management of chronic pain [Internet]. *Anaesth Intensive Care Med*. 2005;6:56–58.
15. Teixeira MJ, de Almeida FF, de Oliveira YS, et al. Microendoscopic stereotactic-guided percutaneous radiofrequency trigeminal nucleotractotomy. *J Neurosurg*. 2012;116: 331–335.
16. Pamir M, Peker S. Microvascular decompression for trigeminal neuralgia: a long-term follow-up study. *Minim Invasive Neurosurg*. 2006;49:342–346.
17. Tyler-Kabara EC, Kassam AB, Horowitz MH, et al. Predictors of outcome in surgically managed patients with typical and atypical trigeminal neuralgia: comparison of results following microvascular decompression. *J Neurosurg*. 2002;96:527–531.
18. Ko AL, Ozpinar A, Lee A, et al. Long-term efficacy and safety of internal neurolysis for trigeminal neuralgia without neurovascular compression. *J Neurosurg*. 2015; 122:1048–1057.
19. Broggi G, Ferroli P, Franzini A, et al. Microvascular decompression for trigeminal neuralgia: comments on a series of 250 cases, including 10 patients with multiple sclerosis. *J Neurol Neurosurg Psychiatry*. 2000;68:59–64.
20. Tronnier VM, Rasche D, Hamer J, et al. Treatment of idiopathic trigeminal neuralgia: comparison of longterm outcome after radiofrequency rhizotomy and microvascular decompression. *Neurosurgery*. 2001;48:1261–1267; discussion 1267–1268.
21. Koopman JSHA, de Vries LM, Dieleman JP, et al. A nationwide study of three invasive treatments for trigeminal neuralgia. *Pain*. 2011;152:507–513.
22. Holland M, Noeller J, Buatti J, et al. The cost-effectiveness of surgery for trigeminal neuralgia in surgically naive patients: a retrospective study. *Clin Neurol Neurosurg*. 2015; 137:34–37.
23. Hitchon PW, Holland M, Noeller J, et al. Options in treating trigeminal neuralgia: expereince with 195 patients. *Clin Neurol Neurosurg*. 2016;149:166–170.
24. Pollock BE, Shoeberl KA. Prospective comparison of posterior fossa exploration and stereotactic radiosurgery dorsal root entry zone target as primary surgery for patients with idiopathic trigeminal neuralgia. *Neurosurgery*. 2010; 67(3):633–639.
25. Zhang X, Zhao H, Tang Y, et al. Comparison of the efficacy of reoperation, percutaneous radiofrequency thermocoagulation when microvascular decompression of trigeminal neuralgia is invalid. *J Craniofac Surg*. 2016; 27:e688–e690.
26. Fraioli B, Esposito V, Guidetti B, et al. Treatment of trigeminal neuralgia by thermocoagulation, glycerolization, and percutaneous compression of the Gasserian ganglion and/or retrogasserian rootlets: long-term results and therapeutic protocol. *Neurosurgery*. 1989;24:239–245.

27. Liu P, Zhong W, Liao C, et al. The role of percutaneous radiofrequency thermocoagulation for persistent or recurrent trigeminal neuralgia after surgery. *J Craniofac Surg.* November 2016;27:e752–e755.
28. Onofrio BM. Radiofrequency percutaneous Gasserian ganglion lesions. Results in 140 patients with trigeminal pain. *J Neurosurg.* February 1975;42:132–139.
29. Tatli M, Satici O, Kanpolat Y, et al. Various surgical modalities for trigeminal neuralgia: literature study of respective long-term outcomes [Internet]. *Acta Neurochir (Wien).* 2008;150:243–255.
30. Noorani I, Lodge A, Vajramani G, et al. Comparing percutaneous treatments of trigeminal neuralgia: 19 years of experience in a single centre. *Stereotact Funct Neurosurg.* 2016;94:75–85.
31. North RB, Kidd DH, Piantadosi S, et al. Percutaneous retrogasserian glycerol rhizotomy. Predictors of success and failure in treatment of trigeminal neuralgia. *J Neurosurg.* 1990;72:851–856.
32. Pollock BE, Phuong LK, Foote RL, et al. High-dose trigeminal neuralgia radiosurgery associated with increased risk of trigeminal nerve dysfunction. *Neurosurgery.* 2001;49: 58–62; discussion 62–64.
33. Zakrzewska JM, Jassim S, Bulman JS. A prospective, longitudinal study on patients with trigeminal neuralgia who underwent radiofrequency thermocoagulation of the Gasserian ganglion. *Pain.* 1999;79:51–58.
34. Maesawa S, Salame C, Flickinger JC, et al. Clinical outcomes after stereotactic radiosurgery for idiopathic trigeminal neuralgia. *J Neurosurg.* 2001;94:14–20.
35. Emril DR, Ho KY. Treatment of trigeminal neuralgia: role of radiofrequency ablation [Internet]. *J Pain Res.* 2010;3: 249–254.
36. Lord SM, Bogduk N. Radiofrequency procedures in chronic pain [Internet]. *Best Pract Res Clin Anaesthesiol.* 2002;16:597–617.
37. Kouzounias K, Schechtmann G, Lind G, et al. Factors that influence outcome of percutaneous balloon compression in the treatment of trigeminal neuralgia. *Neurosurgery.* 2010;67:925–934; discussion 934.
38. Omeis I, Smith D, Kim S, et al. Percutaneous balloon compression for the treatment of recurrent trigeminal neuralgia: long-term outcome in 29 patients. *Stereotact Funct Neurosurg.* 2008;86:259–265.
39. Bergenheim AT, Asplund P, Linderoth B. Percutaneous retrogasserian balloon compression for trigeminal neuralgia: review of critical technical details and outcomes. *World Neurosurg.* 2013;79:359–368.
40. Taha JM, Tew Jr JM. Comparison of surgical treatments for trigeminal neuralgia: reevaluation of radiofrequency rhizotomy. *Neurosurgery.* 1996;38:865–871.
41. Prieto R, Pascual JM, Yus M, et al. Trigeminal neuralgia: assessment of neurovascular decompression by 3D fast imaging employing steady-state acquisition and 3D time of flight multiple overlapping thin slab acquisition magnetic resonance imaging. *Surg Neurol Int.* 2012;3:50.
42. Laghmari M, El Ouahabi A, Arkha Y, et al. Are the destructive neurosurgical techniques as effective as microvascular decompression in the management of trigeminal neuralgia? *Surg Neurol.* 2007;6:505–512.
43. Karol EA, Agner C. Technological advances in the surgical management of trigeminal neuralgia. *Crit Rev Neurosurg.* 1999;9:70–78.
44. Karol EA, Sanz OP, Gonzalez La Riva FN, et al. A micrometric multiple electrode array for the exploration of Gasserian and retrogasserian trigeminal fibers: preliminary report: technical note. *Neurosurgery.* 1993;33: 154–158.
45. Lopez BC, Hamlyn PJ, Zakrzewska JM. Systematic review of ablative neurosurgical techniques for the treatment of trigeminal neuralgia. *Neurosurgery.* 2004;54:973–982; discussion 982–983.
46. Ischia S, Luzzani A, Polati E. Retrogasserian glycerol injection: a retrospective study of 112 patients. *Clin J Pain.* 1990;6:291–296.
47. Lopez BC, Hamlyn PJ, Zakrzewska JM. Stereotactic radiosurgery for primary trigeminal neuralgia: state of the evidence and recommendations for future reports. *J Neurol Neurosurg Psychiatry.* 2004;75:1019–1024.
48. Chatterjee N, Chatterjee S, Roy C. Abducens nerve palsy after percutaneous radiofrequency ablation of Gasserian ganglion. *J Neurosurg Anesthesiol.* 2014;26: 89–90.
49. Madhusudan Reddy KR, Arivazhagan A, Chandramouli BA, et al. Multiple cranial nerve palsies following radiofrequency ablation for trigeminal neuralgia. *Br J Neurosurg.* 2008;22:781–783.
50. Reddy KR, Chandramouli BA, Rao GS. Cardiac asystole during radiofrequency lesioning of the trigeminal ganglion. *J Neurosurg Anesthesiol.* 2006;18:163.
51. Ward L, Khan M, Greig M, et al. Meningitis after percutaneous radiofrequency trigeminal ganglion lesion. Case report and review of literature. *Pain Med.* 2007;8: 835–838.
52. Rath GP, Dash HH, Bithal PK, et al. Intracranial hemorrhage after percutaneous radiofrequency trigeminal rhizotomy. *Pain Pract.* 2009;9:82–84.
53. Meng Q, Zhang W, Yang Y, et al. Cardiovascular responses during percutaneous radiofrequency thermocoagulation therapy in primary trigeminal neuralgia. *J Neurosurg Anesthesiol.* 2008;20:131–135.
54. Chua NH, Halim W, Beems T, et al. Pulsed radiofrequency treatment for trigeminal neuralgia. *Anesth Pain Med.* 2012; 1:257–261.
55. Li X, Ni J, Yang L, et al. A prospective study of Gasserian ganglion pulsed radiofrequency combined with continuous radiofrequency for the treatment of trigeminal neuralgia. *J Clin Neurosci.* 2012;19:824–828.
56. Zhao WX, Wang Q, He MW, et al. Radiofrequency thermocoagulation combined with pulsed radiofrequency helps relieve postoperative complications of trigeminal neuralgia. *Genet Mol Res.* 2015;14:7616–7623.

57. Yao P, Hong T, Zhu YQ, et al. Efficacy and safety of continuous radiofrequency thermocoagulation plus pulsed radiofrequency for treatment of V1 trigeminal neuralgia: a prospective cohort study. *Medicine (Baltimore)*. 2016; 95(44):e5247.
58. Fang L, Tao W, Jingjing L, et al. Comparison of high-voltage- with standard-voltage pulsed radiofrequency of Gasserian ganglion in the treatment of idiopathic trigeminal neuralgia. *Pain Pract*. 2015;15:595–603.
59. Ding W, Chen S, Wang R, et al. Percutaneous radiofrequency thermocoagulation for trigeminal neuralgia using neuronavigation-guided puncture from a mandibular angle. *Medicine (Baltimore)*. 2016;95:e4940.
60. Lai GH, Tang YZ, Wang XP, et al. CT-guided percutaneous radiofrequency thermocoagulation for recurrent trigeminal neuralgia after microvascular decompression. *Medicine (Baltimore)*. 2015;94:e1176.
61. Guo Z, Wu B, Du C, et al. Stereothactic approach combined with 3D CT reconstruction for difficult-to-access foramen ovale on radiofrequency thermocoagulation of the Gasserian ganglion for trigeminal neuralgia. *Pain Med*. 2016;17:1704–1716.
62. Lepski G, Mesquita Filho PM, Ramina K, et al. MRI-based radiation-free method for navigated percutaneous radiofrequency trigeminal rhizotomy. *J Neurol Surg A Cent Eur Neurosurg*. 2015;76:160–167.
63. Chen KT, Lin MH, Tsai YH, et al. Application of MRI and intraoperative CT fusion images with integrated neuronavigation in percutaneous radiofrequency trigeminal rhizotomy. *Acta Neurochir (Wien)*. 2015;157:1443–1448.
64. Telischak NA, Heit JJ, Campos LW, et al. Fluoroscopic C-arm and CT-guided selective radiofrequency ablation for trigeminal and glossopharyngeal facial pain syndromes. *Pain Med*. 2017. https://doi.org/10.1093/pm/pnx088.
65. Zdilla MJ, Hatfield SA, McLean KA, et al. Orientation of the foramen ovale: an anatomic study with neurosurgical considerations. *J Craniofac Surg*. 2016;27:234–237.

FURTHER READING

1. Jin HS, Shin JY, Kim Y-C, et al. Predictive factors associated with success and failure for radiofrequency thermocoagulation in patients with trigeminal neuralgia. *Pain Physician*. 2015;18:537–545.
2. Kosugi S, Shiotani M, Otsuka Y, et al. Long-term outcomes of percutaneous radiofrequency thermocoagulation of Gasserian ganglion for 2nd- and multiple-division trigeminal neuralgia. *Pain Pract*. 2015;15:223–228.
3. Inoue T, Hirai H, Shima A, et al. Long-term outcomes of microvascular decompression and Gamma Knife surgery for trigeminal neuralgia: a retrospective comparison study. *Acta Neurochir (Wien)*. 2017;159.
4. Young B, Shivazad A, Kryscio RJ, et al. Long-term outcome of high-dose Gamma Knife surgery in treatment of trigeminal neuralgia. *J Neurosurg*. 2013;119:1166–1175.
5. Kondziolka D, Zorro O, Lobato-Polo J, et al. Gamma Knife stereotactic radiosurgery for idiopathic trigeminal neuralgia. *J Neurosurg*. 2010;112:758–765.
6. Kalkanis SN, Eskandar EN, Carter BS, et al. Microvascular decompression surgery in the United States, 1996 to 2000: mortality rates, morbidity rates, and the effects of hospital and surgeon volumes. *Neurosurgery*. 2003;52: 1251–1261; discussion 1261–1262.
7. Xu SJ, Zhang WH, Chen T, et al. Neuronavigator-guided percutaneous radiofrequency thermocoagulation in the treatment of intractable trigeminal neuralgia. *Chin Med J (Engl)*. 2006;119:1528–1535.
8. Fraioli MF, Cristino B, Moschettoni L, et al. Validity of percutaneous controlled radiofrequency thermocoagulation in the treatment of isolated third division trigeminal neuralgia. *Surg Neurol*. 2009;71:180–183.

CHAPTER 4

Management of Peripheral Nerve Neuralgia

ANDREW C. ZACEST, MBBS, MS, FRACS, FFPMANZCA

HISTORICAL BACKGROUND

The characteristic clinical features of pain of presumed peripheral nerve origin were described by physicians in the early 19th century and remain accurate to this day.[1] These include the unique quality of neuropathic pain as well as sensory dysfunction and tenderness over the nerve particularly at points of compression. The term "neuralgia" was originally used as a descriptive term for all painful disorders attributed to peripheral nerves and was originally classified as a disease or "neurosis" or "nervous affection." Later in the 19th century, classifications included neuralgia within the "hyperesthesias" and as a "functional" disorder of the nervous system, typically one of exclusion, made in the absence of evidence of a primary lesion of the nervous system. Not surprisingly, the term neuralgia came to be used loosely for a variety of conditions and a psychogenic origin was commonly inferred.[2]

During the course of the American Civil war, Silas Weir Mitchell coined the term "causalgia" to describe severe pain following traumatic nerve injury. Now termed complex regional pain syndrome, Mitchell noted that pain "in the shape of neuralgia" commonly follows nerve injury, is variable in presentation and intensity, often develops in a delayed fashion, and may involve other nerve territories. As noted earlier, Mitchell reported that the severity of the pain may lead some physicians to suspect the patient of "magnifying his pains."[3] Although peripheral nerve surgery was not routinely performed at this time, nerve resection was described with questionable benefit and amputation was frequently requested by patients.

Although neuromas were described in the 17th century, Odier in 1811 described the sensitivity of the bulbous stump of the proximal portion of a transected nerve and Wood in 1828 named the terminal end bulb of an injured nerve a neuroma (cited in Ref. 4). Resection of neuromas back to good nerve was reported in 1886 by Richardson (cited in Ref. 5) and further developed with surgical experience of the treatment of peripheral nerve injury from the World Wars I and II. In 1921, Platt reported his results of "operations for causalgia," including nerve resection and suture, intraneural injection of quinine and urea, and neurolysis, noting the best result for the former and worse for the latter.[6]

In the absence of obvious trauma, the pathophysiology of neuralgia was hypothesized to be due to "inflammation," and the discovery and report of nervi nervorum by Victor Horsley in 1884 furthered this idea and the diagnosis of "neuritis" took favor.[7] Weschler later proposed the term neuropathy as being more appropriate for nerve degeneration in the absence of inflammation in 1938.[8] The current International Association for the Study of Pain (IASP) taxonomy from 1979 defines neuralgia as pain in the distribution of a nerve[9] although, at the present, peripheral neuropathic pain, which may be due to several etiologies including secondary to peripheral nerve injury, is the current term.[10]

A recurring theme throughout the evolution of the concept of neuralgia to neuropathic pain has been the role of psychosocial factors, including Ochoa's "psychogenic pseudoneuropathy"[11] better explained today in terms of the sociopsychobiologic experience of pain. Most importantly, this concept has led to an appreciation of a multidisciplinary approach to assessing and treating patients with complex peripheral neuropathic pain.

PATHOPHYSIOLOGY OF PERIPHERAL NEUROPATHIC PAIN

The pathophysiology of peripheral neuropathic pain following injury is complex and evolving but has been well summarized in recent publications and is the result of both experimental animal models and human data.[10,12,13] After peripheral nerve injury, the key processes occurring at the periphery include ectopic neuronal firing, upregulation of sodium channels on injured fibers, neurogenic inflammation, increased expression of transient receptor potential V1 and adrenoreceptors on uninjured surrounding nerves, and Wallerian degeneration as well as regrowth of nerve fibers due to release of nerve growth factor, leading to peripheral sensitization.

At the dorsal root ganglion (DRG), there is increased neurotransmitter release, proliferation of satellite glial, astrocyte, microglial and Schwann cells, and upregulation of ion channels.[14]

Within the spinal cord, central sensitization of second-order neurones occurs coupled with dysfunction of inhibitory interneurones and descending modulatory control systems. There is proliferation of glial and microglial populations, as well as an increase in membrane channel and excitatory neurotransmitters, resulting in pain in extraterritorial regions.

Within the brain, neoplastic changes have been demonstrated in multiple locations, including the anterior cingulate cortex after experimental peripheral nerve injury in animals and also in patients with chronic neuropathic pain.[15]

An appreciation of this cascade of local, regional, and central pathophysiologic changes, which can arise from a peripheral nerve problem, helps in understanding the clinical presentation of patients and how specific therapies (pharmacology or interventions) may or may not work in treating patients with ostensibly simple peripheral nerve neuralgia.

Neuromas develop as part of the normal repair process after nerve injury or as a result of chronic damage to nerves and may or may not be painful. Factors that appear to be associated with the development of a painful neuroma are the severity of nerve damage, superficial location, mechanosensitivity, and chronic injury or compression, e.g., from scar and contribute to increased nociceptor sensitivity, central sensitization, chemosensitivity to catecholamines due to upregulation of receptors and ectopic firing as discussed above. The high rates of chronic postsurgical pain are highly correlated with nerve damage and neuroma formation, for example, with nerve ingrowth into hernia mesh more likely in patients requiring explants for pain.[16] The typical development of a painful neuroma over time from the onset of injury raises the possibility of prevention particularly with elective surgery and suggests that most neuromas do not cause symptoms and that early intervention including nerve repair or pharmacotherapy may help to prevent development.[17]

The pathology of nerve entrapment, the most common cause of peripheral neuropathic pain in humans, is incompletely understood because of the difficulty in obtaining human tissue. Chronic nerve compression has been associated with Schwann cell proliferation, apoptosis, demyelination, and remyelination in animal models in contrast to nerve injury in which Wallerian degeneration occurs.[18] Other mechanisms include impaired microcirculation, small diameter axonal loss, sensory axon dysfunction, and distal reduction in intraepidermal nerve density.[19] These processes may predate the injury to a peripheral nerve but may be important contributors to ongoing symptoms, including the pain following the injury.

Of the nonsurgical causes of painful peripheral neuralgia or neuropathy, diabetes is the most common in the community, but a long differential diagnosis exists, including inherited channelopathies, neoplastic, metabolic, drugs, toxic, nutritional, infectious, and small fiber neuropathy. The pathophysiology of diabetic neuropathy is multifactorial but involves metabolic, vascular, autoimmune, and altered neurotrophic support and free-radical cascades with chronic hyperglycemia underpinning them all.[13] Given the wide prevalence of diabetes and therefore neuropathy in the community, this is likely to be an important factor in pathology.

PATIENT ASSESSMENT

The key question for a surgeon in assessing a patient with peripheral neuralgia or neuropathic pain is to what degree is the pathophysiology peripheral, e.g., localized neuroma or generalized. In addition, even if there is evidence of central sensitization, is there a significant peripheral component that would benefit from a peripheral intervention, which is usually less invasive and cheaper and may have the prospect of long-term benefit. The assessment involves combining the input from the history, clinical examination, and investigations to formulate a diagnosis of the etiology and pathophysiologic mechanisms involved in the patient's pain syndrome.

The history of the patient with peripheral neuropathic pain needs to be thorough to determine the likely etiology and possible pathophysiology, symptom complex of which pain may or may not be the main problem, a functional or impairment assessment, progression or resolution of symptoms, response to prior treatments, medical history including diabetes and cancer, pain history, patient expectations, and the psychosocial milieu including work.

In the absence of a history of trauma, there is an extensive differential diagnosis of the causes of painful peripheral neuropathy as discussed earlier that should be worked through. Entrapment neurologic syndromes are usually straightforward, of slow onset, and progressive but may be atypical. In the acute setting conditions that mimic peripheral neuropathy including lumbar disc herniation, brachial neuritis, lumbar plexitis, or postherpetic neuralgia should be considered if the diagnosis is not clear and a neurology consult is sought for second opinion.

In the setting of a history of trauma or surgery details of the evolution of symptoms, prior treatment records including operation notes will be essential to isolate the neural structures. Typically, there will be sensory disturbance or dysfunction as part of the nerve injury even if pain is not immediately apparent. In the case of prior nerve surgery, there may have been a period of pain relief before which the current symptoms are returned or not. The separation of nociceptive, neuropathic, or mixed components of pain on history is important in the trauma or postoperative situation, as the treatment of these will be very different. For example, the typical history of a patient with neuroma following hernia surgery, i.e., localized distal numbness, focal tenderness with distal radiation of pain into the nerve territory, or a paroxysmal or burning quality, will be very different to one with periostitis pubis.[20]

Although uncommon, nerve sheath tumors are typically benign and usually minimally symptomatic until large enough. However, if pain without a history of trauma and particularly with progressive neurologic symptoms is a prominent part of the history, a malignant nerve sheath tumor[21] needs to be considered and urgently investigated.

Physical examination of the patient with peripheral neuropathic pain must not only detail the neurologic deficit related to the putative injured peripheral nerve but also consider whether other neurologic diagnoses are present or possible to account for the pain, i.e., is the pain concordant with the one nerve? Even with the same peripheral nerve, two points of pathology may be possible particularly at points of compression. Quantitative sensory testing is being increasingly used particularly in research settings to document sensory and pain thresholds and may give insight into the pathophysiologic mechanisms, e.g., peripheral or central operant in the particular patient.[10,12] They can also be repeated as should all neurologic examinations to document change or response to therapy. Signs beyond the distribution of the peripheral nerve in question, e.g., allodynia, where a normally painless stimulus is painful, suggest central sensitization has occurred.

Typical examination findings for a neuroma are a tender lump along the course of a peripheral nerve, sensitive to percussion with Tinel sign and often associated with distal sensory disturbance in the injured nerve. Combined with relief of symptoms from local anesthetic block, this finding is very supportive of neuroma and may be sufficient to therefore recommend surgery for exploration and removal of neuroma.[20] Tinel sign may also be used at points of nerve compression in suspected entrapment and also to monitor recovery of nerve regrowth at the distal end as the paresthesia evoked implies that sensory axons are continuous with the central nervous system.

INVESTIGATIONS

Electromyography (EMG) and nerve conduction studies can help to support or refute the clinical diagnosis of peripheral nerve dysfunction but have limitations and need to be performed at appropriate time intervals depending on the pattern of injury. The extent of nerve injury, as well as muscle denervation and reinnervation, can be characterized particularly over time. Conduction amplitudes and velocities can assess nerve damage from trauma or entrapment as well as the presence of polyneuropathy with the exception of small fiber neuropathy. Spinal root avulsion, upper motor neurone pathology, and primary muscle disease can also be differentiated by using EMG.

Neuroimaging of the patient with peripheral nerve neuralgia is helpful in supporting the clinical history and examination findings. Ultrasound is an effective, cheap, and real-time tool in demonstrating neuromas and peripheral nerve tumors; however, differentiation may be difficult but is usually based on history.[17] Nerve entrapment, subluxation, and nerve volume can also be assessed reliably. Interestingly, in a recent study, ultrasound was found to be more sensitive and equivalent specificity and better showed multifocal lesions compared with MRI.[22] Ultrasound can also be used preoperatively and intraoperatively to localize lesions.

MRI may be useful for entrapment syndromes, traumas, masses, and acquired or hereditary demyelinating polyneuropathies in peripheral nerve disorders[23] and does have greater resolution for visualizing neural structure using multiplanar reconstruction and showing relationship to adjacent structures. Concomitant spinal imaging can be performed in cases where there is a differential diagnosis. Muscle and joint relations as well as changes in muscle bulk, which may occur in denervation, can be clearly seen. For peripheral nerve tumors, which may be painful, MRI is clearly the modality of choice and can distinguish benign from malignant lesions.[21] With nerve injury, diffusion tensor imaging (DTI) sequences can track axonal degeneration and regeneration following grafting to supplement clinical evaluation.[24] Nerve caliber, flattening or swelling, can also be assessed and be correlated with the clinical syndrome.

TREATMENT

The treatment of peripheral neuropathic pain is directed by the results of the diagnostic formulation and can be broadly considered in terms of pharmacologic, functional, surgical, and neuromodulation options. Management should occur in the context of or with the availability of a multidisciplinary team.

Most patients referred with peripheral neuropathic pain will already be on pharmacotherapy, which may include tricyclic antidepressants, anticonvulsants, gabapentinoids, opioids, norepinephrine reuptake inhibitors, lignocaine, and capsaicin patches as prescribed. A detailed review of pharmacotherapy for peripheral neuropathic pain is beyond the scope of this chapter; however, numerous reviews have determined that many patients do not receive appropriate treatment for neuropathic pain, and only a minority of patients have an adequate response to drug therapy.[25,26] In spite of these limitations and pending results of more specific phenotypically driven pharmacologic trials using Qualitative Sensory Testing (QST), optimization of drug therapy should be attempted in all patients, as this may be sufficient in some patients.

Physical therapy may also be prescribed to minimize deconditioning and retrain muscles in patients with peripheral neuropathic pain with modest but variable benefit according to a recent metaanalysis.[27]

Surgical treatment for pain secondary to nerve entrapment in the nontraumatic setting is usually straightforward, provided the diagnosis is concordant with nerve conduction findings and the nerve decompression is thorough, which are the two most common causes of failure. More difficult situations may arise with a history of trauma, focal pain without neurologic symptoms, advanced axonal damage, workers' compensation or litigation, diabetes, or history of chronic pain. Simple decompression may also be combined with transposition of the nerve if position is an important component of the neural compression. Preoperative screening questionnaires to assess the patient pain experience and evaluate risk factors for poor surgical outcomes may be helpful.[28]

Surgical treatment of peripheral nerve neuroma is based on the premise that a significant proportion of the patient's pain complaint is related to the neuroma or that this peripheral source of the pain is a significant contributor to a centralized process. The latter scenario may occur, for example, in a patient with postamputational pain with a stump neuroma. Successful removal of a neuroma may obviate the need for more complex pain interventions.[4]

Patient selection for surgery is the most important factor in predicting outcomes from neuroma surgery. A discrete clinical nerve syndrome, palpable lump, positive Tinel sign, concordant imaging, distal pain relief following local anesthetic block, and satisfactory psychosocial evaluation will give the best chance of a positive surgical finding and improvement postoperatively.[4,17,20,29,30]

The surgical strategies available for neuroma resection depend on the location of the neuroma in the nerve, particularly if it is on a distal sensory or mixed sensory motor nerve with preserved motor function (neuroma-in-continuity). In the former situation the neuroma can be excised, the distal sensory nerve sacrificed, and the stump reimplanted into a more favorable location but usually bone or muscle. A variety of technical nuances to deal with the sectioned end have been proposed, including ligation alone, diathermy of the cut end, proximal nerve crush, and nerve transposition into muscle or intermuscular planes without tension.[4,17,20,29–31] Neuromas that occur in an amputation stump, the so-called "stump neuromas," are another category of neuroma and may be addressed surgically only if a discrete lesion can be identified, relief can be achieved with local anesthetic block, and sufficient tissue can cover the cut end. In the author's experience, a more diffuse pain syndrome within the stump is more common.

The outcomes from neuroma surgery treatment have been sobering historically with high likelihood of pain recurrence even with initial good outcomes; however, improvements in patient selection and surgical techniques have occurred. Follow-up in the literature has typically been short, and patient populations have been heterogeneous. The trend toward patient-reported outcomes and quality-of-life measures will allow better comparison between studies in the future.

Burchiel reported a 44% surgical success defined by reduction in pain by 50% with mean follow-up of 11 months in a cohort of patients with preoperatively and intraoperatively defined neuroma that could be resected and relocated.[29] Those patients with neuromas-in-continuity who underwent neurolysis alone had no improvement, but those with compression that could be relieved and transposed could improve. Zacest et al. reported 3-year follow-up of patients who underwent resection of ilioinguinal nerve for posthernia pain, most of which had a neuroma identified intraoperatively and noted return of pain was common (68%) although some degree of pain relief was also achieved in 67%.[20]

Domeshek et al. reported improvement in four patient-rated qualities, including pain, depression, disability and quality of life, in 70 patients who underwent neuroma resection, proximal crush, and transposition as well as decompression of associated nerve compression and were followed up at 24 months with a questionnaire and interview. Neuromas attached to large sensorimotor nerves were dissected off the main trunk. For all patients combined, the Visual Analog Pain Score dropped from 6.74 to 5.1 postoperatively ($P < .001$) and the degree of improvement was greater for patients with higher pain scores and depression. Ninety percent of patients had chronic pain for 6 months, suggesting that chronic sensitization was probably present. The authors of the last paper conclude that statistically significant improvements in patient-reported pain and quality of life can occur following surgery in a center with expertise; however, many of the patients will continue to have chronic pain.

The modest results from surgery reported above have led others to avoid surgical intervention altogether or recommend other interventions for patients with intractable peripheral neuropathic pain following trauma or surgery. Moreover, in many patients, perhaps most, in this group, there may be scarce macroscopic evidence of a structural lesion. Available interventions may range from peripheral lesional procedures at the peripheral nerve level or DRG level or neuromodulation strategies from the peripheral nerve level to spinal cord level. Each approach (lesion vs. neuromodulation) presents advantages and disadvantages that need to be carefully weighed in the individual patient. Theoretically, at least, in the likely situation that the patient with peripheral pain has developed some degree of central sensitization neuromodulation strategies would seem the better long-term strategy.

Although a number of local lesional treatments have been trialed for suspected or proven neuromas, including repeated steroid injection, botulinum toxin, tumor necrosis factor inhibitor, phenol, cryotherapy, and radiofrequency (RF), the results are variable with recurrent pain. Their main advantages are low cost, minimal intervention, and repeatability, and if they only reduce the pain from a peripheral pain generator may be a valuable adjuvant to more comprehensive strategies.[17]

Peripheral nerve stimulation (PNS) is a neuromodulation technique in which electrical stimulation is applied to peripheral nerves to ameliorate chronic pain through preferential activation of myelinated fibers inducing long-term depression in synaptic efficiency. Initially developed in the 1960s as a percutaneous technique using an electrode over a peripheral nerve, and later as a surgical electrode, less invasive options include transcutaneous electrical stimulation, percutaneous electrical stimulation (PENS) using electrical stimulation of needles, or most recently noninvasive PENS or external non invasive percutaneous electrical stimulation (PENS). A recent prospective observation study enrolled 76 patients with a variety of conditions (postherpetic neuralgia, causalgia, and postsurgical pain) for a single treatment with a 21-gauge needle with maintenance of pain improvement for 3–6 months.[32] A sham-controlled trial of EN-PENS is currently in progress.[33] The potential advantages of PENS or EN-PENS are its minimally invasive nature, low side effect profile, and ability to be repeated in patients who might not be ideal candidates for implantable neurostimulators. Whether these therapies are capable of providing long-term relief for peripheral-based intractable pain is yet to be determined.

PNS has also been successfully used for pain relief of painful stumps and neuromas in a number of case reports and recent small series.[34–36] In the latter study, high-frequency stimulation (10 kHz) was used, resulting in nerve conduction block without paresthesia from the painful neuroma with patients reporting the greatest degree of pain relief they had ever experienced compared with other therapies. This is further evidence of peripherally mediated central pain and that peripheral therapies may help such patients.

DRG stimulation has recently been demonstrated to be effective in treatment of neuropathic pain, including complex regional pain syndrome,[37] phantom limb pain,[38] and postsurgical pain syndrome[39] with results maintained beyond a year. The relative advantages of this new target include the ability to cover areas difficult to target with conventional spinal cord stimulation (SCS), such as the groin, foot, and back with lower voltages required, minimizing unnecessary limb stimulation and patient preference. Although the present results are very promising, the longer-term outcomes are awaited.

SCS has been the mainstay of neuromodulation therapy for neuropathic pain for the last three decades and has the advantage of being testable, reversible, and adjustable. Moreover, if it can be determined or is suspected that central sensitization has occurred, then the spinal cord would appear to be a logical place to target. Although there have been many technologic advances in lead design and stimulation parameters including conventional tonic, high frequency, and burst, a percutaneous trial with stimulation coverage of the painful area can be performed simply as an outpatient to assess therapeutically whether a permanent system may be an option. Although the highest levels of evidence for benefit of SCS have been for spinal-origin pain,[40,41] phantom limb and neuroma pain have been treated successfully with SCS since 1969; however, the data derived chiefly from case reports and surgical series have been variable.[42,43]

Central neuromodulation, including deep brain stimulation and motor cortex stimulation, has been used for refractory neuropathic pain but is not approved by the Food and Drug Administration because of lack of evidence.[44]

With the explosion of neuromodulation options discussed above and the reluctance of many practitioners to create an irreversible lesion in a patient with neuropathic pain, lesional options including standard RF, root or ganglion section, once practiced historically, have fallen out of favor. An exception may be pulsed RF, which delivers a pulsed RF current of 42°C to the neural target and results in less tissue destruction. Its efficacy in neuropathic pain, despite a recent metaanalysis, suggests a potential benefit in some conditions but little in others.[45]

CONCLUSION

The optimum treatment of the patient with peripheral neuropathic pain, depending on the etiology and pain phenotype, will range from simple pharmacotherapy to consideration of peripheral surgery, including regional lesioning, and then to neuromodulation options within a multidisciplinary framework. Given the pathophysiologic cascade that occurs following peripheral nerve injury, some degree of central sensitization is likely in most patients. In spite of this reality, a peripheral source may be amenable to surgical intervention and is worth considering although the outcomes are modest and the chance of recurrent pain is high. Neuromodulation strategies, if successful, appear to hold the best current hope of longer-term pain control but are rarely curative and require regular maintenance. Such therapies are best provided within a multidisciplinary pain clinic. In the future, better understanding of the pathophysiology of peripherally driven neuropathic pain and how this manifests in clinical pain phenotypes using tools such as QST testing will allow a more personalized approach to obtaining better pain outcomes for our patients.

REFERENCES

1. Armstrong J. On rheumatism and the diagnosis of gout and rheumatism. *Lancet*. 1825;7:65–69.
2. Quintner JL, Bove GM. From neuralgia to peripheral neuropathic pain: evolution of a concept. *Reg Anesth Pain Med*. 2001;26(4):368–372.
3. Mitchell SW, Morehouse GR, Keen WW. The classic. Gunshot wounds and other injuries of nerves by S. Weir Mitchell, M.D., George R. Morehouse, M.D., and William W. Keen, M.D. *Clin Orthop Relat Res*. 1982;(163):2–7.
4. Burchiel KJ, Israel Z,H. Surgical treatment of painful peripheral nerve injuries. In: Burchiel KJ, ed. *Surgical Management of Pain*. New York: Thieme; 2002:654–665.
5. Little KM, et al. An eclectic history of peripheral nerve surgery. *Neurosurg Clin N Am*. 2004;15(2):109–123.
6. Platt H. The surgery of the peripheral nerve injuries of warfare. *Br Med J*. 1921;1(3147):596–600.
7. Horsley V. Preliminary communications on the existence of sensory nerves and nerve endings in nerve trunks, the true "nervi nerorum". *BMJ*. 1884;1(1204):166.
8. Wechsler I. Multiple peripheral neuropathy versus multiple neuritis. *JAMA*. 1938;110(23):1910–1913.
9. Bonica JJ. The need of a taxonomy. *Pain*. 1979;6(3):247–248.
10. Baron R, et al. Peripheral neuropathic pain: a mechanism-related organizing principle based on sensory profiles. *Pain*. 2017;158(2):261–272.
11. Ochoa JL. Essence, investigation, and management of "neuropathic" pains: hopes from acknowledgment of chaos. *Muscle Nerve*. 1993;16(10):997–1008.
12. Baron R, Binder A, Wasner G. Neuropathic pain: diagnosis, pathophysiological mechanisms, and treatment. *Lancet Neurol*. 2010;9(8):807–819.
13. Jay GW, Barkin RL. Neuropathic pain: etiology, pathophysiology, mechanisms, and evaluations. *Dis Mon*. 2014;60(1):6–47.
14. Guha D, Shamji MF. The dorsal root ganglion in the pathogenesis of chronic neuropathic pain. *Neurosurgery*. 2016; 63(suppl 1):118–126.
15. Jaggi AS, Singh N. Role of different brain areas in peripheral nerve injury-induced neuropathic pain. *Brain Res*. 2011;1381:187–201.
16. Bendavid R, et al. A mechanism of mesh-related post-herniorrhaphy neuralgia. *Hernia*. 2016;20(3):357–365.
17. Rajput K, Reddy S, Shankar H. Painful neuromas. *Clin J Pain*. 2012;28(7):639–645.
18. Pham K, Gupta R. Understanding the mechanisms of entrapment neuropathies. Review article. *Neurosurg Focus*. 2009;26(2):E7.
19. Schmid AB, et al. The relationship of nerve fibre pathology to sensory function in entrapment neuropathy. *Brain*. 2014;137(Pt 12):3186–3199.
20. Zacest AC, et al. Long-term outcome following ilioinguinal neurectomy for chronic pain. *J Neurosurg*. 2010;112(4): 784–789.
21. Wasa J, et al. MRI features in the differentiation of malignant peripheral nerve sheath tumors and neurofibromas. *Am J Roentgenol*. 2010;194(6):1568–1574.

22. Zaidman CM, et al. Detection of peripheral nerve pathology: comparison of ultrasound and MRI. *Neurology*. 2013;80(18):1634–1640.
23. Kwee RM, et al. Accuracy of MRI in diagnosing peripheral nerve disease: a systematic review of the literature. *Am J Roentgenol*. 2014;203(6):1303–1309.
24. Simon NG, Kliot M. Diffusion weighted MRI and tractography for evaluating peripheral nerve degeneration and regeneration. *Neural Regen Res*. 2014;9(24):2122–2124.
25. Attal N, Bouhassira D. Pharmacotherapy of neuropathic pain: which drugs, which treatment algorithms? *Pain*. 2015;156(suppl 1):S104–S114.
26. Finnerup NB, et al. Pharmacotherapy for neuropathic pain in adults: a systematic review and meta-analysis. *Lancet Neurol*. 2015;14(2):162–173.
27. Ginnerup-Nielsen E, et al. Physiotherapy for pain: a meta-epidemiological study of randomised trials. *Br J Sports Med*. 2016;50(16):965–971.
28. Tang DT, et al. Nerve entrapment: update. *Plast Reconstr Surg*. 2015;135(1):199e–215e.
29. Burchiel KJ, Johans TJ, Ochoa J. The surgical treatment of painful traumatic neuromas. *J Neurosurg*. 1993;78(5):714–719.
30. Domeshek LF, et al. Surgical treatment of neuromas improves patient-reported pain, depression, and quality of life. *Plast Reconstr Surg*. 2017;139(2):407–418.
31. Brunelli GA. Prevention of damage caused by sural nerve withdrawal for nerve grafting. *Hand Surg*. 2002;7(2):163–166.
32. Rossi M, et al. A novel mini-invasive approach to the treatment of neuropathic pain: the PENS study. *Pain Physician*. 2016;19(1):E121–E128.
33. Johnson S, et al. A randomised, patient-assessor blinded, sham-controlled trial of external non-invasive peripheral nerve stimulation for chronic neuropathic pain following peripheral nerve injury (EN-PENS trial): study protocol for a randomised controlled trial. *Trials*. 2016;17(1):574.
34. Cornish PB. Successful peripheral neuromodulation for phantom limb pain: an update. *Pain Med*. 2016;17(5):991.
35. Meier K, et al. Peripheral neuromodulation for the treatment of postamputation neuroma pain: a case report. *A A Case Rep*. 2017;8(2):29–30.
36. Soin A, Fang ZP, Velasco J. Peripheral neuromodulation to treat postamputation pain. *Prog Neurol Surg*. 2015;29:158–167.
37. Deer TR, et al. Dorsal root ganglion stimulation yielded higher treatment success rate for complex regional pain syndrome and causalgia at 3 and 12 months: a randomized comparative trial. *Pain*. 2017;158(4):669–681.
38. Eldabe S, et al. Dorsal root ganglion (DRG) stimulation in the treatment of phantom limb pain (PLP). *Neuromodulation*. 2015;18(7):610–616; discussion 616–617.
39. Liem L, et al. One-year outcomes of spinal cord stimulation of the dorsal root ganglion in the treatment of chronic neuropathic pain. *Neuromodulation*. 2015;18(1):41–48; discussion 48–49.
40. Kumar K, et al. The effects of spinal cord stimulation in neuropathic pain are sustained: a 24-month follow-up of the prospective randomized controlled multicenter trial of the effectiveness of spinal cord stimulation. *Neurosurgery*. 2008;63(4):762–770; discussion 770.
41. North RB, et al. Spinal cord stimulation versus repeated lumbosacral spine surgery for chronic pain: a randomized, controlled trial. *Neurosurgery*. 2005;56(1):98–106; discussion 106–107.
42. Aiyer R, et al. A systematic review on the treatment of phantom limb pain with spinal cord stimulation. *Pain Manag*. 2017;7(1):59–69.
43. Viswanathan A, Phan PC, Burton AW. Use of spinal cord stimulation in the treatment of phantom limb pain: case series and review of the literature. *Pain Pract*. 2010;10(5):479–484.
44. Moore NZ, Lempka SF, Machado A. Central neuromodulation for refractory pain. *Neurosurg Clin N Am*. 2014;25(1):77–83.
45. Shi Y, Wu W. Treatment of neuropathic pain using pulsed radiofrequency: a meta-analysis. *Pain Physician*. 2016;19(7):429–444.

CHAPTER 5

Peripheral Nerve Stimulation

GARRETT P. BANKS, MD • CHRISTOPHER J. WINFREE, MD, FAANS

INTRODUCTION

Peripheral nerve stimulation (PNS) is the direct electrical stimulation of named nerves outside of the central neuraxis to alleviate pain in the distribution of a targeted peripheral nerve.[1] PNS works by stimulating the nerve that is connected to the area in which the patient is experiencing pain. Because stimulation of the peripheral nervous system was first shown by Sweet and Wall to ameliorate pain,[2] many practitioners have applied neural stimulation for treating various etiologies of pain. Electrical stimulation treatments have shown efficacy in treating various neuropathic,[3,4] musculoskeletal,[5] and visceral refractory pain[6] and are an important part of the treatment repertoire for treating chronic refractory pain. These methods can be implemented in isolation or in addition to other neurostimulation devices such as spinal cord stimulation or deep brain stimulation to best reduce a patient's refractory chronic pain.

MECHANISM OF NEUROSTIMULATION

Our understanding of why neurostimulation is able to alleviate pain has been evolving ever since Sweet and Wall used the principles of gate theory to explain their success with PNS.[2,7] Although we still have much to uncover regarding how the process works, the general principle is thought to involve inhibition and activation of pain-related neural circuitry, including ascending pathways in the dorsal horn nucleus as well as modulatory pathways of the autonomic system.[8] The treatment of pain through neurostimulation has been shown to not simply work by a direct cascade of electrical signals but rather include complex modulatory interactions with several neurotransmitters, such as γ-amino butyric acid and adenosine. In addition, although the original mechanism used to explain pain relief using gate theory suggested the necessity of paresthesias to induce analgesia, new research has shown that high-frequency stimulation (~10 kHz) and burst stimulation using spinal cord stimulation can provide at least similar (if not better) pain relief. As these high-frequency paradigms produce analgesia even when patients are not consciously aware of stimulation, these recent trials suggest that we still do not fully understand the mechanistic underpinnings of electrical stimulation for pain.[9,10]

INDICATIONS

One of the most important principles in neurosurgery for pain is proper patient selection. Any candidate for stimulation must have failed first-line medical conservative therapies. To be eligible for neurostimulation, patients generally should have demonstrated an inadequate response to medications, noninvasive treatment options, and minimally invasive pain management strategies, as appropriate.[11] After failing less invasive treatments, patients should undergo psychologic testing.[12] As many psychologic characteristics and psychiatric pathologies can greatly exacerbate chronic pain, patients should undergo psychiatric evaluation and receive treatment for any psychiatric comorbidity that may be exacerbating their chronic pain.

WORKUP AND ASSESSMENT

The specific distribution of chronic pain is the guiding factor in deciding which specific stimulation is most appropriate. The chosen modality should be able to specifically target the area where pain is experienced, and more invasive modalities should not be chosen over less invasive approaches that are just as efficacious and easier to implement. After selection of an appropriate modality, some institutions proceed directly to a trial of stimulation, whereas other institutions first perform a diagnostic nerve block. The rationale for performing a nerve block is that if the experienced pain improves after chemically blocking the nerve, then the target has been correctly chosen as a stimulation candidate for relieving the patient's pain. Although this practice is helpful in some instances, the necessity of this step is debated.[10] The controversy is due to the unclear use of a negative result. Although a successful nerve block supports treating the nerve in question, many patients have been found to benefit from neurostimulation even if their initial nerve block was negative.

Once the decision has been made to proceed with PNS, the patient must first undergo a stimulation trial.[13] The trial consists of implanting a patient with a temporary electrode that is connected to an external pulse generator. The patient is then discharged home and receives stimulation for a week's duration. At the end of the trial, the level of pain reduction is assessed as well as changes in quality of life. If patients have a 50% or greater reduction in pain and a meaningful improvement in their quality of life, then the trial is considered a success. The temporary device is then replaced with the permanent system. By using this paradigm, only patients who demonstrate benefit from stimulation undergo surgical implantation. Although no set of screening techniques can predict with 100% certainty which patients will ultimately benefit, the combination of judicious screening, careful patient selection, and trialing of the stimulation itself allows for the maximization of the likelihood of success for those who undergo electrical stimulation for chronic pain.

OPEN PLACEMENT OF PERIPHERAL NEUROSTIMULATION

After Sweet and Wall's reported success in 1967, surgeons began to implant battery-powered neurostimulation devices by means of direct implantation.[14] To perform an open implantation, the patient is provided monitored anesthesia and then prepped and draped in the usual fashion. Surgical dissection and exposure is performed of the nerve in question, followed by neurolysis of the nerve from its surrounding tissue. After proper exposure, a lead is placed along the nerve (Fig. 5.1). Although some practitioners have historically wrapped the nerve with a lead, this practice is no longer recommended owing to the scarring and adhesions that result. Early descriptions of paddle lead placement along the nerve recommend the placement of a layer of fascia between the electrode array and the nerve itself. This was done to blunt the intensity of the stimulation, as the early implantable pulse generators did not allow for fine adjustments. Thus, patients could experience dramatic increases in stimulation intensity with the stepwise adjustments available at that time. Current generators can permit fine adjustments, thus obviating the need for a fascial barrier.

The electrodes are then trialed in the operating room using an external pulse generator, and adjustments are made to ensure appropriate coverage. Once satisfactory coverage is achieved, the leads are sutured to the surrounding tissue and then attached to a disposable extension wire that is tunneled out through the skin. The extension lead is then attached to an external pulse generator placed in a sterile sleeve, which is adhered to the outside of the body. The patient leaves the hospital that same day to trial the stimulator for approximately 1 week. If the trial is successful, the patient returns to the operating room for internalization of the device. The disposable extensions are discarded and the leads are tunneled and connected to an implantable pulse generator that is placed in a subfascial pocket. The most commonly used locations to implant the pulse generators are the buttocks, medial thigh, and subclavicular areas.[15]

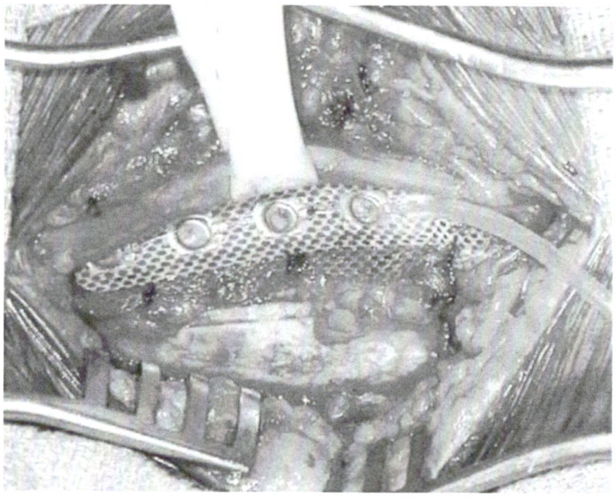

FIG. 5.1 Intraoperative picture showing the direct placement of a tibial nerve stimulator. Whereas in this photo a paddle lead is used, percutaneous electrodes may alternatively be used. (From Stuart RM, Winfree CJ. Neurostimulation techniques for painful peripheral nerve disorders. *Neurosurg Clin N Am*. 2009;20(1):111–120, vii–viii.)

Although efficacious and currently covered by insurance and Medicare, full exposure of the nerve along with placement of the electrode is a procedure that can produce significant pain secondary to the dissection and often results in the buildup of scar tissue when multiple procedures have taken place. In addition, because of the mechanically dynamic nature of the areas where leads are commonly placed, leads occasionally experience mechanical failure and lead migration.[16]

PERCUTANEOUS PLACEMENT OF PERIPHERAL NEUROSTIMULATION

Another method for implanting stimulation leads is percutaneous placement. This alternative implantation technique can be used for both trial electrode placement and permanent placement. Similar to an open approach, the patient is provided monitored anesthesia and then prepped and draped in the usual fashion; however, instead of making an incision and performing a surgical dissection, a needle and tunneling system is used to place four- or eight-contact electrodes in the epifascial plane adjacent to the nerve. For placement of electrodes in shallow areas with obvious external landmarks (such as with craniofacial stimulation), fluoroscopic guidance is generally not required but can be useful for verifying placement and for making adjustments.

After placement, the electrode is similarly connected to an external pulse generator and a stimulation paradigm is chosen that results in adequate coverage. If the placement and coverage is satisfactory, the lead or leads are anchored to the skin with a 3-0 silk to avoid strain or torque on the leads. The external pulse generator is placed in a sterile enclosed adhesive pocket, which is adhered to the patient near the exit site of the lead. The exit site is also covered in sterile dressings, and the patient is sent home for a week to trial the stimulation. Of note, the authors of this paper do not regularly prescribe antibiotics for a stimulation trial. If after the trial a significant decrease in pain and a significant increase in quality of life results, the apparatus is completely removed. A fresh new electrode is then tunneled into position and connected to a pulse generator implanted subcutaneously. If the trial was not a success, a permanent electrode is not placed after removing the trial electrode.

Compared with open surgical placement of the electrode, percutaneous placement is faster, is less traumatic, and usually results in markedly less postoperative pain; however, the technique is only well suited for superficial targets, as placement is performed indirectly. The main drawback of percutaneous placement is that the lead has a higher tendency to migrate.[16] There is minimal tissue friction with the cylindrical lead, and the only things holding the lead in place are the anchor and a stitch. Although the lead only normally migrates deep or superficial and is relatively easy to fix by repositioning, repeated revision of the lead can be burdensome for the patient.

TRIGEMINAL BRANCH STIMULATION

Craniofacial stimulation is one of the most successful indications for PNS because of the inability to use spinal cord stimulation or dorsal root ganglion stimulation to treat pain in craniofacial distributions.[17] One of the patients in the original series published by Wall and Sweet was able to attain chronic facial pain relief using infraorbital stimulation. Since then, many patients have been able to achieve facial pain relief using PNS. Both infraorbital stimulation and supraorbital stimulation have been found to alleviate pain in either postherpetic neuralgia or trigeminal posttraumatic neuropathic pain.[17–21]

Trigeminal branch stimulation is performed using a percutaneous lead insertion technique. The procedure involves first placing the patient supine in the operating room under conscious sedation. (The trial implantation should be performed under conscious sedation, whereas the permanent implant can be placed under general anesthesia, mostly to alleviate tunneling discomfort.) The target starting point is marked behind the hairline and above the zygoma for supraorbital placement or below the zygoma for infraorbital placement. The area is numbed with lidocaine, and a stab incision is made. A large-gauge Tuohy needle is passed subcutaneously under fluoroscopic guidance to the supraorbital or infraorbital region, roughly 1 cm above or below the orbital rim (Fig. 5.2). The lead is passed until the medial border of the orbit is reached. After passage of the needle, the stylet is removed and a four- or eight-contact electrode is passed to the region of interest. For the trial, a temporary electrode is connected to an external pulse generator to confirm coverage, and adjustments are made if necessary. The electrode is anchored in place with a silk suture, hooked up to an external pulse generator. The patient is then sent home to trial the stimulation for a week. If successful, a permanent electrode is implanted. The permanent electrode is connected via extension wires to a pulse generator placed in a subcutaneous infraclavicular pocket.

Interestingly, not only do superficial pains respond well to trigeminal branch stimulation, but a variety of headache etiologies do as well. Chronic cluster headaches have been reported to respond well to supraorbital neurostimulation in patients who gained minimal benefit from an occipital nerve block.[22] The dual usage of both supraorbital and occipital nerve stimulation has also been used to control chronic migraine headaches.[18]

STIMULATION FOR OCCIPITAL NEURALGIA

Neurostimulation is also commonly performed on occipital nerve branches for neuralgias and various headache etiologies to great effect; however, as occipital nerve stimulation is covered in another chapter, it will not be further discussed here.

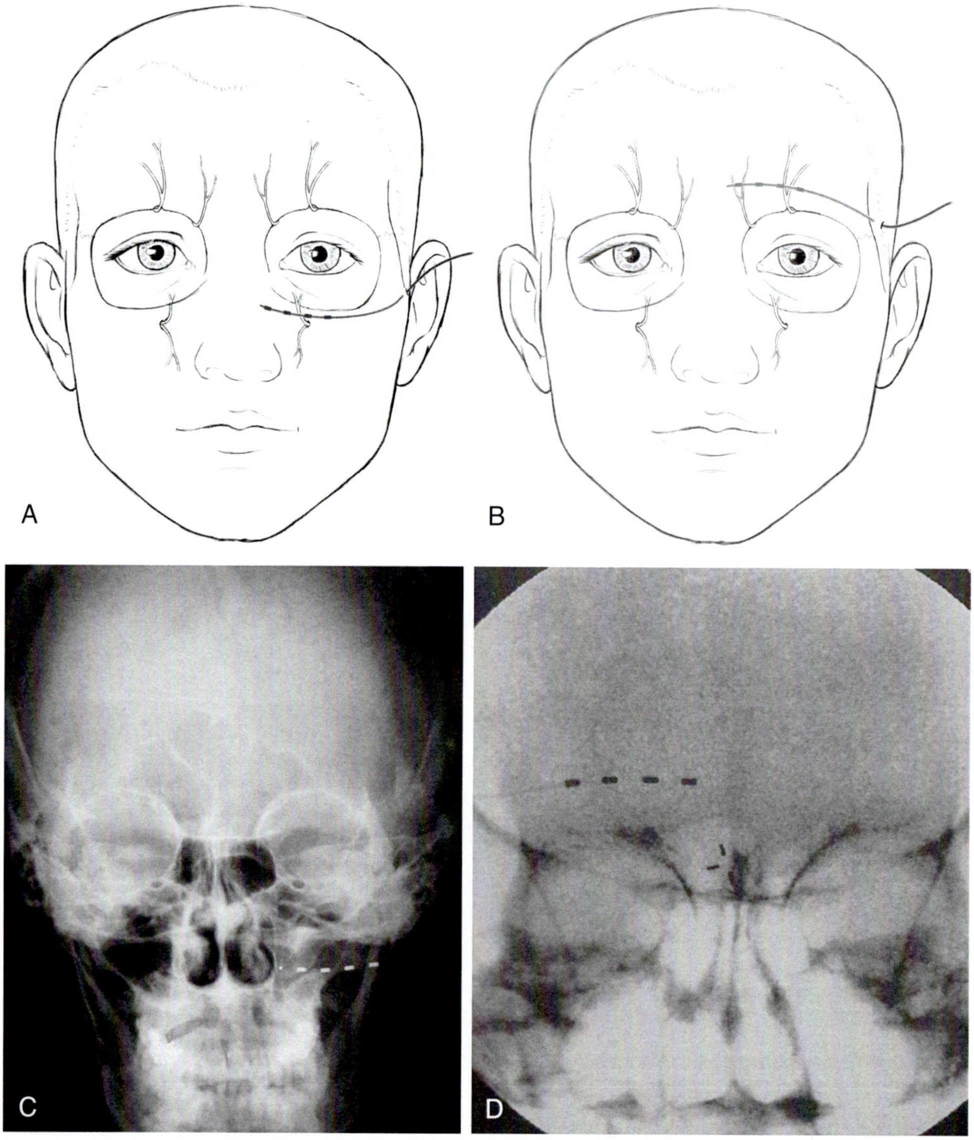

FIG. 5.2 Placement of infraorbital and supraorbital electrodes. **A** and **B** show where infraorbital and supraorbital electrodes are placed, respectively. **C** and **D** show the placement of infraorbital and supraorbital electrodes on plain film X-ray. (From Slavin KV, Wess C. Trigeminal branch stimulation for intractable neuropathic pain: technical note. *Neuromodulation*. 2005;8(1):7–13.)

POSTAMPUTATION LIMB PAIN

PNS has been used for a large variety of indications when other pain treatment modalities have been ineffective. After amputation, up to 70%–80% of patients experience chronic pain, which is either classified as phantom limb pain or residual limb pain. Poorly treated pain syndromes in these patients can further impair their function and even prohibit the use of prosthetics. Additionally, pharmacologic treatment for postamputation pain is frequently inadequate and has the potential for addiction and unwanted side effects. In patients with residual limb pain, PNS of the femoral or sciatic nerve has been shown to significantly reduce pain.[23] In most patients who were implanted for residual limb pain, they experienced a significant decrease in their pain along with improved quality of life.[24]

Recently, some groups are placing PNS leads for postamputation limb pain percutaneously using landmarks. The sciatic nerve can be accessed using a posterior approach, with the greater trochanter and ischial tuberosity as landmarks. The femoral nerve can be accessed using an anterior approach, with the femoral artery and femoral crease as landmarks.

Before placing the lead, a monopolar needle electrode is inserted to within 0.5–3.0 cm of the trunk of the femoral or sciatic nerve to deliver a test stimulation to ascertain proximity to the nerve. The test stimulation is used to confirm that comfortable paresthesias could be produced without evoking muscle contractions or irritating sensations. The paresthesias should be produced in the area of the experienced postamputation pain. If local subcutaneous sensations are experienced, the needle can be advanced and stimulation is again attempted. If muscle contractions are elicited or uncomfortable sensations in the area are supplied by the nerve trunk, the needle is withdrawn slightly. After a satisfactory result is achieved, the stimulation needle is removed, and a fine wire needle is used to place the lead in the same trajectory using ultrasound guidance. Of note, the lead is often advanced approximately a centimeter less than the stimulation electrode, placing the lead slightly farther from the nerve.

PERIPHERAL NERVE/FIELD STIMULATION

When the site of pain to be treated is not clearly localized to a specific nerve, PNS is not the ideal treatment modality. For these patients, if the area of pain is relatively limited in surface area, the area itself rather than the innervating nerve can be stimulated to help ameliorate their pain. This technique is called peripheral nerve/field stimulation (PNFS) and works by directly placing electrodes subcutaneously in the area of pain. For implantation of a PNFS electrode, the same process of placing a percutaneous peripheral nerve lead can be used, but the leads are implanted independent of the nerve path.[11] Cylindrical leads are classically used, with similar tunneling techniques to percutaneously placed PNS leads. In a limited number of cases, paddle leads can be used as well.

In PNFS stimulation, the depth of the placement of the electrode is very important, as electrodes implanted too shallow will cause a stinging or burning sensation and eventually lead to erosion. Alternatively, electrodes implanted too deep will cause unintended muscle stimulation and twitching. Of note, electrodes are placed directly in the area of pain with the exception of when a patient suffers from allodynia. For patients experiencing allodynia, superior outcomes are achieved by bracketing the area off instead. Just like other nerve stimulation techniques, stimulation is first trialed, and a permanent implant is placed if satisfactory criteria are met.

PNFS has been published extensively in the literature, with studies showing decreases in lower back pain,[25,26] chronic abdominal pain, inguinal neuralgia, chronic pancreatitis-related pain, and pain after liver transplant.[6,27] PNFS has even been able to improve thoracic and chest wall pain when implanted at the site of pain.[28] However, although the technique has been shown in many case series to be beneficial, the method is no longer reimbursed in the United States. Because of difficulty attaining reimbursement, PNFS has largely fallen out of favor as a treatment for refractory chronic pain.

ULTRASOUND-GUIDED PERIPHERAL NERVE STIMULATION

The blind placement of percutaneous peripheral nerve stimulator electrode arrays without image guidance can potentially injure any structures, such as blood vessels, in the vicinity of the target nerve. Placing the electrodes with image guidance can substantially ameliorate these risks. Recently, to attain the minimally invasive benefits of percutaneous electrodes placement for deeper targets, practitioners have begun to use ultrasound for the placement of electrodes.

After the patient is administered general anesthesia and antibiotics, the patient is draped in the usual fashion. A small skin nick is made to insert a 14-gauge epidural needle using ultrasound guidance. The needle is advanced deep to the nerve and a few millimeters past it. A standard eight-contact percutaneous epidural neurostimulation electrode is then passed through the needle until resistance is met. The needle is then withdrawn while keeping the electrode in place (Fig. 5.3). After stimulation in the operating room demonstrates paresthesias in the correct location, the lead is anchored in the skin for trials and in the superficial fascia for permanent electrodes. A strain loop is created at the anchoring site to prevent strain-related damage or migration of the lead.[29]

Ultrasound-guided placement of electrodes has the potential to significantly alter the field of neurostimulation for pain. First, ultrasound-guided implantation of percutaneous leads has been advancing

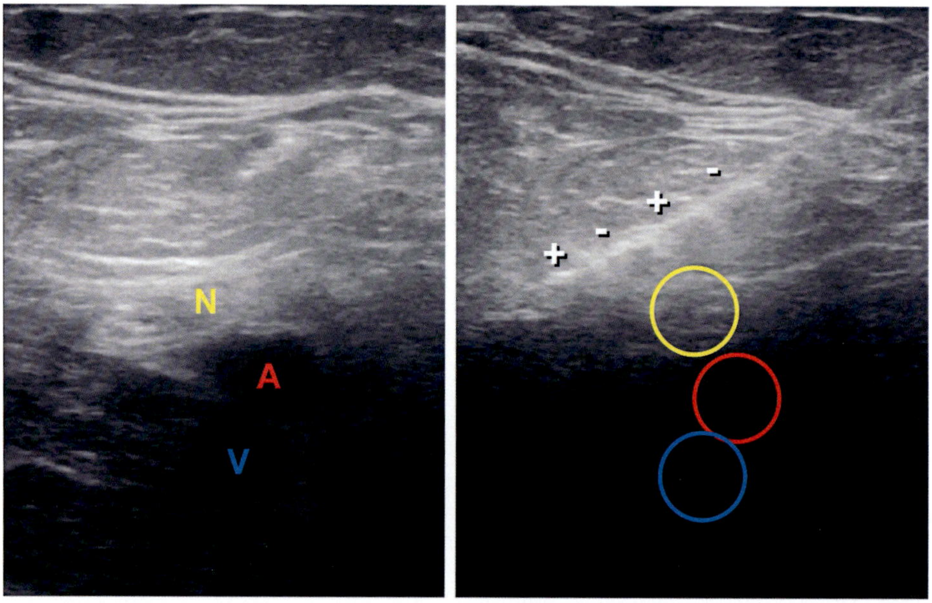

FIG. 5.3 Intraoperative ultrasonogram of the right popliteal region of the patient in the prone position. The left panel shows the relevant anatomy, best seen without the echoic effects of the electrode or needle. The tibial nerve (N, yellow), popliteal artery (A, red), and popliteal vein (V, blue) are all visible. Doppler ultrasonography was used to confirm the vascular anatomy. The right panel shows the percutaneous electrode in position alongside the tibial nerve, away from the great vessels. The appropriate anodes and cathodes are indicated. (From Huntoon MA, Burgher AH. Ultrasound-guided permanent implantation of peripheral nerve stimulation (PNS) system for neuropathic pain of the extremities: original cases and outcomes. *Pain Med.* 2009; 10(8): 1369–1377.)

as practitioners continue to gain expertise. As experience in the field grows, deeper more difficult targets are becoming simple procedures that no longer require incision and neurolysis. Case series have demonstrated that successful implantation of stimulation electrodes adjacent to median, radial, ulnar, peroneal, and posterior tibial nerves is possible.[29] The growing experience with ultrasound has even led practitioners to begin in office trialing of ultrasound-guided electrodes instead of a week-long trial implantations. Preliminary results from this change in treatment paradigm are promising.[30]

EXTERNAL PULSE GENERATORS

Lastly, a new device using a permanently implanted electrode that communicates with an externalized pulse generator recently completed a prospective randomized trial.[31] All previous PNS devices use an implanted pulse generator. This new device does not require an implanted pulse generator and is powered by an external rechargeable device that is worn on the outside of the body. This new technology has also been specifically designed to address many of the limitations of PNS and PNFS, such as having leads manufactured with tines to prevent migration. The device was able to significantly improve pain scores in a randomized clinical trial compared with controls. Additionally, the treatment group demonstrated better improvements in mood, physical activity, and quality of life compared with controls.

CONCLUSION

PNS is an efficacious technique for alleviating chronic refractory pain. Nerve stimulators can be used both in isolation and in combination with other stimulation strategies to tailor neuromodulation therapies to a patient's specific need. Recent technologic advancements are lessening the limitations of these techniques and are making implantation strategies better than ever before. Understanding the indications, benefits, and limitations of PNS for chronic refractory pain is crucial for any practitioner treating chronic pain.

REFERENCES

1. Diwan S, Staats P. *Atlas of Pain Medicine Procedures*. New York: McGraw-Hill Companies, Inc; 2015.
2. Wall PD, Sweet WH. Temporary abolition of pain in man. *Science*. 1967;155(3758):108–109.
3. Al-Jehani H, Jacques L. Peripheral nerve stimulation for chronic neurogenic pain. *Prog Neurol Surg*. 2011;24:27–40.
4. Slavin KV. Peripheral nerve stimulation for neuropathic pain. *Neurotherapeutics*. 2008;5(1):100–106.
5. McRoberts WP, Roche M. Novel approach for peripheral subcutaneous field stimulation for the treatment of severe, chronic knee joint pain after total knee arthroplasty. *Neuromodulation*. 2010;13(2):131–136.
6. Paicius RM, Bernstein CA, Lempert-Cohen C. Peripheral nerve field stimulation in chronic abdominal pain. *Pain Physician*. 2006;9(3):261–266.
7. Melzack R, Wall PD. Pain mechanisms: a new theory. *Science*. 1965;150(3699):971–979.
8. Lee AW, Pilitsis JG. Spinal cord stimulation: indications and outcomes. *Neurosurg Focus*. 2006;21(6):E3.
9. De Ridder D, Plazier M, Kamerling N, Menovsky T, Vanneste S. Burst spinal cord stimulation for limb and back pain. *World Neurosurg*. 2013;80(5): 642–649.e641.
10. Slavin KV, Colpan ME, Munawar N, Wess C, Nersesyan H. Trigeminal and occipital peripheral nerve stimulation for craniofacial pain: a single-institution experience and review of the literature. *Neurosurg Focus*. 2006;21(6):E5.
11. Deogaonkar M, Slavin KV. Peripheral nerve/field stimulation for neuropathic pain. *Neurosurg Clin N Am*. 2014; 25(1):1–10.
12. Campbell CM, Jamison RN, Edwards RR. Psychological screening/phenotyping as predictors for spinal cord stimulation. *Curr Pain Headache Rep*. 2013;17(1):307.
13. Mekhail NA, Mathews M, Nageeb F, Guirguis M, Mekhail MN, Cheng J. Retrospective review of 707 cases of spinal cord stimulation: indications and complications. *Pain Pract*. 2011;11(2):148–153.
14. Campbell JN, Long DM. Peripheral nerve stimulation in the treatment of intractable pain. *J Neurosurg*. 1976; 45(6):692–699.
15. Weiner RL. The future of peripheral nerve neurostimulation. *Neurol Res*. 2000;22(3):299–304.
16. Slavin KV. Technical aspects of peripheral nerve stimulation: hardware and complications. *Prog Neurol Surg*. 2011;24:189–202.
17. Ellis JA, Mejia Munne JC, Winfree CJ. Trigeminal branch stimulation for the treatment of intractable craniofacial pain. *J Neurosurg*. 2015;123(1):283–288.
18. Amin S, Buvanendran A, Park KS, Kroin JS, Moric M. Peripheral nerve stimulator for the treatment of supraorbital neuralgia: a retrospective case series. *Cephalalgia*. 2008;28(4):355–359.
19. Dunteman E. Peripheral nerve stimulation for unremitting ophthalmic postherpetic neuralgia. *Neuromodulation*. 2002;5(1):32–37.
20. Johnson MD, Burchiel KJ. Peripheral stimulation for treatment of trigeminal postherpetic neuralgia and trigeminal posttraumatic neuropathic pain: a pilot study. *Neurosurgery*. 2004;55(1):135–141; discussion 141–132.
21. Slavin KV, Wess C. Trigeminal branch stimulation for intractable neuropathic pain: technical note. *Neuromodulation*. 2005;8(1):7–13.
22. Narouze SN, Kapural L. Supraorbital nerve electric stimulation for the treatment of intractable chronic cluster headache: a case report. *Headache*. 2007;47(7):1100–1102.
23. Rauck RL, Kapural L, Cohen SP, et al. Peripheral nerve stimulation for the treatment of postamputation pain—a case report. *Pain Pract*. 2012;12(8):649–655.
24. Rauck RL, Cohen SP, Gilmore CA, et al. Treatment of post-amputation pain with peripheral nerve stimulation. *Neuromodulation*. 2014;17(2):188–197.
25. Kloimstein H, Likar R, Kern M, et al. Peripheral nerve field stimulation (PNFS) in chronic low back pain: a prospective multicenter study. *Neuromodulation*. 2014;17(2): 180–187.
26. Verrills P, Mitchell B, Vivian D, Sinclair C. Peripheral nerve stimulation: a treatment for chronic low back pain and failed back surgery syndrome? *Neuromodulation*. 2009; 12(1):68–75.
27. Stinson Jr LW, Roderer GT, Cross NE, Davis BE. Peripheral subcutaneous electrostimulation for control of intractable post-operative inguinal pain: a case report series. *Neuromodulation*. 2001;4(3):99–104.
28. Goroszeniuk T, Kothari S, Hamann W. Subcutaneous neuromodulating implant targeted at the site of pain. *Reg Anesth Pain Med*. 2006;31(2):168–171.
29. Huntoon MA, Burgher AH. Ultrasound-guided permanent implantation of peripheral nerve stimulation (PNS) system for neuropathic pain of the extremities: original cases and outcomes. *Pain Med*. 2009;10(8): 1369–1377.
30. Reddy CG, Flouty OE, Holland MT, Rettenmaier LA, Zanaty M, Elahi F. Novel technique for trialing peripheral nerve stimulation: ultrasonography-guided StimuCath trial. *Neurosurg Focus*. 2017;42(3):E5.
31. Deer T, Pope J, Benyamin R, et al. Prospective, multicenter, randomized, double-blinded, partial crossover study to assess the safety and efficacy of the novel neuromodulation system in the treatment of patients with chronic pain of peripheral nerve origin. *Neuromodulation*. 2016; 19(1):91–100.
32. Stuart RM, Winfree CJ. Neurostimulation techniques for painful peripheral nerve disorders. *Neurosurg Clin N Am*. 2009;20(1):111–120, vii–viii.

CHAPTER 6

Spinal Cord Stimulation

NATALY RAVIV, MD • JULIE G. PILITSIS, MD, PHD

SPINAL CORD STIMULATION FOR PAIN

The use of electric current in pain management originated in the 1st century AD, when a member of the Roman court stepped on and was shocked by a torpedo fish and found that he was cured of gout. Scribonius, the Roman physician, began to promote the torpedo's sting as a remedy for arthritis and headache, citing this fortuitous accident. Electric discharge continued to be employed in the treatment of various medical ailments, including muscle spasm, pain, and wound healing,[1] culminating in the implantation of the first unipolar spinal cord stimulator in 1967 by Dr. Norman Shealy at Case Western Reserve University.[2] Today, spinal cord stimulation (SCS) is the most used and successful electric stimulation modality in the treatment of pain.

Mechanism of Neuromodulation

The exact mechanism by which SCS modulates the pain experience is still undetermined, but several theories exist. The gate control theory of pain was published by Ron Melzack and Patrick Wall in 1965, which stated that pain is transmitted by transmission (T) cells in the dorsal horns. The theory holds that T cells are stimulated by small fibers and inhibited by large fibers acting through the substantia gelatinosa (SG). Dorsal column stimulation in relation to this theory acts by stimulating large cells and SG cells, thereby obstructing the transmission of pain.[3] Other theories have explored its effects on neurotransmitters and their pathways, as well as its influence on the autonomic nervous system.[4,5]

Clinical Use

Indications

Today, spinal cord stimulators are one of the most commonly used and well-researched modalities in the management of pain. The US Food and Drug Administration (FDA) has approved SCS for several indications, the most common of which are failed back surgery syndrome (FBSS), chronic peripheral neuropathy or plexopathy, neuropathic pain, and complex regional pain syndrome (CRPS). Other indications that have also received FDA approval, though are less responsive to SCS, include postherpetic neuralgia, phantom limb pain, intercostal neuralgia, multiple sclerosis pain, and spinal cord injury with variable motor and sensory deficits.[6] SCS has been used in off-label indications such as peripheral vascular disease, refractory angina, cervicalgia, and other vascular and visceral pain conditions.[4,6]

Several randomized controlled studies have demonstrated the efficacy of SCS. Kemler et al. performed a randomized control trial on CRPS patients, in which patients were assigned to undergo SCS and physical therapy (PT) or PT alone. These patients all reported impaired function in addition to intractable pain, and all were unable to work as a result of their conditions. The two groups were followed up to 6 months, and SCS was found to be effective in reducing pain and enhancing quality of life, although it was ineffectual in improving function.[7]

North et al. performed the first prospective, randomized control study for FBSS, in which 50 patients were assigned to receive SCS implantation or undergo lumbosacral spine reoperation. At follow-up of about 3 years, SCS patients reported significantly greater levels of pain relief than those who underwent reoperation, with decreased use of narcotic analgesics. Further studies continued to demonstrate the efficacy of SCS in the management of chronic pain.[8] Cost-effectiveness of SCS in selected patients has also been shown,[8–10] although was found to be limited when workers' compensation patients were examined.[11]

Contraindications

Contraindications may include anatomy that renders conditions unfavorable, such as prior surgery with epidural scarring, severe stenosis or scoliosis, or spine instability. Treatable causes of neuropathy must be excluded. Comorbidities such as infection, requirement for antithrombotic therapy, and coagulopathy must be addressed before surgery, and any medical setting in which surgical risk outweighs benefit may preclude a patient from SCS. All patients undergo psychiatric and pain psychologic evaluation before surgery to identify psychosocial factors such as secondary gain, suspicion of somatoform disorders, or unstable axis I or II disorders, which would limit efficacy.[5,6] An open working relationship with pain psychologists is essential to determine which patients need additional psychotherapy, coaching on expectations, and psychiatric treatment before proceeding.

Complications and Risks

SCS is a relatively safe and reversible method of pain management; however, there may be both technical and clinical complications. Technical complications include lead failure, migration or disconnection, device malfunction, current leakage, and battery failure or inability to recharge. Clinical complications include intraoperative trauma to the neuraxis, such as dural puncture or tissue damage, as well as the subsequent development of bleeding, paresthesias, epidural scarring, hematoma, or infection. Mekhail et al. conducted a retrospective review of 707 cases of SCS performed for a variety of indications at the Cleveland Clinic between 2000 and 2005. No permanent neurologic deficits or deaths were reported as a complication of SCS implantation; however, device-related complications were reported in 38% of patients who underwent permanent implantation. These complications included lead migration (22.6%), lead connection failure (9.5%), and lead breakage (6%), all of which required revision. Other complications included pain at the generator site (12%) and clinical infection (4.5%), the latter of which required explantation and an antibiotic regimen, as well as bleeding and paresthesias.[12]

Protocol

Spinal cord stimulation trial

Placement of a spinal cord stimulator is preceded by a trial procedure, giving the patient and surgeon the opportunity to determine whether a permanent implant would adequately alleviate pain and improve quality of life. The goal of the trial is to achieve 50% pain relief or 50% improvement in performing activities of daily living. We tell our patients that they must do everything possible during the trial to make this a "black and white" decision. Patients who do not clearly know that this is the answer for them should be seen during the trial period and alternative waveforms and programming settings are attempted.

Trials are generally performed on awake patients in an aseptic setting outside of the operating room. The implants are placed percutaneously into the epidural space and attached to an external programmable pulse generator. The trial is performed in the outpatient setting for 3–10 days or so, allowing the patient to better evaluate the effects of the stimulator in their daily lives.

The trial additionally provides insight into the optimal location of electrodes and number of electrodes and leads for pain coverage, as well as waveforms. One or more trial leads may be placed. Trial leads are generally single-columned, cylindrical in shape, and percutaneous, with a versatility that allows for more precise positioning along the dorsal columns as well as the ability to reprogram stimulation if lead migration occurs during the trial. Two leads may be employed to allow for redundant coverage given the possibility of lead migration and to allow for more programming options and information gathering. The trial allows for better evaluation of the patient anatomy and potential obstacles to stimulator placement or function, such as epidural space capacity and CSF depth, which may affect signal dispersion.[6]

The information gathered during the trial includes preferred settings, such as electrode geometry, signal intensity and frequency, and the efficacy of different levels of voltage, current, amplitude, pulse width and duration, frequency, and waveform. This information allows for better battery selection, as low energy requirements may be well supported by a primary cell battery and higher requirements may necessitate use of a rechargeable battery. The latter may pose an additional burden of time and compliance on the patient, which overall should be taken into account when weighing the desirability of permanent stimulator placement.[6] The patient's ability to recharge must also be considered. Paddle trials may be attempted in cases where percutaneous leads cannot be easily placed (i.e., patient has Harrington rods for scoliosis) or in cases where a percutaneous trial has led to stimulation of the ligamentum flavum, which causes intrascapular pain and precludes the patient's ability to feel relief from the stimulator.

Permanent implantation

Permanent leads may be percutaneous or paddle leads. The percutaneous leads are similar to those placed during the trial—single-columned and cylindrical in shape. The electrode number and spacing vary depending on the model and manufacturer. Paddle leads contain one to five columns, the number and spacing again differ according to make and manufacturer.

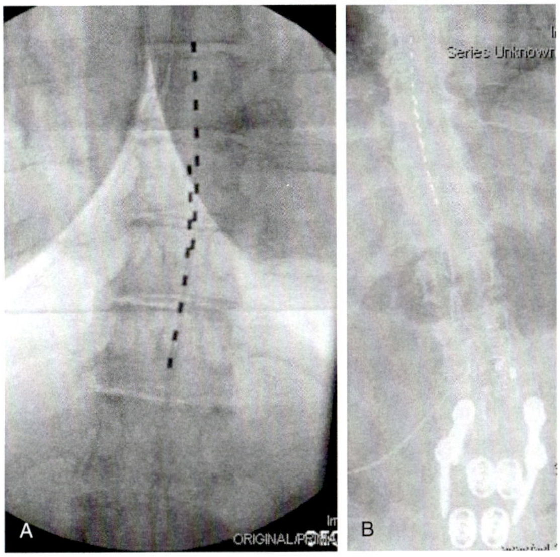

FIG. 6.1 **(A)** Intraoperative X-ray from the placement of percutaneous leads in a 57-year-old with failed back surgery syndrome; **(B)** Postoperative imaging of lead placement.

Percutaneous leads emit 360 degrees of stimulation. Their placement is less invasive, but these leads do have a greater tendency to migrate than the paddle leads and often migrate a greater distance. Percutaneous leads have a more limited span, as they only provide one column of stimulation, and so the placement of more than one lead may be needed to increase the field of stimulation and provide redundancy (Fig. 6.1).

Paddle leads are multicolumned and only provide ventrally directed stimulation directed toward the dorsal columns. The outer columns may provide stimulation and enlarge the region of possible stimulation, but may also be used to provide anodal blocking to focus stimulation to the midline in the case of refractory back pain. Paddle leads may allow for prolonged battery life, given their more focused direction of stimulation, but require a laminotomy for placement[6] (Fig. 6.2).

The selection of lead type may be determined by patient preference regarding invasiveness of surgery and battery type, as well as by the body habitus, anatomy, medical comorbidities, and stimulation requirements of a patient. A randomized control trial comparing percutaneous and paddle electrodes demonstrated comparable long-term outcomes.[8]

Follow-up

Postoperative follow-up is highly variable. In our practice, we follow patients at 2 weeks, 6 weeks, 3 months, 6 months, 1 year, and then annually. Patients' pain is evaluated using a standardized method of assessment and a review of current medications. Evaluations may vary between clinics; however, responses are generally categorized as excellent (>75% pain relief), good (≥50% relief), and poor (<50% relief).[5]

Developments in Spinal Cord Stimulation

Despite the success of traditional SCS in the management of chronic pain and the careful patient selection process, the benefits of this treatment modality may

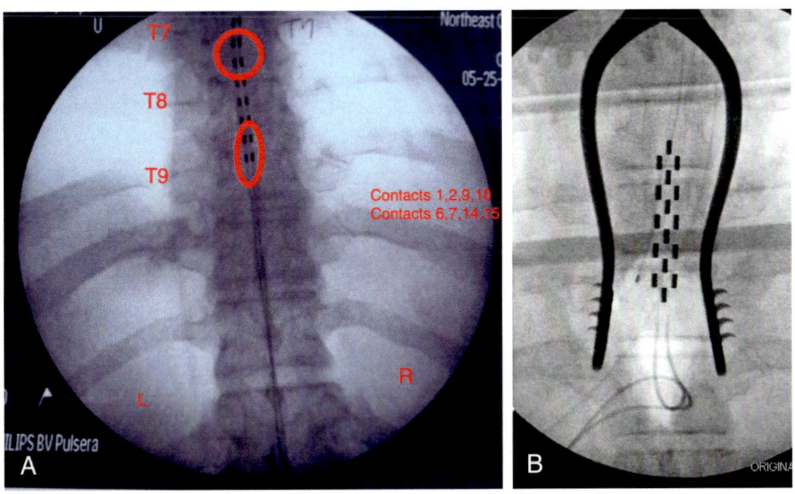

FIG. 6.2 **(A)** Image from a stimulator trial for a 43-year-old man with failed back surgery syndrome. "Sweet spots" of stimulation were identified at T7 and T9 during the trial; **(B)** Intraoperative X-ray of paddle placement.

be limited. Approximately 40% of patients with SCS implants report inadequate pain relief.[13] Over time, treatment may lose effectiveness in 50% of patients who initially received good pain control, and long-term efficacy may be affected by the development of tolerance, which was reported to occur in one study in 29% of patients over a 10-year period.[14,15] Neuroplasticity of pain pathways, cellular or fibrotic changes in tissue, the altered perception of pain over time, and concomitant psychologic or psychiatric social factors and disorders have been identified as possible etiologies of this phenomenon.[6] Additionally, patients may be unable to tolerate the paresthesias that accompany traditional SCS or find that certain anatomic areas are insufficiently covered. The value and limitations of SCS continue to promote the exploration and development of this field, and new mechanisms of stimulation have been developed. These include new waveforms, different programming algorithms, and stimulation of connected neural tissue.

Waveforms

Most notably over the last 5 years, changes in waveforms have led to clinical efficacy. These waveforms include high frequency and burst paradigms.

High-frequency SCS at 10 kHz (HF10 therapy) has been shown to be an effective paresthesia-free alternative to traditional SCS and may even provide pain relief in distributions that are typically difficult to treat or attain sustained relief with traditional SCS, such as isolated back pain. Russo et al. performed a retrospective, multicenter observational case series study in which 256 patients underwent a trial of HF10 SCS. Thirty percent had undergone traditional SCS without success, and the remaining patients were considered to be highly refractory to treatment or were not recommended for traditional SCS. A total of 189 patients received a permanent implant and then were reassessed 3 and 6 month postimplant. Trial success rates were highest for patients with both back and leg pain (81%), followed by patients with isolated back pain (72%). A mean level of pain relief of 50% was sustained at 6 months for the entire patient population. Sixty-eight percent of patients who had previously failed traditional SCS experienced a mean pain reduction of 49% at 6 months with HF10 therapy.[16] The SENZA trial was a randomized control trial that compared patients treated with traditional, albeit last generation SCS, and HF SCS. The patients were followed for 24 months. The study demonstrated noninferiority of HF 10. At 24-month follow-up, more patients responded to HF10 therapy than traditional SCS for both back pain and leg pain (76.5% and 72.9% vs. 49.3%) and the extent of pain relief was greater with HF10.[17]

Burst stimulation likewise has been shown to be effective in the management of chronic pain while reducing or even eliminating paresthesias. One trial involved 100 patients with chronic, intractable pain who received both traditional and burst SCS in a randomized crossover paradigm. Each patient had previously undergone a traditional SCS trial with tonic stimulation and experienced greater than 50% reduction in pain. The study revealed the noninferiority of burst stimulation, and at 24 weeks, 69% of participants preferred burst stimulation, with 91% reporting decreased paresthesias.[18]

Advanced algorithmic and positional stimulation

SCS outcome has further been improved by anatomic algorithms and position-sensing devices. When SCS equipped with anatomic algorithmic programming was compared with devices with traditional programming in a retrospective observational study, algorithmic targeting provided improved pain relief over traditional SCS (overall pain responder rate 74% vs. 51%, axial low back pain 71% vs. 41%, leg pain 81% vs. 63%). The ability to demonstrate therapeutic effect in patients with isolated low back pain, which has traditionally been difficult to address using previous SCS models, was particularly notable.[19]

The intensity of stimulation is dependent on body position; perception of paresthesias varies by the volume of the cerebral spinal fluid surrounding the spinal cord, with more intensity experienced in the supine position. Traditional devices require manual programming adjustment to compensate for the variability. Position-adaptive stimulation adjusts for changes in body position according to patient preferences. One study implanted 79 patients with a neurostimulation device that allowed for both automatic position-adaptive stimulation and manual adjustment. 86.5% of patients reported improved pain relief with increased convenience when using the position-adaptive setting.[20]

Targets

Recently, dorsal root ganglion (DRG) stimulation has come to the forefront. It is believed to more directly activate the neurons that innervate the area of pain distribution than traditional dorsal column stimulation, which is thought to recruit multiple fiber types in addition to primary sensory neurons. It has been suggested that more direct recruitment of specific sensory cell bodies may allow for more precise targeting. This may be particularly useful in distributions where traditional SCS has been shown to have limited benefit, such as in the foot or groin, while limiting the paresthesias in unwanted regions. In a recent study, 51 patients, some of whom had undergone previous unsuccessful stimulation therapies, including peripheral nerve stimulation (n = 3) and SCS (n = 9), underwent a trial of DRG-SCS. 76.5% (n = 39) experienced a good response with reported average pain relief of 74.2%. Thirty-two patients were implanted with permanent devices, and these patients were reevaluated at 12-month follow-up. Overall pain had improved by 56.3% from baseline, with relief of back pain by 41.9%, leg pain by 62.4%, and, most notably, foot pain by 79.5%. Sixty percent of patients reported at least 50% improvement in their overall pain, with 37.5%, 68.4%, and 87.5% reporting alleviation of their back, leg, and foot pain, respectively, by at least 50%. Quality-of-life ratings were improved at 12 months, with a 64% increase in EQ-5D VAS score.[21]

A large randomized controlled trial comparing the efficacy and safety of DRG stimulation to a traditional SCS system randomized 152 patients with CRPS and peripheral causalgia to a DRG or control SCS group across 22 sites. At 1 year follow-up, DRG-SCS was reportedly effective in 74.2% of the patients, compared with 53% of traditional SCS patients. Ninety-two percent of DRG patients who experienced paresthesias reported that the sensation was limited to only the area of pain distribution in comparison with 61.2% of control patients.[22]

Future of spinal cord stimulation

SCS has been used for pain relief historically, with little effect on isolated function. However, a potential role for SCS in this capacity has been identified. Buonocore et al. reported a case involving a patient with FBSS who experienced both chronic pain and muscle weakness. SCS provided only transient and minimal analgesic effect; however, the patient obtained improvement in lower extremity muscle strength and gait.[23] Harkema et al. published the case of a 23-year-old paraplegic man who was able to stand and achieve locomotor-like patterns during epidural stimulation.[24] Rejc et al. demonstrated that lumbosacral SCS could generate motor patterns in two clinically sensory and motor complete spinal cord injury patients that would allow for standing.[25] The role of SCS in the treatment of brain and spinal cord injury and tumors is currently a potent area of investigation.

The indications and methods of SCS continue to evolve, as it remains a compelling domain of research and patient care. SCS has been used for approximately 50 years. During this time, outcomes have improved as technique and patient selection criteria have been modified. The role of spinal neuromodulation will continue to grow with improvement of our technique and understanding of this modality.

REFERENCES

1. Tsoucalas G, Karamanou M, Lymperi M, Gennimata V, Androutsos G. The "torpedo" effect in medicine. *Int Marit Health*. 2014;65(2):65–67. https://doi.org/10.5603/imh.2014.0015.
2. Sinclair C, Verrills P, Barnard A. A review of spinal cord stimulation systems for chronic pain. *J Pain Res*. 2016;9:481–492. https://doi.org/10.2147/jpr.s108884.
3. Melzack R, Wall PAD. Pain mechanism: a new theory. *Science*. 1965;150(3699):971–979.
4. Compton AK, Shah B, Hayek SM. Spinal cord stimulation: a review. *Curr Pain Headache Rep*. 2012;16:35–42.
5. Lee AW, Pilitsis JG. Spinal cord stimulation: indications and outcomes. *Neurosurg Focus*. 2006;21(6). http://www.medscape.com/viewarticle/554863_4.
6. Wheeler AH. *Spinal Cord Stimulation*. Medscape; January 7, 2015. http://emedicine.medscape.com/article/1980819-overview.
7. Kemler MA, Barendse GAM, van Kleef M. Spinal cord stimulation in patients with chronic reflex sympathetic dystrophy. *N Engl J Med*. 2000;343:618–624. https://doi.org/10.1056/NEJM200008313430904.
8. North RB, Kidd DH, Dorsi MJ. Spinal cord stimulation electrode design: a prospective, randomized, controlled trial comparing percutaneous with laminectomy electrodes: part II-clinical outcomes. *Neurosurgery*. 2005;57(5):990–996.
9. Simpson EL, Duenas A, Holmes MW, et al. Spinal cord stimulation for chronic pain of neuropathic or ischaemic origin: systematic review and economic evaluation. *Health Technol Assess*. 2009;13(17):1–154. iii, ix–x.
10. Taylor RS, Ryan J, O'Donnell R, et al. The cost-effectiveness of spinal cord stimulation in the treatment of failed back surgery syndrome. *Clin J Pain*. 2010;26:463–469.
11. Hollingworth W, Turner JA, Welton NJ, Comstock BA, Deyo RA. Costs and cost-effectiveness of spinal cord stimulation (SCS) for failed back surgery syndrome: an observational study in a workers' compensation population. *Spine*. 2011;36:2076–2083. https://doi.org/10.1097/BRS.0b013e31822a867c.
12. Mekhail NA, Mathews M, Nageeb F, Guirguis M, Mekhail MN, Cheng J. Retrospective review of 707 cases of spinal cord stimulation: indications and complications. *Pain Pract*. 2011;11:148–153.
13. Frey ME, Manchikanti L, Benyamin RM, Schultz DM, Smith HS, Cohen SP. Spinal cord stimulation for patients with failed back surgery syndrome: a systematic review. *Pain Physician*. 2009;12:379–397.

14. Kumar K, Wilson JR, Taylor RS, Gupta S. Complications of spinal cord stimulation, suggestions to improve outcome, and financial impact. *J Neurosurg Spine*. 2006;5(3): 191–203.
15. Sears NC, Machado AG, Nagel SJ, et al. Long-term outcomes of spinal cord stimulation with paddle leads in the treatment of complex regional pain syndrome and failed back surgery syndrome. *Neuromodulation*. 2011;14: 213–218.
16. Russo M, Verrills P, Mitchell B, Salmon J, Barnard A, Santarelli D. High frequency spinal cord stimulation at 10 kHz for the treatment of chronic pain: 6-month Australian clinical experience. *Neuromodulation Pain Physician*. 2016;19(4):267–280.
17. Kapural L, Yu C, Doust MW, et al. Comparison of 10-kHz high-frequency and traditional low-frequency spinal cord stimulation for the treatment of chronic back and leg pain: 24-month results from a multicenter, randomized, controlled pivotal trial. *Neurosurgery*. 2016;79(5):667–677. https://doi.org/10.1227/NEU.0000000000001418.
18. Courtney P, Espinet A, Mitchell B, et al. Improved pain relief with burst spinal cord stimulation for two weeks in patients using tonic stimulation: results from a small clinical study. *Neuromodulation*. 2015;18:361–366. https://doi.org/10.1111/ner.12294.
19. Veizi E, Hayek SM, North J, et al. Spinal cord stimulation (SCS) with anatomically guided (3D) neural targeting shows superior chronic axial low back pain relief compared to traditional SCS-LUMINA study. *Pain Med*. 2017. https://doi.org/10.1093/pm/pnw286.
20. Schultz DM, Webster L, Kosek P, Dar U, Tan Y, Sun M. Sensor-driven position-adaptive spinal cord stimulation for chronic pain. *Pain Physician*. 2012;15(1):1–12.
21. Liem L, Russo M, Huygen FJ, et al. One-year outcomes of spinal cord stimulation of the dorsal root ganglion in the treatment of chronic neuropathic pain. *Neuromodulation*. 2015;18(1):41–49.
22. Levy R, Deer T. *A Prospective, Randomized, Multi-center, Controlled Clinical Trial to Assess the Safety and Efficacy of the Spinal Modulation AxiumTM Neurostimulator System in the Treatment of Chronic Pain*. Presented at NANS. 2015.
23. Buonocore M, Bonezzi C, Barolat G. Neurophysiological evidence of antidromic activation of large myelinated fibres in lower limbs during spinal cord stimulation. *Spine*. 2008;33:90–93.
24. Harkema S. Effect of epidural stimulation of the lumbosacral spinal cord on voluntary movement, standing, and assisted stepping after motor complete paraplegia: a case study. *Lancet*. 2011;377(9781):1938–1947. https://doi.org/10.1016/S0140-6736(11)60547-3.
25. Rejc E, Angeli C, Harkema S. Effects of lumbosacral spinal cord epidural stimulation for standing after chronic complete paralysis in humansDi Giovanni S, ed. *PLoS One*. 2015;10(7):e0133998. https://doi.org/10.1371/journal.pone.0133998.

FURTHER READING

1. North RB, Kidd D, Shipley J, Taylor RS. Spinal cord stimulation versus reoperation for failed back surgery syndrome: a cost effectiveness and cost utility analysis based on a randomized, controlled trial. *Neurosurgery*. 2007;61: 361–368.
2. Verrills P, Sinclair C, Barnard A. A review of spinal cord stimulation systems for chronic pain. *J Pain Res*. 2016;9:481.

CHAPTER 7

Advances in Spinal Modulation: New Stimulation Waveforms and Dorsal Root Ganglion Stimulation

GEOFFREY STRICSEK, MD • STEVEN M. FALOWSKI, MD, FAANS

INTRODUCTION

Chronic pain affects more than 100 million people. The direct costs of medical care and the indirect costs of lost productivity were estimated at $560–635 billion in a report released in 2011, which clearly places this as a health crisis.[1] Although these numbers are staggering, chronic pain is not an affliction unique to today's society. The use of spinal cord stimulation (SCS) for the treatment of pain traces its origin to the work of Shealy and colleagues in 1967 with an implant that produced resolution of a patient's chest and abdominal pain.[2] The theoretical basis of the results seen in 1967 is rooted in the gate control mechanism of Melzack and Wall, which states that activity in Aβ fibers of large diameter inhibits transmission of noxious information to the brain by small C and Aδ fibers.[3] It is believed that exogenous stimulation of the larger fibers inhibits transmission of painful sensation by the smaller fibers. This belief has led to the foundation of the therapeutic effect of SCS being based on the generation of paresthesias concordant with the distribution of pain. Although much of the early advancement in SCS centered on hardware improvement, recent innovation has been focused on improving pain relief through different stimulation patterns, as well as with new stimulation targets.

CONVENTIONAL SPINAL CORD STIMULATION

Conventional SCS relies on the generation of paresthesias in somatotopic distributions overlapping a patient's pain.[4] Leads are placed in the epidural space overlying the posterior columns of the spinal cord with final positioning adjusted to achieve appropriate paresthesia coverage; an implanted pulse generator delivers tonic stimulation at a frequency between 40 and 100 Hz[5] (Fig. 7.1). Randomized controlled studies have demonstrated significant improvement in neuropathic radicular pain and health-related quality of life metrics when comparing conventional SCS with best medical therapy[6,7] and even repeat lumbar spine surgery.[8,9] Kumar et al. found that nearly 50% of patients derived at least a 50% improvement in lower extremity neuropathic pain after SCS implantation compared with only 9% of patients undergoing medical management at 6 months.[6] This treatment effect was shown to be durable at 12 months[6] and even out to 24 months; however, other research has shown that there is a subset of SCS patients who experience decreasing efficacy of stimulation over time.[7] Similar benefits were observed in a randomized controlled study comparing SCS with reoperation in patients with signs of recurrent neural compression; nearly 50% of subjects had a minimum of 50% pain relief at 6 months with SCS compared with only 12% in the reoperation group.[9] Conventional SCS has also been shown to be an effective treatment for diabetic neuropathy with patients deriving significant reduction in pain compared with medical therapy.[10]

Given the successes of conventional SCS in the aforementioned studies, ongoing development has been encouraged with a goal of improving pain control for those who did not experience significant relief or had decreasing relief over time, as well as those with chronic pain who fell outside the inclusion criteria in the early clinical studies. One approach has targeted delivery of electrical current to the spinal cord. Early SCS systems delivered the same current across all the electrodes within an implanted stimulator lead, whereas recent technological advances have allowed current to be adjusted at the level of each contact within an electrode, rather than at the level of the battery. Fractionalization

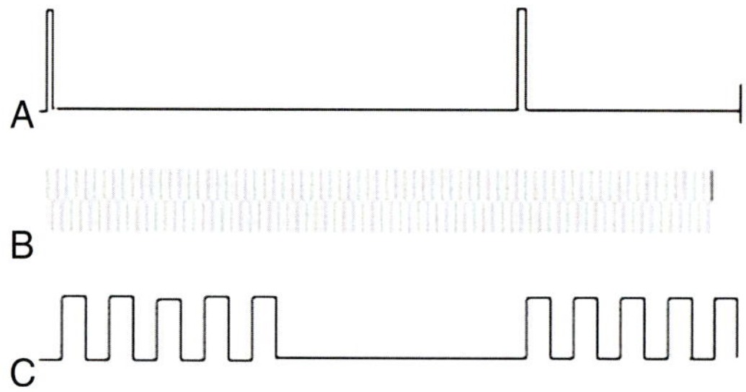

FIG. 7.1 Stimulation strategies: **(A)** Tonic stimulation 40 Hz; **(B)** High frequency 10,000 Hz; **(C)** Burst stimulation.

of current across individual contacts allows the electric field to be directed toward a specific region based on patient feedback, thereby improving paresthesia coverage.[11] Trial data suggested good response to steerable current with 75% of patients undergoing permanent implant after having received at least 50% pain relief.[12] Unfortunately, long-term data from that study are limited owing to receipt of FDA premarket approval; however, 38 of the 49 implanted patients demonstrated an average of 60% pain relief at 3 months, decreasing slightly to an average of 53% pain relief in 34 patients followed out to 6 months.[12]

HIGH-FREQUENCY SPINAL CORD STIMULATION

The works of North[8,9] and Kumar[6,7] were an exciting advancement, which demonstrated SCS could deliver significant pain relief in patients with persistent or recurrent lower extremity pain after previous lumbosacral spine surgery. However, despite observing positive outcomes in almost 50% of their study population, a significant amount who did not receive adequate pain relief as well as those patients with predominant back pain were excluded in the initial studies. Modification of conventional SCS hardware and software permitted investigation of a new form of tonic stimulation: high-frequency stimulation at 10,000 Hz (HF10 Nevro, Redwood City, CA) (Fig. 7.1). An early prospective cohort study focusing on chronic low back pain in 25 patients observed greater improvement in visual analog scale (VAS) scores with high-frequency stimulation as compared with conventional SCS while also demonstrating the ability to achieve paresthesia-free pain relief, thereby challenging the previous paradigm of paresthesia-dependent pain control.[13] Larger prospective trials demonstrated significant improvement of pain scores in 74% of patients with chronic, predominantly low back pain at 6 months[14] and in 60% of patients at 24 months[15]; significant improvements in leg pain were also noted.[14,15] The observed efficacy of high-frequency stimulation led to a prospective randomized controlled trial (SENZA-RCT) comparing it with conventional SCS. Results of the SENZA-RCT showed that significantly more patients treated with 10,000-Hz stimulation derived a significant improvement in both back and leg pain at 3 and 12 months as compared with traditional SCS.[16] These findings were found to be durable with significant differences remaining for both back and leg pain with patients followed to 24 months (Table 7.1).[17] Recently released data at a large national meeting demonstrated efficacy of high-frequency stimulation for treatment of chronic neck and upper extremity pain as well.[18] The stimulation frequency of 10,000 Hz may hold particular significance as another study found no difference when comparing sham to high-frequency stimulation at 5000 Hz in a patient population stabilized on conventional SCS.[19]

BURST SPINAL CORD STIMULATION

Divergent from tonic stimulation, the most recent waveform to receive FDA approval is burst stimulation (Figs. 7.1 and 7.2). Research suggests that sensory information from a unique stimulus may be transmitted by parallel systems: one employing a tonic pattern of neuron firing and the other employing a burst pattern.[20–22] Translational work in an animal model demonstrated burst firing of the thalamocortical

TABLE 7.1
Positive Response Rate From SENZA-RCT Comparing High-Frequency Stimulation (HF10) With Conventional SCS

	HF10 (%)	Traditional SCS (%)
3 MONTHS		
Back pain	84.5	43.8
Leg Pain	83.1	55.5
12 MONTHS		
Back pain	80	50
Leg pain	80	50–55
24 MONTHS		
Back pain	76.5	49.3
Leg Pain	72.9	49.3

Positive response defined as at least a 50% improvement in pain from baseline. *SCS*, spinal cord stimulation.

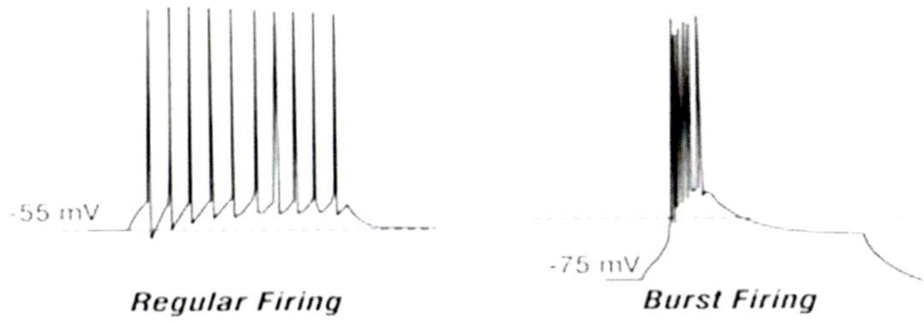

FIG. 7.2 Burst stimulation firing pattern.[35]

synapse to be a more potent activator of the cerebral cortex than tonic firing.[23–25] Discovery of the role of burst stimulation in the activation of pain pathways led to two early studies investigating the effect of exogenously applied burst stimulation in patients with chronic low back and leg pain. By using 40-Hz bursts with five spikes at 500 Hz per burst, results were found to be equivocal in terms of pain control compared with conventional tonic SCS but did demonstrate a significant improvement versus placebo and an overwhelming patient preference for burst compared with SCS.[26,27] It is possible that the preference for burst is a result of its limited incidence of paresthesias.[26,28]

The initial burst studies looked at differences in pain relief during a 28-day trial period, but subsequent studies have evaluated the impact of burst stimulation in patients who already had a conventional SCS implanted and had received treatment for at least 6 months. In follow-up, burst was shown to significantly reduce foot pain in patients with diabetic neuropathy, back and leg pain in patients with failed back surgery syndrome, and even further decrease leg and back pain in patients who had reduced efficacy of their conventional SCS.[28–30] Burst appears to have significant pain control benefits compared with conventional SCS and may be able to function as a salvage therapy addressing the concerns for sustainability of the therapy.

Given the positive results, a prospective RCT was undertaken to further evaluate burst versus tonic stimulation: SUNBURST IDE. Specifically designed as a crossover study, patients with medically refractory chronic back and/or limb pain underwent a trial with conventional SCS and then were randomized to either a burst or conventional SCS treatment arm. Following 12 weeks of treatment, each patient would then be switched to the other therapy form so that each patient would serve as his/her own control. Final data have not yet been published, but preliminary results and presentations at large society meetings indicate a significant improvement in back, leg, and overall pain scores when comparing burst with conventional SCS.[31] Similar to previous studies, a significant proportion of patients preferred burst stimulation to conventional tonic stimulation.[31] These findings have led to an FDA approval with superiority labeling.

A SUNBURST substudy looked at brain activation using Fluorodeoxyglucose(FDG-PET) scan while patients were receiving either tonic or burst stimulation. Increased activation of the sensorimotor, dorsal anterior cingulate, and posterior cingulate cortex indicating greater modulation of lateral and medial pain pathways with burst stimulation as compared with tonic was noted.[32] Both the lateral and medial pathways involve transmission of pain information via the spinothalamic tract; but the lateral pathway projects to the somatosensory cortex and is responsible for the discriminatory aspects of pain,[33] whereas the medial pathway projects to the dorsal anterior cingulate cortex and is responsible for the motivational, affective, and attention components of pain.[33,34] Thus, in addition to modulating the transmission of pain signals in the lateral pathway, burst stimulation also influences the medial pathway and the attention paid to pain as well as its impact on mood.[22,26,27]

HIGH-DENSITY SIMULATION

As conventional SCS pulse generators improved through successive iterations, their programming now permits stimulation frequencies up to 1200 Hz, even though standard programming paradigms remained in the 40–60 Hz range. Recognizing the benefit of a higher rate of energy delivery in burst and high-frequency stimulation for the treatment of chronic pain, the question arose whether maximizing energy utilization from a conventional SCS generator would yield similar results. One study did show a significant improvement in back and leg pain after transition to high-density stimulation from SCS; however, their sample size was small and only followed prospectively for 8 weeks.[36] This has subsequently been followed up with a multicenter pivotal trial in which the results have not been published but are promising. This further demonstrates that patients may need to have options and a single waveform may not be universal for patients.

DORSAL ROOT GANGLION STIMULATION

Although there have been many gains in the treatment of chronic pain using SCS, improvements in the management of chronic regional pain syndrome (CRPS) have remained elusive. Five-year follow-up data from a prospective RCT demonstrated no difference in pain-related outcomes when comparing SCS and physical therapy with physical therapy alone; however, results were very positive in the initial few years following SCS.[37]

The dorsal root ganglion (DRG) is the site of the cell bodies for sensory neurons, acting as a relay point for sensory information as it travels from the periphery to the spinal cord and on to the brain. Accordingly, the DRG has been shown to play a role in the generation of chronic pain[38,39] through a combination of ectopic DRG firing,[40–42] altered gene expression causing upregulation of ion channels and signaling molecules,[43–48] and increased activity of growth factors and growth factor–associated proteins,[49,50] all contributing to a pathologic electrochemical environment. Given the evidence supporting the use of SCS in the treatment of chronic pain and an increased understanding of the role of the DRG in the generation of chronic pain, a prospective clinical study was undertaken to examine the clinical benefits of DRG stimulation. Patients with chronic, medically intractable pain of the trunk, limbs, and/or sacral region were selected as candidates for trial implantation. Stimulator leads (Fig. 7.3) were inserted percutaneously and directed with fluoroscopic guidance to rest along the DRG in the dorsal neural foramina between adjacent pedicles (Fig. 7.4). The waveform for DRG stimulation is similar to conventional tonic stimulation with a frequency between 40 and 50 Hz[51] and therefore relies on the generation of paresthesias overlapping the area of pain, which must be confirmed at the time of placement. However, subsequent programming is usually subthreshold. Results at 6-months postimplantation were encouraging: 52% of implanted patients had at least 50% pain relief.[51] The ability to selectively isolate regions of pain is one of the great strengths of DRG stimulation, evidenced by back pain relief of 58.1% on the VAS, leg pain relief of 69.3%, and foot pain relief of 84.5% compared with baseline.[51] These initial results from 6 months were shown to be durable at 1-year follow-up (Table 7.2).[52] The ACCURATE trial was a prospective, randomized, multicenter study designed to compare efficacy of DRG stimulation with convention SCS in patients with CRPS of the lower limbs. Patient follow-up at 12 months demonstrated 74.2% patients implanted with DRG stimulator having at least 50% improvement in pain symptoms as opposed to only 53% of patients with conventional SCS, a statistically significant difference.[53] Final results are expected to be released in 2017.

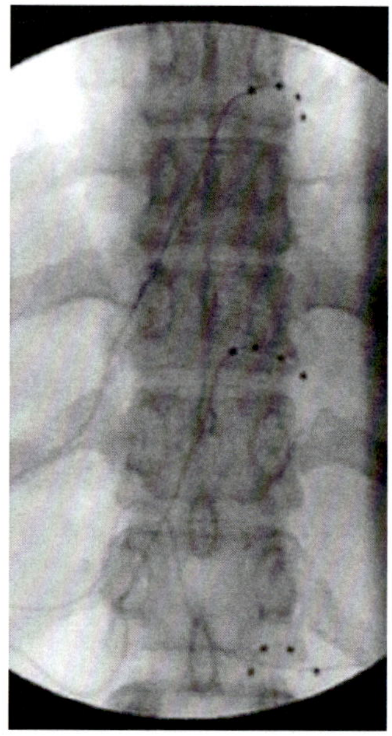

FIG. 7.3 Dorsal root ganglion stimulator electrode, St. Jude Medical (permission pending).

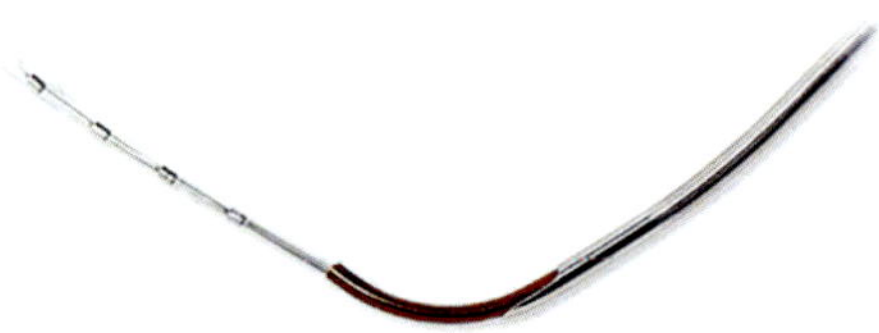

FIG. 7.4 Anteropostetior X-ray following implantation of dorsal root ganglion stimulators in neural foramina.

SUMMARY

The treatment of pain has evolved tremendously since the first spinal cord stimulator implantation in 1967. Multiple options are now available from current directionality and improved targeting in conventional SCS systems to high-frequency to burst to targeted

TABLE 7.2
Average Reduction in VAS Score Following DRG stimulator Implant

	6 months (%)	1 year (%)
Overall pain	56.3	56
Back pain	58.1	42
Leg pain	69.3	62
Foot pain	84.5	80

DRG, dorsal root ganglion; *VAS*, visual analog scale.

stimulation with DRG stimulators. The supporting research behind each technology demonstrates a significant benefit, but when looking closely, there are subsets of patients in each study who do not obtain relief or experience decreasing relief over time. Despite this, it is also clear that different stimulation modalities may provide a benefit where others have failed. Although our understanding of pain is not refined enough to understand the mechanisms underpinning success versus not, it is clear that a single form of SCS is not the answer to everyone's pain; different forms of pain require different therapeutic modalities.

DISCLOSURE STATEMENT

Dr. Falowski is a consultant for St. Jude, Medtronic, and Nevro.

Dr. Stricsek has no relevant disclosures.

REFERENCES

1. Committee on Advancing Pain Research, Care, and Education, Institute of Medicine. *Relieving Pain in America: A Blueprint for Transforming Prevention, Care, Education, and Research*. Washington, DC: The National Academies Press; 2011.
2. Shealy C, Mortimer J, Reswick J. Electrical inhibition of pain by stimulation of the dorsal columns: preliminary clinical report. *Anesth Analg*. 1967;46(4):489–491.
3. Melzack R, Wall P. Pain mechanisms: a new theory. *Science*. 1965;150:971–979.
4. North R, Ewend M, Lawton M, Piantadosi S. Spinal cord stimulation for chronic, intractable pain: superiority of "multi-channel" devices. *Pain*. 1991;44(2):119–130.
5. Falowski S, Pope J, eds. *Integrating Pain Treatment into Your Spine Practice*. Springer International Publishing; 2016.
6. Kumar K, Taylor R, Jacques L, et al. Spinal cord stimulation versus conventional medical management for neuropathic pain: a multicentre randomised controlled trial in patients with failed back surgery syndrome. *Pain*. 2007;132: 179–188.
7. Kumar K, Taylor R, Jacques L, et al. The effects of spinal cord stimulation in neuropahtic pain are sustained: a 24-month follow-up of the prospective randomized controleld multicenter trial of the effectiveness of spinal cord stimulation. *Neurosurgery*. 2008;63:762–770.
8. North R, Kidd D, Piantodosi S. A prospective, randomized study of spinal cord stimulation versus reoperation for failed back surgery syndrome: initial results. *Stereotact Funct Neurosurg*. 1994;62:267–272.
9. North R, Kidd D, Farrokhi F, Piantadosi S. Spinal cord stimulation versus repeated lumbosacral spine surgery for chronic pain: a randomized, controlled trial. *Neurosurgery*. 2005;56:98–107.
10. Duarte R, Andronis L, Lenders M, de Vos C. Quality of life increases in patients with painful diabetic neuropathy following treatment with spinal cord stimulation. *Qual Life Res*. 2016;25:1771–1777.
11. Oakley J, Varga C, Krames E, Bradley K. Real-time paresthesia steering using continuous electric field adjustment. Part I: intraoperative performance. *Neuromodulation*. 2004;7:157–167.
12. Oakley J, Krames E, Prager J, et al. A new spinal cord stimulation system effectively relieves chronic, intractable pain: a multicenter prospective clinical study. *Neuromodulation*. 2007;10(3):262–278.
13. Tiede J, Brown L, Gekht G, Vallejo J, Yearwood T, Morgan D. Novel spinal cord stimulation parameters in patients with predominant back pain. *Neuromodulation*. 2013;16(4):370–375.
14. Van Buyten J, Al-Kaisy A, Smet I, Palmisani S, Smith T. High-frequency spinal cord stimulation for the treatment of chronic back pain patients: results of a prospective multicenter European clinical study. *Neuromodulation*. 2013;16:59–66.
15. Al-Kaisy A, Van Buyten J, Smet I, Palmisani S, Pang D, Smith T. Sustained effectiveness of 10 kHz high-frequency spinal cord stimulation for patients with chronic, low back pain: 24-month results of a prospective multicenter study. *Pain Med*. 2014;15:347–354.
16. Kapural L, Yu C, Doust M, et al. Novel 10-kHz high-frequency therapy (HF10 therapy) is superior to traditional low-frequency spinal cord stimulation for the treatment of chronic back and leg pain. The SENZA-RCT randomized controlled trial. *Anesthesiology*. 2015;123(4): 851–860.
17. Kapural L, Cong Y, Doust M, et al. Comparison of 10-kHz high-frequency and traditional low-frequency spinal cord stimulation for the treatment of chronic back and leg pain: 24-month results from a multicenter, randomized, controlled pivotal trial. *Neurosurgery*. 2016;79(5): 667–677.
18. Amirdelfan K. In: *Plenary Presentation*. Las Vegas, NV; 2017.
19. Perruchoud C, Eldabe S, Batterham A, et al. Analgesic efficacy of high-frequency spinal cord stimulation: a randomized double-blind placebo-controlled study. *Neuromodulation*. 2013;16:363–369.
20. Chacron M, Longtin A, Maler L. To burst or not to burst? *J Comput Neurosci*. 2004;17(2):127–136.

21. Oswald A, Chacron M, Doiron B, Bastian J, Maler L. Parallel processing of sensory input by bursts and isolated spikes. *J Neurosci*. 2004;24(18):4351–4362.
22. De Ridder D, Vanneste S. Burst and tonic spinal cord stimulation: different and common brain mechanisms. *Neuromodulation*. 2016;19:47–59.
23. Lisman J. Bursts as a unit of neural information: making unreliable synapses reliable. *Trends Neurosci*. 1997;20(1): 38–43.
24. Swadlow H, Gusev A. The impact of "bursting" thalamic impulses at a neocortical synapse. *Nat Neurosci*. 2001; 4(4):402–408.
25. Murray S. Tonic and burst firing: dual modes of thalamocortical relay. *Trends Neurosci*. 2001;24(2):122–126.
26. De Ridder D, Vanneste S, Plaizer M, van der Loo E, Menovsky T. Burst spinal cord stimulation: toward paresthesia-free pain suppression. *Neurosurgery*. 2010; 66(5):986–990.
27. De Ridder D, Plaizer M, Kamerling N, Menovsky T, Vanneste S. Burst spinal cord stimulation for limb and back pain. *World Neurosurg*. 2013;80(5):642–649.
28. de Vos C, Bom M, Vanneste S, Lenders M, de Ridder D. Burst spinal cord stimulation evaluated in patients with failed back surgery syndrome and painful diabetic neuropathy. *Neuromodulation*. 2014;17:152–159.
29. de Ridder D, Lenders M, de Vos C, et al. A 2-center comparative study on tonic versus burst spinal cord stimulation: amount of responders and amount of pain suppression. *Clin J Pain*. 2015;31:433–437.
30. Schu S, Slotty P, Bara G, von Knop M, Edgar D, Vesper J. A prospective, randomised, double-blind, placebo-controlled study to examine the effectiveness of burst spinal cord stimulation patterns for the treatment of failed back surgery syndrome. *Neuromodulation*. 2014;17:443–450.
31. Deer T. In: *Plenary Presentation*. Las Vegas, NV; 2015.
32. Yearwood T, Falowski S, Venkatesan L, Vanneste S. In: *Comparison of Neural Activity in Chronic Pain Patients during Tonic and Burst Spinal Cord Stimulation: A SUNBURST Substudy*. Baltimore; 2016.
33. Bushnell M, Ceko M, Low L. Cognitive and emotional control of pain and its disruption in chronic pain. *Nat Rev Neurosci*. 2013;14:502–511.
34. Price D. Psychological and neural mechanisms of the affective dimension of pain. *Science*. 2000;288:1769–1772.
35. Pope J, Falowski S, Deer T. Advanced waveforms and frequency with spinal cord stimulation: burst and high-frequency energy delivery. *Expert Rev Med Devices*. 2015; 12(4):431–437.
36. Sweet J, Badjatiya A, Tan D, Miller J. Paresthesia-free high-density spinal cord stimulation for postlaminectomy syndrome in a prescreened population: a prospective case series. *Neuromodulation*. 2016;19:260–267.
37. Kemler M, de Vet H, Barendse G, van den Wildenberg F, van Kleef M. Effect of spinal cord stimulation for chronic complex regional pain syndrome type I: five-year final follow-up of patients in a randomized controlled trial. *J Neurosurg*. 2008;108:292–298.
38. Sapunar D, Kostic S, Banozic A, Puljak L. Dorsal root ganglion-a potential new therapeutic target for neuropathic pain. *J Pain Res*. 2012;5:31–38.
39. Van Zundert J, Patijn J, Kessels A, Lame I, van Suijlekom H, van Kleef M. Pulsed radiofrequency adjacent to the cervical dorsal root ganglion in chronic cervical radicular pain: a double blind sham controlled randomized clinical trial. *Pain*. 2007;127:173–182.
40. Wu G, Ringkamp M, Murinson B, et al. Degeneration of myelinated efferent fibers induces spontaneous activity in uninjured C-fiber afferents. *J Neurosci*. 2002;22(17): 7746–7753.
41. Devor M. Ectopic discharge in AB afferent as a source of neuropathic pain. *Exp Brain Res*. 2009;195:115–128.
42. Sukhotinsky I, Ben-Dor E, Raber P, Devor M. Key role of the dorsal root ganglion in neuropathic tactile hypersensibility. *Eur J Pain*. 2004;8:135–143.
43. Xiao H, Huang Q, Zhang F, et al. Identification of gene expression profile of dorsal root ganglion in the rat peripheral axotomy model of neuropathic pain. *Proc Natl Acad Sci USA*. 2002;99(12):8360–8365.
44. Waxman S, Cummins T, Dib-Haj S, Fjell J, Black J. Sodium channels, excitability of primary sensory neurons, and the molecular basis of pain. *Muscle Nerve*. 1999;22: 1177–1187.
45. Devor M, Govrin-Lippmann R, Angelides K. Na+ channel immunolocalization in peripheral mammalian axons and changes following nerve injury and neuroma formation. *J Neurosci*. 1993;13:1976–1992.
46. McCallum J, Kwok W, Sapunar D, Fuchs A, Hogan Q. Painful peripheral nerve injury decreases calcium current in axotomized sensory neurons. *Anesthesiology*. 2006;105: 160–168.
47. Rush A, Dib-Hajj S, Liu S, Cummins T, Black J, Waxman S. A single sodium channel mutation produces hyper- or hypoexcitability in different types of neurons. *Proc Natl Acad Sci USA*. 2006;103:8245–8250.
48. Fields R. New culprits in chronic pain. *Sci Am*. 2009;301: 50–57.
49. Krames E. The dorsal root ganglion in chronic pain and as a target for neuromodulation: a review. *Neuromodulation*. 2015;18:24–32.
50. Aaron R, Boyan B, Ciombor D, Schwartz Z, Simon B. Stimulation of growth factor synthesis by electric and electromagnetic fields. *Clin Orthop Relat Res*. 2004;429:30–37.
51. Liem L, Russo M, Huygen F, Van Buyten J, Smet I. A multicenter, prospective trial to assess the safety and performance of the spinal modulation dorsal root ganglion. *Neuromodulation*. 2013;16(5).
52. Liem L, Russo M, Huygen F, et al. One-year outcomes of spinal cord stimulation of the dorsal root ganglion in the treatment of chronic neuropathic pain. *Neuromodulation*. 2015;18:41–49.
53. Levy R. In: *Plenary Presentation*. Las Vegas, NV; 2015.

CHAPTER 8

Occipital Nerve Stimulation

MICHAEL D. STAUDT, MD, MSc • JENNIFER A. SWEET, MD

INTRODUCTION

The treatment of chronic headaches and craniofacial pain syndromes with neuromodulation techniques can be traced back to 1967, when Wall and Sweet stimulated their own infraorbital nerves to test the gate control theory of pain.[1] This early application of peripheral nerve stimulation (PNS) was used to suppress pain signals in patients with "chronic cutaneous pain" syndromes. Subsequently, there have been numerous attempts at defining a variety of indications for PNS because of the diversity of pain syndromes attributed to peripheral nerve etiology. The early era of peripheral neuromodulation involved open surgery for placement of stimulation devices, and the introduction of percutaneous lead placement has resulted in significant and sustained interest in PNS techniques.[2] In their landmark 1999 paper, Weiner and Reed described placement of a percutaneous lead in the proximity of the greater occipital nerve for the treatment of occipital neuralgia (ON).[2] In contemporary practice, occipital nerve stimulation (ONS) for ON continues to be the most commonly performed PNS procedure. However, despite its common use, ONS unfortunately is not yet FDA-approved and thus remains an off-label use of stimulation.

ON is a pain disorder characterized as sharp, shooting, or stabbing paroxysmal pain, which manifests unilaterally or bilaterally along the distribution of the greater (GON), lesser (LON), and/or third occipital nerve.[3] Typically, ON presents with recurring episodes of lancinating pain lasting for a seconds to minutes and may or may not be associated with a more chronic and dull component of pain. Palpation of the affected nerve branch often elicits the painful symptoms. Additionally, pain may be spontaneous or triggered with certain movements of the head and neck. Dysesthesias or allodynia may also be present within the same distribution.

The use of ONS for the treatment of headache disorders, including ON, is well described. There is evidence demonstrating the benefit of ONS in the management of occipital migraines and occipital neuropathic pain, cluster headaches,[4,5] cervicogenic pain,[6] hemicrania continua,[7] and posttraumatic headaches.[8] The treatment of intractable chronic migraines with ONS has received particular attention, with mixed results.[9–11] The diversity of headache presentations and pain distributions treated by ONS may perhaps be explained by the convergence between cervical and trigeminal afferents in the pars caudalis of the spinal trigeminal nucleus, suggesting a common overlap from occipital afferents at the C2 level.[12,13]

Conservative management with medications is considered first-line treatment for craniofacial pain syndromes, including ON. However, many cases are refractory to medical management, thus requiring more invasive treatment options. ONS has emerged as an additional treatment modality for patients with medically refractory pain. ONS is also a reversible and adjustable treatment that does not produce numbness, unlike more invasive and permanent lesioning procedures. The aim of this chapter is to understand the patient selection rationale and surgical technique of ONS, with a review of clinical efficacy and outcomes. Although ONS techniques are applicable to various headaches and craniofacial pain syndromes, the primary focus of this chapter will be on medically refractory ON, for which ONS has been demonstrated to provide excellent and sustained pain relief with low complication rates.[2,14]

ANATOMICAL AND CLINICAL FEATURES

A number of headache and nonheadache disorders may present with pain in the posterior scalp region (Table 8.1). Symptoms associated with ON are characterized by localized tenderness and pain in the distribution of the occipital nerves. As such, it is essential to have familiarity with the anatomy of the occipital nerves to understand the diagnosis and treatment of ON. The

TABLE 8.1
Differential Diagnosis of Posterior Scalp Pain

Occipital neuralgia
Migraine headache
Tension headache
Cluster headache
Cervicogenic headache
Hemicrania continua
Myofascial pain
CHIARI malformation
Atlanto-axial degenerative arthritis
Whiplash
Giant cell arteritis
Systemic vasculitis
Post-herpetic neuralgia
Neoplasm
Infection
Diabetes

C2 ganglion, unlike other cervical ganglia, emerges posteriorly between the atlas and axis and is not encased behind bone.[15] Thus, it is more susceptible to compression than other ganglia. The dorsal ramus of C2 curves obliquely and inferiorly, before its medial fibers contribute to the GON. The GON traverses through the trapezius and semispinalis capitis and then courses superficially to supply the occipital skin toward the scalp vertex.[12] It is often accompanied by the occipital artery. The C2 dorsal ramus similarly gives rise to the LON, which ascends the posterior border of the sternocleidomastoid before piercing the posterior triangle of the neck to innervate the mastoid region.[12,16] Occasionally, the LON receives a contribution from the C3 dorsal ramus as well. The superficial medial branch of the C3 dorsal ramus is the origin of the third occipital nerve, which innervates the suboccipital region.[17] It is important to recognize the functional connections between occipital nerve and meningeal afferents in the upper spinal cord, termed the "trigeminocervical complex," as this may explain the therapeutic benefit of ONS for the treatment of diverse migrainous and cervicogenic headache disorders.[18–20]

The clinical history of a patient is also important in distinguishing ON from other headache disorders, primarily based on the distribution and characteristics of pain. True ON pain is described as sharp and stabbing with paroxysmal attacks. It can be elicited with palpation of the neck or occiput in the distribution of the occipital nerves and can be triggered with neck movements. In contrast, diffuse nonlocalizable pain that is described as dull, aching, and throbbing is less likely to be ON. Patients may report that they avoid wearing hats and minimize washing or brushing their hair. It is important to obtain a detailed history and ask about prior head or neck trauma, neck surgery or other systemic disorders.

Most presentations of ON tend to be idiopathic.[16] However, there are a variety of potential etiologies, and ON can occur as a result of compression of or trauma to the occipital nerves, resulting in fibrous tissue entrapment or bony compression of the upper cervical dorsal root ganglia.[21] Rarely, a neoplastic process with infiltration or compression of the nerve or ganglion is implicated. In addition to a thorough history and physical examination, radiographic imaging such as flexion/extension X-rays or a cervical MRI may be useful as well. Local occipital nerve blocks are commonly performed for diagnostic and therapeutic purposes and may provide temporary symptoms relief; however, the lack of efficacy of a block does not necessarily exclude ON as a diagnosis.[22–24]

CONSERVATIVE AND SURGICAL TREATMENTS

There have been numerous treatment measures described in the management of ON. Initial treatment options are conservative and may include alternating warm or cold compresses, massage or physical therapy to alleviate muscle tension, and pharmacologic therapy.[25] The regular use of antiepileptic and antidepressant medications may decrease the frequency and severity of ON pain, and the use of antiinflammatories often alleviates pain during acute episodes.[25] Local anesthetic blocks and steroid injections can be both diagnostic and therapeutic; however, the benefit tends to be transient. The injection of botulinum toxin into neck muscles has reportedly resulted in some effectiveness for ON secondary to a cervicogenic pathology.[26] Pulsed radiofrequency has also been described as an alternative nondestructive treatment, but these effects are also short-lived.[27]

There are various surgical treatment options for medically refractory ON; however, these procedures tend to be invasive and confer variable benefit.[28] Such measures include occipital nerve decompression, occipital neurectomy, C2 ganglionectomy, and rhizotomy.[29–32] Occipital nerve decompression for entrapment has been found to produce benefit in carefully selected patients; however, localization of the nerve can be challenging.[33,34] Occipital neurectomy of the GON and/or LON results in numbness in the distribution of the nerve and has a high rate of pain recurrence. In addition, the proximal nerve stump may develop a painful neuroma.[29,35] Ganglionectomy also results in complete sensory loss in the C2 distribution but avoids the issue of nerve regeneration and neuroma formation that occur with neurectomy because the entire cell body is removed.[30,36] However, this procedure is more invasive and technically complex and can occasionally result in a painful deafferentation syndrome.[30] Rhizotomy is the most invasive and complex of the ablative procedures.[37] Selective dorsal rhizotomies are usually attempted to minimize sensory loss.[31,32] In contrast to the above techniques, ONS is a minimally invasive, reversible, and adjustable alternative that avoids many of the limitations of conservative and ablative therapies, making it the procedure of choice for selected patients with medically refractory ON.[2,14]

PATIENT SELECTION

Although numerous trials describing the efficacy of ONS have been performed, many of the current prospective, randomized clinical trials have not exclusively focused on medically refractory ON and have included other headache pathologies as well.[9,11] As such, neurosurgical guidelines for the use of ONS in the treatment of medically refractory ON have been established with level III evidence.[14] Although the neurosurgical guidelines address the use of ONS specifically for ON, ONS may also be considered for the treatment of chronic migraines and other craniofacial pain syndromes or headache disorders with a primary occipital pain distribution.[2,4–7,9,11,12,28,38] Notably, ONS is not FDA-approved for the treatment of headache and craniofacial pain and thus represents an off-label use.

Perhaps the most important predictor of success with ONS is patient selection based on neuropsychologic factors. Chronic pain syndromes are disabling conditions, which confer enormous personal, social, and economic burden. Patients that may not benefit from ONS are those with a history of psychiatric comorbidities, such as depression, drug seeking, or addiction, or a history of multiple pain procedures.[28,39,40] It is imperative to have a realistic discussion regarding expectations of therapeutic benefit, as the goal of neuromodulation is to manage but not eliminate pain. Some practitioners may choose to refer prospective patients to specialized pain psychologists who are part of the routine preoperative assessment.

During assessment of ON, a physical examination should demonstrate pain on palpation of the occipital region. There may also be allodynia with stimulation of other scalp regions or manipulation of the hair. A positive Tinel sign over the affected nerve is frequently elicited. The occipital region and neck should be examined for scars or irregularities from previous trauma or surgery; such anatomic variation may result in altered pain distributions.

An initial diagnostic workup commonly includes head and neck CT or MRI imaging to rule out a structural cause for the patient's symptoms, such as degenerative cervical spine disease, Chiari malformation, or tumor, as treatment of these pathologies may be indicated first. Flexion and extension X-rays should be performed when abnormal cervical motion or instability is suspected, as this may also require intervention. If the clinical history is suggestive of systemic metabolic or inflammatory etiologies, additional blood work may be taken. Local anesthetic blockade of the GON and/or LON has been reported to be both diagnostic and therapeutic. However, it is important to recognize that the absence of benefit does not exclude ON as a potential pathology and that other headache pathologies may also respond to occipital nerve blocks.[24,41]

In general, patients who may be considered candidates for an ONS trial are those with ongoing ON who have failed conventional medical therapy and who possess realistic expectations regarding pain management. Patients with other headache presentations may also be considered suitable candidates for an ONS trial if their pain has been refractory. In general, a successful ONS trial is defined as 50% or greater pain reduction with adequate coverage of the painful area with paresthesias. The trial period is variable based on practitioner experience and is generally 1 week or less.

OCCIPITAL NERVE STIMULATION TECHNIQUE

The surgical technique for ONS implantation can vary substantially. However, like all forms of neuromodulation, it is advantageous for patients to first undergo an ONS trial before ONS implantation. Patients can be implanted either asleep, with general anesthesia, or awake, with conscious sedation.[2,12,14,38,40,42] The latter allows for intraoperative awake testing of the lead to ensure adequate positioning for coverage of the patient's pain. Intraoperative fluoroscopy is an important tool, particularly for asleep patients, to ensure that the electrode lead is in the appropriate location.[9,28]

Positioning can be supine with a shoulder bump and the head turned, lateral decubitus, or prone.[14] The generator can be placed in the infraclavicular region, the abdomen, or the buttocks, depending on the position of the patient.[2,12,28,38,42–44]

There are also several options for electrode location. Leads can be placed unilaterally or bilaterally, depending on the distribution of pain. Placement of the lead at the level of the posterior arch of C1, using fluoroscopy for intraoperative guidance, is ideal for stimulation the LON, which exits the muscle more laterally and inferiorly, while still reaching fibers from the GON and LON.[2,38,42,44] Alternatively, the leads can also be placed just below the level of the occipital protuberance, targeting the GON medially after it emerges from the muscle more superiorly or reaching the LON laterally.[12] Occasionally the ideal lead position is along the course of the nerve, according to the location of a positive Tinel sign marked preoperatively, or as seen with an open dissection and direct placement of the lead.[45] Intraoperative awake testing of the lead can be beneficial to ensure that a patient's symptoms are adequately covered by the electrode; however, this can be difficult to do in the prone position. Decision of the lead location should ultimately depend on the distribution of a patient's pain and the results from the trial.[14]

Once the lead location is decided, the approach must also be determined. Electrode leads can be passed from a lateral entry site and directed medially toward the midline or past the midline to the contralateral side (Fig. 8.1A).[2,28,38,43] Alternatively, electrodes can be passed from a midline incision extending laterally on one or both sides, which some surgeons prefer for bilateral lead placement (Fig. 8.1B).[12,28,42–44] It may also be possible to combine approaches if patients are supine or lateral, such that the ipsilateral lead is placed from lateral to medial and the contralateral lead is placed from midline to the contralateral side.

When choosing which electrode to use for the procedure, it is important to note that ONS is still considered an "off-label" use of stimulation, and there is thus no single stimulator that is designed specifically for ONS. As such, spinal cord stimulator leads are most commonly used for ONS. This includes percutaneous and paddle electrode leads, quadrapolar and octapolar leads, and leads with tightly spaced or widely spaced contacts, and there are insufficient data to suggest one type over another.[9] The paddle electrodes can be placed via direct dissection into the subcutaneous space with insertion of the lead. Placement of the percutaneous electrodes is done using a spinal needle, which is often curved slightly with the bevel down to better facilitate passage into the subcutaneous tissue along the contour of the skull without breaching through the skin. Although subfascial lead insertion can also be done, this tends to result in unintended activation of the muscle fibers, which can result in discomfort for the patient.[46]

The most common complication reported in the literature is migration of the leads.[47] Lead migration can result in loss of efficacy and the need for more

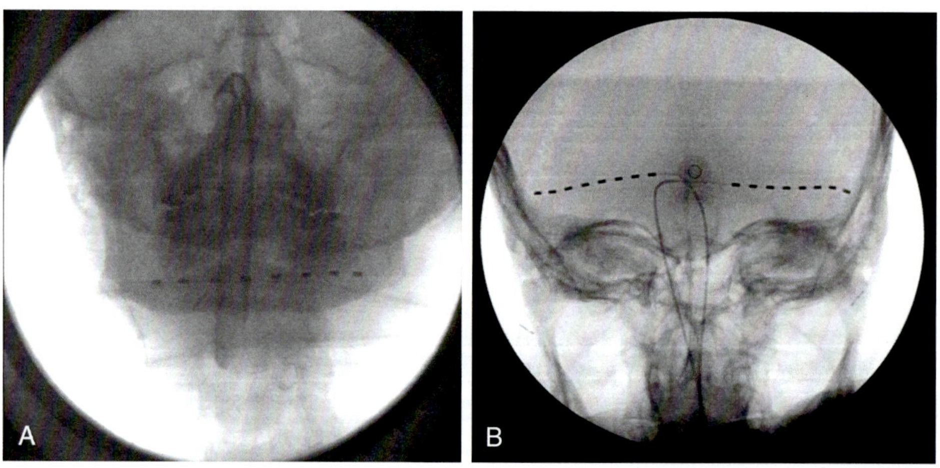

FIG. 8.1 Intraoperative X-rays during trial occipital nerve stimulator electrode implantation. The electrode can be inserted through a lateral approach projecting to the contralateral side **(A)** or through a midline incision extending laterally on either side **(B)**.

complex programming or even surgical revision or replacement of the lead. The risk of migration can be reduced by the use of an anchor attached to cervical fascia to hold the lead in position and placement of one or more strain relief loops to reduce direct pull on the lead.[47] Some reports suggest that paddle leads may also reduce migration compared with percutaneous leads.[38,47] Finally, avoiding the placement of leads and incisions in areas with increased mobility, as well as minimizing the distance between the lead and the generator site, may also reduce migration.[38,47] As such, some authors prefer placement of the lead via a midline incision and/or placement of the generator in the chest rather than the buttocks. However, a review of the literature did not show any statistically significant difference in such techniques, and thus the ONS guidelines do not provide recommendations regarding these variations.[14] Other complications reported in the literature include infection, wound dehiscence, pain at the incisions, loss of efficacy, and breakage of the leads.[2,12,14,28,38,40,43–45,47]

OUTCOMES

Despite the popularity of ONS for the treatment of ON, the literature lacks robust, prospective comparative studies describing long-term outcomes. In comparison, there have been randomized control trials evaluating the effectiveness of ONS for other headache disorders; however, these studies and their interpretations are limited by variations in outcome reporting and trial methodology.

Regarding medically refractory ON, there have been numerous case series in the literature providing Class III Level evidence.[14] Three articles detail prospective case series without a corresponding control. The largest was a 12-week pilot study of 11 patients, with 91% of patients reporting decreased medication usage and 64% reporting reduction in the number of headaches.[43] One study of six patients reported decreased pain scores and opioid use,[44] whereas another study of seven patients reported 75%–100% reduction in pain scores.[45] The patients in this latter study did not undergo trial stimulation, and the high success rate was attributed to an open surgical technique with direct visualization of the occipital nerve for lead placement.[45] However, both of these studies are limited by their short follow-up of 3 months.

The retrospective case series of ONS for medically refractory ON generally describe larger patient cohorts and longer follow-up. The seminal Weiner and Reed paper reviewed 13 patients who underwent trial stimulation followed by permanent implantation, with all 13 patients reporting greater than 50% pain relief, including two-thirds with greater than 75% pain relief, with a mean follow-up of 2.4 years.[2] Other studies have reported similarly excellent clinical results, with significant pain relief sustained with follow-up durations of 5–47 months.[12,28,38,40,42]

The more robust, but also controversial, data for the use of ONS for headache disorders are in the treatment of chronic migraines. Like many studies of peripheral neuromodulation, initially promising reports of clinical effectiveness from open-label studies have difficulty transitioning into subsequent controlled trials. For example, the Occipital Nerve Stimulation for the Treatment of Chronic Migraine Headache feasibility study reported 39% of patients with adjustable stimulation to be responders at 3-month follow-up[9]; a responder was defined as achieving 50% or greater reduction in number of headache days per month or a reduction in average overall pain intensity by 3 points or greater. A larger randomized study of 157 patients did not identify a significant difference in responders receiving either active or control (sham) stimulation at 3 months; however, there was a significant reduction in the number of headache days and improvement in migraine-related disability and pain relief.[10] Clinical efficacy regarding these secondary outcomes was maintained at 1-year follow-up; however, an astounding 183 device or procedure-related adverse events were identified, representing 70% of patients.[11] Common adverse events included hardware-related complications (lead migration or fracture, battery failure) and biologic (erosion, infection) complications. Interestingly, other studies have also reported a high rate of adverse events.[48] It has been suggested that a lower rate of adverse events may be associated with improved practitioner experience and familiarity with PNS procedures.[49]

It has been suggested that the evidence for the use of ONS for the treatment of chronic migraine is mixed because of different definitions of clinical success. Outcomes are equivocal with regard to "responder rates," with no studies reaching this primary endpoint; however, there may be meaningful clinical differences with regard to additional quality of life measures such as number of headache days and patient satisfaction.[50,51] In addition to the high complication rate, concerns have also been raised regarding the costs related to ONS implantation in this patient population.[52] As such, its use in the treatment of chronic migraine should be considered on a case-by-case basis.

CONCLUSION

ONS for medically refractory headache and craniofacial pain syndromes can be an effective treatment option in appropriately selected patients. These patient populations experience debilitating daily pain, resulting in personal, social, and economic burden. Treatment failure is high with conventional measures, necessitating consideration for alternative modalities such as ONS. Proper patient selection is essential, as is practitioner experience with PNS techniques. As both ONS technology and implantation techniques evolve, improvements should be realized with regard to clinical effectiveness and complication rates. Larger and well-designed studies with extended follow-up are essential to establish an ongoing role for ONS in the treatment of these pain syndromes.

REFERENCES

1. Wall PD, Sweet WH. Temporary abolition of pain in man. *Science*. 1967;155:108–109.
2. Weiner RL, Reed KL. Peripheral neurostimulation for control of intractable occipital neuralgia. *Neuromodulation*. 1999;2:217–221. https://doi.org/10.1046/j.1525-1403.1999.00217.x.
3. The international classification of headache disorders, 3rd edition (beta version). *Cephalalgia*. 2013;33:629–808. https://doi.org/10.1177/0333102413485658.
4. Burns B, Watkins L, Goadsby PJ. Treatment of medically intractable cluster headache by occipital nerve stimulation: long-term follow-up of eight patients. *Lancet*. 2007;369:1099–1106. https://doi.org/10.1016/S0140-6736(07)60328-6.
5. Leone M, Franzini A, Cecchini AP, Broggi G, Bussone G. Stimulation of occipital nerve for drug-resistant chronic cluster headache. *Lancet Neurol*. 2007;6:289–291. https://doi.org/10.1016/S1474-4422(07)70061-3.
6. Rodrigo-Royo MD, Azcona JM, Quero J, Lorente MC, Acin P, Azcona J. Peripheral neurostimulation in the management of cervicogenic headache: four case reports. *Neuromodulation*. 2005;8:241–248. https://doi.org/10.1111/j.1525-1403.2005.00032.x.
7. Burns B, Watkins L, Goadsby PJ. Treatment of hemicrania continua by occipital nerve stimulation with a bion device: long-term follow-up of a crossover study. *Lancet Neurol*. 2008;7:1001–1012. https://doi.org/10.1016/S1474-4422(08)70217-5.
8. Schwedt TJ, Dodick DW, Hentz J, Trentman TL, Zimmerman RS. Occipital nerve stimulation for chronic headache–long-term safety and efficacy. *Cephalalgia*. 2007;27:153–157. https://doi.org/10.1111/j.1468-2982.2007.01272.x.
9. Saper JR, Dodick DW, Silberstein SD, McCarville S, Sun M, Goadsby PJ. Occipital nerve stimulation for the treatment of intractable chronic migraine headache: ONSTIM feasibility study. *Cephalalgia*. 2011;31:271–285. https://doi.org/10.1177/0333102410381142.
10. Silberstein SD, Dodick DW, Saper J, et al. Safety and efficacy of peripheral nerve stimulation of the occipital nerves for the management of chronic migraine: results from a randomized, multicenter, double-blinded, controlled study. *Cephalalgia*. 2012;32:1165–1179. https://doi.org/10.1177/0333102412462642.
11. Dodick DW, Silberstein SD, Reed KL, et al. Safety and efficacy of peripheral nerve stimulation of the occipital nerves for the management of chronic migraine: long-term results from a randomized, multicenter, double-blinded, controlled study. *Cephalalgia*. 2015;35:344–358. https://doi.org/10.1177/0333102414543331.
12. Johnstone CS, Sundaraj R. Occipital nerve stimulation for the treatment of occipital neuralgia-eight case studies. *Neuromodulation*. 2006;9:41–47. https://doi.org/10.1111/j.1525-1403.2006.00041.x.
13. Mueller O, Hagel V, Wrede K, et al. Stimulation of the greater occipital nerve: anatomical considerations and clinical implications. *Pain Physician*. 2013;16:E181–E189.
14. Sweet JA, Mitchell LS, Narouze S, et al. Occipital nerve stimulation for the treatment of patients with medically refractory occipital neuralgia: congress of neurological surgeons systematic review and evidence-based guideline. *Neurosurgery*. 2015;77:332–341. https://doi.org/10.1227/NEU.0000000000000872.
15. Acar F, Miller J, Golshani KJ, Israel ZH, McCartney S, Burchiel KJ. Pain relief after cervical ganglionectomy (C2 and C3) for the treatment of medically intractable occipital neuralgia. *Stereotact Funct Neurosurg*. 2008;86:106–112. https://doi.org/10.1159/000113872.
16. Cesmebasi A, Muhleman MA, Hulsberg P, et al. Occipital neuralgia: anatomic considerations. *Clin Anat*. 2015;28:101–108. https://doi.org/10.1002/ca.22468.
17. Bogduk N. Cervicogenic headache: anatomic basis and pathophysiologic mechanisms. *Curr Pain Headache Rep*. 2001;5:382–386.
18. Bartsch T, Goadsby PJ. The trigeminocervical complex and migraine: current concepts and synthesis. *Curr Pain Headache Rep*. 2003;7:371–376.
19. Goadsby PJ, Knight YE, Hoskin KL. Stimulation of the greater occipital nerve increases metabolic activity in the trigeminal nucleus caudalis and cervical dorsal horn of the cat. *Pain*. 1997;73:23–28.
20. Matharu MS, Bartsch T, Ward N, Frackowiak RS, Weiner R, Goadsby PJ. Central neuromodulation in chronic migraine patients with suboccipital stimulators: a PET study. *Brain*. 2004;127:220–230. https://doi.org/10.1093/brain/awh022.

21. Ehni G, Benner B. Occipital neuralgia and C1-C2 arthrosis. *N Engl J Med*. 1984;310:127. https://doi.org/10.1056/NEJM198401123100220.
22. Tobin JA, Flitman SS. Occipital nerve blocks: effect of symptomatic medication: overuse and headache type on failure rate. *Headache*. 2009;49:1479–1485. https://doi.org/10.1111/j.1526-4610.2009.01549.x.
23. Tobin J, Flitman S. Occipital nerve blocks: when and what to inject? *Headache*. 2009;49:1521–1533. https://doi.org/10.1111/j.1526-4610.2009.01493.x.
24. Kinfe TM, Schuss P, Vatter H. Occipital nerve block prior to occipital nerve stimulation for refractory chronic migraine and chronic cluster headache: myth or prediction? *Cephalalgia*. 2015;35:359–362. https://doi.org/10.1177/0333102414541685.
25. Vanelderen P, Lataster A, Levy R, Mekhail N, van Kleef M, Van Zundert J. 8. Occipital neuralgia. *Pain Pract*. 2010;10:137–144. https://doi.org/10.1111/j.1533-2500.2009.00355.x.
26. Freund BJ, Schwartz M. Treatment of chronic cervical-associated headache with botulinum toxin A: a pilot study. *Headache*. 2000;40:231–236.
27. Cohen SP, Peterlin BL, Fulton L, et al. Randomized, double-blind, comparative-effectiveness study comparing pulsed radiofrequency to steroid injections for occipital neuralgia or migraine with occipital nerve tenderness. *Pain*. 2015;156:2585–2594. https://doi.org/10.1097/j.pain.0000000000000373.
28. Slavin KV, Nersesyan H, Wess C. Peripheral neurostimulation for treatment of intractable occipital neuralgia. *Neurosurgery*. 2006;58:112–119; discussion 112–119.
29. Gille O, Lavignolle B, Vital JM. Surgical treatment of greater occipital neuralgia by neurolysis of the greater occipital nerve and sectioning of the inferior oblique muscle. *Spine*. 2004;29:828–832.
30. Lozano AM, Vanderlinden G, Bachoo R, Rothbart P. Microsurgical C-2 ganglionectomy for chronic intractable occipital pain. *J Neurosurg*. 1998;89:359–365. https://doi.org/10.3171/jns.1998.89.3.0359.
31. Dubuisson D. Treatment of occipital neuralgia by partial posterior rhizotomy at C1-3. *J Neurosurg*. 1995;82:581–586. https://doi.org/10.3171/jns.1995.82.4.0581.
32. Rasskazoff S, Kaufmann AM. Ventrolateral partial dorsal root entry zone rhizotomy for occipital neuralgia. *Pain Res Manag*. 2005;10:43–45.
33. Junewicz A, Katira K, Guyuron B. Intraoperative anatomical variations during greater occipital nerve decompression. *J Plast Reconstr Aesthet Surg*. 2013;66:1340–1345. https://doi.org/10.1016/j.bjps.2013.06.016.
34. Li F, Ma Y, Zou J, et al. Micro-surgical decompression for greater occipital neuralgia. *Turk Neurosurg*. 2012;22:427–429. https://doi.org/10.5137/1019-5149.JTN.5234-11.1.
35. Bovim G, Fredriksen TA, Stolt-Nielsen A, Sjaastad O. Neurolysis of the greater occipital nerve in cervicogenic headache. A follow up study. *Headache*. 1992;32:175–179.
36. Wang MY, Levi AD. Ganglionectomy of C-2 for the treatment of medically refractory occipital neuralgia. *Neurosurg Focus*. 2002;12:E14.
37. Chambers WR. Posterior rhizotomy of the second and third cervical nerves for occipital pain. *J Am Med Assoc*. 1954;155:431–432.
38. Oh MY, Ortega J, Bellotte JB, Whiting DM, Alo K. Peripheral nerve stimulation for the treatment of occipital neuralgia and transformed migraine using a c1-2-3 subcutaneous paddle style electrode: a technical report. *Neuromodulation*. 2004;7:103–112. https://doi.org/10.1111/j.1094-7159.2004.04014.x.
39. Notaro P, Buratti E, Meroni A, Montagna MC, Rubino FG, Voltolini A. The effects of peripheral occipital nerve stimulation for the treatment of patients suffering from chronic migraine: a single center experience. *Pain Physician*. 2014;17:E369–E374.
40. Palmisani S, Al-Kaisy A, Arcioni R, et al. A six year retrospective review of occipital nerve stimulation practice—controversies and challenges of an emerging technique for treating refractory headache syndromes. *J Headache Pain*. 2013;14:67. https://doi.org/10.1186/1129-2377-14-67.
41. Bovim G, Sand T. Cervicogenic headache, migraine without aura and tension-type headache. Diagnostic blockade of greater occipital and supra-orbital nerves. *Pain*. 1992;51:43–48.
42. Abhinav K, Park ND, Prakash SK, Love-Jones S, Patel NK. Novel use of narrow paddle electrodes for occipital nerve stimulation—technical note. *Neuromodulation*. 2013;16:607–609. https://doi.org/10.1111/j.1525-1403.2012.00524.x.
43. Melvin Jr EA, Jordan FR, Weiner RL, Primm D. Using peripheral stimulation to reduce the pain of C2-mediated occipital headaches: a preliminary report. *Pain Physician*. 2007;10:453–460.
44. Kapural L, Mekhail N, Hayek SM, Stanton-Hicks M, Malak O. Occipital nerve electrical stimulation via the midline approach and subcutaneous surgical leads for treatment of severe occipital neuralgia: a pilot study. *Anesth Analg*. 2005;101:171–174. https://doi.org/10.1213/01.ANE.0000156207.73396.8E.
45. Magown P, Garcia R, Beauprie I, Mendez IM. Occipital nerve stimulation for intractable occipital neuralgia: an open surgical technique. *Clin Neurosurg*. 2009;56:119–124.
46. Hayek SM, Jasper JF, Deer TR, Narouze SN. Occipital neurostimulation-induced muscle spasms: implications for lead placement. *Pain Physician*. 2009;12:867–876.
47. Falowski S, Wang D, Sabesan A, Sharan A. Occipital nerve stimulator systems: review of complications and surgical techniques. *Neuromodulation*. 2010;13:121–125. https://doi.org/10.1111/j.1525-1403.2009.00261.x.
48. Mekhail NA, Estemalik E, Azer G, Davis K, Tepper SJ. Safety and efficacy of occipital nerves stimulation for the treatment of chronic migraines: randomized, double-blind, controlled single-center experience. *Pain Pract*. 2017;17:669–677. https://doi.org/10.1111/papr.12504.

49. Sharan A, Huh B, Narouze S, et al. Analysis of adverse events in the management of chronic migraine by peripheral nerve stimulation. *Neuromodulation*. 2015;18: 305–312; discussion 312. https://doi.org/10.1111/ner.12243.
50. Chen YF, Bramley G, Unwin G, et al. Occipital nerve stimulation for chronic migraine—a systematic review and meta-analysis. *PLoS One*. 2015;10:e0116786. https://doi.org/10.1371/journal.pone.0116786.
51. Yang Y, Song M, Fan Y, Ma K. Occipital nerve stimulation for migraine: a systematic review. *Pain Pract*. 2016;16: 509–517. https://doi.org/10.1111/papr.12303.
52. Mueller O, Diener HC, Dammann P, et al. Occipital nerve stimulation for intractable chronic cluster headache or migraine: a critical analysis of direct treatment costs and complications. *Cephalalgia*. 2013;33:1283–1291. https://doi.org/10.1177/0333102413493193.

CHAPTER 9

Spinal Ablation for Cancer Pain (Cordotomy and Myelotomy)

ASHWIN VISWANATHAN, MD

INTRODUCTION

Spinal ablation remains a relevant and important technique for the treatment of medically refractory cancer pain. Interruption of the spinothalamic tract (cordotomy) or the dorsal columns' visceral pain pathway (myelotomy) can be achieved either through open surgical techniques, including laminectomy, or percutaneously. Advantages of these techniques as compared with intrathecal drug delivery include immediate onset relief, no ongoing medical visits for maintenance of therapy, and cost-effectiveness. In this chapter, we will review cordotomy and myelotomy with an emphasis on surgical technique.

CORDOTOMY

Two important neurosurgical series of CT-guided cordotomy have been published. In a prospective study of 41 patients who underwent cordotomy, 80% of the patients had no pain postoperatively and for 1 month postprocedure.[1] At 6 months postprocedure, 32% of the patients had no pain and another 48% of the patients had partial satisfactory pain relief. Similarly, in Kanpolat's[2] series of 207 cordotomies, a significant improvement in the pain intensity from a mean of 7.6 (preoperatively) to a mean of 1.3 (postoperatively) was achieved. When Kanpolat reported his subset of 108 patients with lung cancer, 89% of the patients had no pain postoperatively.

Indications

Cordotomy is highly effective for the treatment of nociceptive pain due to cancer. Nociceptive pain is pain due to direct tissue involvement of tumor. Cordotomy is safest when performed unilaterally, so as to avoid Ondine's curse by the bilateral interruption of reticulospinal fibers.[3,4] Owing to the decussation of spinothalamic fibers, cordotomy is effective for pain arising 2–5 segments below the targeted spinal level. Hence, a C1-2 percutaneous cordotomy can usually have an effect on pain arising from the C5 or C6 dermatome and below.

There are variable reports of the effectiveness of cordotomy in the treatment of neuropathic pain. At least in the author's experience, cordotomy is very effective for purely nociceptive pain and is much less effective in patients with pain associated with complete deafferentation. However, in the treatment of cancer pain, most pain conditions are a mixture of nociceptive and neuropathic pains. In this mixed pain population, we have experienced some variability in pain outcomes with cordotomy. The exact reasons for this variability in outcomes are unclear; however, an incomplete ablation of the spinothalamic tract is likely one relevant variable.

Intraprocedural Imaging Considerations

Although fluoroscopy can be used as the standalone imaging modality for cordotomy, we would argue that the additional safety and accuracy afforded by three-dimensional intraoperative imaging has improved outcomes for this procedure. There are two principal imaging modalities to which neurosurgeons have access. The first is a conventional CT scanner. This is available in either a diagnostic radiology suite or can be available in the operating room (OR). A CT scanner with a movable table is highly advantageous for this procedure, as the patient can be moved quickly in and out of the scanner to adjust the needle position, and scanning is very fast.

The O-arm is another intraoperative imager that is available in many modern ORs. The advantage of the O-arm is that X-rays can be performed during the advancement of the spinal needle, as opposed to performing short-segment CT scans. This may lead to time-saving and lower radiation dose during needle insertion as compared with a traditional CT scanner.

However, to limit the extent of the scan to working area (i.e., C1-C2 region) is not possible, and instead complete images of the craniocervical junction are acquired with each O-arm spin. However, the myelogram quality obtained with an O-arm is adequate for cordotomy (Fig. 9.1).

Endoscopy is another modality for performing cordotomy, and we refer the reader to Fonoff et al.[5] who have described this technique.

Surgical Techniques

A preoperative cranial CT scan should be obtained to rule out any mass lesion and to prevent herniation during the C1-2 puncture. On the day of the procedure, the patient is transported to the diagnostic CT scanning area. A lumbar puncture is performed and intrathecal contrast is administered to obtain an adequate cervical myelogram. The patient is placed in Trendelenburg position for 15–20 min to allow adequate dispersion of the contrast.

Intravenous sedation is provided through intermittent propofol boluses, along with a continuous infusion. Lidocaine (1%) is used to anesthetize the region approximately 1 cm inferior and posterior to the tip of the mastoid. A CT scan of the cervical spine is obtained, focusing on the C1-2 region. The skin to dura distance is measured and is noted on the 20-gauge spinal needle provided with the disposable percutaneous cordotomy electrode (LCED, Cosman Medical). The 20-gauge spinal needle is advanced toward the C1-2 interspace, and multiple short CT scans spanning 15 mm are used to direct the needle toward the dura. For lower extremity pain, the target for the spinal needle is just anterior to the anterior-posterior midpoint of the spinal cord. For pain in the chest or upper extremities, a target 1–2 mm more anteriorly is chosen. The tip of the spinal needle is advanced further until it is adjacent to the spinal cord. At this point the stylet is replaced with the LCED electrode. Impedance measurement along with tactile feel is used to determine the location of the electrode. When the electrode is in cerebrospinal fluid (CSF), the impedance will measure a few hundred ohms (<300 Ω). As the electrode abuts and presses into the pia of the spinal cord, the impedance will increase significantly into the range of several hundred ohms (300–500 Ω). Entrance of the electrode into the spinal cord is met with a clear popping sensation, and the impedance will increase dramatically to greater than 700 Ω. At this point, another CT scan is obtained; the electrode may be beyond the midpoint of the spinal cord, as it requires some pressure for the electrode to penetrate the pia. The electrode is withdrawn if necessary until it sits within the radiographically expected location of the spinothalamic tract (Fig. 9.2).

Intraoperative physiologic testing is then performed to test for both sensory and motor effects. Sensory testing is performed at 100 Hz and 0.1 msec pulse width, whereas motor testing is performed at 2 Hz. At this point in the procedure, the patient's cooperation is needed, and hence the sedation is lightened until the patient can intelligibly answer questions. Sensory testing is performed to ensure physiologic presence within the spinothalamic tract. Testing for motor contractions is also performed up to 1 V stimulation, indicating a safe distance from the corticospinal tract.

When the radiofrequency (RF) electrode is in an appropriate radiologic and physiologic location, lesioning is performed using increasing levels of temperature starting at 60°C for 60 s and proceeding up to 80°C for 60 s. As lesioning the spinothalamic tract is not painful,

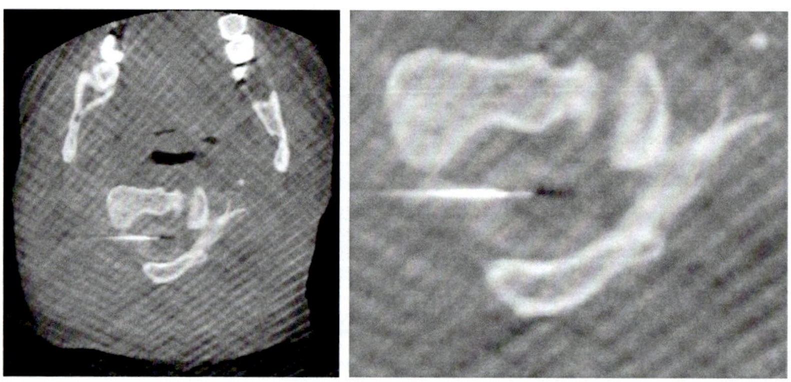

FIG. 9.1 Axial O-arm (Medtronic, MN) images of the C1-C2 region obtained after contrast administration and after placement of the cordotomy RF electrode. Good visualization of the spinal cord parenchyma and electrode position is achieved.

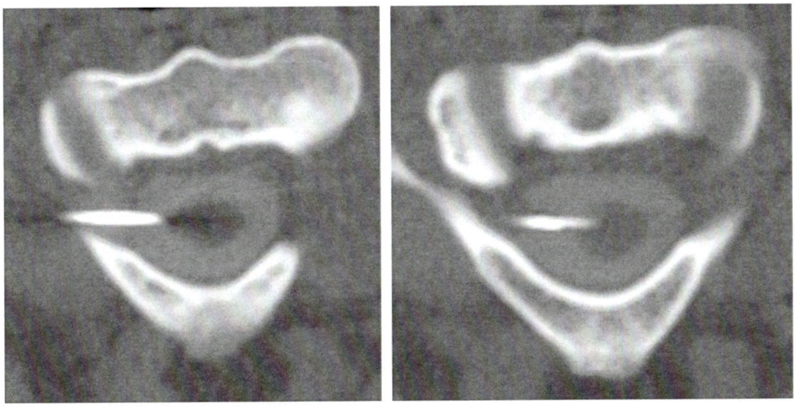

FIG. 9.2 Axial CT scan images obtained with intrathecal contrast obtained after the placement of spinal needle abutting spinal cord (left) and after the insertion of radiofrequency electrode into the spinal cord (right).

additional sedation is not required for the ablation. Between lesions, testing for the development of hypesthesia is helpful, as an additional lesion may be required if the patient has no decreased pinprick sensation. The goal of the cordotomy is to create a moderate hypalgesia.

Complications

Cordotomy is a safe procedure, especially in the era of CT guidance. The risk associated with spinal needle insertion and penetration of the RF electrode into the pia of the spinal cord appears to be very small. In the author's experience of more than 50 cordotomies, no complication has been attributable to insertion of the spinal needle or introduction of the RF electrode, even in patients undergoing multiple pial penetrations to map the somatotopy of the spinothalamic tract.

The RF ablation itself can be a source of complication for cordotomy. Hence the art of cordotomy is determining the appropriate balance between an aggressive lesion to optimize a durable pain outcome and a safe lesion to avoid undesired side effects. The author has moved toward performing two lesions at 80°C for 60 s each, as these parameters seem to provide an adequate ablation of the spinothalamic target. In select cases, the author has made three lesions at 80°C for 60 s each. With increasing ablation, the risk of bothersome dysesthesia increases. Two lesions at 70°C for 60 s are very unlikely to produce bothersome dysesthesia.

Motor complications, and specifically ipsilateral weakness, are an avoidable complication of cordotomy when using a CT-guided approach. When performing cordotomy, if the RF electrode is anterior to the midpoint of the spinal cord, and no motor contractions are elicited at 1V when performing motor stimulation (2Hz, 0.1ms pulse width), it is highly unlikely that the patient will experience any motor deficit. Occasionally, however, in the pursuit of an adequate lesion of the spinothalamic tract, placing the RF electrode at the midpoint of the spinal cord is desirable. We have had an incidence of 2%–6% of transient ipsilateral lower extremity weakness in our series of 50 patients. In these patients, the leg weakness was at least 4/5 strength, and the patients could ambulate with a walker. The weakness improved over the course of 3 weeks postoperatively.

Other complications of cordotomy include bothersome dysesthesias, seen in 2% of our series. We, and others, have not seen a case of respiratory complications or serious neurologic injury when using a CT-guided approach.

Data from more than 200 CT-guided cordotomies have been published in the literature.[1,2] In 2008, Raslan reported his series of 41 patients who underwent cordotomy, and no patients were found to have new neurologic deficits. In Kanpolat's[2] series of 207 cordotomies, five patients (2.4%) developed temporary weakness and five patients (2.4%) developed temporary ataxia. These symptoms resolved within 3 weeks after the procedure. In the 251 CT-guided cordotomies reported in the literature, four patients (1.6%) had dysesthetic pains. Importantly, there has been no other major morbidity.

MYELOTOMY

Surgical interventions for the management of visceral pain have focused on interrupting either commissural fibers associated with the anterolateral system,[6] midline fibers associated with the visceral pain pathways, or both. Various surgical techniques have been proposed for performing a myelotomy for pain control, including open midline myelotomy,[7] stereotactic percutaneous myelotomy,[8] CT-guided percutaneous myelotomy,[9] and punctate midline myelotomy.[10] The midline commissural myelotomy was introduced by Armour,[11] and in 1968, Hitchcock performed the first stereotactic percutaneous myelotomy. With Hitchcock's approach, the patient was seated with the head flexed within a stereotactic headframe. A myelogram was performed via a puncture in the atlantooccipital membrane to delineate the spinal cord. A spark gap diathermy machine was then used to make a lesion within the spinal commissure.[8] Following myelotomy, Hitchcock noted a far greater degree of pain relief than would have been expected by only lesioning (as opposed to dividing) the commissural fibers, supporting previous hypotheses of another spinal pathway for visceral pain.

Preclinical studies have augmented our understanding of the midline dorsal columns' visceral pain pathway. The primary afferents for this dorsal columns' visceral pain pathway travel to cell bodies situated in the nucleus proprius and in the region of the spinal gray matter dorsal to the central canal of the spinal cord. From here, the axons ascend ipsilaterally along the midline portion of the dorsal columns before synapsing in the nucleus gracilis.[12–14]

Candidates for midline myelotomy include patients with intractable pain associated with malignancy in the abdominal or pelvic region.

Surgical Techniques

Myelotomy can be performed using three different techniques: open punctate myelotomy, percutaneous RF myelotomy, and percutaneous mechanical myelotomy.

Open limited myelotomy

A technique initially described by Nauta[10,15] and others[16–18] can be used to perform an open punctate myelotomy. Under general anesthesia, patients are placed in the prone position, and the surgical level is confirmed using fluoroscopy. With the understanding that the goal of surgery is the interruption of an ascending pain pathway, a spinal level is chosen which is rostral to the source of pain. Based on previous reports, the T3 or T4 level is chosen for upper abdominal pain, and the T6 to T8 levels are chosen for perineal pain. A single-level thoracic laminectomy is performed at the intended level of lesioning. As the procedure is performed in the thoracic spine which is stabilized by the rib cage, a wide laminectomy is performed to allow visualization of the root entry zone bilaterally. Visualization of the root entry zone bilaterally helps to confirm the midpoint of the spinal cord. A midline dural incision is made, and dural retention sutures are placed. Preservation of the midline dorsal vein is attempted in all cases by mobilization of the vein if it obscured the dorsal median sulcus. Once the midline is confirmed, the pia is coagulated with a microbipolar. A 16-gauge angiocatheter is used to create the lesion. The catheter portion of the angiocatheter assembly is cut to allow an exposed tip of 5 mm, the desired lesion depth. Four lesions are made in one location by rotating the angiocatheter 90 degrees between lesions (Fig. 9.3). The goal is to create a lesion that extends 0.5 mm from the midline bilaterally, with a lesion depth of 5 mm. Hemostasis is obtained with the use of gelfoam soaked with thrombin. The dura is closed with running sutures without the use of dural sealants, relaying on an excellent fascial closure to prevent CSF leak. The patient is mobilized on the evening of surgery.

Percutaneous radiofrequency lesioning

Our center is following Kanpolat's[9] technique for performing percutaneous RF myelotomy. This procedure can be performed either at the occiput-C1 level or in the thoracic spine. As Kanpolat has reported better experience using a larger diameter electrode for myelotomy, we have chosen a custom 26G RF electrode of diameter 0.46 mm (Cosman Medical, MA). This compares with the cordotomy electrode of 0.33 mm diameter, which has also been explored for myelotomy.

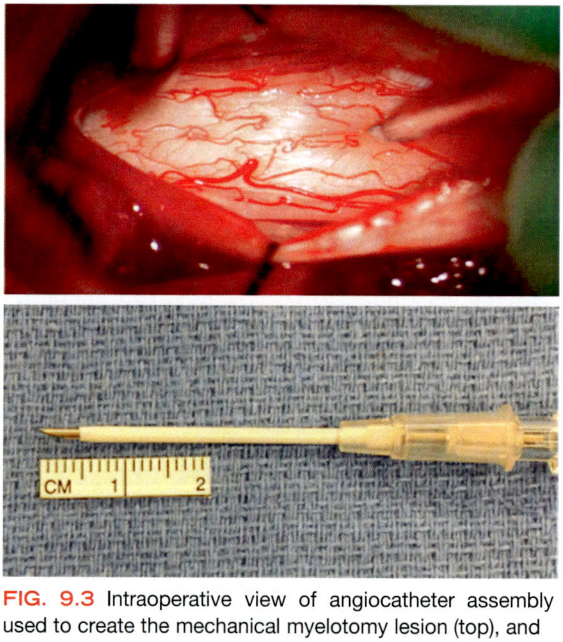

FIG. 9.3 Intraoperative view of angiocatheter assembly used to create the mechanical myelotomy lesion (top), and magnified view of the angiocatheter cut to expose a 5-mm tip (bottom).

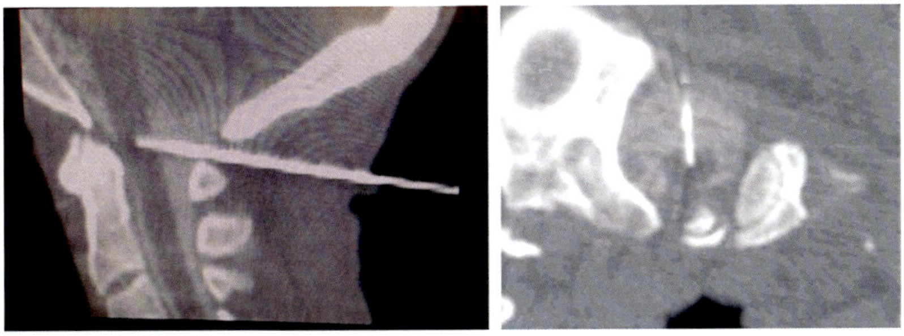

FIG. 9.4 Intraoperative view of a percutaneous radiofrequency (RF) myelotomy performed at the occiput-C1 level using a 26G RF electrode (Cosman, MA). Left: Sagittal CT scan image demonstrating the trajectory of the spinal needle and depth of RF electrode. Right: Axial CT image demonstrating the desired midline trajectory of the spinal needle and RF electrode.

A spinal myelogram is performed before the procedure to visualize the spinal cord, and the patient is positioned prone with head flexed. Intraoperative CT guidance is used to target the space between the occiput and C1 level or the relevant thoracic level. The spinal needle is advanced toward the midline of the spinal cord from a posterior approach. The RF electrode is introduced into the spinal cord parenchyma with the goal of advancing the electrode to the anteroposterior midpoint of the spinal cord (Fig. 9.4). Impedance measurements are used to confirm the presence of electrode in the spinal cord parenchyma, and sensory stimulation (100 Hz, 100 μs) is performed, which can elicit lower limb paresthesias, usually at voltages less than 0.2 V. Two RF ablations at 70–80°C for 60 s are performed.

Percutaneous mechanical lesioning

Our technique for the percutaneous mechanical myelotomy is similar to that published by Vilela Filho,[19] with the exception that we have used contrast myelography as opposed to air myelography. After performing a spinal myelogram, the patient is positioned prone, and intraoperative CT imaging is used to find the target thoracic spinal level. A 16-gauge angiocatheter assembly is inserted into the interspinous space and advanced intrathecally until cerebrospinal fluid is obtained. Care is taken to ensure the trajectory of the needle remains in the midline as best as possible. Using CT guidance, the needle is introduced into the spinal cord parenchyma. The needle is inserted into posterior midline of the spinal cord to a depth of 5 mm and confirmed on CT imaging. Only one penetration of the spinal cord is performed.

Complications

Motor complications when using image-guided percutaneous techniques are rare, given the opportunity for intraoperative motor stimulation and the relative distance of the corticospinal tract from the midline of the spinal cord. Using an open surgical technique is similarly safe, provided that care is taken to ensure the lesion is made in the midline. We have found spinal cord motor and sensory monitoring to be a valuable adjunct to open punctate myelotomy.

As the lesion in myelotomy is between the dorsal columns, transient dysfunction of the dorsal columns can occur. This may manifest as decreased proprioception, sensations of coolness, or tingling. These side effects are generally mild and well tolerated.

CONCLUSION

Spinal ablation remains a safe and effective means for treating medically refractory cancer pain. A small learning curve exists to develop comfort with these techniques, but proficiency can be developed within 5–10 cases. These techniques are safe and well tolerated by patients even in advanced stages of disease.

REFERENCES

1. Raslan AM. Percutaneous computed tomography-guided radiofrequency ablation of upper spinal cord pain pathways for cancer-related pain. *Neurosurgery*. 2008;62(3 suppl 1):226–234.
2. Kanpolat Y, Ugur HC, Ayten M, Elhan AH. Computed tomography-guided percutaneous cordotomy for intractable pain in malignancy. *Neurosurgery*. 2009;64(suppl 3):ons187–ons194.
3. Krieger AJ, Rosomoff HL. Sleep-induced apnea. Part 1: a respiratory and autonomic dysfunction syndrome following bilateral percutaneous cervical cordotomy. *J Neurosurg*. 1974;40:168–180.
4. Nannapaneni R, Behari S, Todd NV, Mendelow AD. Retracing "Ondine's curse". *Neurosurgery*. 2005;57:354–363.

5. Fonoff ET, de Oliveira YS, Lopez WO, Alho EJ, Lara NA, Teixeira MJ. Endoscopic-guided percutaneous radiofrequency cordotomy [Technical note]. *J Neurosurg.* 2010; 113:524–527.
6. Sourek K. Commissural myelotomy. *J Neurosurg.* 1969;31: 524–527.
7. Gildenberg PL, Hirshberg R. Limited myelotomy for the treatment of intractable cancer. *J Neurol Neurosurg Psychiatry.* 1984;47:94–96.
8. Hitchcock E. Stereotactic cervical myelotomy. *J Neurol Neurosurg Psychiatry.* 1970;33:224.
9. Kanpolat Y, Savas A, Caglar S, Akyar S. Computerized tomography-guided percutaneous extralemniscal myelotomy. *Neurosurg Focus.* 1997;2:e5.
10. Nauta HJW, Soukup VM, Fabian RH, et al. Punctate midline myelotomy for the relief of visceral cancer pain. *J Neurosurg.* 2000;92(suppl):125–130.
11. Armour D. Surgery of the spinal cord and its membranes. *Lancet.* 1927;i:691–697.
12. Al Chaer ED, Lawand NB, Westlund KN, Willis WD. Pelvic visceral input into the nucleus gracilis is largely mediated by the postsynaptic dorsal column pathway. *J Neurophysiol.* 1996;76:2675–2690.
13. Wang Y, Wu J, Lin Q, Nauta HJ, Yue Y, Fang L. Effects of general anesthetics on visceral pain transmission in the spinal cord. *Mol Pain.* 2008;4:50.
14. Willis WD, Al Chaer ED, Quast MJ, Westlund KN. A visceral pain pathway in the dorsal column of the spinal cord. *Proc Natl Acad Sci USA.* 1999;96:7675–7679.
15. Nauta HJW, Hewitt E, Westlund KN, Willis WD. Surgical interruption of a midline dorsal column visceral pain pathway. *J Neurosurg.* 1997;86:538–542.
16. Hong D, Andren-Sandberg A. Punctate midline myelotomy: a minimally invasive procedure for the treatment of pain in inextirpable abdominal and pelvic cancer. *J Pain Symptom Manage.* 2007;33:99–109.
17. Hwang SL, Lin CL, Lieu AS, et al. Punctate midline myelotomy for intractable visceral pain caused by hepatobiliary or pancreatic cancer. *J Pain Symptom Manage.* 2004;27: 79–84.
18. Kim YS, Joon KS. High thoracic midline dorsal column myelotomy for severe visceral pain due to advanced stomach cancer. *Neurosurgery.* 2000;46:85–92.
19. Vilela Filho O, Araujo MR, Florencio RS, Silva MAC, Silveira MT. CT-guided percutaneous punctuate midline myelotomy for the treatment of intractable visceral pain: a technical note. *Stereotact Funct Neurosurg.* 2001;77:177–182.

FURTHER READING

1. Schvarcz JR. Stereotactic extralemniscal myelotomy. *J Neurol Neurosurg Psychiatry.* 1976;39:53–57.

CHAPTER 10

Intrathecal Drug Delivery Systems for Pain: A Case-Based Approach

CHRISTOPHER MILLER, MD • MICHAEL KINSMAN, MD

Case 1: Mrs. Smith is a 65-year-old woman with a medical history of metastatic breast cancer. She has undergone bilateral mastectomy with lymph nodes biopsy 2 years before. She follows regularly with an oncologist who has been treating with chemotherapy. She recently underwent radiation for a T9 spinal metastasis. Previously the oncologist was able to control her pain with opioids, but since the radiation therapy, she has been complaining of midback pain. Increases in pain medication have been unproductive, and she is complaining that her level of pain medication is also making her too lethargic to function throughout the day. The oncologist has sent her to your clinic to evaluate for any potential surgical treatments that could reduce her systemic opioid dose. She complains of a dull achy pain over her midback without any radiation. You are told her life expectancy is over a year. Neuro examination is intact. On imaging, she has a stable lesion in the T9 vertebral body without any fracture and T10–12 rib head lesions. She is asking what her options are.

KEY QUESTIONS

1. What is the most appropriate surgical pain management modality for this patient?
2. How should the patient be screened and counseled before implantation of a device?
3. What are the key considerations when placing the pump?
4. How should the pump be managed after implantation?

PREOPERATIVE

This patient has been referred to your surgical clinic because of intractable pain related to cancer diagnosis and treatment. She notes that her opioid requirement has been increasing recently because of pain in her midback where she is known to have boney metastasis. She reports that her thinking has become increasingly cloudy and that she is too tired to perform her normal activities.

Based on these clinical findings, she is appropriate for surgical evaluation for pain control. The goal of any intervention is to reduce the systemic dose of opioid medications. In turn, she will reduce the risk of high systemic opioid doses and decrease the side effects on her mental status and energy levels. There are a number of surgical modalities available, including spinal cord stimulation (SCS), dorsal root entry zonelesion, intrathecal pain medications, and peripheral nerve stimulation.[2] Given this patient has localized, stable, nociceptive cancer-related pain, she is a good candidate for intrathecal pain pump (ITPP) placement (Fig. 10.1). The patient agrees and she is consented to surgery.

PATIENT SELECTION

Treating a patient with chronic pain requires particular attention to patient selection. The Polyanalgesic Consensus Conference (PACC) has produced in-depth best practices and guidelines for ITPPs. Appropriate patient selection begins with an understanding of how ITPPs fit within the global pain care algorithm.

There are a number of modalities for treatment of cancer pain. The PACC outlines a specific algorithm to help guide practitioners when selecting the best modality. Oral, local, or transdermal pain medication should be used as first-line therapy. If the pain is refractory, then surgical evaluation is appropriate. Refractory pain for device implantation is defined as:

> *Pain is defined as refractory, regardless of etiology, when 1) multiple evidence-based biomedical therapies used in a clinically appropriate and acceptable fashion have failed to reach treatment goals that may include adequate pain reduction and/or improvement in daily functioning or have resulted in intolerable adverse effects, and when 2) psychiatric disorders and psychosocial factors that could influence pain outcomes have been assessed and appropriately optimized.*[2]

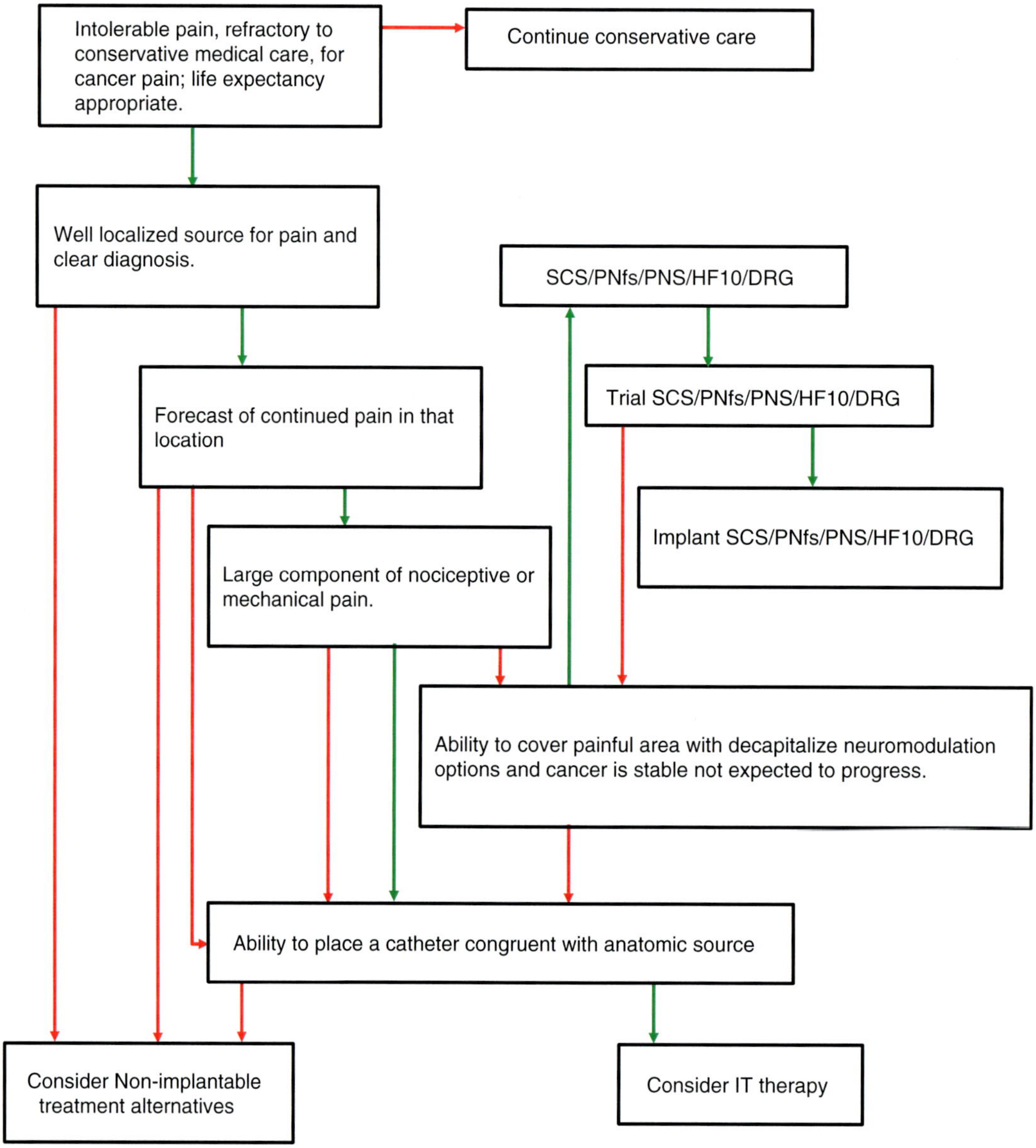

FIG. 10.1 2017 Polyanalgesic Consensus Conference Algorithm for cancer pain. *Green arrows* indicate positive; *red arrows* indicate negative response. *DRG*, dorsal root ganglion; *HF10*, high-frequency stimulation; *PNfs*, peripheral nerve field stimulation; *PNS*, peripheral nerve stimulation; *SCS*, spinal cord stimulation. (From Deer TR, Pope JE, Hayek SM, et al. The Polyanalgesic Consensus Conference (PACC): recommendations on intrathecal drug infusion systems best practices and guidelines. *Neuromodulation*. 2017; 20(2):96–132.)

Once the patient's pain is classified as refractory, there are a number of key questions that help decipher whether an implantable device is appropriate:

1. Does the pain localize to a single region?

Pain localization is described as global, diffuse, or localized. Global pain is defined as pain throughout the body. Implantable devices can be used for global pain, but the evidence is limited and practitioners should use caution and exhaust other options before considering implantation. Diffuse pain is limited to a given region such as an arm or a leg. Localized pain is specific to one area such as a dermatome, abdominal quadrant, or single vertebral level. A more specific location of pain and a clear diagnosis for why the pain is occurring increases the likelihood of success with an implantable device.

2. Is the pain expected to remain in the localized region?
   If the pain is expected to progress to other regions of the body, then an implantable device will likely have limited benefit. If the pain moves beyond the region targeted by the implant, the efficacy would be impaired and another procedure would be required to cover the new area. The patient described earlier is therefore a good candidate for surgical pain intervention: she has a localized anatomical region of pain (T9–T12), a known cause of the metastatic lesion, and stability of the lesion on serial imaging after radiation.
3. How is the pain best classified? (i.e., mechanical, nociceptive, radicular)
   At this point the type of pain should be considered to further delineate what type of device should be implanted. Cancer pain that is mechanical or nociceptive in nature should be considered for ITPP at the same level as implantation of a SCS. Radicular or neuropathic pain is likely better treated by SCS, and ITPP should be a later consideration.
4. Is the severity of the pain expected to be stable?
   Assessing the stability of the pain should be performed next. If the pain is expected to increase intensity, then an implantable device should be considered. However, intrathecal therapy becomes more attractive. One-time surgical procedures such as dorsal root ablation are not adjustable, and any loss of therapeutic value would require another procedure. Spinal cord or peripheral nerve stimulators are able to adjust through programming; however, the modality is only electrical stimulation and only frequency and intensity can be adjusted. ITPPs offer the highest level of flexibility. Programming can adjust the rate of dosing, timing of dosing, and bolus dosing all of which can be patient-controlled. Furthermore, the medication used in the pump can be changed, thus allowing flexibility in therapeutic modality. The flexibility in ITPP therapy makes the modality particularly appealing when treating cancer pain. For example, in the patient described, although the lesion is thought to be stable after radiation and stable imaging, there continues to be the possibility that the lesion will progress and the pain intensity will increase. In these situations, being able to adjust medications and dosing strategy can be particularly useful.
5. Can a catheter be placed at an appropriate spinal level?
   The final step in the algorithm is to consider if the pain is in a location such that a catheter can be placed at a spinal level congruent with the pain. This may require obtaining imaging to ensure that there are no spinal canal blocks or unusual anatomy that would prevent appropriate placement of the catheter.

OTHER SCREENING

Even if the patient appears appropriate for ITPP placement based on the PACC algorithm, there are further screening criteria that should be assessed before intervention. These extra layers of screening are to ensure that patient will tolerate the surgery and will be likely to benefit from surgical pain control.

Implantation of a pain pump requires that a patient be able to tolerate the standard risks of surgery as well as the risks of having a relatively large implant. The standard risks of surgery should be weighed including anesthesia, bleeding risk, and wound healing. Any necessary medicine, cardiology, pulmonology, or anesthesia consultations should be completed. Furthermore, in cancer patients, particular attention should be paid to their health status, including Karnofsky performance scale, current status of their underlying disease, and any treatment that could affect bleeding risk, pulmonary risk, and overall health. Particular attention should also be paid to a patient's skin quality and ability to heal. The pain pump is a foreign body that carries an increased risk for developing an infection. Furthermore, the pump is relatively large compared with many implantable devices such that skin with poor integrity or reduced ability to heal is at high risk for wound breakdown.[3,4]

Respiratory status is also an important consideration for ITPP implant. The respiratory status must be strong enough to tolerate anesthesia and the medications that will be used for intrathecal therapy. Any history of central or obstructive sleep apnea, advanced age, pulmonary disease, and cardiac disease should be investigated for risk of opioid-induced respiratory depression. This is particularly true for patients being treated in upper thoracic or cervical region. However, a practitioner should be aware of the potential advantages of using intrathecal opioids in difficult respiratory patients, as the systemic dose of opioids is likely to be reduced. There is a particular advantage when treating midthoracic or lower pain, as the drug is unlikely to travel superior enough to cause respiratory depression. Regardless, there is still the risk of overdose and respiratory depression when using intrathecal opioids and physician discretion is an important tool.[2,3,5]

Psychologic status of the patient should be well understood and used for screening patients preoperatively. Patients with severe depression and posttraumatic stress disorder are noted by the PACC to be at high risk of failure with intrathecal therapy. Positive factors such as support system, coping skills, and appropriate expectations should also be considered. The PACC additionally makes an exception for psychologic screening of terminally ill patients, as the overall goal is palliation. In these situations, psychologic counseling should still be used.[1,6]

Preoperative evaluation of patients for ITPP placement requires a solid understanding of the various methods for pain control as well as what modality would best serve a patient. The PACC has provided algorithms to assist surgeons in modality selection. Beyond modality selection, additional screening should be performed to further increase the likelihood of success for the patient. The extensive preoperative evaluation is important to select patients who will benefit from taking on the risk of surgery and avoid patient and practitioner frustrations with failure of adequate analgesia.

PREOPERATIVE PLANNING

After successfully selecting an appropriate patient for therapy and localizing the source of the pain, attention should be turned to planning. The patient should undergo an intrathecal trial of medication to ensure the desired effect can be obtained. In addition, there needs to be consideration of who will manage the pump after implantation. Appropriate conversations with the patient are needed as to what should be expected, concerning symptoms, and how to inform medical practitioners of their device. The planning phase also includes decisions on pump type, medication type, and medication dosage.

An intrathecal trial is most commonly accomplished with a single bolus dose; however, an externalized catheter could be used if a longer-term continuous trial period is desired. For a new patient who is naive to intrathecal medications, the most common and recommended monotherapy is morphine. Therefore, most trials are performed with a bolus of morphine to the targeted level. The PACC recommends 0.075–0.15 mg of morphine for a single intrathecal dose regardless of prior therapy based on the literature demonstrating this to be a well-tolerated dose. After bolus dose is administered the patient should be closely observed for at least 23 h to ensure there are no side effects. There should be particular attention paid to respiratory status. Ziconotide is another potential first-line therapy that has well-known efficacy. Trialing ziconotide can be a challenging because of the drug requiring a relatively slow titration. Bolus dosing can be used for trialing, but the patient will be more likely to experience unwanted side effects that may cloud the physician's judgment in medication selection. A patient only requires 6 h of observation after dosing. A physician could consider using an externalized catheter to better mimic the continuous dosing of ziconotide. When transitioning to continuous therapy with an implanted pump, a starting dose of 50% of the trial dose over the first 24 h is recommended.[6] When selecting a pump, there are a number of features to consider. The two most common pumps on the market are the Medtronic Synchromed II and the Prometra Flowonix pump. Medtronic Synchromed is a programmable pump that comes with a patient programmer that allows for dose adjustments and bolus dosing. The pump uses a peristaltic rotor method for delivery of medications. There is conditional labeling for up to 3T magnetic resonance imaging (MRI), but the pump needs to be interrogated after any MRI. The Prometra Flowonix pump is a propellant-powered pump that has a gated valve to control dosing. It also features programmability, a patient programmer, and 1.5 T MRI conditional labeling that similarly requires post-MRI interrogation.[7,8] The gated valve does allow for the pump to be entirely shut off, whereas the Medtronic valve has a lowest dose of 0.048 mL/day. Both pumps are battery-powered; Medtronic has a 5- to 7-year battery life, whereas Prometra has a 10-year battery life.

Before initiation of intrathecal morphine therapy, patients should be counseled on reducing their current oral dose of opioids. Multiple studies have shown that tapering of opioid dose can be performed safely and without significant changes in a patient visual analog score (VAS).[9,10] There is limited evidence that reducing the pretrial dose of opioids results in lower oral doses of opioids for analgesic efficacy after implantation of ITPP. Grider et al. reported 20 sequential patients undergoing ITPP implantation with a pretrial opioid cessation. They demonstrated reduced intrathecal dose necessary for acceptable anesthesia and acceptable anesthesia without opioid therapy during the trialing period. They argue that by tapering preoperatively the patient opioid tolerance would be reduced allowing for greater efficacy of intrathecal medications.[9] Because of the demonstrated safety and tolerability of opioid cessation before trialing, a practitioner should consider reduction or cessation in oral opioids before trialing and implantation.

As noted in the patient selection and screening section, a localized or diffuse (i.e., single limb) pain allows for the best results. The spinal cord must also be accessible such that a catheter can be placed at a level referable to the pain. The reason for these screening criteria is the cerebrospinal fluid (CSF) flow dynamics. The CSF space should not be considered a simple column of fluid. The arachnoid layers, pia layer, and spinal cord all act as barriers for the medications to reach the target receptors. Furthermore, the increased research in the CSF dynamics revealed that there is little bulk flow and mostly oscillatory flow within the spinal cord. Ultimately, the drug delivery is reliant on the kinetic energy of the drug, as it exits the catheter, and the solubility characteristics of the drug. In addition, consider that because of crossover of pain fibers at the spinal cord levels, there is some need to cover levels above and below the specific dermatomal target. Therefore, there are no specific guidelines on where a catheter should be placed in the spinal cord. The PACC accepts the general teaching of targeting the spinal level that best approximates the dermatome of the patient's pain, thus allowing the best chance for drug delivery to the target receptors at the necessary levels in the spinal cord for analgesia.[1,4]

SURGICAL PROCEDURE

The patient is positioned in the lateral decubitus position with appropriate padding and an axillary role. The skin is prepped and draped exposing the lower back for needle insertion, abdomen for the pump pocket, and lateral aspect of the abdomen for passing the catheter. The pump pocket can be created before or after the spinal catheter placement. It should be made large enough to house the pump without any hardware directly under the incision. It is generally placed in the subcutaneous fat but can be placed subfascially in patients with thin skin or little fat layer. When ready to place the catheter a 2 to 3-inch incision is made down to the fascia. Next a Tuohy needle is passed from the fascia through the interlaminar space and into the CSF space, typically at the L3-4 or L4-5 level. Higher levels can be used if necessary for high catheter placement, but caution should be taken with regard to cord injury. Once CSF is noted to be coming from the Tuohy needle, the catheter is inserted to the appropriate level. Fluoroscopy and careful counting of spinal level should be used. Anteroposterior and lateral views are used for confirmation that the catheter is dorsal to the cord. Once positioned, the catheter should be secured to the fascia. The distal catheter is then tunneled to the pump pocket. A small incision can be made on the lateral aspect of the abdomen if the anatomy does not allow for a single pass. The distal catheter is then connected to the pump. Any length of catheter that is cut or removed should be reported to the programmer, so appropriate priming and dosing can be performed postoperatively. Incisions are closed in layers making an effort to avoid hardware directly under the incision.

POSTIMPLANTATION MANAGEMENT

Postimplantation multiple members of the medical team are involved in the ongoing care of the pain pump. The PACC has recommended a number of specific roles to ensure patient care needs are met. The principal member of the team is the pump manager. This is a physician role whose key responsibilities include central oversight of pump management, diagnosis and treatment of overdose or withdrawal, understanding of intrathecal drug dose dynamics, and medication managements. The physician manager is often separate from the physician implanter of the drug delivery system. The implanter should be a pain medicine or surgery physician with adequate training to plan and execute the surgery, assess a patient's ability to tolerate implantation, and control any ongoing complications. Programmers and pump maintainers have also an important role. They are responsible for interrogating and refilling the pump at appropriate intervals. They should be supervised by the pump manager and be educated to recognize problems with the pump such as excessive residual volume, pump failure, and granuloma formation. Pump interrogators are personnel available at a hospital to assess the pump and run diagnostic programs to assess whether the pump is working correctly. Their primary role is to relay any information to the pump manager. First responders can become involved in pump management if an emergency occurs with an implanted patient. Their role is primarily recognition of the presence of an implantable device, collection of any information that can help identify the device, and contacting the appropriate pump interrogator or manager. Because of the wide range of personnel involved, a practitioner who installs or manages pain pumps should be prepared to educate the patient and the community about implanted pain pumps.

A comprehensive discussion of medications is beyond the scope of this chapter. In brief, the recommendation of the PACC is to start with FDA-approved modalities at the lowest dose capable of achieving a reasonable level of analgesia before initiating other therapies. For cancer pain, morphine or ziconotide should be trialed first as monotherapy.[1,10–15] From there, other opioids (fentanyl and hydromorphone) can be trialed as monotherapy or in combination with local anesthetics (i.e., bupivacaine) and ziconotide. Clonidine has also been used successfully as combination therapy with opioids.[16–18] Baclofen is often added if spasticity is a component of the patient's pain. All compounded medications are currently not approved by the FDA and should be used with caution. All intrathecal pain medications noted are generally found to have good neurotoxicity profiles; however, with any opioid medications, catheter tip granulomas are a possibility and the risk of formation increases with increased dose.[19–22]

TREATMENT OF NONCANCER PAIN

ITPP should also be a consideration for localized and diffuse noncancer pain such as failed back surgery syndrome. If an appropriate target can be isolated that allows for treatment with an accurately placed catheter, then ITPP treatment is similar as in cancer patients with some notable exceptions. First, in the algorithm the use of SCS is slightly preferred over ITPP, especially in cases of neuropathic pain. There is limited research in this area, and therefore clinical judgment should be used in deciding between the two therapeutic modalities. Furthermore, after processing a patient through the modality algorithm, the psychologic screening is a more important factor. A noncancer pain patient is not being treated for palliation; therefore, any psychologic factors that may affect outcomes need to be investigated and considered. This is to avoid adding risk and morbidity to a patient who does not receive adequate analgesia after implantation.[1,23]

Medication selection for noncancer pain patients is similar to cancer pain patients, but ziconotide should be trialed first in patients taking high doses of systemic opioid therapy (>120 morphine equivalents). Otherwise, the medication selection should be similar to cancer patients with initial trialing of monotherapy and addition of other medications and combinations with rapid dose increase or medication failure.[1]

CONCLUSION

ITPP represents a significant tool in the treatment of cancer and noncancer pain. The use of intrathecal therapy should not be considered as salvage therapy but instead as on par with other implantable devices such as SCS. Careful patient selection is key for successful analgesia and requires decision-making on appropriate modality as well as screening. Localized or diffuse pain is most appropriate to ITPP, and catheters should be placed as close as possible to the vertebral level congruent with the pain symptoms. An appropriate team should be assembled for the ongoing care and management of the pump. If the appropriate steps are taken, the goal of increasing patient quality of life while reducing systemic opioid medications can be achieved.

REFERENCES

1. Deer TR, Pope JE, Hayek SM, et al. The Polyanalgesic Consensus Conference (PACC): recommendations on intrathecal drug infusion systems best practices and guidelines. *Neuromodulation*. 2017;20(2):96–132.
2. Blomstedt P, Hariz GM, Hariz MI, Koskinen LO. Thalamic deep brain stimulation in the treatment of essential tremor: a long-term follow-up. *Br J Neurosurg*. 2007; 21(5):504–509.
3. Coffey RJ, Owens ML, Broste SK, et al. Medical practice perspective: identification and mitigation of risk factors for mortality associated with intrathecal opioids for noncancer pain. *Pain Med*. 2010;11(7):1001–1009.
4. Deer TR, Levy R, Prager J, et al. Polyanalgesic Consensus Conference-2012: recommendations to reduce morbidity and mortality in intrathecal drug delivery in the treatment of chronic pain. *Neuromodulation*. 2012;15(5):467–482.
5. Coffey RJ, Owens ML, Broste SK, et al. Mortality associated with implantation and management of intrathecal opioid drug infusion systems to treat noncancer pain. *Anesthesiology*. 2009;111(4):881–891.
6. Deer TR, Hayek SM, Pope JE, et al. The Polyanalgesic Consensus Conference (PACC): recommendations for trialing of intrathecal drug delivery infusion therapy. *Neuromodulation*. 2017;20(2):133–154.
7. De Andres J, Villanueva V, Palmisani S, et al. The safety of magnetic resonance imaging in patients with programmable implanted intrathecal drug delivery systems: a 3-year prospective study. *Anesth Analg*. 2011;112(5):1124–1129.
8. Diehn FE, Wood CP, Watson Jr RE, Mauck WD, Burke MM, Hunt CH. Clinical safety of magnetic resonance imaging in patients with implanted SynchroMed EL infusion pumps. *Neuroradiology*. 2011;53(2):117–122.
9. Grider JS, Harned ME, Etscheidt MA. Patient selection and outcomes using a low-dose intrathecal opioid trialing method for chronic nonmalignant pain. *Pain Physician*. 2011;14(4):343–351.
10. Hamza M, Doleys D, Wells M, et al. Prospective study of 3-year follow-up of low-dose intrathecal opioids in the management of chronic nonmalignant pain. *Pain Med*. 2012;13(10):1304–1313.
11. Pope JE, Deer TR. Ziconotide: a clinical update and pharmacologic review. *Expert Opin Pharmacother*. 2013;14(7): 957–966.

12. Schmidtko A, Loetsch J, Freynhagen R, Geisslinger G. Ziconotide for treatment of severe chronic pain. *Lancet*. 2010;375(9725):1569–1577.
13. Wallace MS, Charapata SG, Fisher R, et al. Intrathecal ziconotide in the treatment of chronic nonmalignant pain: a randomized, double-blind, placebo-controlled clinical trial. *Neuromodulation*. 2006;9(2):75–86.
14. Wallace MS, Rauck R, Fisher R, et al. Intrathecal ziconotide for severe chronic pain: safety and tolerability results of an open-label, long-term trial. *Anesth Analg*. 2008;106(2):628–637.
15. Gradert TL, Baze WB, Satterfield WC, Hildebrand KR, Johansen MJ, Hassenbusch SJ. Safety of chronic intrathecal morphine infusion in a sheep model. *Anesthesiology*. 2003;99(1):188–198.
16. Classen AM, Wimbish GH, Kupiec TC. Stability of admixture containing morphine sulfate, bupivacaine hydrochloride, and clonidine hydrochloride in an implantable infusion system. *J Pain Symptom Manag*. 2004;28(6):603–611.
17. Eisenach JC, DeKock M, Klimscha W. Alpha(2)-adrenergic agonists for regional anesthesia – a clinical review of clonidine (1984-1995). *Anesthesiology*. 1996;85(3):655–674.
18. Uhle EI, Becker R, Gatscher S, Bertalanffy H. Continuous intrathecal clonidine administration for the treatment of neuropathic pain. *Stereotact Funct Neurosurg*. 2000;75(4):167–175.
19. Abejon D, del Saz JM, Ley L, Sanchez MR, del Pozo C. Spinal granuloma in a patient receiving a spinal infusion of morphine and clonidine. *Rev Esp Anestesiol Reanim*. 2009;56(6):380–384.
20. Anderson SR, Orbegozo M, Racz G, Raj PP. Intrathecal granuloma in patients receiving high-dose intrathecal morphine therapy: a report of two cases. *Pain Pract*. 2001;1(1):61–67.
21. Bejjani GK, Karim NO, Tzortzidis F. Intrathecal granuloma after implantation of a morphine pump: case report and review of the literature. *Surg Neurol*. 1997;48(3):288–291.
22. Blount JP, Remley KB, Yue SK, Erickson DL. Intrathecal granuloma complicating chronic spinal infusion of morphine – report of three cases. *J Neurosurg*. 1996;84(2):272–276.
23. Raffaeli W, Righetti D, Caminiti A, et al. Implantable intrathecal pumps for the treatment of noncancer chronic pain in elderly population: drug dose and clinical efficacy. *Neuromodulation*. 2008;11(1):33–39.

CHAPTER 11

Dorsal Root Entry Zone Lesioning for Brachial Plexus Avulsion Pain

CHRISTOPHER C. YOUNG, MBCHB, DPhil • ANDREW L. KO, MD

INTRODUCTION

Brachial plexus avulsion (BPA) injuries occur in about 1% of polytrauma victims, predominantly in young males between 18 and 25 years of age, most commonly after motorcycle accidents (Fig. 11.1).[1] Avulsion of the preganglionic dorsal nerve roots between the dorsal root ganglion and the spinal cord results in erratic firing of second-order sensory neurons in the dorsal horn and causes both paroxysmal and continuous pain.[2] Both components may present immediately after trauma or months to years later and respond poorly to conventional treatments, including analgesics, antidepressants, and anticonvulsants. Neuromodulation via deep brain stimulation (DBS) and spinal cord stimulators has had statistically significant but unsatisfactory pain reduction, whereas ablative procedures such as medial thalamotomy, spinothalamic tractotomy, and anterolateral cordotomy have not demonstrated long-term benefits and are associated with disabling side effects.[3]

Microsurgical dorsal root entry zone (DREZ) lesioning, or DREZotomy, is a surgical procedure that has been used with success for the treatment of pain syndromes, spasticity, hyperactive bladder, and, in particular, chronic pain after BPA. The procedure consists of a microsurgical incision and bipolar coagulation of the lateral part of DREZ, the medial part of the tract of Lissauer, and extends to the apex of the dorsal horn.[4] First performed by Sindou and colleagues in the 1970s, the purpose of DREZotomy is the selective destruction of nociceptive fibers grouped in the lateral bundle of the dorsal root, the excitatory fibers of medial tract of Lissauer, and the deafferented hyperactive neurons of the dorsal Rexed laminae (Fig. 11.3).[2]

Based on improved understanding of neuroanatomic pathways and neurophysiologic conduction of pain in the 1950s and 1960s, there was great interest in anatomic lesioning for the treatment of pain.[5] The gate control theory published in 1965 highlighted the possibility that the DREZ may be a suitable target for surgical lesioning for the treatment of chronic pain syndromes.[6] The theory debunked the notion that pain is a simple transmission of nociceptive signals from peripheral receptors and the conduction of "pain" through the nervous system sensory apparatus. Instead, it hypothesized that pain is a patterned response that correlated to magnitude and pattern of sensory/nociceptive receptor stimulation.

Peripheral stimulation evokes nerve impulses that are transmitted to the dorsal horn of the spinal cord and synapse with second-order sensory neurons of the ascending sensory pathway. The peripheral impulses are "gated" by a group of densely packed neurons known as the substantia gelatinosa (SG). SG has an inhibitory effect on the second-order afferents, and depending on the quality and magnitude of the peripheral nerve impulses, the SG regulates second-order afferent transmission via both positive and negative feedback loops and thus determines the nature of excitatory signal that is transmitted in the nociceptive spinothalamic pathway. In pathologic pain states, such as denervation hypersensitivity, the normal balance of peripheral nerve impulses arriving at the dorsal horn, i.e., SG, is disrupted and results in hyperactive firing of the deafferented second-order neurons.[7] The DREZ is recognized as a complex network of neuronal connections, and disruption of this delicately balanced environment leads to abhorrent pain augmentation and transmission. DREZotomy thus involves the surgical destruction of erratically firing SG and second-order afferents to prevent the transmission of pain, analogous to the surgical resection of an epileptic cortical tissue to abolish seizure activity.[3,8]

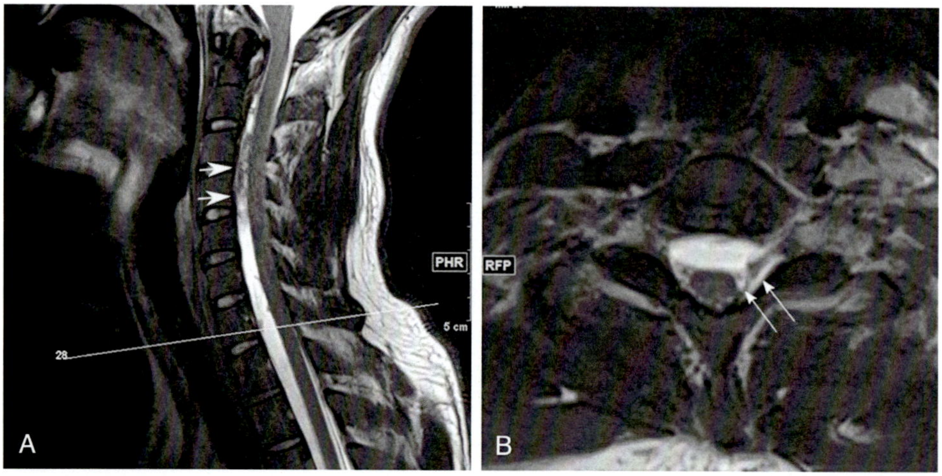

FIG. 11.1 T2-weighted magnetic resonance imaging (MRI) of the cervical spine in a patient involved in a high-speed motor vehicle collision. The patient sustained brachial plexus avulsion on the left with weakness in the C5-T1 myotomes. **(A)** The sagittal MRI shows evidence of ventral subdural blood product (*large arrowheads*). Additionally, there is elevation of the posterior longitudinal ligament along the posterior aspect of the dens. **(B)** The axial image shows displaced spinal cord with a ventral fluid collection concerning for a pseudomeningocele. The left aspect of the spinal cord at C7 is blunted with T2 signal abnormalities and the irregular nerve roots suggestive of nerve root avulsion (*small arrowheads*).

ANATOMY

The DREZ is situated lateral to the midline in the dorsal spinal cord where cervical dorsal roots insert into the dorsal intermediolateral sulcus (Fig. 11.2). The normal DREZ is easily identified at the respective cervical level by the 6−11 rootlets that insert into the sulcus and can be found 2.2−3.5 mm lateral of the posterior median sulcus.[9]

The DREZ consists of three parts, including (1) the central grouping of dorsal rootlets, which enter the dorsal horn proximal to the pial ring within 1 mm of the dorsal intermediolateral sulcus, (2) the medial part of the tract of Lissauer, and (3) the Rexed laminae I-V of the dorsal horn, which include nucleus proprius and the SG where the afferent fibers synapse with second-order spinothalamic and spinoreticular afferents with input from the SG (Fig. 11.3).

Microsurgically, DREZotomy targets the lateral grouping of central dorsal rootlets (small-diameter nociceptive fibers), the excitatory medial tract of Lissauer, as well as the nucleus proprius, the SG, and dorsal Rexed laminae, which contain deafferented hyperactive neurons.

PREOPERATIVE EVALUATION

Before surgical intervention, patients must be thoroughly evaluated with regards to symptoms, etiology, treatments attempted thus far and response, and appropriate diagnostic studies to ascertain whether the patients are suitable candidates for the procedure with a reasonable likelihood of deriving significant benefit from it. In the case of BPA injury, a careful history will reveal the mechanism of injury and the level of injury,

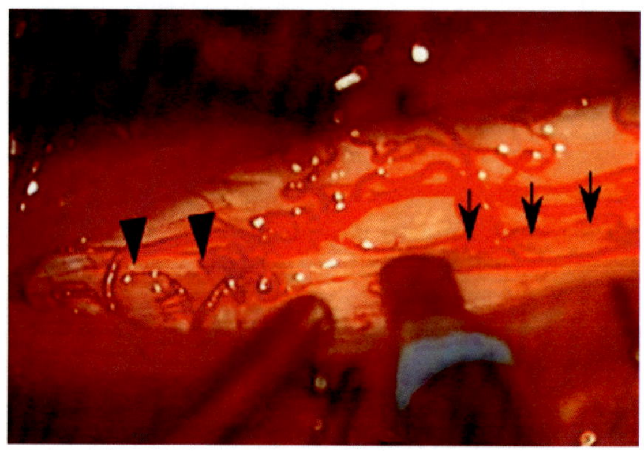

FIG. 11.2 Intraoperative photograph during DREZotomy. Note the normal nerve roots (*triangles*), which should be visualized above and below levels to be lesioned. This can be useful in locating the DREZ when anatomy is distorted by scarring. Also, note the pitting and scarring within the dorsal intermediolateral sulcus (*arrows*). An incision is being made at 45 degrees angle into the pia arachnoid of the spinal cord; this is continued in a staccato fashion along the length of the sulcus. Microbipolar cautery is used to complete the lesion through these openings in the pia arachnoid.

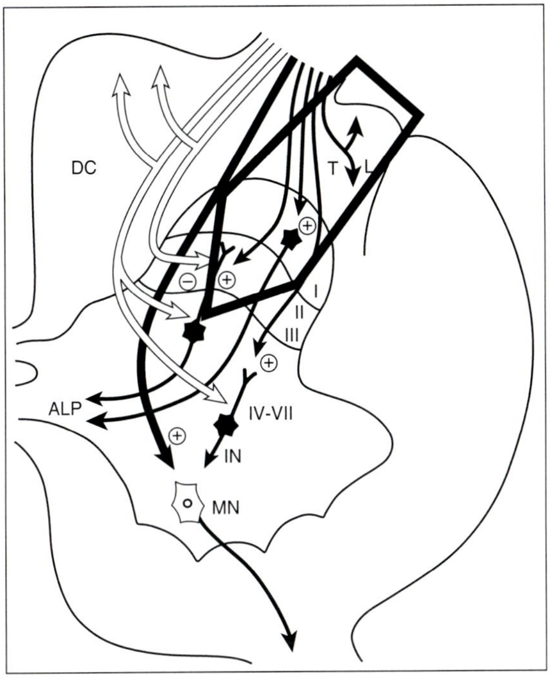

FIG. 11.3 Cross-sectional view of the cervical spinal cord showing the DREZ and microsurgical anatomy of DREZotomy. The DREZ consists of three parts, including (1) the central grouping of dorsal rootlets, which enter the dorsal horn proximal to the pial ring within 1 mm of the intermediolateral sulcus, (2) the medial part of the tract of Lissauer, and (3) the Rexed laminae I-V of the dorsal horn, which include nucleus proprius and the SG where the afferent fibers synapse with second-order spinothalamic and spinoreticular afferents with input from the SG. (Adopted from Sindou M. Microsurgical DREZotomy (MDT) for pain, spasticity, and hyperactive bladder: a 20-year experience. *Acta Neurochir (Wien)*. 1995; 137(1–2):1–5; with permission.)

which can be confirmed on physical examination by focal neurological findings at the affected dermatome and myotome levels. Electrodiagnostic studies, such as nerve conductions, somatosensory-evoked potentials (SSEP), motor-evoked potentials (MEP) and electromyography, provide functional confirmation of injury. In BPA, somatosensory-evoked potential is obtained at the Erb's point with absent cervical and cortical responses. Preganglionic BPA can be differentiated from postganglionic injuries by evaluating sensory nerve action potentials, which are disrupted by postganglionic lesions and preserved in BPA.[10] Magnetic resonance imaging (MRI) of the brachial plexus and spine may provide additional information regarding localization of the injury, although up to 50% of patients with partial or complete root avulsion may have no observable meningeal alterations on MRI.[4] However, we have shown recently that normal DREZ morphology on MRI may in fact be a positive predictive factor of a favorable response to DREZotomy in BPA pain.[3] Furthermore, anatomical avulsion and sensory deficits do not always clinically correlate. In Sindou's series, dorsal root avulsion seen at surgery and sensory deficits correlates only in 52% of patients. In 30% of patients, a larger sensory deficit is observed, whereas 14% of patients have a smaller deficit, and in 4%, the deficit is at an adjacent level. Nevertheless, there appears to be good correlation between the preganglionic root avulsion and pain territory and can be adequately treated by DREZotomy.[11] Preganglionic root avulsion is much more likely to be associated with chronic pain compared with postganglionic root avulsion (82 vs. 33%), and the percentage of patients with chronic pain increases with the number of avulsed roots (71%, 82%, 85%, and 90% for two, three, four, and five avulsed roots, respectively) and approaching 100% for patients with total avulsion of all five levels.[12]

SURGICAL TECHNIQUE

After endotracheal intubation, the patient is placed under general anesthesia. If using neurophysiological monitoring, total intravenous anesthesia is employed. Prophylactic antibiotics are administered. The patient is positioned prone on gel rolls, and a Mayfield head clamp is applied. For unilateral pathology, a midline incision is made, and a unilateral subperiosteal paraspinal muscle elevation is performed. Intraoperative fluoroscopy is used to confirm the correct spinal levels. Owing to the additional C8 cervical root and the topographic arrangement of the spinal segment in relation to the cervical vertebrae, the cervical spinal segment usually corresponds to the cervical lamina one level above; in other words, the C5-T1 nerve roots are found below the C4-C7 laminae. Hemilaminectomies are performed for operative exposure and are preferred for unilateral pathology as this technique allows the preservation of the spinous process and midline tension bands. Care is taken to avoid disruption of facet joint capsules to minimize mechanical sequelae from the procedure. Adequate exposure to allow visualization of the DREZ above and below the intended surgical target is essential as the normal anatomy at these levels often provide important reference for the localization of DREZ at the pathologic level which can be disrupted by scarring. The thecal sac is exposed by careful dissection of soft tissue. The operative microscope is brought in for durotomy and the remainder of the procedure.

Under the operative microscope, durotomy is performed and the dural leaflets are retracted with holding sutures. Arachnoid adhesions, if present, may need to be freed. Microsurgical release of arachnoid tethering is important for correct anatomical localization of DREZ, and furthermore, it is postulated that arachnoid adhesions may cause meningeal irritation and contribute to pain symptoms. Pseudomeningoceles of the radicular dural sleeve are often encountered and can further distort the underlying spinal cord anatomy. The DREZ is carefully identified and inspected with reference to adjacent normal levels. In BPA, the affected DREZ may have pits, which mark the location of avulsed roots, or have a gray atrophic appearance. The dorsal intermediolateral sulcus is a critical anatomical landmark, which often contains a small radicular vessel within the sulcus. DREZotomies are made with staccato lesions using a sharp incision with a Beaver knife inserted ventromedially at 45 degrees angle into the intermediolateral sulcus to a depth of 2–3 mm (Figs. 11.2 and 11.4). This is followed by microbipolar cautery and targets the lateral dorsal rootlets, the medial portion of Lissauer's tract, the nucleus proprius, and the SG in the dorsal horn. The lesions should span the intermediolateral sulcus from the normal rootlets above to those below the targeted level.

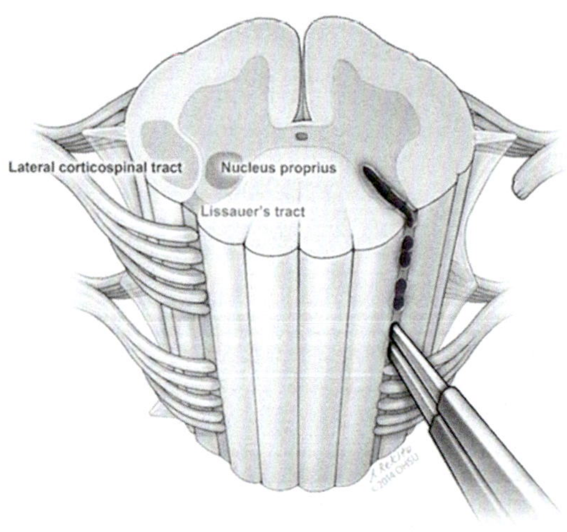

FIG. 11.4 Schematic depiction of DREZotomy viewed from the dorsal spinal cord. Note the intermediolateral sulcus with avulsed cervical rootlets. Staccato lesions are created in the DREZ using microbipolar cautery. The target for lesion creation is the medal portion of Lissauer's tract and the nucleus proprius to a depth of 2–3 mm. Entry into the cord at 45 degrees angle prevents damage to the adjacent lateral corticospinal tract.[3]

Surgeons have used variations of the above technique, with different types of microsurgical techniques, incorporating other modalities such as radiofrequency thermocoagulation,[13] carbon dioxide laser,[14] or ultrasound.[15] Although direct comparisons of techniques have not been made, reported efficacy rates are similar without obvious advantages or disadvantages of one technique over the others.

After the DREZotomy, the dura is closed primarily to prevent cerebrospinal fluid (CSF) egress, and the soft tissues are closed in standard fashion in layers. The presence of pseudomeningoceles at avulsed levels is important, as these can be the source of occult CSF leak; if found, care should be taken to primarily close any openings in the dura that are seen.

Neurophysiologic monitoring with SSEP and MEPs is a useful adjunct in confirming spinal levels and providing an additional level of accuracy and safety. Intrafield stimulation can be used for the stimulation of ventral roots, if present, to confirm operative levels, as well as location of the midline if there is uncertainty regarding orientation of the spinal cord in the operative field.

POTENTIAL COMPLICATIONS

As an invasive neurosurgical procedure, DREZotomy for BPA is for the most part a well-tolerated procedure. There are general surgical risks and potential complications associated with cervical spine surgery such as infection, CSF leakage, formation of pseudomeningoceles, and neural damage. Because of the traumatic etiology of BPA, the underlying anatomy may be abnormal and the presence of scar tissue may increase the risk of CSF leak and pseudomeningocele formation. Given the manipulation and lesioning of the cervical spinal cord, there is also the risk of permanent neurological damage, which includes motor weakness and sensory loss depending on the location of injury. For example, a lateral incision can damage the corticospinal tract with resultant ipsilateral hemiparesis. Similarly, the spinocerebellar tract may result in dysfunction of motor coordination. Damage to the posterior column in a lesion that is too medial can result in difficulties with balance and proprioception. A lesion that is too deep may sever sacral fibers and result in urinary dysfunction.

In published series, motor weakness and sensory abnormalities are the most common complications. In Nashold's and Ostdahl's original series, 11 of the 21 patients (52%) had varying degree of persistent motor weakness, whereas 15 of the 21 patients experienced sensory changes after the procedure.[8] More recent series reports significant lower rates of complication, and in one series 2 out of the 19 (11%) patients reported mild weakness at an average follow-up of 5 years.[16] In a large single-center series followed for a mean of 6 years, neurologic complications were low, with 3 out of the 55 patients (5.4%) experiencing permanent disabling neurologic deficits, with 2 patients reporting disabling ipsilateral lower extremity weakness and a third patient with permanent genitourinary disturbances.[4]

OUTCOMES

Efficacy and Durability of DREZotomy for BPA Pain

Several single-center series have been published reporting outcomes after DREZotomy for BPA. Overall, DREZotomy provides significant and lasting alleviation of pain after BPA in approximately two-thirds of patients, and this has been replicated in a number of case series at centers around the world (Table 11.1).

The single most important outcome measure in a treatment for pain is naturally the successful resolution of pain. However, successful treatment of pain or the definition of a "good" outcome is not always clear. A reasonable and commonly used definition is 50% improvement in pain with or without additional analgesics as measured on the visual analog scale. Using this criterion and analyzing published case series consisting of at least 10 patients followed for a minimum of 5 years, the reported rate of treatment success ranges from 54% to 90% (Table 11.1). In Sindou's series consisting of 44 patients with a mean follow-up of 6 years, 65.9% of the patients experienced pain improvement by at least 50% with 71% reporting good quality of life.[4] In our own experience, we reported a long-term success rate of 66% using the above criteria, which is commensurate with published results.[3]

Pain relief after DREZotomy for BPA appears to be lasting. The early series by Nashold and Ostadahl in the United States with a mean follow-up of 1.8 years reported very good or fair outcome in 55.6% and 16.7% of patients, respectively.[8] When the follow-up times were extended and the results were reviewed a decade later in 1988, the rate of pain relief remained comparable with good outcome in 54% and fair outcome in 13% of patients.[17] Sindou demonstrated excellent early outcome after the procedure with 94.6% of patients not requiring additional analgesic medication at the time of discharge from hospital after DREZotomy. This number dropped to 81.8% at 3 months follow-up, and at final follow-up at a mean of 6 years, 65.9% of patients experienced excellent or good outcome, with or without additional analgesics.[4] Similarly, in a German series of 39 patients followed for a mean of 14 years, good pain reduction was achieved in 86% of the patients immediately postoperatively, 68% at 3 months, and 63% at 6 months, which remained stable at long-term follow-up, with an average pain reduction of 63% (SD 34%).[18] In another series of 40 patients followed up for 10 years in Taiwan, rate of excellent or good pain control decreased from 80% early in the postoperative period to 60% at 5 year follow-up and 50% at 10 years.[19]

Prognostic Factors

Several prognostic factors for successful pain relief after DREZotomy have been described, including the duration of pain, the characteristics of pain, and the presence of anatomic and imaging evidence of structural spinal cord abnormality (Table 11.2).

A lengthier preoperative duration of pain has been correlated with better long-term results from DREZotomy. Interestingly, in one study, better results and sustained pain alleviation were obtained in patients with deafferentiation pain of more than 5 years at long-term follow-up, even though there was no difference noted postoperatively and at short-term (1 year) follow-up.[20] In our own experience, the duration of pain before DREZotomy was significantly correlated with a better outcome, and all the patients in our study who had a poor pain outcome underwent DREZotomy within 36 months of the onset of deafferentiation pain.[3] The duration of preoperative pain remained significant even after multivariable analysis with linear regression modeling. On the other hand, several other series did not find the duration of pain to be a significant prognostic factor.[4,18]

Clinical observations have suggested that different components of BPA pain may respond differently to DREZotomy and that it may have a more pronounced effect on paroxysmal pain. In a prospective case series, relief from paroxysmal pain is more likely than relief from constant pain after DREZotomy.[21] There was a 11.5% statistically significant improved pain outcome in patients treated with paroxysmal pain compared with those treated with chronic pain. Similar favorable outcome for paroxysmal pain has been obtained for other destructive procedures treating pain of a spinal cord origin.[22]

Anatomic alterations to the spinal cord are common after BPA. Marked rotation or lateral deviation of the spinal cord was observed in a third to a half of patients, with associated gliosis and arachnoid adhesions.

TABLE 11.1
Review of Reported Case Series After DREZotomy

Author	Country	Surgical Technique	Number of Patients	Collected Years	Mean Follow-up Years (Range)	PAIN RELIEF OUTCOME % OF PATIENTS				COMPLICATIONS % OF PATIENTS	
						Excellent	Good	Fair	Poor	Motor	Sensory
Friedman et al. (1988)	USA	RF-Th	39	NA	5 (1–10)	54		13	33	40	40
Thomas and Kitchen (1994)	UK	RF-Th	44	10	5 (1–12)	68		11	21	22	18
Rath et al. (1996)	Germany	RF-Th	14	16	6 (3–12)	57		14	29	43	NA
Samii et al. (2001)	Germany	RF-Th	39	18	14 (2–18)	63		31	17	17	NA
Sindou et al. (2005)	France	MS	44	15	6 (1–27)	34	32	34		1.8	3.6
Prestor (2006)	Slovenia	MS	17	15	5	47	29	24		4	11
Aichaoui et al. (2011)	France	MS	26	10	5 (1–10)	77		23		3	7
Awad et al. (2013)	USA	RF-Th	13	25	5	37	32	16	16	NA	NA
Haninec et al. (2014)	Croatia	RF-Th	48	17	7 (2–14)	71	21	8		NA	NA
Ko et al. (2016)	USA	MS	27	18	8 (1–18)	66		34		0	0

These include series which contain at least 10 patients followed for more than 5 years. Pain reduction outcomes: *Excellent* = 75%–100% pain reduction, *Good* = 50%–75%, *Fair* = <50%, *Poor* = minimal effect. *MS*, microsurgery; *NA*, not available; *RF-Th*, radiofrequency thermocoagulation.

TABLE 11.2
Prognostic Factors of Favorable Response to DREZotomy

Longer duration of pain before surgery
Paroxysmal pain
Absence of spinal cord abnormality on MRI

Pseudomeningoceles are present in half of avulsed roots and are almost pathognomonic of BPA. Microscopically, focal gliosis and microcysts can be observed within the DREZ and dorsal horn in a third of cases, although the functional significance of these findings in relation to pain generation and response to DREZotomy is not well understood.

MRI may have value in predicting immediate and long-term outcome after DREZotomy. Pain alleviation significantly and negatively correlated with the degree of abnormality seen on imaging of the spinal cord. An increase in the number of abnormalities (either intrinsic cord signal or DREZ avulsion) was correlated with a poorer outcome score. In a series of 27 patients followed for a mean of 8 years, all patients with MRI showing a normal spinal cord, without intrinsic signal abnormality or damage to the DREZ, had excellent or pain-free outcomes. In contrast, only 2 of the 12 patients with cord abnormalities on MRI had excellent relief from pain, and none were completely pain-free. One hypothesis to explain this phenomenon may be that if the success of DREZotomy is predicated based on the successful ablation of abnormally hyperactive interneurons within the DREZ, the extent of injury to the spinal cord may impact the success rate of this procedure. In other words, if the DREZ is injured to the point that the secondary nociceptive pathways are already inactive, then the procedure may be less successful. This may be because the pain is not the result of aberrant signaling within the spinal cord but the result of a more central process.

Other Treatment Modalities

Spinal cord and DBS have been shown to provide pain relief after BPA. In Europe, DBS is approved for the treatment of neuropathic pain, and in a series of seven patients who underwent thalamic DBS for BPA pain, there was 52% reduction in pain at 1 year as measured by the visual analog scale.[23] Spinal cord stimulators have also gained popularity because of the nonlesional and reversible nature of the procedure; however, its efficacy is thought to be lower when compared with DREZ.[24] In a small series of 10 patients, different techniques for treating BPA pain were compared. Dorsal column stimulation and thalamic DBS were largely ineffective in comparison with DREZotomy.[25] Other surgical ablative procedures such as medial thalamotomy, spinothalamic tractotomy, and anterolateral cordotomy have not demonstrated long-term benefits and have disabling side effects. Furthermore, within the existing literature that examines the efficacy of BPA treatment, there are no documented control groups when comparing outcomes. This is particularly relevant, given that the natural history of BPA pain is largely undetermined. One long-term study of patients with BPA who did not undergo surgical treatment reports that after 4 years, 25% of patients continued to have severe pain that was considered unacceptable and after 11 years this number dropped to 17%.[11] However, within this cohort of patients, only 6% had spontaneous and complete remission of pain. It seems that the natural history of BPA pain is unremitting pain, but this becomes tolerable in a majority of patients; whether the rate of acceptable pain levels after surgical intervention is better than the rate of 75% after 4 years achieved by conservative observation is an open question.

CONCLUSION

DREZotomy is a safe, effective, and durable treatment for pain resulting from BPA. Over the past 40 years, centers around the world have reported successful treatment of pain in two-thirds of patients undergoing the procedure. With refinement of microsurgical techniques and the availability of intraoperative neuromonitoring, success rates have improved and disabling complications are rare. Functional modalities such as spinal cord stimulation and thalamic DBS yield promise, and the nonlesional nature of these modalities are favored by many, although current results are inferior in comparison with DREZotomy.

REFERENCES

1. Midha R. Epidemiology of brachial plexus injuries in a multitrauma population. *Neurosurgery*. 1997;40(6): 1182–1188; discussion 1188–1189.
2. Sindou M. Microsurgical DREZotomy (MDT) for pain, spasticity, and hyperactive bladder: a 20-year experience. *Acta Neurochir (Wien)*. 1995;137(1–2):1–5.
3. Ko AL, Ozpinar A, Raskin JS, Magill ST, Raslan AM, Burchiel KJ. Correlation of preoperative MRI with the long-term outcomes of dorsal root entry zone lesioning for brachial plexus avulsion pain. *J Neurosurg*. 2016; 124(5):1470–1478.

4. Sindou MP, Blondet E, Emery E, Mertens P. Microsurgical lesioning in the dorsal root entry zone for pain due to brachial plexus avulsion: a prospective series of 55 patients. *J Neurosurg.* 2005;102(6):1018–1028.
5. Maccarty CS, Drake RL. Neurosurgical procedures for the control of pain. *Proc Staff Meet Mayo Clin.* 1956;31(7): 208–214.
6. Melzack R, Wall PD. Pain mechanisms: a new theory. *Science.* 1965;150(3699):971–979.
7. Loeser JD, Ward AA, White LE. Chronic deafferentation of human spinal cord neurons. *J Neurosurg.* 1968;29(1):48–50.
8. Nashold Jr BS, Ostdahl RH. Dorsal root entry zone lesions for pain relief. *J Neurosurg.* 1979;51(1):59–69.
9. Xiang J-P, Liu X-L, Xu Y-B, Wang J-Y, Hu J. Microsurgical anatomy of dorsal root entry zone of brachial plexus. *Microsurgery.* 2008;28(1):17–20.
10. Mansukhani KA. Electrodiagnosis in traumatic brachial plexus injury. *Ann Indian Acad Neurol.* 2013;16(1):19–25.
11. Parry CB. Pain in avulsion lesions of the brachial plexus. *Pain.* 1980;9(1):41–53.
12. Narakas A. Surgical treatment of traction injuries of the brachial plexus. *Clin Orthop Relat Res.* 1978;(133):71–90.
13. Rawlings 3rd CE, el-Naggar AO, Nashold Jr BS. The DREZ procedure: an update on technique. *Br J Neurosurg.* 1989; 3(6):633–642.
14. Young RF. Clinical experience with radiofrequency and laser DREZ lesions. *J Neurosurg.* 1990;72(5):715–720.
15. Dreval ON. Ultrasonic DREZ-operations for treatment of pain due to brachial plexus avulsion. *Acta Neurochir (Wien).* 1993;122(1–2):76–81.
16. Awad AJ, Forbes JA, Jermakowicz W, Eli IM, Blumenkopf B, Konrad P. Experience with 25 years of dorsal root entry zone lesioning at a single institution. *Surg Neurol Int.* 2013;4:64.
17. Friedman AH, Nashold BS, Bronec PR. Dorsal root entry zone lesions for the treatment of brachial plexus avulsion injuries: a follow-up study. *Neurosurgery.* 1988;22(2): 369–373.
18. Samii M, Bear-Henney S, Lüdemann W, Tatagiba M, Blömer U. Treatment of refractory pain after brachial plexus avulsion with dorsal root entry zone lesions. *Neurosurgery.* 2001;48(6):1269–1275; discussion 1275–1277.
19. Chen HJ, Tu YK. Long term follow-up results of dorsal root entry zone lesions for intractable pain after brachial plexus avulsion injuries. *Acta Neurochir Suppl.* 2006;99:73–75.
20. Prestor B. Microcoagulation of junctional dorsal root entry zone is effective treatment of brachial plexus avulsion pain: long-term follow-up study. *Croat Med J.* 2006; 47(2):271–278.
21. Aichaoui F, Mertens P, Sindou M. Dorsal root entry zone lesioning for pain after brachial plexus avulsion: results with special emphasis on differential effects on the paroxysmal versus the continuous components. A prospective study in a 29-patient consecutive series. *Pain.* 2011; 152(8):1923–1930.
22. Tasker RR, DeCarvalho GT, Dolan EJ. Intractable pain of spinal cord origin: clinical features and implications for surgery. *J Neurosurg.* 1992;77(3):373–378.
23. Pereira EAC, Boccard SG, Linhares P, et al. Thalamic deep brain stimulation for neuropathic pain after amputation or brachial plexus avulsion. *Neurosurg Focus.* 2013;35(3): E7.
24. Brill S, Aryeh IG. Neuromodulation in the management of pain from brachial plexus injury. *Pain Physician.* 2008; 11(1):81–85.
25. Teixeira MJ, De Souza EC, Yeng LT, Pereira WC. Lesion of the Lissauer tract and of the posterior horn of the gray substance of the spinal cord and the electrical stimulation of the central nervous system for the treatment of brachial plexus avulsion pain. *Arq Neuropsiquiatr.* 1999;57(1): 56–62.
26. Thomas DG, Kitchen ND. Long-term follow up of dorsal root entry zone lesions in brachial plexus avulsion. *J Neurol Neurosurg Psychiatr.* 1994;57(6):737–738.
27. Rath SA, Seitz K, Soliman N, Kahamba JF, Antoniadis G, Richter HP. DREZ coagulations for deafferentation pain related to spinal and peripheral nerve lesions: indication and results of 79 consecutive procedures. *Stereotact Funct Neurosurg.* 1997;68(1–4 Pt 1):161–167.
28. Haninec P, Kaiser R, Mencl L, Waldauf P. Usefulness of screening tools in the evaluation of long-term effectiveness of DREZ lesioning in the treatment of neuropathic pain after brachial plexus injury. *BMC Neurol.* 2014;14: 225.

CHAPTER 12

Trigeminal Tractotomy-Nucleotomy

ABIGAIL RAO, MD • AHMED M. RASLAN, MD, FAANS

INTRODUCTION

Central nervous system ablation for pain is an old and deeply rooted principle.[1,2] It had been a common practice by neurosurgeons for many years before the introduction of opioids in their various formulations (oral, IV, and intrathecal). There has been a general departure of practitioners from ablation, with few exceptions; trigeminal tractotomy would be one of those exceptions.[3]

Trigeminal tractotomy-nucleotomy (TR-NC) is one ablative procedure used for control of facial pain. As with other spinal ablation procedures such as cordotomy and midline myelotomy, the underlying principle is creation of a discrete lesion in a compact bundle of fibers or nucleus of cell bodies that transmits or processes pain from a defined area of the body. The target of TR-NC is the lateral descending trigeminal tract and nucleus caudalis of the spinal trigeminal nucleus, located in the posterolateral aspect of the cervicomedullary junction and accessed between the occiput and C1. The primary diagnoses that are good candidates for this procedure are types of trigeminal neuropathic pain, craniofacial cancer pain (including glossopharyngeal or geniculate neuralgia), postherpetic neuralgia, and poststroke pain. Here we will outline the background, indications, procedural details, and our studied outcomes from TR-NC.

RELEVANT ANATOMY

The trigeminal or Gasserian ganglion, located in Meckel's cave of the petrous temporal bone, contains pseudounipolar neurons. These neurons extend distal projections to the face, from nearly the vertex of the head to above the angle of the jaw and posteriorly to just into the auricle. There are three central nuclei that the central processes segregate to: the mesencephalic nucleus, where proprioceptive fibers synapse; the chief sensory nucleus in the pons, where light touch, pressure, and vibration are conveyed; and the spinal nucleus, which carries pain and temperature fibers. From the spinal nucleus, the pain and temperature fibers decussate in the brainstem and travel in the ventral trigeminothalamic tract to VPM of the thalamus.[4]

In the medulla, the descending trigeminal tract is dorsal to the spinal trigeminal nucleus at the level of the craniocervical junction. Sensory inputs from the head carried by cranial nerves V, VII, IX, and X also travel in the descending trigeminal tract and join the spinal nucleus. Within the descending trigeminal tract, there is topographic organization of the three trigeminal divisions. The spinal trigeminal nucleus extends from the pons down to C2 and has three subdivisions: (1) the nucleus oralis between the pons and medulla, (2) the nucleus interpolaris, and (3) the nucleus caudalis. The nucleus caudalis extends from the medullospinal junction down to C2 and has similar cytoarchitecture and neurochemistry to the substantia gelatinosa of the spinal cord, highlighting it as a pain and temperature processing area. Lesioning of the entire nucleus caudalis at the dorsal root entry zone (DREZ) represents a more extensive version of the trigeminal nucleotomy and is performed via open approach after suboccipital craniectomy and C1 hemilaminectomy.[5] Here, however, we focus on percutaneous TR-NC, a sort of "mini caudalis DREZ."

From a technical perspective, the location of the trigeminal tract shifts lateral from caudal to rostral, as such the trigeminal tract at C1 is more medial to its location at craniocervical junction (Fig. 12.1).

HISTORY AND BACKGROUND

The compact nature of the sensory information contained in the trigeminal tract made it an ideal target for surgical intervention. Lesioning of the trigeminal tract was first reported by Sjoqvist in 1938, after a transverse stab incision in the dorsal medulla at the level of the inferior olive led to interruption of the trigeminal tract.[1] Falconer then modified the technique to treat V1-V2 trigeminal neuralgia.[6] In the late 1960s, Crue et al. and Hitchcock independently developed a stereotactic radiofrequency electrode for lesioning of the

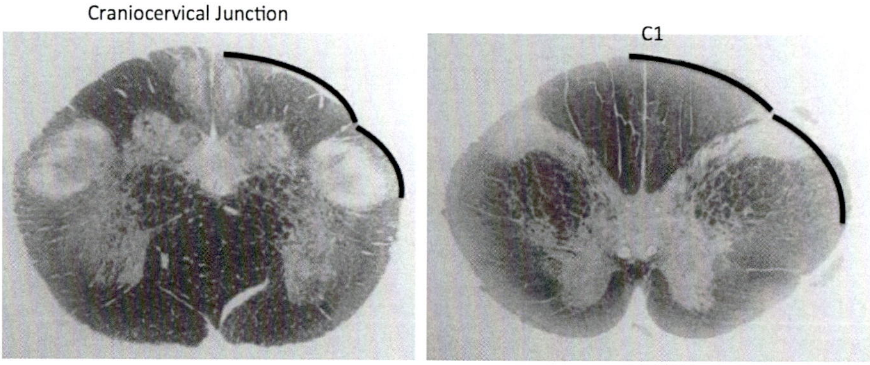

FIG. 12.1 The location of the trigeminal tract at both craniocervical junction and below C1. The trigeminal tract is more lateral caudally.

trigeminal tract.[7–9] Fox in 1971[9] reported a series of percutaneous trigeminal tractotomy. About a decade after Hitchcock's report, Schvarcz used the same procedure for lesioning the nucleus caudalis at the craniocervical junction and named this trigeminal nucleotomy.[10] In the late 1980s, Nashold described open craniotomy for multiple lesion creation with radiofrequency between the dorsal root of C2 and obex, termed caudalis DREZ.[5] In 1989, Dr. Kanpolat developed and reported CT-guided percutaneous trigeminal tractotomy. Since that time, he has been the most prolific surgeon performing this surgery, and it is his basic technique that has shaped current iterations of the procedure.

INDICATIONS

Trigeminal tractotomy is an effective operation in conditions where peripheral ablation would not be effective or could exacerbate the condition. Moreover, it is effective when the pain is due to involvement of multiple cranial nerves such as cancer pain of the tongue or the face. Bilateral trigeminal V3 pain that is not a candidate for MVD (microvascular decompression) would be a good candidate for TR-NC, given the risk of severe masticatory muscle weakness if peripheral ablation is contemplated.[3,4,11,12]

Patients falling into the following diagnoses can be considered good candidates for TR-NC: cancer- or tumor-related craniofacial pain, trigeminal neuropathic pain, poststroke pain, postherpetic neuralgia, glossopharyngeal neuralgia, and geniculate neuralgia. Anesthesia dolorosa may not be an ideal indication for trigeminal tractotomy, given the need for an extensive lesioning of the trigeminal nucleus, which would not be possible with the current approach of needle-based trigeminal tractotomy.[13]

TECHNIQUE

Radiofrequency lesioning of the descending trigeminal tract and nucleus caudalis is performed percutaneously under CT guidance. Dr. Kanpolat first described CT-guided percutaneous TR-NC and mentored the senior author in this procedure. As such, many case series of this procedure come from the experience of Drs. Kanpolat and Raslan. Currently, we perform the procedure under general anesthesia, given the challenge of maintaining patients with sensitive facial pain prone while awake. The patient first undergoes lumbar puncture for injection of intrathecal contrast such as 300 iohexol (Omnipaque, GE Health Care). This is performed under local anesthetic while the patient is in the preoperative holding area. Care must be taken to properly label the local anesthetic and contrast and so prevent inadvertent intrathecal local anesthetic injection. The patient is then kept in slight Trendelenburg position for 30–45 min. During that period, the patient is transported to the CT suite, and general anesthesia is induced. The patient is positioned prone on the CT table, with the head resting on a foam headrest, with care taken to keep the head neutral or in slight flexion. We have found that monitoring somatosensory or motor evoked potentials is not helpful, given the electrical artifact produced by the radiofrequency generator during lesioning. We recommend the procedure be performed with a wide bore CT, be it in the diagnostic or operating suite, to avoid collision of the electrode with the scanner.

An initial localization CT is taken, centered around the craniocervical junction, from the foramen magnum to caudal aspect of C1. Care is taken to avoid any metal fillings or dentures in the mouth that would create imaging artifact; typical slice thickness is 1–1.25 mm. The planned entry point into the skin, between the occiput and C1, is identified, and the distances from

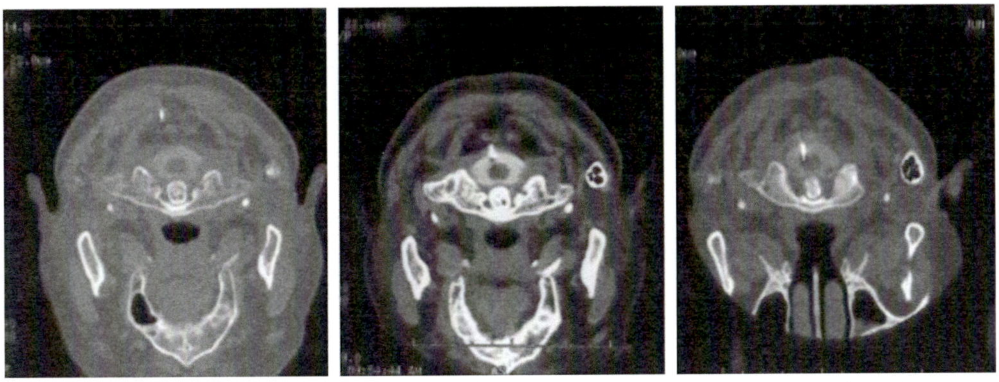

FIG. 12.2 Illustration of the lesioning electrode in the trigeminal tract using CT myelography.

the skin to the dura and skin to the cord pia are measured. The target is identified, typically two-thirds of the distance from the midline to the equator of the spinal cord, which targets the trigeminal tract dorsally and the nucleus caudalis ventrally. The skin-to-dura distance is marked on the introducer cannula for the Levin-Cosman cordotomy electrode system (Cosman Medical, Burlington, MA). The electrode depth is adjusted to project 3 mm from the introducer metal cannula. The laser of the CT scanner is used to mark the entry point on the skin, and the site is prepped and draped sterilely. Serial CT scans are used to guide the tip of the introducer needle to target. Once the subarachnoid space is entered, impedance, as measured by the Radionics RFG-3C generator (formerly Radionics Inc.), is 300–400 Ω. As the spinal cord is entered, impedance should increase to over 1000 Ω. After correct cannula positioning is confirmed on CT, the stylet is removed and the electrode is introduced. Another scan is used to confirm positioning (Fig. 12.2).

Recently, we have switched to a version of the procedure that is completely performed under general anesthesia. We have found it to be very difficult to perform such a procedure in patients with severe facial hypersensitivity. Under general anesthesia, sensory stimulation is not possible; therefore anatomic verification using CT scan and electrophysiologic verification using motor stimulation are performed instead.

Sensory stimulation is performed at 50 Hz up to 0.1 V, which results in tachycardia, suggesting pain. Motor stimulation at 2 Hz should show no motor activity in the ipsilateral leg. We often make two tandem lesions. Given that TR-NC lesioning can be very painful, and that pain severity correlates directly with temperature used, we recommend a lower lesion temperature of 55° for up to 120 s if the procedure is to be performed awake; higher lesion temperatures for shorter duration (similar to cordotomy parameters), such as up to 80° for 60 s, also can be used. After lesioning, the needle with electrode is removed and a final scan is obtained to examine the cord for any tract or contrast penetration.

Postoperatively, we observe the patient in the intensive care unit for serial neurologic examinations overnight. Typically, patients discharge home the next day.

ADVERSE EFFECTS

The most commonly reported adverse effect is transient ataxia of the ipsilateral upper extremity, from edema of the dorsal spinocerebellar tract. Rates reported range from 5% to 10%. Ipsilateral and contralateral paresthesias due to involvement of the dorsal column or the spinothalamic tract are possible side effects of the tractotomy procedure. Motor weakness is very unlikely owing to the very ventral location of motor pathways at the level of the lesioning at the craniocervical junction.

OUTCOMES

The majority of outcome literature comes from the experiences of Drs. Kanpolat and Raslan.[3,4,12] Kanpolat's largest series describes 65 patients over a follow-up period of 20 years: 21 with atypical facial pain, 13 with craniofacial malignancies, and 17 with vagoglossopharyngeal neuralgia, and the remainder with geniculate neuralgia, postherpetic neuralgia, cluster headache, anesthesia dolorosa, or failed trigeminal neuralgia. They report that early pain relief was obtained in 84% of patients, with a statistically significant immediate postoperative reduction in Visual Analog Scale (VAS) score of 5.4.[4] The best results were obtained in the vagoglossopharyngeal neuralgia patients and geniculate neuralgia patients. Of 21 patients, 19 patients with atypical facial pain achieved pain relief, and of 13 patients, 11 patients with craniofacial or oral cancer pain achieved relief. In these 65 patients, the procedure was performed 73 times. There were no mortalities; there was a 6% rate of transient ataxia due to large lesions affecting the spinocerebellar tract, and these resolved within 2 weeks.

Another large series of patients who underwent TR-NC was reported by Raslan in 2008.[3] All these 10 patients had facial pain secondary to malignancy and are reported together with a cohort of 41 patients who underwent unilateral cordotomy (lesioning of the spinothalamic tract between C1 and C2) for localized body pain. These 10 patients underwent the procedure while awake and underwent sensory test stimulation at 100 Hz for 0.1 ms until severe ipsilateral face or throat pain was reproduced at less than 0.5 V. This aided in confirmation of proper electrode placement. Voltage threshold above 0.5 V or sensory response in a limb implies inaccurate electrode placement. Motor test stimulation at 2 Hz for 0.1 ms also was performed, and if no motor response was obtained in the ipsilateral hemibody other than local contraction of the neck musculature, with voltages above 1 V, lesioning was performed. Two lesions were performed: typically first at 45° for 180 s and then at 55° for 120 s. This article provides useful parameters for relevant CT measurements (i.e., mean skin-to-dura distance is 51.4 mm) and impedance (mean 1272.9 Ω). Mean age was 52.1 years, with time from pain onset to surgical procedure ranging from 1 to 9 months. 98% of patients reported no pain or partial satisfactory pain relief postprocedure, with the rate still high at 80% at 6 months. Average sleeping hours and mean Karnofsky Performance Score both increased. Since this large initial case series, we have transitioned to performing the procedure under general anesthesia.

In a large review of ablative procedures for cancer pain, such as trigeminal tractotomy, although the results generally ranged around 80% initial pain relief, the numbers of both published papers as well as published treated patients were small. They were all case series with only one prospective open label trial. There was no level I or level II evidence behind the therapy.[3]

FUTURE DIRECTIONS

An endoscopic version of this procedure had been tried using small pen endoscope (personal communication). The potential advantage is a staggered-multiple-lesions approach would be helpful in conditions such as anesthesia dolorosa.

CONCLUSIONS

Modern-day approaches to TR-NC are performed with percutaneous radiofrequency lesioning under CT guidance. In select patient populations, careful lesion creation can be highly effective in providing immediate and long-lasting pain relief, with minimal adverse effects, cost, risks, and hospital length of stay. Although modulatory or pharmacologic treatments may be favored over ablative procedures, ablative procedures should be considered for patients with economic or logistic limitations that make intrathecal infusions challenging. Ablative TR-NC also is effective in patients with craniofacial pain syndromes or anesthesia dolorosa who wish to undergo a procedure relatively less invasive than open craniotomy and caudalis DREZ.

REFERENCES

1. Sjogvist O. *Studies on pain conduction in the trigeminal nerve. A contribution to the surgical treatment of facial pain*. In: *Acta Psychiatr Neural Scand Suppl XVII*. Helsingfors: Mercators Tryckeri; 1938:93–122.
2. Spiller W, Martin E. The treatment of persistent pain of organic origin in the lower part of the body by division of the anterolateral column of the spinal cord. *JAMA*. 1912;58:1489–1490.
3. Raslan AM, Cetas JS, McCartney S, Burchiel KJ. Destructive procedures for control of cancer pain: the case for cordotomy. *J Neurosurg*. 2011;114:155–170.
4. Kanpolat Y, Kahilogullari G, Ugur HC, Elhan AH. Computed tomography-guided percutaneous trigeminal tractotomy-nucleotomy. *Neurosurgery*. 2008;63(1 suppl 1): ONS147–153.
5. Bernard Jr EJ, Nashold Jr BS, Caputi F, Moossy JJ. Nucleus caudalis DREZ lesions for facial pain. *Br J Neurosurg*. 1987; 1(1):81–91.
6. Falconer MA. First and second division trigeminal neuralgia treated by intramedullary trigeminal tractotomy. *Proc R Soc Med*. 1954;47(4):299–300.
7. Hitchcock E. Stereotactic trigeminal tractotomy. *Farmatsiia*. 1970;19:131–135.
8. Crue BL, Carregal EJA, Felsoory A. Percutaneous stereotactic radiofrequency trigeminal tractotomy with neurophysiological recording. *Stereotact Funct Neurosurg*. 1972;34: 389–397.
9. Fox JL. Intractable facial pain relieved by percutaneous trigeminal tractotomy. *JAMA*. 1971;218:1940–1941.
10. Schvarcz JR. Stereotactic trigeminal tractotomy. *Confin Neurol*. 1975;37:73–77.
11. Raslan AM. Percutaneous computed tomography-guided radiofrequency ablation of upper spinal cord pain pathways for cancer-related pain. *Neurosurgery*. 2008;62: 226–233, discussion 233–224.
12. Kanpolat Y, Deda H, Akyar S, Caglar S, Biglic S. CT-guided trigeminal tractotomy. *Acta Neurochir(Wien)*. 1989; 100(3–4):112–114.
13. Thompson EM, Burchiel KJ, Raslan AM. Percutaneous trigeminal tractotomy-nucelotomy with use of intraoperative computed tomography and general anesthesia: report of 2 cases. *Neurosurg Focus*. 2013;35(3):E5.

FURTHER READING

1. Hitchcock E. Stereotactic trigeminal tractotomy. *Ann Clin Res*. 1970;2:131–135.

CHAPTER 13

Presurgical Localization of Epilepsy

DAVID C. SPENCER, MD

INTRODUCTION

Effective epilepsy surgery depends heavily on the foundational work of localizing the epileptogenic zone. This meticulous process must be undertaken before a specific surgical approach can be entertained.

Early approaches to epilepsy surgery did not circumvent this process. Sir Victor Horsley, considered to be the father of modern epilepsy surgery, reported his initial findings from three epilepsy surgeries in 1886.[1] Localization of the epileptogenic zone was crude but was nonetheless an essential element of the process. He localized seizure onset in two patients by identification of focal skull fractures and in the third by careful observation of the ictal semiology (focal motor symptoms). Later pioneering work by Herbert Jasper and Wilder Penfield emphasized the importance of localization of both ictal onsets and neighboring eloquent cortex. Jasper, the neurologist, took the lead in determining epilepsy localization, using EEG as a primary tool. Of Jasper, the neurosurgeon Penfield reported, "He could, he said, localize the focus of an epileptic seizure by the disturbance of brain rhythms outside the skull. I doubted that but hoped it might be true."[2] Verification of this truth formed the basis for their long collaboration. Since these early explorations of localization, many new techniques, especially in the area of neuroimaging, have revolutionized the evaluation of patients for epilepsy surgery, but many basic principles remain unchanged.

Presurgical Localization: Scope of Discussion, Prerequisites, and Definitions

This chapter will center on treatment of focal epilepsy and will not address disconnection procedures such as corpus callosotomy. The principal subject of these discussions will be localization before "epilepsy surgery"—a procedure in which treatment of epilepsy is the primary consideration, regardless of the specific surgical technique that is used. Similar principles of localization may apply to patients undergoing surgery for a different primary indication (e.g., tumor resection) in whom treatment of tumor-related epilepsy is a secondary consideration. Additionally, focal responsive neurostimulation, which has recently emerged as an FDA-approved therapy, has a similar imperative for accurate seizure localization before implantation of recording and stimulating electrodes.

Thus, effective surgical treatment of epilepsy depends on identification of the epileptogenic zone. The term "epileptogenic zone" deserves further definition, as it is a theoretical construct. The epileptogenic zone can be defined as the region from which the patient's typical seizures arise, and removal of which results in seizure freedom. This is distinguished from the concept of the "irritative zone"—the region that generates spikes—which may be larger than the epileptogenic zone or even multifocal, and the "lesional zone"—the area defined by imaging in patients with radiologically visible lesions—which is often related to, but not synonymous with, the epileptogenic zone. As our understanding of epilepsy has matured, our thinking of epilepsy as a network disease has diverged from the simplistic notion of a "spot in the brain causing seizures" that we may use as a shorthand description with patients. In a more nuanced view, the epileptogenic zone might be considered a node in the network that is critical to seizure generation.

For patients to be considered candidates for epilepsy surgery, the benefit must outweigh the risk. Thus, most patients entering the process of presurgical localization have disabling focal-onset seizures that are not controlled by antiseizure medications. In select cases, epilepsy surgery may be considered in patients whose seizures *are* controlled with medications, particularly when medications are producing problematic side effects and circumstances suggest a high success rate of epilepsy surgery.

The concept of drug-resistant epilepsy (DRE) was recently refined by the International League Against Epilepsy (ILAE).[3] The ILAE definition includes the possible outcomes of an appropriate AED trial (seizure-free, treatment failure, or undetermined) and establishes a definition of seizure freedom: three times the longest preintervention interseizure interval or 1 year, whichever is longer. With these parameters established, the definition states that "failure of adequate trials of two tolerated and appropriately chosen and used AED schedules to achieve seizure freedom" constitutes DRE.

If patients with DRE who have well-localized seizures are selected for intervention, epilepsy surgery can have tremendous benefits on seizure control and quality of life.[4–6] A randomized controlled trial of temporal lobectomy for treatment of DRE showed marked benefits relative to continued antiseizure medication trials.[7] On the basis of this and other studies, epilepsy surgery guidelines have been established by professional societies, including the American Academy of Neurology and the American Epilepsy Society.[8]

To realize the full benefits of epilepsy surgery, the process of presurgical localization must be thorough and precise.

PRESURGICAL LOCALIZATION OF EPILEPSY: STANDARD EVALUATION

Although some elements of the presurgical localization process vary between patients and among centers on the basis of unique characteristics of each, certain components can be considered essential to the evaluation of all patients considered for epilepsy surgery. These components include a neurologic history and examination, video-EEG monitoring, brain magnetic resonance imaging (MRI), and neuropsychologic testing. This is a broad and intensively studied area, and the following discussion, with focus on the approach to localization rather than the details of each technique, is necessarily limited.

History and Physical Examination

Similar to the approach to other neurologic conditions, the history and physical examination form the basis of evaluation.

A detailed description of the seizures is an important initial step of establishing the diagnosis of epilepsy and excluding its mimics. A clear description of the sequence of events during a seizure may be the strongest initial clue to seizure localization and may indicate the hemisphere, lobe, or even sublobar location of the ictal onset. See also the discussion of the ictal semiology in the section on video-EEG monitoring.

Assessment of historical risk factors may direct a search for a specific pathology in some instances (e.g., hippocampal sclerosis in a patient with a history of complex febrile seizures; traumatic encephalomalacia in a patient with a history of closed head injury). Careful review of prior trials of antiseizure medications is necessary to establish a diagnosis of DRE, the entry point and necessary prerequisite for presurgical evaluation. It is important to assess not only the number of drugs tried but also whether they were appropriate for the epilepsy type and whether adequate doses and levels were achieved. Some patients who underwent inadequate antiseizure medication trials that were limited by adverse effects may achieve complete seizure control with an alternative drug.

Identification of comorbidities is another important function of a detailed neurologic and medical history. In addition to identifying comorbidities that might directly influence surgical risk (e.g., cardiopulmonary disease, bleeding or clotting issues), other conditions frequently associated with epilepsy—especially, depression and anxiety—should be identified and treated before consideration of epilepsy surgery. Cognitive comorbidities may present additional surgical risk and should be carefully assessed before any proposed surgery. Although the examination may be normal in many patients with chronic epilepsy, some findings on general examination (e.g., skin findings in the phacomatoses) may suggest a specific underlying diagnosis, and lateralized findings on examination may be an initial clue to lateralization of the epilepsy.

Video-EEG Monitoring

Video-EEG monitoring is central to the presurgical localization process, and both the video and EEG components may contribute complementary information.

Video recording of ictal events is essentially an extension of the neurologic history and physical examination. It may clarify and allow detailed analysis of the seizure description provided by the patient or other observers, and these observations constitute a sort of neurologic examination during the paroxysmal event, aided by assessment performed at the bedside by an epilepsy-trained nurse. The regional specialization of brain function may allow localization of onset of focal seizures based on initial symptoms and signs. In some instances, scalp-recorded EEG may not show changes during the ictal event or may be obscured by artifact, and ictal semiology may be the major indicator of localization.

Much has been written about the localizing significance of various features of the ictal semiology. Although analysis of the ictal semiology may allow a master clinician to develop a strong hypothesis regarding ictal localization on the basis of observation alone, it is also an area fraught with pitfalls. Several points regarding the localizing ability of the ictal semiology should be considered including the following:

- The first clinical symptoms of a seizure may not accurately reflect the ictal onset zone. Seizures may arise from "silent" or noneloquent cortex, and initial clinical symptoms may reflect manifestations of spread of the ictal discharge to neighboring or remote, connected brain regions. For example, seizures beginning in the posterior cingulate gyrus may produce symptoms suggestive of a temporal lobe or frontal lobe seizure on the basis of ictal propagation.[9]
- The localizing value of ictal semiological signs varies in its reliability, and localization should not rest too heavily on any single feature.
- Semiological features that appear late in the seizure may reflect ictal spread and have less localizing value.
- Seizures precipitated by abrupt withdrawal of antiseizure medications may not faithfully represent the patient's habitual seizures (both by semiology and by EEG findings).
- Developmental characteristics may lead to different ictal semiology in children than in adults despite similar ictal localization.[10–12]

A detailed review of ictal semiology signs is not the focus of this chapter, and there are too many nuances to do justice to the topic here. The interested reader is directed to several excellent reviews in this area.[13–15]

The full value of video analysis of the ictal semiology is realized when reviewed in conjunction with simultaneously recorded EEG during video-EEG monitoring.

EEG monitoring for presurgical localization has been widely used and reviewed for decades, and a comprehensive review of the technique is beyond the scope of this chapter. Similar to seizure semiology, ictal recording by use of scalp EEG is a powerful tool that also comes with limitations and known pitfalls.

Much as ictal semiology may be misleading when it represents propagated spread from silent to eloquent cortex, scalp-recorded EEG may mislead or falsely localize when ictal discharges first appear as propagated signals that initially arose from deep or electrophysiologically inaccessible epileptogenic areas. This concern is especially acute when a scalp-recorded EEG pattern appears late after clinical onset.

In some cases, propagation pathways are relatively consistent, as with hippocampal-onset seizures that usually propagate to and are detected by scalp EEG in ipsilateral temporal neocortex. In a small proportion of cases, however, preferential spread to contralateral temporal neocortex can produce a false lateralization pattern.[16] If laterality (or bilaterality) of ictal onsets is in question, invasive or semiinvasive (e.g., foramen ovale electrode) EEG recording is usually needed to resolve the uncertainty. In other cases, such as seizures arising from deep-seated hypothalamic hamartomas, scalp EEG is notoriously misleading, and seizures arising from the hamartoma frequently appear on scalp EEG as temporal lobe or frontal lobe seizures, but resection of temporal or frontal lobe structures does not target the epileptogenic zone and is ineffective in controlling seizures.[17]

Many of the limitations of scalp EEG recording directly relate to technical limitations of EEG recording:

- The EEG signal drops off as a function of distance from the recording electrodes (limiting detection of deep foci).
- The EEG signal depends on production of synchronous activity from an adequate volume of cortex (limiting detection of very focal simple partial seizures).
- The amplitude of the EEG signal recorded depends on orientation of the electrodes to the dipole source (dipoles parallel to recording electrodes may not be detected).
- The EEG signal is substantially filtered by intervening tissues (scalp, skull, meninges).

Despite these caveats, video analysis of ictal behavior and examination of scalp-recorded EEG during ictal events are among the core localization tools used by epileptologists.

Magnetic Resonance Imaging

More than any other technology, MRI has revolutionized the presurgical localization of epilepsy. A summary of the enormous scope of literature in this area will not be attempted here, and most readers will be familiar with the basics of MRI. Identification of an epileptogenic lesion on MRI is one of the strongest predictors of surgical success, and complete resection of the lesion is associated with superior seizure outcomes.[18–20] Patients without an identified lesion on MRI have lower success rates with epilepsy surgery overall; however, further investigations with functional imaging and intracranial EEG monitoring can predict good outcomes in selected cases.[21]

Both in patients with and without an MRI lesion, it is important to keep in mind several principles and potential pitfalls when applying findings from MRI imaging to presurgical localization of epilepsy.

- Not all MRI studies are equivalent, and optimal identification of an epileptogenic lesion depends on both scanner technology and expertise of the reader.[22,23] Joint review of epilepsy protocol MRI studies by the epileptologist and neuroradiologist may produce the highest yield.

- Several technical factors influence yield of MRI, including slice thickness, orientation, and pulse sequence. Optimal pulse sequence parameters can aid the detection of epileptogenic lesions, and some specific sequences (e.g., FLAIR images) produce the highest yield.[24]
- The high spatial resolution of MRI imaging may lead to identification of MRI lesions that are unrelated to the epilepsy—a "red herring" (e.g., arachnoid cyst).
- In other cases, a lesion with true epileptogenic potential may be identified in a patient with non-epileptic events or mixed epileptic and non-epileptic events. (e.g., identification of a small cavernous hemangioma in a patient with psychogenic seizures). Thus even highly epileptogenic lesions identified by imaging should not be considered in isolation.
- Multiple MRI lesions may be detected, and additional testing may be needed to determine whether a single lesion or multiple lesions are responsible for seizures.
- Large, sometimes multilobar lesions may be identified by MRI. Further testing is often needed to determine what aspect(s) of the lesion may be epileptogenic, and thus MRI represents more of a starting point than an end point for localization in such cases.
- As previously noted, in many cases, no epileptogenic lesion may be identified on MRI.

Thus MRI, although often the linchpin of the presurgical localization of epilepsy, may not always be revealing, and findings must be considered carefully in the context of the entire clinical scenario.

Neuropsychological Testing

Neuropsychologic testing is the final component of the standard presurgical evaluation. The goals of testing are at least twofold.

First, in the context of a discussion of presurgical localization, neuropsychologic testing can be thought of as an additional localizing tool.[25,26] The highly ordered functional organization of the brain permits a correlation between specific areas of cognitive dysfunction and regional anatomic or functional deficits that may be tied to the epileptogenic region. Although less spatially precise than some other tools such as MRI, neuropsychologic testing can nonetheless provide additional concordant localizing information (e.g., identification of verbal memory dysfunction in a right-handed patient with left temporal lobe epilepsy) or identify potentially discordant findings that require further investigation (e.g., marked verbal and visuospatial memory impairment in a patient thought to have unilateral nondominant temporal lobe epilepsy). Deficits in functions ascribed to areas outside of the epileptogenic zone are common and may represent dysfunction in connected networks (e.g., signs of frontal lobe dysfunction in patients with temporal lobe epilepsy). However, global cognitive impairment may reflect more widely distributed disease and is a relative negative predictor of surgical success.[27]

Second, in addition to providing additional localizing information, neuropsychologic testing also offers an assessment of psychiatric comorbidities and may highlight areas of potential cognitive risk in patients being considered for epilepsy surgery. In many cases, additional testing may be needed to address neurocognitive risk of epilepsy surgery using the intracarotid amobarbital procedure (IAP) (Wada test) or functional MRI (fMRI) as discussed below. Finally, neuropsychologic testing establishes a baseline of cognitive functioning to which postoperative function may be compared.

Summation and Integration of Findings From the Standard Evaluation

At most epilepsy surgical centers, a multidisciplinary group representing neurology, neurosurgery, neuroradiology, and neuropsychology meets to discuss and integrate the findings of the standard epilepsy surgery evaluation.

Review of these findings often results in one of the following three outcomes (Fig. 13.1):

1. Decision to not pursue surgical resection. Common reasons for exclusion are
   - predominant or exclusive nonepileptic events,
   - generalized epilepsy, and
   - multifocal epilepsy.
2. Decision to pursue resection of the defined epileptogenic zone without further testing. This decision is most often made on the basis of concordant data from testing, usually in the case of an identified epileptogenic lesion on MRI with concordant EEG and other findings.
3. Decision that patient may be a candidate for epilepsy surgery, but further testing is required to determine the bounds of the epileptogenic zone or safety of resection in the vicinity of eloquent cortex. Common scenarios include
   - nonlesional temporal lobe epilepsy,
   - nonlesional extratemporal epilepsy,
   - vague lesion,
   - multiple lesions,
   - lesion near eloquent cortex,

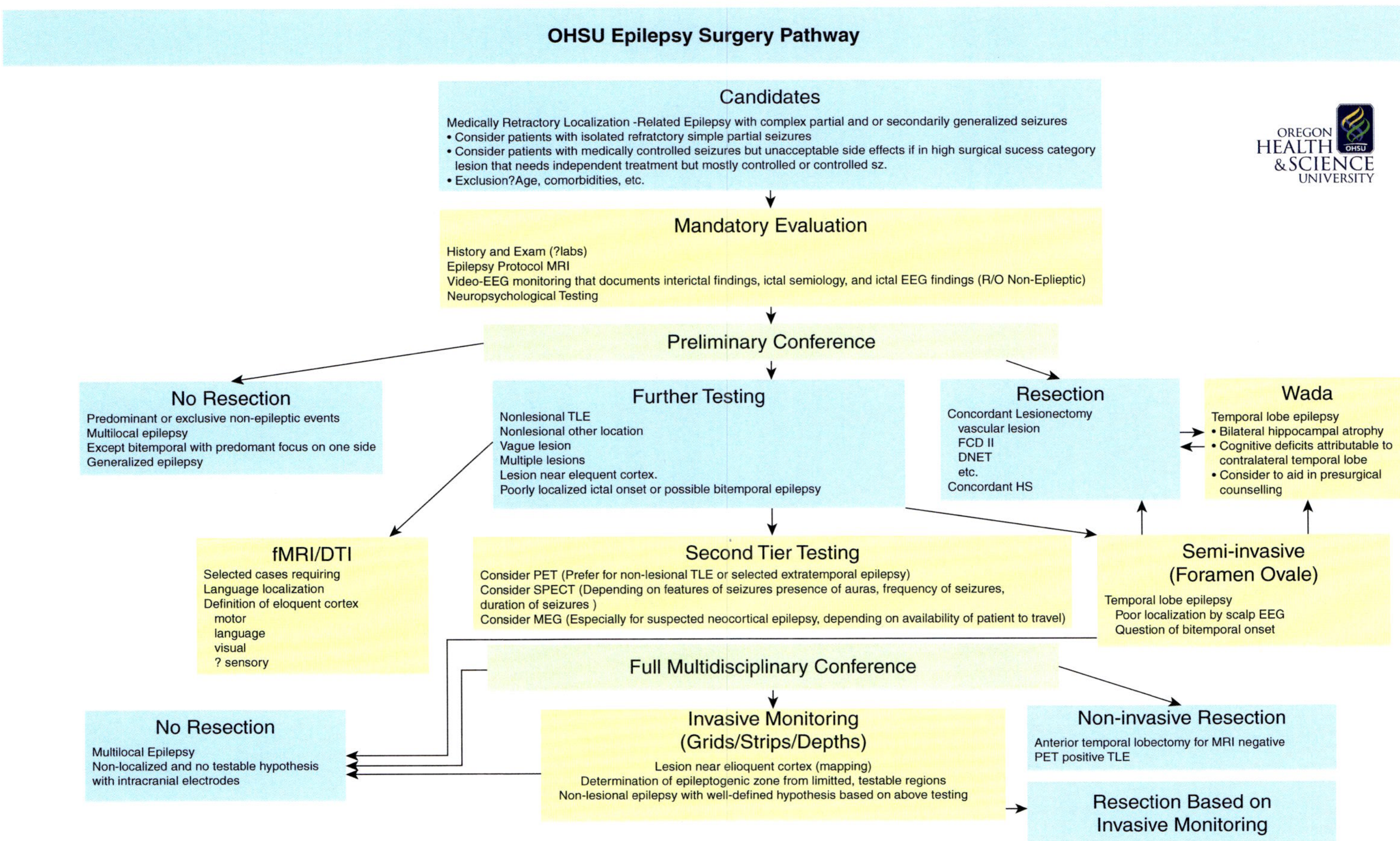

FIG. 13.1 Epilepsy surgery localization pathway.

- poorly localized ictal onset, and
- possible bitemporal epilepsy.

There may be exceptions to these general categories. For example, not all patients with multifocal epilepsy are excluded from consideration of epilepsy surgery. Some may be candidates for palliative resection, and emerging technologies such as laser thermal ablation and responsive neurostimulation may allow greater latitude to treat epilepsy that does not arise from a single focus.

PRESURGICAL LOCALIZATION OF EPILEPSY: TAILORED EVALUATION

In the event that the standard presurgical evaluation neither excludes the patient from surgery nor adequately localizes ictal onset to permit resection or device implantation (situation #3 above), additional evaluation is indicated.

Substantial variation in the path to ultimate ictal localization is seen among epilepsy surgical programs. Differences in access to technology and experience in interpreting the findings are one source of variation. Some centers take a more aggressive approach and are willing to attempt to localize and surgically treat epilepsy patients who have lower odds of successful outcome. The threshold of certainty in presurgical localization may vary; some centers may persevere to exclude any shadow of doubt about localization with extensive use of technology and invasive testing, whereas others may take a relatively less invasive approach, aiming for adequate localization with lower morbidity and cost, while keeping open the possibility of further assessment and intervention if the initial approach were incompletely effective.

Despite these differences, the guiding principles are similar. The goal is to obtain additional localizing information that can generate a hypothesis, or limited set of hypotheses that can be directly tested by intracranial monitoring, or that rarely may lead directly to epilepsy surgery without invasive, intracranial EEG monitoring. The following section outlines this process in general terms, while at times describing the specific approach used in our own epilepsy surgery program.

Positron Emission Tomography

Fluorodeoxyglucose-positron emission tomography (FDG-PET) maps glucose metabolism in the brain and is commonly used in cases in which the standard epilepsy evaluation has not yielded a clear localization and surgical plan. Use of other PET receptor–binding ligands to identify the epileptogenic zone has been investigated, but these are not in widespread use.

In the epilepsy presurgical evaluation, FDG-PET is performed as an interictal study, and areas of PET hypometabolism correlate with the region of ictal onset.[28] Localized PET findings are more common in temporal than extratemporal epilepsy.[29] The hypometabolic region, which can be identified visually or by quantitative techniques, is often larger than the epileptogenic zone but may establish regional localization. Thus FDG-PET studies do not have adequate spatial resolution to define the bounds of the epileptogenic region or surgical resection but may be an important guide to planning intracranial electrode studies for ictal localization before resection. In some cases, closer examination of MR images in the region of hypometabolism may lead to identification of previously unrecognized structural abnormalities such as cortical dysplasia.

The specific use of FDG-PET in cases of "MRI-negative" temporal lobe epilepsy merits discussion. Not infrequently, ictal semiology and interictal and ictal EEG studies implicate the temporal lobe, yet MRI studies at high field strength, with dedicated epilepsy protocols and with expert interpretation, still fail to yield a finding of hippocampal sclerosis or other epileptogenic lesion. Several studies have demonstrated that temporal lobe PET hypometabolism concordant with semiology and EEG findings predicts surgical success following anterior temporal lobectomy, with surgical outcomes approaching those in patients with well-defined hippocampal sclerosis.[30–32] At our center, MRI-negative patients with concordant clinical, EEG, and PET findings often proceed directly to temporal lobe resection, particularly if lateralized to the nondominant temporal lobe. Other centers may routinely pursue invasive intracranial monitoring in these situations. Further investigation is needed particularly if there are features that suggest extratemporal onset with secondary temporal lobe involvement or if further testing might refine the surgical plan and permit a more targeted resection (e.g., selective amygdalohippocampectomy or focal corticectomy), especially in the dominant temporal lobe.

There is considerable variation between programs with respect to the use of PET. At some centers, PET studies are considered part of the standard evaluation, whereas at other sites, PET is used much more selectively. At our center, we have found that PET often adds little incremental value to cases that are well localized by the described "standard" evaluation, and we use PET imaging more selectively, especially in cases of "MRI-negative" epilepsy.

Single Photon Emission Tomography

Single photon emission tomography (SPECT) can be a useful tool when the standard presurgical evaluation is unable to provide adequate localization. SPECT creates brain perfusion images following intravenous administration of a radionuclide that is taken up in the brain in proportion to cerebral blood flow. Because focal seizures create increased local metabolic demand and consequently increased cerebral blood flow, areas of ictal hyperperfusion are closely linked to the epileptogenic zone. SPECT isotope is taken up rapidly and not redistributed, creating a "first-pass" snapshot of brain perfusion that remains stable for a period of hours, permitting imaging after recovery from a seizure.

Interictal SPECT (evaluating interictal hypoperfusion) is relatively insensitive for detection of the epileptogenic region. The primary virtue of SPECT in epilepsy localization comes from the ability to perform SPECT as an ictal study. Typically executed in an epilepsy monitoring unit with concurrent EEG monitoring, ictal SPECT has as its goal the injection of isotope as early as possible after seizure onset—ideally within 30 s. Ictal SPECT images can be examined visually or quantitatively for areas of ictal hyperperfusion. Because the epileptogenic region may be relatively hypoperfused interictally, subtraction images created from paired ictal-interictal SPECT scans, overlaid on MRI—the so called SISCOM (subtraction ictal SPECT coregistered to MRI)—can be especially powerful and provide advantages over review of the raw images alone.[33] SISCOM studies have been demonstrated to accurately localize the epileptogenic region and can provide critical localizing information, especially in cases of "MRI-negative" and extratemporal epilepsy.[34,35] Although extent of resection of the SISCOM-positive region is positively correlated with surgical outcome,[35] the identified area of ictal hyperperfusion is not generally used to define the bounds of resection but rather may identify the epileptogenic lesion in a patient with multiple MRI lesions or identify a region to implant with intracranial electrodes in a patient with no MRI lesion.

The major drawback to ictal SPECT is that it is resource-intensive, and the ability to successfully obtain an ictal injection is uncertain. Success rates are highest in patients with high seizure frequency and a reliable aura.

In the interpretation of SPECT and SISCOM images, it is important to be mindful of factors that may influence results, most importantly the timing of injection with respect to seizure onset. Seizure type, intensity, and propagation are also important. There is a sort of "Goldilocks" principle, in which limited focal seizures or auras may not be detected by SPECT imaging,[36] and secondarily, generalized seizures may also be less informative.[37] The "just right" seizure is often a complex partial seizure that remains focal and ongoing, as the ictal injection is performed.

Magnetoencephalography

Application of magnetoencephalography (MEG) to the presurgical evaluation of epilepsy is perhaps one of the areas of greatest variation between surgical programs. This is in part due to the relatively more limited availability of the technology. MEG detects fluxes in magnetic fields generated by electrical activity in the brain and is used as an interictal test to detect and localize the source of interictal epileptiform discharges (source localization).

Because MEG is used as an interictal study, it can help identify the irritative zone, which is often associated with, but not synonymous with, the epileptogenic zone. Thus direct resection of modeled dipoles identified by MEG is not usually undertaken, but rather this information may be used to generate or confirm a hypothesis regarding the epileptogenic zone that can be tested with intracranial monitoring. Another limitation of MEG is that it is more sensitive to detecting and localizing discharges in superficial areas of cortex and less effective at identifying and localizing deep sources.

MEG can be particularly useful in cases in which no epileptogenic lesion is identified on MRI ("MRI-negative" cases) and can potentially contribute in cases in which there is no clear hypothesis regarding seizure onset, in cases in which there is a large lesional zone on MRI, or in cases of multifocal imaging abnormalities.

The limitations discussed above explain two major pitfalls with use of MEG. First, in patients with large or multifocal lesions, MEG may preferentially identify superficial sources over deep ones. Second, MEG is an interictal, not ictal, study. In patients with a single epileptogenic zone, it may identify a larger irritative zone or more than one irritative zone, with the potential to mislead.

Semiinvasive evaluation

A limited number of localization questions can be addressed with the use of semiinvasive EEG monitoring techniques that do not breach the integrity of the skull, such as the use of foramen ovale electrodes. The distal contacts of percutaneously placed foramen ovale electrodes lie in the ambient cistern, in close proximity to medial temporal lobe structures. Foramen ovale recordings are particularly useful in the determination of laterality in cases of suspected independent bitemporal epileptogenic regions.

Although the presence of a bilateral irritative zone—bitemporal independent interictal epileptiform discharges—is very common in patients with a unilateral epileptogenic zone, other features may raise greater concern for bilateral independent ictal onsets. These could include more than one aura type, bilateral hippocampal atrophy or other bilateral pathology on MRI, equal or greater interictal activity on the anticipated nonsurgical side, or ictal EEG with discordant or ambiguous laterality. Discordant asymmetries in memory performance on neuropsychologic testing or intracarotid amobarbital (Wada) test may also raise concerns. Although many centers use intracranial monitoring—specifically bilateral hippocampal depth electrodes—to address this question, the use of foramen ovale electrodes placed under fluoroscopic guidance can often resolve the question semiinvasively. Clearly, given the limitations of scalp-recorded ictal EEG in recording from deep foci, findings of bilateral or poorly lateralized onsets by scalp EEG should not terminate a presurgical evaluation, and the specific question of laterality in temporal lobe epilepsy can often be effectively answered by this semiinvasive technique.[38]

Intracarotid amobarbital procedure (Wada test), functional magnetic resonance imaging, and diffusion tensor imaging

Although these studies are often an important part of the presurgical evaluation, they are most often used as part of a safety assessment before surgery rather than a critical part of the localization process, and thus will receive only brief mention here.

The intracarotid amobarbital, or Wada test, was developed to assist in determining hemispheric language dominance and later adapted to assess lateralized memory function before surgery.[39] Information pertaining to these two functions can supplement data from neuropsychologic testing and may guide decisions about the extent of resection in the language-dominant hemisphere, prompt further investigations to localize language function before resection, or inform decision-making and counseling regarding risk to memory with temporal lobe resection. The IAP is invasive, carries risks and discomforts, and is not standardized across centers, and its reliability has been questioned from a number of perspectives, including variable distribution of drug and limited data from healthy controls.

The ability of fMRI to substitute for the IAP has been debated for at least a decade, and a recent practice guideline from the American Academy of Neurology reviews the data bearing on this question and supports the consideration of fMRI in place of the IAP in many instances in the epilepsy presurgical evaluation.[40] Diffusion tensor imaging has had limited application in the epilepsy presurgical evaluation and is primarily used to map white matter tracts as part of presurgical safety planning; however, there is potential for information about white matter disturbances to contribute to localization and understanding of cognitive comorbidities.[41–43]

Functional deficits identified by IAP or fMRI, like those found by neuropsychologic testing, may provide additional indirect clues to the epileptogenic region but are not primary localizing tools. There are other advanced imaging techniques that may be used in selected cases or in certain institutions, including magnetic resonance spectroscopy, and a variety of digital imaging postprocessing tools, discussion of which is beyond the scope of this chapter.

Assessment and integration of findings from the expanded noninvasive evaluation

At most centers, data from the expanded, tailored presurgical localization investigation are reconsidered in a multidisciplinary case conference. Review of these findings often results in one of the three outcomes (Fig. 13.1):

1. Decision to not pursue surgical resection. Common reasons for exclusion at this stage include
   - multifocal epilepsy and
   - nonlocalized seizures and no testable hypothesis with intracranial electrodes.
2. Decision to proceed to resection without invasive intracranial monitoring (including the specific case of MRI-negative, PET-positive temporal lobe epilepsy discussed above).
3. Decision to proceed with invasive intracranial monitoring with grid, strip, and/or depth electrodes. Common scenarios include
   - lesion near eloquent cortex requiring mapping,
   - determination of epileptogenic zone from limited, testable regions, and
   - nonlesional epilepsy with well-defined hypothesis based on prior testing.

Intracranial monitoring

The techniques of intracranial monitoring have been refined over decades of use and have been well reviewed.[44–47] A detailed discussion of these techniques is beyond the scope of this chapter, and the following will instead focus on principles of localization using intracranial monitoring.

A variety of techniques can be used for intracranial EEG sampling, including the use of subdural grid or strip electrodes and stereotactically placed depth electrodes.

In general, depth electrodes are best suited to sample deep foci (e.g., mesial temporal lobe, periventricular nodular heterotopia, deep frontal regions). Recent advances in technology have facilitated more rapid, accurate placement of depth electrodes in multiple bilateral brain regions, which can allow greater sampling from disparate brain regions; however, this does not eliminate the need for a carefully thought-out hypothesis that can be tested with depth electrodes. If detailed mapping of neighboring cortical regions is a critical part of the evaluation, subdural electrodes are often better suited to address this need.

Subdural grid or strip electrodes are generally used to assess suspected neocortical foci; however, the medial contacts of well-placed subtemporal strip electrodes can sample the parahippocampal gyrus and detect hippocampal-onset seizures, albeit, with less sensitivity than hippocampal depth electrodes.[48]

The study of high-frequency signals in interictal and ictal intracranial recordings is now well established as an additional localizing tool for identification of the epileptogenic zone; however, care must be taken to distinguish pathologic from physiologic high-frequency oscillations.[49,50]

Intracranial monitoring using any of these techniques has certain limitations that must be considered before embarking on a plan of electrode implantation. In contrast to scalp EEG recordings that provide broad sampling from bihemispheric brain regions, intracranial electrode implantations are necessarily limited and sample targeted brain regions. The more restricted "visual field" with intracranial recordings means that poorly planned or placed intracranial electrodes may fail to accurately identify ictal onset in neighboring cortex. Some brain regions may be more or less accessible to safe electrode implantation or ultimate resection.

With intracranial studies, an ictal pattern on EEG is expected to precede or appear simultaneously with clinical onset and to show high-frequency or repetitive spiking pattern at onset; late appearance of slower-frequency ictal activity or simultaneous appearance of ictal patterns on widespread contacts of intracranial electrodes suggests that a propagated signal is being recorded that may provide limited or misleading localizing information.

Despite these limitations, well-planned intracranial EEG studies can lead to successful epilepsy surgery in cases that are inadequately localized by non-invasive means.

CONCLUSION: SYNTHESIS OF FINDINGS, LOCALIZATION, AND SURGICAL DECISION-MAKING

Localization before functional neurosurgical or other directed surgical treatment plays a larger role in epilepsy than in other neurologic conditions such as Parkinson disease, where the anatomic substrate of the disease is more uniform.

For epilepsy presurgical localization, the described "standard" evaluation may provide sufficient information to proceed to a directed neurosurgical procedure without additional invasive, intracranial monitoring. A subset of patients will lack adequate localization after these initial steps and will not meet "skip criteria" to proceed directly to surgery and instead will require further evaluation. Specialized neuroimaging or neurophysiology studies such as PET, SPECT, and MEG may provide critical additional localizing information that rarely may resolve ambiguities of localization and permit direct surgical targeting of the epileptogenic zone; more commonly, these additional studies may permit secure identification of a region or regions of suspected seizure onset that can be tested by invasive, intracranial monitoring.

It is important to keep in mind that localization is not the end point but rather the starting point in surgical decision-making. Once localization is established, an informed discussion can be undertaken with the patient that outlines the estimated benefit and risk of a proposed resective procedure or device implantation. This includes a quantitative estimate of the likelihood of seizure freedom and a qualitative estimate of the impact on quality of life.

Experienced clinicians will recognize that optimal decision-making represents a partnership between the epilepsy team and the patient that is not overly paternalistic but that also does not disproportionately place the burden of decision-making on the patient.

REFERENCES

1. Horsley V. Brain surgery. *Br Med J.* 1886;2:670–675.
2. Penfield WJH. Recent contributions to clinical neurophysiology: international symposium in neurosciences in honor of Herbert H. Jasper. *EEG Clin Neurophysiol.* 1972;31:9–12.
3. Kwan P, Arzimanoglou A, Berg AT, et al. Definition of drug resistant epilepsy: consensus proposal by the ad hoc task force of the ILAE Commission on Therapeutic Strategies. *Epilepsia.* 2010;51:1069–1077.
4. Seiam AH, Dhaliwal H, Wiebe S. Determinants of quality of life after epilepsy surgery: systematic review and evidence summary. *Epilepsy Behav.* 2011;21:441–445.

5. Mohammed HS, Kaufman CB, Limbrick DD, et al. Impact of epilepsy surgery on seizure control and quality of life: a 26-year follow-up study. *Epilepsia*. 2012;53:712–720.
6. Spencer SS, Berg AT, Vickrey BG, et al. Health-related quality of life over time since resective epilepsy surgery. *Ann Neurol*. 2007;62:327–334.
7. Wiebe S, Blume WT, Girvin JP, Eliasziw M, Effectiveness, Efficiency of Surgery for Temporal Lobe Epilepsy Study G. A randomized, controlled trial of surgery for temporal-lobe epilepsy. *N Engl J Med*. 2001;345:311–318.
8. Engel J Jr, Wiebe S, French J, et al. Practice parameter: temporal lobe and localized neocortical resections for epilepsy. *Epilepsia*. 2003;44:741–751.
9. Enatsu R, Bulacio J, Nair DR, Bingaman W, Najm I, Gonzalez-Martinez J. Posterior cingulate epilepsy: clinical and neurophysiological analysis. *J Neurol Neurosurg Psychiatry*. 2014;85:44–50.
10. Nordli DR Jr, Kuroda MM, Hirsch LJ. The ontogeny of partial seizures in infants and young children. *Epilepsia*. 2001; 42:986–990.
11. Fogarasi A, Janszky J, Faveret E, Pieper T, Tuxhorn I. A detailed analysis of frontal lobe seizure semiology in children younger than 7 years. *Epilepsia*. 2001;42:80–85.
12. Fogarasi A, Jokeit H, Faveret E, Janszky J, Tuxhorn I. The effect of age on seizure semiology in childhood temporal lobe epilepsy. *Epilepsia*. 2002;43:638–643.
13. Stoyke C, Bilgin O, Noachtar S. Video atlas of lateralising and localising seizure phenomena. *Epileptic Disord*. 2011; 13:113–124.
14. Rossetti AO, Kaplan PW. Seizure semiology: an overview of the 'inverse problem'. *Eur Neurol*. 2010;63:3–10.
15. So EL. Value and limitations of seizure semiology in localizing seizure onset. *J Clin Neurophysiol*. 2006;23:353–357.
16. Sammaritano M, de Lotbiniere A, Andermann F, Olivier A, Gloor P, Quesney LF. False lateralization by surface EEG of seizure onset in patients with temporal lobe epilepsy and gross focal cerebral lesions. *Ann Neurol*. 1987;21:361–369.
17. Cascino GD, Andermann F, Berkovic SF, et al. Gelastic seizures and hypothalamic hamartomas: evaluation of patients undergoing chronic intracranial EEG monitoring and outcome of surgical treatment. *Neurology*. 1993;43: 747–750.
18. McIntosh AM, Averill CA, Kalnins RM, et al. Long-term seizure outcome and risk factors for recurrence after extratemporal epilepsy surgery. *Epilepsia*. 2012;53:970–978.
19. Tellez-Zenteno JF, Hernandez Ronquillo L, Moien-Afshari F, Wiebe S. Surgical outcomes in lesional and non-lesional epilepsy: a systematic review and meta-analysis. *Epilepsy Res*. 2010;89:310–318.
20. Bien CG, Szinay M, Wagner J, Clusmann H, Becker AJ, Urbach H. Characteristics and surgical outcomes of patients with refractory magnetic resonance imaging-negative epilepsies. *Arch Neurol*. 2009;66:1491–1499.
21. So EL, Lee RW. Epilepsy surgery in MRI-negative epilepsies. *Curr Opin Neurol*. 2014;27:206–212.
22. Von Oertzen J, Urbach H, Jungbluth S, et al. Standard magnetic resonance imaging is inadequate for patients with refractory focal epilepsy. *J Neurol Neurosurg Psychiatry*. 2002; 73:643–647.
23. Phal PM, Usmanov A, Nesbit GM, et al. Qualitative comparison of 3-T and 1.5-T MRI in the evaluation of epilepsy. *Am J Roentgenol*. 2008;191:890–895.
24. Wellmer J, Quesada CM, Rothe L, Elger CE, Bien CG, Urbach H. Proposal for a magnetic resonance imaging protocol for the detection of epileptogenic lesions at early outpatient stages. *Epilepsia*. 2013;54:1977–1987.
25. Helmstaedter C. Neuropsychological aspects of epilepsy surgery. *Epilepsy Behav*. 2004;5(suppl 1):S45–S55.
26. Jones-Gotman M, Smith ML, Risse GL, et al. The contribution of neuropsychology to diagnostic assessment in epilepsy. *Epilepsy Behav*. 2010;18:3–12.
27. Malmgren K, Olsson I, Engman E, Flink R, Rydenhag B. Seizure outcome after resective epilepsy surgery in patients with low IQ. *Brain*. 2008;131:535–542.
28. Vinton AB, Carne R, Hicks RJ, et al. The extent of resection of FDG-PET hypometabolism relates to outcome of temporal lobectomy. *Brain*. 2007;130:548–560.
29. Engel J Jr. PET scanning in partial epilepsy. *Can J Neurol Sci*. 1991;18:588–592.
30. Gok B, Jallo G, Hayeri R, Wahl R, Aygun N. The evaluation of FDG-PET imaging for epileptogenic focus localization in patients with MRI positive and MRI negative temporal lobe epilepsy. *Neuroradiology*. 2013;55:541–550.
31. LoPinto-Khoury C, Sperling MR, Skidmore C, et al. Surgical outcome in PET-positive, MRI-negative patients with temporal lobe epilepsy. *Epilepsia*. 2012;53:342–348.
32. Yang PF, Pei JS, Zhang HJ, et al. Long-term epilepsy surgery outcomes in patients with PET-positive, MRI-negative temporal lobe epilepsy. *Epilepsy Behav*. 2014;41:91–97.
33. O'Brien TJ, So EL, Mullan BP, et al. Subtraction ictal SPECT co-registered to MRI improves clinical usefulness of SPECT in localizing the surgical seizure focus. *Neurology*. 1998;50: 445–454.
34. Bell ML, Rao S, So EL, et al. Epilepsy surgery outcomes in temporal lobe epilepsy with a normal MRI. *Epilepsia*. 2009; 50:2053–2060.
35. O'Brien TJ, So EL, Mullan BP, et al. Subtraction peri-ictal SPECT is predictive of extratemporal epilepsy surgery outcome. *Neurology*. 2000;55:1668–1677.
36. Elwan SA, Wu G, Huang SS, Najm IM, So NK. Ictal single photon emission computed tomography in epileptic auras. *Epilepsia*. 2014;55:133–136.
37. Varghese GI, Purcaro MJ, Motelow JE, et al. Clinical use of ictal SPECT in secondarily generalized tonic-clonic seizures. *Brain*. 2009;132:2102–2113.
38. Alarcon G, Kissani N, Dad M, et al. Lateralizing and localizing values of ictal onset recorded on the scalp: evidence from simultaneous recordings with intracranial foramen ovale electrodes. *Epilepsia*. 2001;42:1426–1437.
39. Wada J, Rasmussen T. Intracarotid injection of sodium amytal for the lateralization of cerebral speech dominance. 1960. *J Neurosurg*. 2007;106:1117–1133.
40. Szaflarski JP, Gloss D, Binder JR, et al. Practice guideline summary: use of fMRI in the presurgical evaluation of patients with epilepsy: Report of the Guideline Development, Dissemination, and Implementation Subcommittee of the American Academy of Neurology. *Neurology*. 2017; 88:395–402.

41. Winston GP. The potential role of novel diffusion imaging techniques in the understanding and treatment of epilepsy. *Quant Imaging Med Surg*. 2015;5:279–287.
42. Gross DW. Diffusion tensor imaging in temporal lobe epilepsy. *Epilepsia*. 2011;52(suppl 4):32–34.
43. Luat AF, Chugani HT. Molecular and diffusion tensor imaging of epileptic networks. *Epilepsia*. 2008;49(suppl 3): 15–22.
44. Kovac S, Vakharia VN, Scott C, Diehl B. Invasive epilepsy surgery evaluation. *Seizure*. 2017;44:125–136.
45. Fernandez IS, Loddenkemper T. Electrocorticography for seizure foci mapping in epilepsy surgery. *J Clin Neurophysiol*. 2013;30:554–570.
46. Sperling MR. Clinical challenges in invasive monitoring in epilepsy surgery. *Epilepsia*. 1997;38(suppl 4):S6–S12.
47. Risinger MW, Gumnit RJ. Intracranial electrophysiologic studies. *Neuroimaging Clin N Am*. 1995;5:559–573.
48. Spencer SS, Spencer DD, Williamson PD, Mattson R. Combined depth and subdural electrode investigation in uncontrolled epilepsy. *Neurology*. 1990;40:74–79.
49. Jacobs J, Staba R, Asano E, et al. High-frequency oscillations (HFOs) in clinical epilepsy. *Prog Neurobiol*. 2012; 98:302–315.
50. Menendez de la Prida L, Staba RJ, Dian JA. Conundrums of high-frequency oscillations (80-800 Hz) in the epileptic brain. *J Clin Neurophysiol*. 2015;32:207–219.

CHAPTER 14

Intraoperative Functional Cortical Localization

ERIK C. BROWN, MD, PHD • AHMED M. RASLAN, MD, FAANS

INTRODUCTION

By the time of Aelius Galenus (also known simply as Galen; AD 130–210), the brain had become accepted as the seat of voluntary movement, sensation, and even intelligence.[1] Exactly how it performs these functions remained a mystery, as it still does in many ways today. It would be thousands of years before any progress was made in beginning to unravel the highly complex relationships between structure and function in the brain.

The localization of brain function was originally studied primarily by observing the effects of various structural lesions on function.[2–4] John Hughlings Jackson (1835–1911) was able to infer that seizures were a cortical phenomenon and also lay out a rudimentary but revolutionary map of motor and language functions on the brain's surface based on such observations[1]; the term "Jacksonian March" originates from this work. Many of Dr. Jackson's findings were later confirmed by David Ferrier (1843–1928) with some of the earliest experiments with electric brain stimulation[1] largely using animal models. With these developments, the foundation of the localizationist view of the brain was born,[5] identifying links between brain structure and function. This first enabled the ability to explain and predict neurologic abnormalities of functions based on structural changes. As the rudiments of neurologic surgery progressed, it enabled the confidence to pursue resective surgery. Based on the location of a lesion, a proposed resection could be planned and the postoperative deficits predicted. The first successful brain tumor removal was performed by Sir William Macewen (1848–1924) in a young woman in 1881.[1,6] The lesion was dural-based, likely a meningioma, and his localization was performed seemingly entirely by clinical examination,[7] which was significantly aided by hyperostosis of the skull over the left orbit causing a cosmetic defect. After 3 years, in 1884, Dr. Rickman Godlee (1849–1925) performed a successful cerebral tumor resection via a small craniotomy after localizing the lesion to the middle third of the right precentral gyrus based entirely on his description of the pattern of evolution of left-sided focal seizures correlating with right retinal hemorrhages.[1] This was a revolution in the application of the localizationist method of inferring the involved brain matter from the constellation of neurologic and other clinical findings.

The Wernicke-Lichtheim model of language structure and function, formulated in 1885,[3] had brilliantly converted Wernicke's ideas of language organization into a diagrammatic form that was both easy to understand and predictive of both known and unknown disorders of language. The power of the theories put forth by Pierre Paul Broca (1824–80) and Carl Wernicke (1848–1905) entrenched the localizationist view that there existed a static organization of the cerebral cortex into "eloquent" regions essential for a specific function and "noneloquent" regions playing a largely supporting but nonessential role in carrying out the cortical processes that manifest function.[5] Despite the power and durability of these models, it is incomplete in its degree of detail and also fails to provide a robust method of localization in individuals, particularly the function of language. Indeed, the exact localization of different language functions has high interindividual localization variability.[8–12] Evidence suggests the topography of language function to be so highly variable that precise localization cannot be reliably inferred from anatomic landmarks.[10,11] As we learn more about the brain and its underlying processes, the localizationist view appears too rigid and modular. Indeed, localizationist theories fail to account for the improvement that can frequently be demonstrated in patients with lesions to "eloquent" areas as their cortex reorganizes as well as the important contributions of underlying white matter pathways to cerebral function.[5]

The overall movement of the field of neuroscience is away from a rigid localizationist view of cerebral organization to a dynamic, connectomal view that accounts for wide variability, neuroplasticity, and the large-scale neuronetworks that allow multiple and sometimes distant cortical regions to interact both directly and indirectly.[5] Experience and data accumulate with time to resolve that the brain indeed is not organized into precise anatamo-functional relationships that may be inferred strictly from anatomic landmarks.

Glioma is likely to be the best-studied intracranial pathology in regard to intraparenchymal lesions and their surgical treatment. As these lesions are frequently intimately enmeshed with normal cortical tissue, resection always involves the destruction of some degree of normal cortex and/or white matter. Thus much can be generalized from what has been learned in this realm to other indications for resection involving cortical tissue. In regard to glioma, it has been shown that maximal resection improves not only overall survival but also progression-free survival. However, when a lesion lies within "eloquent" cortex, a fine balance must be sought between the competing ideals of maximal resection and minimal postoperative neurologic deficit.[14] The "eloquent" cortex is that cortex which is necessary to preserve to minimize risk of clinically significant neurologic deficits. As aforementioned, in many instances, anatomic localization alone is insufficient to optimize the balance that will enable the longest possible survival with the greatest possible function. Indeed, herein lies the necessity for cortical mapping in resective surgery of the cerebral cortex.

It is also equally important to map white matter tracts involved in various cognitive and motor functions. White matter fibers provide the connectivity between various brain structures and in certain instances are essential for functions, such as the case with motor fibers in corona radiata or internal capsule. A recent review of contemporary language models had described the complexity of language networks and described at least eight distinct white matter pathways involved in language processing with distinct neurologic deficits associated with each.[13] In fact, recovery from cortical injury after surgery is more likely than recovery for white matter tract injury given the condensed nature of white matter and the relative lack of plasticity or redundancy.

INDICATIONS

The ultimate goal of resective brain surgery for any lesion is to maximize removal of the target pathology while minimizing the risk of any postoperative functional decline attributable to the surgical procedure itself. The maximal removal of target pathology is critical in multiple disease paradigms. In glioma surgery, whether it is a low grade or high grade, maximal resection will either achieve cure or prolong survival. In epilepsy surgery, maximal resection can provide life-long seizure freedom. In vascular pathologies, maximal resection will prevent future—possibly fatal bleeds.

It is equally important to preserve functions while achieving maximal resection. In fact, performance status may have a more profound impact on survival if it is to be diminished; therefore, preserving functional status is just as important for patient survival as maximal resection.

The indications of cortical and/or subcortical mapping are a to colocalized brain pathology to eloquent cortex or subcortical detrimental white matter tract, or more commonly juxtapositioning of a brain pathology with eloquent cortex and/or subcortical white matter bundle. The ultimate indication of cortical and/or subcortical mapping is then to localize both brain pathology and eloquent cortex and white matter, juxtaposing the functional with the pathological in order to maximize the chance of a good outcome.

The concept of eloquence itself is relative; while motor functions, language functions, and visual functions are clear domains of eloquence, other 'higher order' skills might be individually important as well. For example, the right parietal lobe is critical for individuals with visuospatial skills important to their quality of life; the same is true for musicians. In other words, eloquence as determined on an individual basis.

PREOPERATIVE AND EXTRAOPERATIVE METHODS

Preoperative mapping has previously been dominated for several decades by use of the intracarotid sodium amobarbital procedure, also known as the Wada test, for lateralizing language and memory functions; indeed, in the early 1990s, nearly all centers used the procedure leading up to epilepsy surgery.[15] The procedure uses an intraarterial catheter to inject sodium amobarbital into a selected internal carotid artery to temporarily anesthetize a hemisphere of the brain, during which the patient is subjected to a series of language and memory tasks; the minimal dose to induce hemianesthesia is used, as measured empirically per clinical exam and electroencephalography (EEG). A lateralization index is calculated based on the scoring of the task in each hemisphere and compared between the hemispheres to provide a semiquantitative indicator of the strength of lateralization of function; there is some variability between institutions in exactly how this is performed, but it is generally a percentage of maximal score for one hemisphere subtracted from that of the other. Specifically, with the advent of noninvasive functional magnetic resonance imaging (fMRI), this modality of presurgical planning has seen a great decline in use, although, there are select clinical scenarios in which it may still enjoy employment, as described below.

fMRI has been a breakthrough imaging modality in the study of brain structure and function. Leveraging the high spatial resolution of magnetic resonance imaging (MRI), fMRI is capable of mapping sites of presumed cortical function to brain regions in four dimensions, including time; it is clear why this modality has garnered interest for its use in preoperative functional mapping in preparation for resective cerebral surgery. The fMRI modality relies on a phenomenon known as the blood-oxygen-level-dependent (BOLD) signal in which the radiofrequency signal detected by MRI from hydrogen atoms is influenced by local changes in the blood flow and oxygenation. Although it is an indirect measure of cortical processing with dynamic changes occurring on the order of approximately 4 s rather than milliseconds, the BOLD signal has been shown to correlate with local field potentials, defined as neurophysiologic activity below 300 Hz and related electrophysiologic phenomena, such as the electroencephalogram (EEG), magnetoencephalogram (MEG), and electrocorticogram (ECoG).[16] Task-based fMRI typically comes in one of the two designs: block and event related. The details of these fMRI designs are beyond the scope of this chapter, although the block designs are typically employed in the clinical setting because of time constraints. A higher statistical power may be achieved with a block design, although the functional information obtained is expected to be less detailed. When compared with intraoperative direct electric stimulation, fMRI has unfortunately been deemed to possess low reliability; with a sensitivity of only 37.1% and a specificity of 83.4%.[5] On a more coarse scale, fMRI has proven clinically useful, that is, in lateralizing language function to the left or the right hemisphere. Indeed, it has been shown that when fMRI lateralizes language to the left hemisphere preoperatively, its performance may obviate the need for the Wada test in many cases[17]; when a semantic decision task and tone decision task subtraction is performed with fMRI, it has been shown that fMRI and Wada are concordant 94% of the time when fMRI demonstrates left language dominance.[15]

Diffusion tensor imaging (DTI) is another MRI modality that is capable of approximating the size and shape of major white matter pathways in the brain. Although this modality does not directly localize brain function, it does identify the important white matter substrates associated with important brain functions; e.g., the arcuate fasciculus for language, the corticospinal tract for motor. Indeed, the emerging connectomal view of the brain identifies that axonal connectivity between brain regions is required to ensure maximal postoperative cortical plasticity to maximize potential to compensate for neurologic deficits induced by the surgical resection of cortical lesions.[5] Thus, there is a growing awareness of a necessity to "respect" the white matter pathways during resective procedures, and with this is a growing use for preoperative DTI tractography.

The extraoperatively setting presented the opportunity for long duration deployment of invasive methods. Predominantly, these are electrical brain stimulation and passive ECoG recording. These are further described below in the section on awake mapping, but are important to mention here as their utility is further explanded in the extraoperative setting due to the expansion of time and potential combination with non-invasive imaging modalities mentioned here. The extraoperative setting is that period following placement of invasive devices, such as electrodes, but prior to the ultimate surgical goal, which is often resection of pathological tissue. This period may last for days to weeks, depending on clinical circumstances, along for prolonged mapping sessions combining multiple modalities. Task-related ECoG has particularly shown promise for both clinical utility and scientific study of the cortical function, especially in the realm of language.[5a]

INTRAOPERATIVE METHODS

During Sleep/Anesthesia

1. Somatosensory Evoked Potential (SSEP) phase reversal
   This is a commonly used technique to observe the shift of N20/P20 waves across the central sulcus. It is attractive given its utility under general anesthesia. However, it is not a very specific or sensitive test, and in conditions where anatomy is altered, it's utility can be lost entirely. However, it provides a quick and simple algorithm for determination of sensory and motor areas under anesthesia.
2. Motor stimulation mapping
   Electric stimulation is a methodology elaborated later when discussing the awake patient. In a sleeping patient, this "gold standard" methodology is limited to the mapping of functions that can be visibly observed without the patient's conscious report of findings, or lack thereof. Indeed, this leaves

only the realm of primary motor function, as the stimulation of a region of cortex leading to activation of an upper motor neuron will lead to the physical and visible contraction of skeletal muscle. Asleep motor mapping usually requires a higher amplitude of stimulation compared with awake motor mapping. Amplitudes up to 15 mA had been described in the literature for both cortical and subcortical motor mapping.[18] This reduced sensitivity of asleep motor mapping is due the effect of anesthetic, with minimum alveolar concentration (MAC) often at 0.3-0.5. ECoG can be used to evaluate both level of anesthesia and potential induction of epileptic activities, such as after discharges that may occur with stimulation.

3. Other methods for the sleeping patient
   Other methods to map cortical function in the sleeping patient are under development. The advent of the intraoperative MRI has brought the MRI into the operating room for the primary purpose of ensuring that maximal resection of a lesion has been achieved. Its presence opens the door to explore the utility of other MRI-based modalities. Functional MRI (fMRI) does not require a patient to be awake when a resting state network is being assessed, thereby overcoming the limitation of task-based fMRI for intraoperative mapping. The resting state fMRI (RS-fMRI) technique analyzes the synchronous low-frequency fluctuations of the BOLD signal between spatially distinct regions to identify "networks" that exist when the brain is "at rest." Resting state networks of the brain are multiple, are associated with various functional processes, and have been shown to be remarkably stable.[19] RS-fMRI has been little examined in the intraoperative setting, although feasibility has been demonstrated. Roder et al. demonstrated that intraoperative RS-MRI was not only able to identify a stable resting state motor network despite propofol anesthesia but also able to predict postoperative deficits at the time of discharge after resective surgery.[20] Although the duration of the scan is only 7 min, the clinical applicability is limited by long processing times on the order of hours to days. It can be expected that with technological advances that shorten processing times of these data, intraoperative RS-MRI may become useful in the clinical setting.

Awake Mapping

1. Stimulation mapping
   Direct electric stimulation in the awake patient (Fig. 14.1) is widely regarded as the gold standard functional mapping technique of the brain and is employed as such in the clinical setting, even though the mechanisms precisely responsible for inactivation of functions (speech and motor mapping) or activation of functions (motor mapping) are not entirely understood. As aforementioned, early methods of stimulation became available well over a century ago. The basic principle is to generate a "transitory virtual lesion"[21] in cerebral tissue by applying a current, typically biphasic at a frequency of 50−60 Hz and from 3 to 9 mA for a period ranging from 1 to 10 s or more, and observing alterations in neurologic function.[5] In regard to motor, the action is typically "positive" in that stimulation of eloquent motor cortex will induce contraction of associated muscle groups, as aforementioned. However, in other functional realms such as language, the action of stimulation is typically "negative" in that to observe for a change in function, that patient must be actively engaged in a task; for example, stimulation associated with inability to respond to a question, although the question is clearly understood, may identify a site associated with expressive language function. Sites of electric stimulation associated with either a positive or negative functional effect observed is said to be "eloquent," i.e., "essential," for that realm of function, and often resection of such sites is avoided. Although direct electric stimulation is applied over and directly interacts with only a very small region of cortex, the focal perturbation will disrupt the entire corresponding subnetwork[5] via the associated white matter pathways. Indeed, direct electric stimulation of the brain is the only existing modality to test the

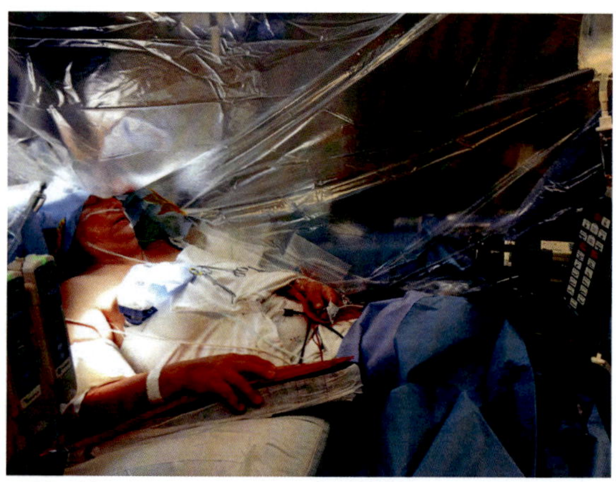

FIG. 14.1 Awake patient in semisitting position with transparent draping.

function of white matter fascicles. This can be performed either by direct stimulation of the white matter or more indirectly by assessing for cortico-cortical propagation of the electric discharge to more distant sites. The primary limitations of the procedure relate to the occurrence of "after-discharges," which represent a sustained synchronization of stimulated cortex that may at times evolve into a seizure, and the discomfort often experienced by the patient; indeed, either or both of these limitations may entirely preclude the use of the technique in some patients. Methods do exist to minimize the occurrence of after-discharges as well as terminate them when they are discovered, such as EEG recording from surrounding brain (Fig. 14.2), stepwise increases in stimulation intensity and/or frequency, and application of cold saline to the cortex, among others.[14]

Awake craniotomy is clearly not suitable for all patients. Absolute contraindications include uncontrollable coughing or other frequent paroxysmal phenomena that would physically interfere with the surgical procedure, severe aphasia preventing effective communication with the awake patient, severe motor weakness or hemiplegia preventing awake motor mapping, and lack of willingness. Relative contraindications include developmental delay or cognitive impairment; communication difficulties such as deafness; age less than 12 years;[14] and significant morphologic abnormalities of the brain such as midline shift, extensive cerebral edema, and concern for elevated intracranial pressure that may benefit from the use of general anesthesia for improved control. However, when appropriately pursued, evidence exists to show that awake craniotomies may have both cost and outcome benefits over use of general anesthesia. Although there are no randomized clinical trials to date for direct and unbiased comparisons, strong evidence in the field of surgical resection of gliomas associated with primary motor cortex suggests that awake craniotomy may have improved functional outcomes at 2 months postoperatively, greater incidence of gross total resection, shorter hospital stays, and reduced nausea and vomiting in the immediate postoperative period when compared with the use of general anesthesia in similar patients. Indeed, to achieve these excellent outcomes, an institutional investment is necessary to develop specialized teams, as the learning curve is steep in the application of awake craniotomy due to complexity.

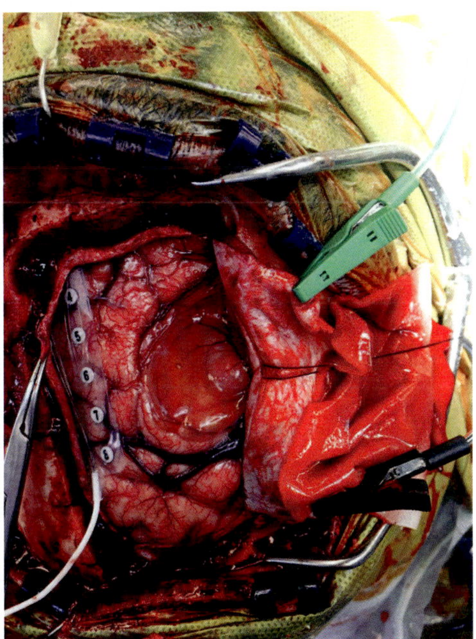

FIG. 14.2 Electrocorticogram grid placed over adjacent brain to the stimulation zone to detect after-discharges.

2. Passive mapping

Passive detection of cortical field potential power fluctuation—specifically γ power fluctuations—had been described in relation to a wide array of cortical activation paradigms (movement,[22,23] speech production and perception,[24] auditory stimulation,[25] visual stimulation,[26] cognitive processing,[27,28] and pain[29]). The γ power activity is the main focus of passive mapping given its surrogate nature to functional cortical activation. The electrocorticographic (ECoG) signals provide the opportunity of a better signal to noise ratio over scalp EEG and allows the mapping of higher frequency bands >70 Hz, which are typically filtered in routine EEG; therefore, ECoG signals are currently widely researched in relation to cortical functional mapping,[30–32] brain-machine interface applications,[33] and cognitive neuropsychology.[34,35] These ECoG signal characteristics render them very suitable for analysis of different frequency bands as well as broadband analysis. It also allows both the online and the off-line analysis of ECoG signals in relation to different functions. The potential advantage of ECoG mapping over electrical brain stimulation is the avoidance of after-discharges and stimulation-induced seizures, which were reported in up to 9.5% of patients.[36]

With recent designs of cortical grids, high-density mapping is possible using grids with small electrode pitch. Several studies have demonstrated a broadband increase in local field potential power measured by ECoG or by EEG in relation to cortical activation, which showed that broadband activation was originally thought to be specific to the γ band. Subsequent studies examined the ECoG correlates of cortical activity using recording systems with faster sampling rates. These studies found that this signal was a broadband ECoG power increase that appeared simultaneously at all frequencies[37,38] rather than being limited to a particular frequency band. Indeed the broadband activity correlated more closely with neuronal firing than narrowband activity. However, for practical purposes, broad γ band power alteration mapping is considered a surrogate marker of cortical activation that could reliably be examined to determine cortical functions.

It was demonstrated that intraoperative ECoG mapping using a high-density electrode grid over the inferior frontal gyrus and employing only two functional tasks, verb generation and word repetition, was able to identify sites of expressive language function within a time period that is operatively useful. These intraoperative findings are correlated with both extraoperative ECoG and extraoperative electric stimulation mapping[39] in a patient undergoing resection of a left frontal mass associated with seizures. Although there are few large-scale studies confirming the utility of broad application, intraoperative ECoG is a rapidly developing tool that may prove a complement and in some instances a replacement to intraoperative electric stimulation mapping.

Additional potential advantages of passive mapping include the incorporation of passive mapping with stimulation mapping to allow for a smaller more precise or 'targeted' stimulation. It also allows mapping of sensory phenomena as well as complex tasks such as solving a Rubik's cube or playing a musical instrument.

REFERENCES

1. Kerr PB, Caputy AJ, Horwitz NH. A history of cerebral localization. *Neurosurg Focus*. 2005;18(4):e1.
2. Dronkers NF, et al. Paul Broca's historic cases: high resolution MR imaging of the brains of Leborgne and Lelong. *Brain*. 2007;130(Pt 5):1432–1441.
3. Graves RE. The legacy of the Wernicke-Lichtheim model. *J Hist Neurosci*. 1997;6(1):3–20.
4. Lichtheim L. On aphasia. *Brain*. 1885;7:433–484.
5. Duffau H. The error of Broca: from the traditional localizationist concept to a connectomal anatomy of human brain. *J Chem Neuroanat*. 2017;89:73–81.

5a. Nakai Y, Jeong JW, Brown EC, Rothermel R, Kojima K, Kambara T, Shah A, Mittal S, Sood S, Asano E. Three- and four-dimensional mapping of speech and language in patients with epilepsy. *Brain*. 2017;140(5):1351–1370.

6. Preul MC. History of brain tumor surgery. *Neurosurg Focus*. 2005;18(4):1.
7. Macmillan M. Localization and William Macewen's early brain surgery Part II: the cases. *J Hist Neurosci*. 2005; 14(1):24–56.
8. Berger MS, et al. Brain mapping techniques to maximize resection, safety, and seizure control in children with brain tumors. *Neurosurgery*. 1989;25(5):786–792.
9. Duchowny M, et al. Language cortex representation: effects of developmental versus acquired pathology. *Ann Neurol*. 1996;40(1):31–38.
10. Hamberger MJ, et al. Distribution of auditory and visual naming sites in nonlesional temporal lobe epilepsy patients and patients with space-occupying temporal lobe lesions. *Epilepsia*. 2007;48(3):531–538.
11. Ojemann G, et al. Cortical language localization in left, dominant hemisphere. An electrical stimulation mapping investigation in 117 patients. *J Neurosurg*. 1989;71(3): 316–326.
12. Ojemann SG, et al. Localization of language function in children: results of electrical stimulation mapping. *J Neurosurg*. 2003;98(3):465–470.
13. Chang EF, Raygor KP, Berger MS. Contemporary model of language organization: an overview for neurosurgeons. *J Neurosurg*. 2015;122:250–261.
14. Eseonu CI, et al. Awake craniotomy vs craniotomy under general anesthesia for perirolandic gliomas: evaluating perioperative complications and extent of resection. *Neurosurgery*. 2017;81(3):481–489.
15. Janecek JK, et al. Language lateralization by fMRI and Wada testing in 229 patients with epilepsy: rates and predictors of discordance. *Epilepsia*. 2013;54(2):314–322.
16. Logothetis NK. The underpinnings of the BOLD functional magnetic resonance imaging signal. *J Neurosci*. 2003; 23(10):3963–3971.
17. Massot-Tarrus A, Mousavi SR, Mirsattari SM. Comparing the intracarotid amobarbital test and functional MRI for the presurgical evaluation of language in epilepsy. *Curr Neurol Neurosci Rep*. 2017;17(7):54.
18. Bertani G, et al. Intraoperative mapping and monitoring of brain functions for the resection of low-grade gliomas: technical considerations. *Neurosurg Focus*. 2009; 27(4):E4.
19. Barkhof F, Haller S, Rombouts SA. Resting-state functional MR imaging: a new window to the brain. *Radiology*. 2014; 272(1):29–49.
20. Roder C, et al. Resting-state functional MRI in an intraoperative MRI setting: proof of feasibility and correlation to clinical outcome of patients. *J Neurosurg*. 2016;125(2): 401–409.

21. Ojemann GA. The neurobiology of language and verbal memory: observations from awake neurosurgery. *Int J Psychophysiol.* 2003;48(2):141–146.
22. Crone NE, Miglioretti DL, Gordon B, Lesser RP. Functional mapping of human senosrimotor cortex electrocorticographic spectral analysis. II. Event-related synchronization in the gamma band. *Brain.* 1998;121:2301–2315.
23. Crone NE, Miglioretti DL, Gordon B, et al. Functional mapping of human senosrimotor cortex electrocorticographic spectral analysis. I. Alpha and beta event-related desynchronization. *Brain.* 1998;121:2271–2299.
24. Sinai A, Bowers CW, Crainiceanu CM, et al. Electrocorticographic high gamma activity versus electrical cortical stimulation mapping of naming. *Brain.* 2005;128: 1556–1570.
25. Haenschel C, Baldeweg T, Croft RJ, Whittington M, Gruzelier J. Gamma and beta frequency oscillations in response to novel auditory stimuli: a comparison of human electroencephalogram (EEG) data with in vitro models. *Proc Natl Acad Sci USA.* 2000;97:7645–7650.
26. Tallon-baudry C. The roles of gamma-band oscillatory synchrony in human visual cognition. *Front Biosci.* 2009; 14:321–332.
27. Wang XJ. Neurophysiological and computational principles of cortical rhythms in cognition. *Physiol Rev.* 2010; 90:1195–1268.
28. Bartos M, Vida I, Jonas P. Synpatic mechanisms of synchronized gamma oscillation in inhibitory interneuron networks. *Nat Rev Neurosci.* 2007;8:45–57.
29. Tiemann L, Schulz E, Gross J, Ploner M. Gamma oscillations as a neural correlate of the attentional effects of pain. *Pain.* 2010;150:302–308.
30. Miller KJ, Leuthart EC, Schalk G, et al. Spectral changes in cortical surface potentials during motor movement. *J Neurosci.* 2007;27:2424–2432.
31. Schalk G, Leuthardt E, Brunner P, et al. Real-time detection of event-related brain activity. *Neuroimage.* 2008;43: 245–249.
32. Roland J, Brunner P, Johnston J, Schalk G, Leuthart E. Passive real-time identification of speech and motor cortex during an awake craniotomy. *Epilepsy Behav.* 2010;18:123–128.
33. Leuthardt E, Shalk G, Wolpaw J, Ojemann J, Moran D. A brain-computer interface using electrocorticographic signals in humans. *J Neural Eng.* 2004;1:63–71.
34. Canolty RT, Edwards E, Dalal SS, et al. High gamma power is phase-locked to theta oscillations in human neocortex. *Science.* 2006;313:1626–1628.
35. Fries P. Neuronal gamma-band synchronization as a fundamental process in cortical computation. *Annu Rev Neurosci.* 2009;32:209–224.
36. Szelenyi A, Joksimovic B, Seifert V. Intraoperative risk of seizures associated with transient direct cortical stimulation in patients with symptomatic epilepsy. *J Clin Neurophysiol.* 2007;24:39–43.
37. Miller KJ, denNijs M, Shenvoy P, et al. Real-time functional brain mapping using electrocorticography. *Neuroimage.* 2007;37:504–507.
38. Manning JR, Jacobs J, Fried I, Kahana M. Broadband shifts in local field potential power spectra are correlated with single-neuron spiking in humans. *J Neurosci.* 2009;29: 13613–13620.
39. Taplin AM, et al. Intraoperative mapping of expressive language cortex using passive real-time electrocorticography. *Epilepsy Behav Case Rep.* 2016;5:46–51.

CHAPTER 15

Vagus Nerve Stimulation

COLIN ROBERTS, MD • CARLI BULLIS, MD

INTRODUCTION

Vagus nerve stimulation (VNS) is a palliative treatment modality for refractory epilepsy. It involves the placement of electrodes coiled around the cervical vagus nerve. The electrodes are connected to a generator that sits on the chest wall and gives off chronic intermittent stimulation. The history of vagus nerve stimulation and its relation to seizures dates back at least a century. Stimulation of the vagus nerve and its effects on cerebral activity were first documented in 1938 by Bailey and Bremmer. This was followed in 1951 by Dell and Olson, who discovered that stimulating the vagus nerve causes an evoked response at the ventroposterior complex and intralaminar regions of the thalamus.[1] In 1952, Zanchetti et al. used a chemically induced seizure model in cats and found that stimulation of the vagus nerve stopped the seizures. The first human implantation of a vagus nerve stimulator was done in 1988 by William Bell. The patient was a 25-year-old man with medically refractory epilepsy.[2] It was not until 1997 that vagus nerve stimulation was approved by the US FDA as an adjunctive therapy for patients above 12 years with partial-onset and medically refractory epilepsy.[3] Difficult-to-treat partial epilepsy affects between 150,000 and 300,000 people in the United States. As an effective treatment modality for these patients, VNS has become a very common procedure.[4] As of January 2016, there had been 133,000 vagus nerve stimulator implantations in a total of 85,000 patients. This chapter will highlight the proposed mechanisms of vagus nerve stimulation and give a brief overview of the implantation process and the indications (both on- and off-label) and outcomes of implantation.

MECHANISM

The mechanism of vagus nerve stimulation is not fully understood. There have been a number of hypotheses of its mechanism. We do know that the vagus nerve communicates with the nucleus tractus solitarius (NTS). The NTS then has numerous projections, including the locus ceruleus and raphe magnus.[2] Stimulation to these areas via the vagus nerve suggests that modulation of norepinephrine and serotonin release may play a role. Multiple studies have shown that stimulation of the vagus nerve increases blood flow to bilateral thalami. Krahl et al. found that lesioning of the locus ceruleus in rats decreased the efficacy of VNS, another suggestion that the locus ceruleus is involved in the mechanism. Cukiert et al. noted that there is typically not a significant effect on electroencephalography (EEG) postimplantation. This would suggest that the action of VNS is likely modulatory rather than affecting the seizure generation itself.[5]

In terms of the VNS system (Fig. 15.1), the stimulator functions by a programmable pulse generator delivering a chronic intermittent electric stimulation to the vagus nerve. This can be set to different intensities and rates. A very common therapeutic setting is 30 s of stimulation, followed by 5 min of off time. If there is a suspected aura or seizure occurring, a magnet can be swiped over the generator, which causes it to deliver an extra dose of stimulation, hopefully aborting the seizure in the process.

The FDA-approved VNS implantation is for patients aged >12 years who have refractory partial epilepsy with no option for resective surgery. Focal disorders, such as mass lesions or mesial temporal sclerosis should be surgically treated with resection or ablation. Lesions that are unresectable, such as in eloquent areas, can be treated with VNS. Patients who have failed prior epilepsy surgery, such as resection of seizure focus or corpus callosotomy, may also be candidates for VNS. They may or may not meet FDA criteria based on their age or seizure type, but studies do show an improvement in seizure frequency for many of these patients with refractory epilepsy. There are also a number of off-label indications that are frequently associated with VNS placement. Many children aged <12 years undergo placement. In fact, it has been suggested in some literature that implanting children at a younger age may be a greater benefit than waiting until they are older.[1] Uncontrolled seizures can lead to a cognitive decline over time. It is likely that children implanted at an earlier age have a lesser period of time

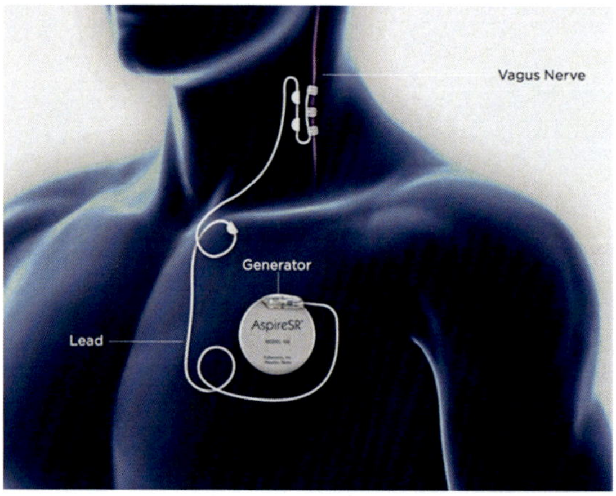

FIG. 15.1 VNS therapy, as depicted in photo Model 10 6 (https://us.livanova.cyberonics.com).

of inadequately controlled seizures, and therefore do not experience as much cognitive decline. This theory could explain the trend of improved cognition in children implanted at a younger age. Patients with generalized seizures, such as in Lennox-Gastaut syndrome (LGS), are also being treated with VNS with a relative amount of success. Treatment for refractory depression has now also become an FDA-approved indication for VNS placement.

The latest versions of the VNS device are capable of delivering automatic stimulation in response to detection of acceleration of heart rate that precedes seizure activity while delivering the chronic duty cycle chronic stimulation.

PROCEDURE

The patient is placed under general endotracheal anesthesia. Preoperative antibiotics are given. They are positioned in the supine position on a standard table. A shoulder roll is placed beneath the scapula, and the head is rotated about 15 degrees to the right to expose the left side of the neck. Approximately halfway between the sternal notch and mandible, a transverse incision is drawn from the sternocleidomastoid to approximately the midline. Local anesthetic is infiltrated. The incision is sharply incised. The platysma is undermined and overmined with scissors and then opened transversely with monopolar electrocautery. Blunt dissection is used to dissect down to the carotid sheath. The carotid sheath is opened sharply. The vagus nerve is encountered deep and lateral to the carotid artery and deep and medial to the jugular vein at approximately the level of the thyroid cartilage. Vessel loops are placed around the vagus nerve to help isolate and elevate it. At this point, we then perform the pocket incision. An approximately 5-cm transverse incision is made 1 cm below the clavicle. Monopolar electrocautery is used to dissect down to the pectoralis fascia. The pocket is made inferiorly in a suprafascial plane. The test generator can be used to help for sizing. Once the pocket is made, a tunneling device is then used to tunnel from the neck incision to the pocket. The leads are then passed through the tunnel. The helical electrodes are then opened by the strings at their ends and wrapped around the vagus nerve. The generator end of the leads is then connected to the generator. Excess lead length is coiled behind the generator, and the generator is placed in the pocket. The device is then interrogated. Upon successful interrogation, the incisions are then irrigated, a small amount of vancomycin powder (<1 g) is placed within them, and they are closed in the usual fashion with absorbable sutures. The patient is woken from general anesthesia and is ultimately taken to the ward where he or she recovers overnight.

OUTCOMES

VNS has demonstrated a reduction in seizures in both adults and children across a number of studies. Greater than 50% reduction of seizures has been considered a positive outcome, with patients known as "responders," in most studies.[5,6] How meaningful this is to the individual patient, however, can vary, depending on their seizure severity and type. For instance, drop seizures can pose a danger to those patients secondary to trauma. Any reduction in the amount of these seizures will decrease the risk of trauma. Unless a person is completely seizure free, however, a reduction in seizures will still leave them with an impaired quality of life, unable to drive, perform certain jobs and activities, and leave the possibility for mild seizure-related cognitive impairment. Although only about 5% of patients will be completely seizure free after VNS placement, many will have a significant reduction in their number and severity of seizures, which, depending on the seizure type, may have a profound impact on their quality of life. In studying the effects of VNS, and seizure treatments in general, it is very meaningful to study not just the number of seizures a patient has but their improvement in quality of life after treatment.[5]

Sirven et al. published a study in 2000, which analyzed 45 patients above 50 years. Twenty of these patients were in randomized controlled trials. Twenty-five of them received the device open label after FDA approval. Sixty-seven percent of the patients had at least 50% reduction in their seizures with the device on high stimulation (35 mA for 30 s every 5 min). This study also showed a significant increase in the seizure reduction rate over time. Twenty-seven percent of people had greater than 50% seizure reduction at 3 months. Sixty-seven percent of people had greater than 50% reduction at 1 year.[7] In that particular study, they used low stimulation as a control group. High stimulation has been shown in some studies, such as Handforth et al. in 1998, to have a significantly increased seizure frequency reduction over low stimulation.[4] García-Navarrete et al. performed a prospective trial of 43 patients, followed them for 18 months, and found that 62% of the patients had >50% reduction in number of seizures. There was no significant correlation with age of onset, duration of onset, stimulation intensity, previous surgery, or seizure type.[8] Benifla et al. also studied 41 children, aged 3–19 years, and found that 38% had a seizure reduction of >90%. Forty-one percent had >50% seizure reduction. The same number had no response to VNS. They also found no correlation with age of onset, duration, prior surgeries, or seizure type.[9] A 2015 Cochran Review analyzed the results of five randomized controlled trials of patients with different VNS frequencies and found that patients with high frequency were 1.73 times more likely to be responders than those on low frequency (which in many studies is considered a placebo setting).[6] Degiorgio et al. performed a randomized prospective trial of 64 patients, placing all the patients in three different high-frequency groups, and found that there was no difference between these groups. These results have been echoed in other studies, finding no significant difference in the responder rate between different high-frequency settings.[10]

In addition to helping seizure frequency, studies have also shown a significant improvement with mood in adults treated with VNS. Elger et al. in 2000 published a randomized, double-blinded study, which analyzed mood in adults with medically refractory seizures treated with VNS. They found a significant improvement in mood within the first 3 months after implantation. This benefit was unrelated to any decrease or change in seizure frequency. This benefit was maintained at 6 months postimplantation, and it did not seem to be dose-dependent.[11] The FDA has now approved the use of VNS as an adjunctive treatment for refractory depression in patients above 18 years who have not responded to at least four other treatment options.

Although not originally indicated for treatment in the pediatric population, VNS has become very widely used in this setting. In 1999, the Pediatric VNS Study Group published a landmark study that showed an improvement in seizure frequency in children. Sixty-six children, aged 3–18 years, with medically refractory epilepsy underwent VNS placement under a compassionate protocol. At 1 year, 46% of the children had a 42% reduction in seizure frequency.[1] In a literature review, Morris et al. found that out of the 470 children with VNS placed, 55% of them saw at least a 50% reduction in seizures.[3] There have not, however, been randomized controlled trials to study its impact on children. As noted in other studies, they also found that the effectiveness of VNS increased over time, 7% in years 1–5 after implantation.[1,12] Healy et al. did retrospective review of 16 patients below 12 years and found that 56% had >50% reduction in seizures. They also found a significant decrease in the use of AEDs after VNS implantation.[13]

LGS has become another increasing off-label use for VNS in both children and adults. LGS consists of multiple seizure types in affected patients. It is refractory to multiple medications and is not amenable to any respective surgery. Often, imaging for these patients will appear normal or be associated with diffuse gliosis, but there is generally no discrete lesion.[5] Morris et al. studied 113 patients with LGS and found that 55% of these patients had at least a 50% decrease in the number of their seizures.[3] Cukiert et al. prospectively studied 24 patients with LGS or LGS-like syndrome and found that there was >50% reduction in 35 seizure types. Seventeen of the seizure types were stopped entirely with VNS. They found that the seizure types with the highest rates of success with VNS were atypical absence, generalized tonic-clonic, and myoclonic seizures. They found VNS less affective at treating atonic, or drop, seizures, although other studies have shown differing results.[5] Benifla et al. found in a retrospective review that 4 of their 10 patients with LGS had >50% decrease in seizure frequency.

COMPLICATIONS

VNS implantation is generally an uncomplicated surgery. Aside from the standard risks in surgery of infection and bleeding, there are the risks of minimal or no seizure improvement, hoarse voice, headache, cough, and dysphagia.[6,14] Infection is a very significant risk in these surgeries because a surgical site infection often necessitates the removal of the entire system and treatment with long-term antibiotics. The risk of infection is typically quoted to be 3%–5%, although this varies between institutions and patient populations.[1] Some have reported rates as high as 11%.[15] Headaches, cough, and hoarseness or voice alteration are common and generally transient side effects caused by decreased adduction of the left vocal fold via the left recurrent and left superior laryngeal nerves.[16] Those side effects will generally diminish between the first and third years after implantation.[17] For the same reason, patients can also have worsening of obstructive sleep apnea and dysphagia.[9] In general, VNS is very well tolerated by the majority of patients, and hoarseness of voice is the most common postoperative complaint.

REFERENCES

1. Hauptman J, Mathern G. Vagal nerve stimulation for pharmacoresistant epilepsy in children. *Surg Neurol Int*. 2012; 3(5):269. https://doi.org/10.4103/2152-7806.103017.
2. Lulic D, Ahmadian A, Baaj AA, Benbadis SR, Vale FL. Vagus nerve stimulation. *Neurosurg Focus*. 2009;27(3):E5. https://doi.org/10.3171/2009.6.FOCUS09126.
3. Morris GL, Gloss D, Buchhalter J, Mack KJ, Nickels K, Harden C. Evidence-based guideline update: vagus nerve stimulation for the treatment of epilepsy. *Epilepsy Curr*. 2013;13(6):297–303. https://doi.org/10.5698/1535-7597-13.6.297.
4. Handforth A, DeGiorgio CM, Schachter SC, et al. Vagus nerve stimulation therapy for partial-onset seizures: a randomized active-control trial. *Neurology*. 1998;51(1):48–55. https://doi.org/10.1212/WNL.51.1.48.
5. Cukiert A, Cukiert CM, Burattini JA, et al. A prospective long-term study on the outcome after vagus nerve stimulation at maximally tolerated current intensity in a cohort of children with refractory secondary generalized epilepsy. *Neuromodulation*. 2013;16(6):551–555. https://doi.org/10.1111/j.1525-1403.2012.00522.x.
6. Panebianco M, Rigby A, Weston J, Ag M. Vagus nerve stimulation for partial seizures. *Cochrane Database Syst Rev*. 2015;(4). https://doi.org/10.1002/14651858.CD002896. www.cochranelibrary.com.
7. Sirven J, Sperling M, Naritoku D, Schachter S. Vagus nerve stimulation therapy for epilepsy in older adults. *Neurology*. 2000:1179–1182. http://www.neurology.org/content/54/5/1179.short.
8. García-Navarrete E, Torres CV, Gallego I, Navas M, Pastor J, Sola RG. Long-term results of vagal nerve stimulation for adults with medication-resistant epilepsy who have been on unchanged antiepileptic medication. *Seizure*. 2013; 22(1):9–13. https://doi.org/10.1016/j.seizure.2012.09.008.
9. Benifla M, Rutka JT, Logan W, Donner EJ. Vagal nerve stimulation for refractory epilepsy in children: indications and experience at The Hospital for Sick Children. *Childs Nerv Syst*. 2006;22(8):1018–1026. https://doi.org/10.1007/s00381-006-0123-6.
10. Degiorgio C, Heck C, Bunch S, et al. Vagus nerve stimulation for epilepsy: randomized comparison of three stimulation paradigms. *Neurology*. 2005;65(2):317–319.
11. Elger G, Hoppe C, Falkai P, Rush AJ, Elger CE. Vagus nerve stimulation is associated with mood improvements in epilepsy patients. *Epilepsy Res*. 2000;42(2–3):203–210. https://doi.org/10.1016/S0920-1211(00)00181-9.
12. Dodrill CB, Morris GL. Effects of vagal nerve stimulation on cognition and quality of life in epilepsy. *Epilepsy Behav*. 2001;2:46–53. https://doi.org/10.1006/ebeh.2000.0148.
13. Healy S, Lang J, Te Water Naude J, Gibbon F, Leach P. Vagal nerve stimulation in children under 12 years old with medically intractable epilepsy. *Childs Nerv Syst*. 2013;29(11): 2095–2099. https://doi.org/10.1007/s00381-013-2143-3.
14. The Vagus Nerve Stimulation Study Group. A randomized controlled trial of chronic vagus nerve stimulation for treatment of medically intractable seizures. *Neurology*. 1995;45: 224–230. https://doi.org/10.1212/WNL.45.2.224.
15. Rossignol E, Lortie A, Thomas T, et al. Vagus nerve stimulation in pediatric epileptic syndromes. *Seizure*. 2009;18(1): 34–37. https://doi.org/10.1016/j.seizure.2008.06.010.
16. Klinkenberg S, Aalbers MW, Vles JSH, et al. Vagus nerve stimulation in children with intractable epilepsy: a randomized controlled trial. *Dev Med Child Neurol*. 2012;54(9):855–861. https://doi.org/10.1111/j.1469-8749.2012.04305.x.
17. Morris GL, Mueller WM. Long-term treatment with vagus nerve stimulation in patients with refractory epilepsy. *Neurology*. 1999;53(8):1731. https://doi.org/10.1212/WNL.53.8.1731.

CHAPTER 16

Stereoelectroencephalography (sEEG) Versus Grids and Strips

GEOFFREY STRICSEK, MD • MICHAEL J. LANG, MD • CHENGYUAN WU, MD, MSBmE

INTRODUCTION

In the United States, almost 150,000 people are diagnosed with epilepsy each year, adding to the approximately 3 million people who already carry the diagnosis[1]; internationally, the prevalence swells to more than 50 million.[1,2] Of those with epilepsy, up to one-third will not have satisfactory seizure control, even with appropriate medical management.[3–8] Fortunately, evidence from randomized clinical trials has demonstrated that surgery can have a significant impact on seizure control in patients with drug-resistant epilepsy.[9–11] Evaluation of candidates for resective epilepsy surgery begins with a detailed history, physical examination, and advanced neuroimaging, followed by long-term noninvasive (phase I) electroencephalography (EEG) recording. Although the technologies for each noninvasive modality continue to improve and their diagnostic efficacy climbs, there are still situations where the seizure onset zone (SOZ) cannot be adequately localized. In roughly 25% of cases, long-term intracranial monitoring (phase II) using subdural electrodes (SDEs), intraparenchymal depth electrodes, or a combination of both is required to further define the area from which seizures originate and their spatial relationship with eloquent regions of the brain.[12,13]

INTRACRANIAL MONITORING: SUBDURAL ELECTRODES

Intracranial electrode recording was first described by Wilder Penfield in the 1930s[14]; however, the technique was not used regularly until the 1970s.[15,16] SDEs can provide generous coverage of the cortical surface (Fig. 16.1), and they offer higher resolution of electric activity than scalp EEG by eliminating the interference of the skull.[17] Enhanced recording fidelity and a reduced distance between the SOZ and recording electrodes enable more precise EEG localization of seizure foci in contrast with scalp EEG, which captures signal as it begins to dissipate which can reduce resolution and anatomic accuracy.[15,18,19]

Hardware Specifications

SDEs come in two different forms: *strips* containing a single row of up to 8 contacts or *grids* arranged in multiple rows of up to 64 contacts (Fig. 16.2). Contacts can be made of either stainless steel or a platinum-iridium alloy and are embedded in a thin, flexible, and biologically inert material such as Silastic or Teflon.[20] Stainless steel contacts are less expensive, but platinum-iridium contacts are magnetic resonance imaging (MRI) compatible and have a lower resistance, which offers signal recording with less interference.[21] Contacts used in SDEs are typically placed 10 mm apart when measured from the center of one electrode contact to the center of the adjacent contact. The electrode contacts themselves are usually 2–5 mm in diameter, although some manufacturers offer smaller contacts, ranging from 1 to 4.5 mm. Microwires can also be interspersed between macro contacts to provide single-unit recordings for research purposes. Each contact in a grid or strip is electrically isolated from the other to limit interference and improve accuracy.[20] Double-sided electrodes are also available commercially, enabling interhemispheric recording while reducing implant burden.

Implantation Procedure

The recommendation for long-term (phase II) intracranial monitoring is usually made on a case-by-case basis in the setting of a multidisciplinary conference based on the review of a patient's seizure semiology, video-EEG data, neuroimaging, and neuropsychologic testing results.

SDEs are implanted under general anesthesia and require either multiple burr holes for strip electrodes,

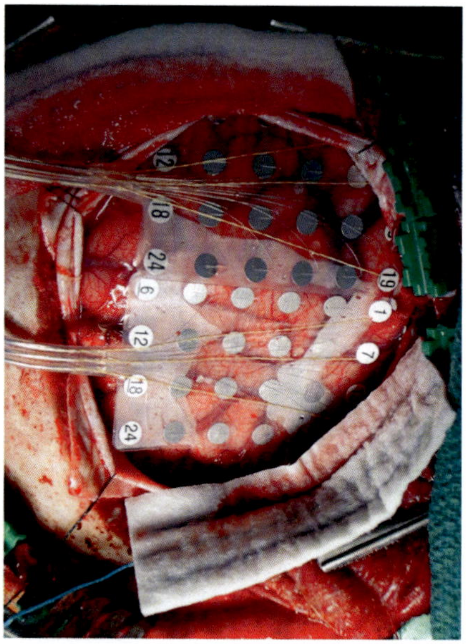

FIG. 16.1 Intraoperative photograph of two 24-contact subdural grid electrodes implanted via an open craniotomy.

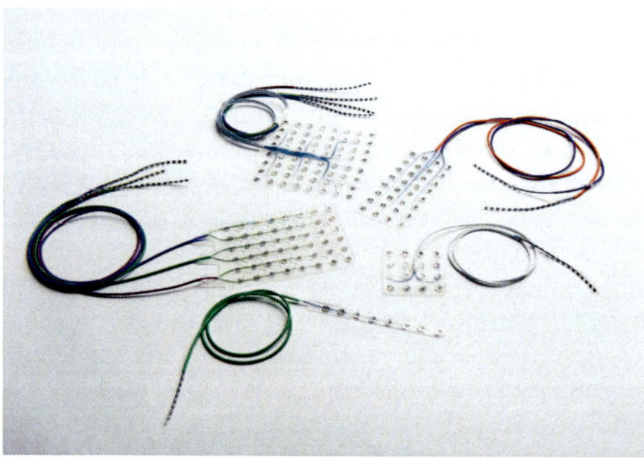

FIG. 16.2 Subdural grid electrodes (top) with 16–64 electrode contacts arranged in multiple rows; and a subdural strip electrode (bottom) with 8 contacts in a single row. (From PMT Corporation; with permission.)

a craniotomy for grid and strip placement, or a combination of the two depending on the recording paradigm and designated electrode array. Once the implantation strategy has been determined, the head is positioned in a manner that allows for access to all targets of implantation. The head is then prepped and draped in a standard sterile fashion. Once the craniotomy flap has been elevated and the dura is opened, the planned montage of SDEs is placed over the cortical convexity. Subdural grids are placed under direct visualization, whereas subdural strip electrodes may be advanced in the subdural space over cortex that may not be directly visible. The wires for each electrode may be sutured to the dura to minimize the possibility of electrode migration.

The wires are then tunneled to a site remote from the incision to minimize the risk of infection; the amount of tissue disrupted at the electrode exit site is minimized, and a purse-string suture is used to limit the risk of both cerebrospinal fluid (CSF) leak and electrode dislodgement.[20–23] Once all SDEs have been implanted and secured in this manner, the skull flap may be replaced and secured with titanium plates and screws. Some institutions elect to withhold replacement of a patient's bone flap until intracranial monitoring has concluded because of concerns about mass effect from subdural implants or interference with EEG recording from the flap.[22,23] A nonsterile assistant in the operating room will usually construct a diagram of lead placement, which serves as an aid for the anatomic mapping of the SOZ and neighboring eloquent cortex, both of which are performed during the postoperative course in the epilepsy monitoring unit (Fig. 16.3).[24]

Postoperative Course

Postoperatively, patients typically spend at least one evening in the ICU before being transferred to a specialized epilepsy monitoring unit for continuous video-EEG recording and mapping. Functional mapping is a critical part of the monitoring process, as precisely identifying eloquent cortex can reduce the risk of adverse events in the event a patient is able to undergo resective surgery.[21] An immediate postoperative CT or MRI scan may be obtained to evaluate lead placement and to rule out hemorrhage. Postoperative steroids and antibiotics may be administered. The duration of postoperative antibiotics varies between institutions from none, to 24 hours of coverage, to continuous administration throughout the duration of recording. However, a meta-analysis of the available literature demonstrated only a trend toward reduced complications with antibiotic use in patients having 67 or more implanted contacts.[25]

Monitoring concludes once sufficient data have been obtained to localize and characterize the SOZ or at any time the risks of ongoing monitoring are deemed to outweigh the benefits as longer duration of monitoring is associated with a significantly increased risk of adverse event.[15,25,26] Although some institutions may elect to remove subdural strip electrodes at the bedside, SDE explantation typically requires a return to the operating room. The electrodes are typically cut at the skin surface, which allows the head to be prepped and draped in a standard sterile fashion. Under general

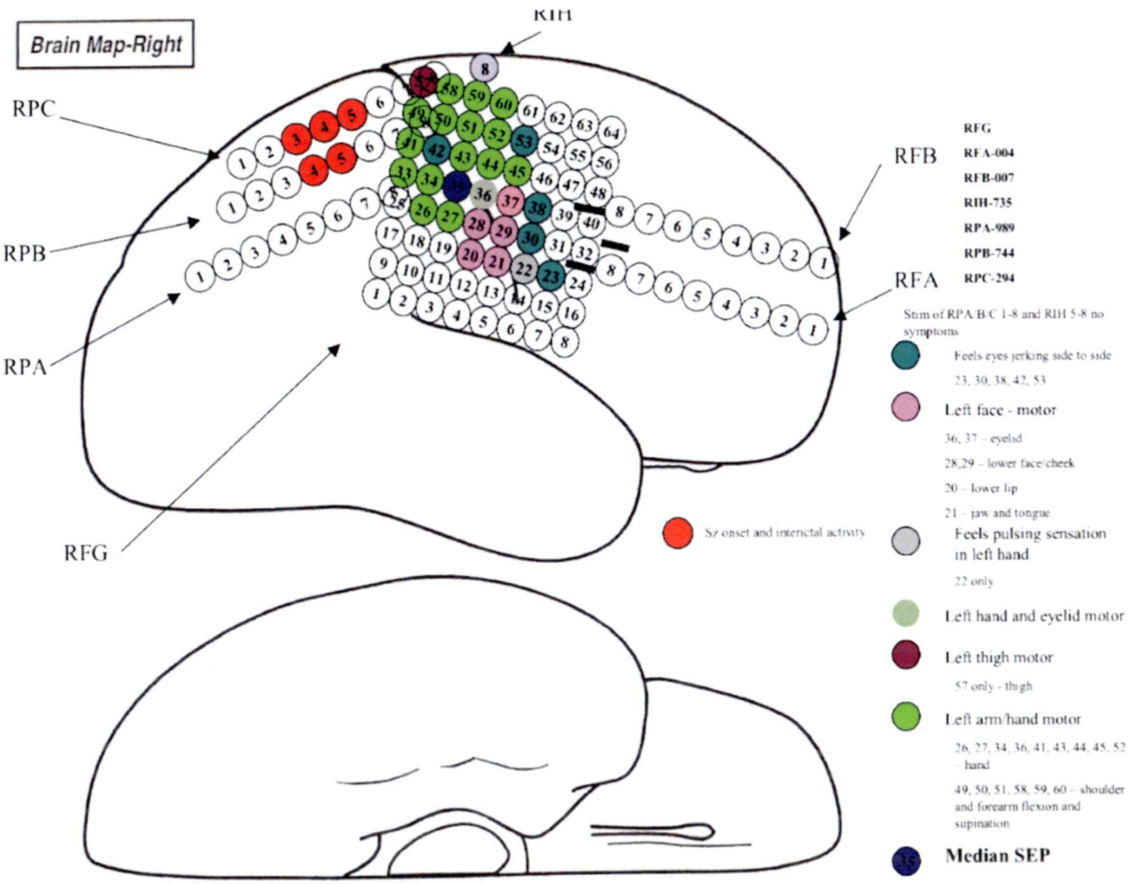

FIG. 16.3 Two-dimensional cartoon of implanted subdural electrodes **(A)**, and the corresponding postimplantation skull X-ray **(B)** for a patient implanted with a 64-contact grid and six 8-contact strip electrodes. As shown on the left, the map serves as an aid for the anatomic mapping of the seizure onset zone and neighboring eloquent cortex, both of which are performed during the postoperative course in the epilepsy monitoring unit.

anesthesia, the prior incision or incisions are reopened. If a bone flap was replaced at the time of implantation, it is removed to allow for direct visualization of the electrodes, which can then be explanted. The number of contacts is carefully counted to ensure complete removal of all implanted electrodes. A postoperative CT scan is also performed to evaluate for any postoperative complications and to ensure that all hardware was successfully removed.

Because the electrodes are typically removed in the operating room, resection of the epileptogenic focus can proceed concurrently if an appropriate target was identified during the recording period. Before electrode explantation, the completed diagram illustrating the SOZ and its relationship with the results of stimulation testing is used to help identify the appropriate areas for surgical resection.

Complications

Although a valuable tool in localization, SDEs are not without risk, with a rate of clinically significant complications of roughly 10%.[27] Electrode placement in the subdural space generates mass effect on adjacent parenchyma, which can cause midline shift,[21,28] elevated intracranial pressure (2.4%),[25] and headache. It is for these reasons that some institutions choose to delay replacement of the bone flap until after surgery.[22,23] At the same time, there are conflicting data as to whether delayed reimplantation increases the risk of infection.[23,28] Other potential complications include

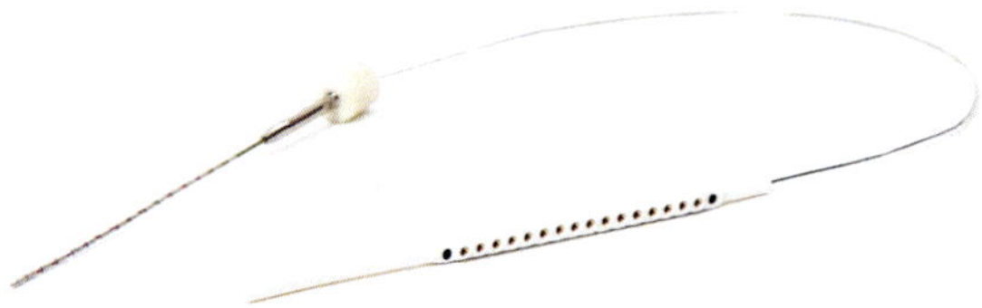

FIG. 16.4 A 16-contact stereoelectroencephalography electrode with its accompanying anchor bolt and locking screw. (From PMT Corporation; with permission.)

hemorrhage (3%–16.4%), infection (2.3%–12.1%), inadvertent placement into parenchyma (3.2%), cerebral edema (2.5%), cerebral infarction (2.2%), and CSF leak (12.1%).[23,25,27,29] Although the potential for adverse events is an inherent part of any surgical procedure, it should be noted that the placement of SDEs is associated with a significantly higher rate of complication when compared with depth electrodes.[27]

INTRACRANIAL MONITORING: STEREOELECTROENCEPHALOGRAPHY

Stereoelectroencephalography (sEEG), first introduced in 1962, relies on the stereotactic placement of multiple depth electrodes to record ictal and interictal activity with the goal of identifying a SOZ amenable to surgical resection.[30–32] Interestingly, although sEEG relies on the use of stereotactic principles, the "stereo" of sEEG actually refers to the three-dimensional nature of sEEG recording.

Hardware Specifications

sEEG leads typically have a diameter of 0.8 mm and can have up to 16 cylindrical platinum-iridium contacts, each 2 mm in length and spaced from 3 to 8 mm apart (Fig. 16.4). As with selection of different SDEs, decisions about specific lead use are dependent on monitoring goals and target area.

Implantation Procedure

Similar to SDEs, recommendation for long-term (phase II) intracranial monitoring with sEEG leads should come from the conclusions of a multidisciplinary conference. sEEG implantation demands a significant commitment to the preoperative planning phase: data gleaned from noninvasive monitoring, MRI, functional magnetic resonance imaging, and positron emission tomography imaging help inform decision-making regarding depth electrode targets. Furthermore, because sEEG electrodes are equipped electrode contacts that can extend from the lateral cortical convexity to the

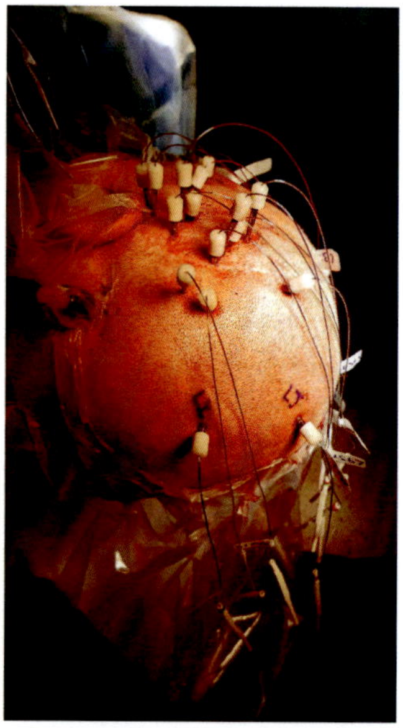

FIG. 16.5 A left-sided stereoelectroencephalography implantation in a patient with a prior craniotomy and resection, who continued to suffer from drug-resistant epilepsy. The implantation scheme shown here covers the posterior temporal lobe, the parietal lobe, the insula and has dense coverage of the temporal lobe immediately posterior to the prior resection.

medial cortex, the surgeon must consider not only the target but also the entry point and the course of the trajectory in stereotactic planning of sEEG implants. As with other stereotactic procedures, a gadolinium-enhanced MRI with or without additional vascular imaging modalities is used to map trajectories that enter on the crest of gyri and avoid sulci, vessels, and the ventricular system. Furthermore, when dealing with several intracranial trajectories in sEEG implants, one must also ensure that no collisions between electrodes occur. Similarly, entry points should be planned at least 1 cm apart to provide adequate space for adjacent anchor bolts to be placed.

Implantation of sEEG leads occurs in the operating room with the patient under general anesthesia. Typically, a stereotactic headframe is placed in the preoperative area, which can be paired with a ring and an arc system or a stereotactic robot for lead implantation. In the operating room, the patient is intubated and typically placed in a supine position The presence of the headframe increases both the difficulty of intubation and the potential for complication; the anesthesia team must therefore have a comprehensive plan in place before surgery to minimize adverse events.[33]

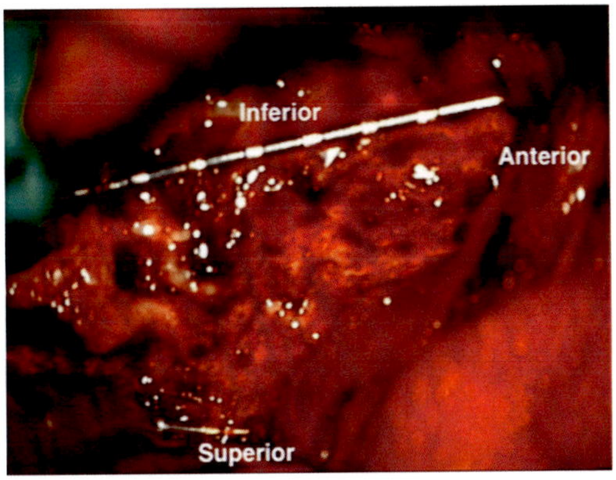

FIG. 16.6 One scenario in patients performing a resection before electrode explantation is with extensive insular resections. As shown here, after resection of the insula, the previously implanted stereoelectroencephalography electrodes help delineate the borders of the insular triangle during surgery.

Once the patient is properly positioned, the head is prepped and draped in the standard surgical fashion.

The chosen stereotactic system is then used to determine the desired trajectory for the implanted electrode. Once the starting for a given lead is identified on the scalp, a small nick is made and a 2- to 3-mm burr hole is made in the skull. The dura and pia are sharply opened and cauterized. Next an anchor bolt is placed and the trajectory is cannulated with a stylet before the electrode is inserted and secured in place to the anchor bolt with a locking screw. Electrode position is confirmed by matching its final position with the position of the stylet using intraoperative fluoroscopy. This process is repeated for each electrode (Fig. 16.5). Once all electrodes have been implanted, an intraoperative CT scan may be performed to confirm appropriate positioning of all electrodes before completion of the procedure.

Postoperative Course

As with SDE implantations, patients typically spend at least one evening in the ICU before being transferred to a specialized epilepsy monitoring unit for continuous video-EEG recording and mapping. A postoperative MRI scan is obtained to rule out occult hemorrhage and to map electrode placement for the purpose of facilitating anatomic localization of seizure onset. Given the more complex nature of having to localize electrodes in three-dimensional space—in comparison to the two-dimensional diagrams that can be created with SDE implantation—specialized software may be used to assist in the interpretation of sEEG data.

Once again, monitoring concludes once adequate data have been obtained to localize and characterize the SOZ or at any time the risks of ongoing monitoring outweigh the benefits. Unlike SDEs, however, electrode removal can be performed at the bedside, rather requiring a return trip to the operating room and general anesthesia. Similar to SDEs, a CT scan is performed after electrode removal to evaluate for potential complications and to ensure that all hardware was successfully removed. In the scenario of patients with an SOZ within the insula, however, there may be a benefit to performing operative resection of seizure focus with the leads in place to help delineate the borders of the insular triangle during surgery (Fig. 16.6).[34]

Complications

The risk of complication with sEEG is significantly lower when compared with that of SDE.[27,35] The rate of hemorrhage is 4%–7.5% with less than 1% being clinically significant; infection is 1%–3.8%; CSF leak is 1.3%; and infarct is less than 0.5%.[27,36,37] As a stereotactic procedure, sEEG also carries with it risks associated with placement of the stereotactic frame including pin site infection, bleeding from pin sites, skull fracture, and disruption of a prior craniotomy site.[38] The reduced risk of adverse events with sEEG as compared with SDE implantation can be attributed to its minimally invasive nature, which decreases the risk of infection, CSF leak, and overall implant burden (Table 16.1). The most common patient concern is discomfort associated with the anchor bolts, which can be effectively managed with adequate padding underneath a headwrap and mild pain medications.

TABLE 16.1
Summary of Rate of Complications Associated With Subdural Electrode (SDE) Implantation and Stereoelectroencephalography (sEEG) Electrode Implantation

	SDE (%)	sEEG (%)
Overall	19.6	6.9
Hemorrhage	4–16.4	4%–7.5
Infection	2.3–5.7	1–3.8
Contusion	4.4	2.5
Edema	2.5	1.9
Infarct	2.2	0.3
CSF leak	0.9–12.1	1.3

SELECTION OF SUBDURAL ELECTRODES VERSUS STEREOELECTROENCEPHALOGRAPHY

Where surgery had previously been shown to be an effective tool for the treatment of refractory epilepsy,[9–11] intracranial monitoring has expanded its application. Ultimately, these two methods of phase II monitoring should be viewed as complimentary. It is therefore important to understand the strengths and weaknesses of each modality to select the best approach to long-term intracranial monitoring.

For the patient with ictal onset located either in or near eloquent cortex, SDEs are the suggested first option[39] as most clinicians are familiar with using this option for purposes of mapping functions of the cortical surface. However, despite improved sensitivity and spatial resolution when compared with scalp recording, SDEs still have difficulty providing coverage of deep cortical and interhemispheric structures, gray matter within a sulcus, and bilateral or multilobar targets.[39] Bilateral SDE implantation can be a logistic challenge, and electrode placement along basal frontal, basal temporal, and mesial frontal cortex can carry an increased risk of bleeding from bridging veins if passage corridors are insufficiently visualized.[40] Additionally, SDEs fall short in the localization of a three-dimensional target as they are only a two-dimensional tool. SDEs are highly adept at sampling gray matter along the convexity, but nearly 70% of cortical gray matter lies within sulci.[41] In addition to a reduced ability to record from sulcal gray matter, this tissue is oriented tangentially to the plane of a grid and as such, precise localization of seizure activity can be compromised.[42]

Unlike SDEs, sEEG directly provides a three-dimensional representation of an epileptic network from the site or sites of onset and its continuation through propagation pathways.[43] sEEG lead placement has been shown to be highly accurate[44] and enables direct recording from sulcal gray matter and deep gray matter, including the insula[34]; cingulate gyrus; and medial frontal, temporal, and parietal gyri.[42] It has also been successfully used in patients who have recurrent or persistent epilepsy after prior surgery; the strength of sEEG in this clinical scenario springs both from its ability to provide additional information about seizure focus localization and its ability to avoid scar tissue dissection during lead placement.[43,45] Furthermore, sEEG can be a successful salvage technique when other invasive techniques have been unable to localize SOZ.[46–49] Successful SOZ localization occurs in 75% –97% of patients[37,43,46,48,50] who undergo sEEG implantation, and nearly 70% of those undergoing resection surgery will have Engel I outcomes at 2 years.[37,43]

TABLE 16.2
Summary of Preferred and Secondary Methods of Long-Term (Phase II) Invasive Monitoring in Various Clinical Scenarios

Clinical Scenario	Preferred Method	Secondary Method
Lesion or hypothetical SOZ near or in eloquent cortex	SDE	sEEG
Lesion or hypothetical SOZ has a deep location or is not near eloquent cortex		
Need for bilateral explorations and reoperation	sEEG	SDE and depth electrodes
Prior failure of SDE to localize SOZ		
Need to map epileptogenic network		

SDE, subdural electrode; *sEEG*, stereoelectroencephalography; *SOZ*, seizure onset zone.

Although it has many strengths, sEEG also has limitations. Improved sampling of deep structures comes at the expense of superficial coverage which in turn limits functional mapping; however, speech mapping has been demonstrated with lead positioning in the pars opercularis.[51] sEEG is also a "blind" procedure in the sense that any intraoperative bleed, although uncommon,[27,36] may not be immediately identified and can be difficult to control given that access is severely constrained unless a larger burr hole is made (Table 16.1).

In summary, deep-seated lesions, possible bilateral onset, failure of SDE, or history of refractory or recurrent epilepsy after prior surgery favor sEEG.[39] Additionally, if everything else is equal in the clinical balance, it is important to keep in mind that SDEs carry a significantly higher risk of adverse event compared with sEEG[27] (Table 16.2).

SUMMARY

Epilepsy is a serious and significant health issue impacting millions of people across the globe. The costs associated with refractory epilepsy are high, both in terms of absolute medical costs and reduced quality of life and lost productivity.[52–55] Nearly 30% of patients diagnosed with epilepsy will have poor seizure control despite adequate medical therapy. Fortunately, surgery has been shown to have a positive impact on patients with refractory epilepsy with postoperative seizure freedom rates between 58% and 73%.[9,10,37] Although advanced neuroimaging and scalp EEG recording are often sufficient to identify a surgical target, localization of seizure onset remains unclear in up to 25% of cases.[12] Of those in whom a seizure focus cannot be identified using noninvasive techniques, definitive characterization can be obtained in more than 75% using intracranial monitoring techniques such as SDEs, stereotactic implantation of depth electrodes, or a combination of the two.[37,43,46,48] Although not a universal solution, electrode implantation has conferred a significant benefit on the epilepsy population by providing improved seizure control for many patients who previously had refractory seizures. As such, it is important to understand the different methods of intracranial monitoring to select the most appropriate options for phase II monitoring.

REFERENCES

1. Epilepsy Foundation. Epilepsy Statistics. Available at: http://www.epilepsy.com/learn/epilepsy-statistics.
2. WHO. Epilepsy Fact Sheet. Available at: http://www.who.int/mediacentre/factsheets/fs999/en/.
3. Kwan P, Brodie M. Early identification of refractory epilepsy. *N Engl J Med*. 2000;342:314–319.
4. Brodie M, Dichter M. Antiepileptic drugs. *N Engl J Med*. 1994;340:168–175.
5. Sander J. Some aspects of prognosis in the epilepses: a review. *Epilepsia*. 1993;34:1007–1016.
6. Schmidt D, Gram L. Monotherapy versus polytherapy in epilepsy: a reappraisal. *CNS Drugs*. 1995;3:194–208.
7. Rosenow F. Presurgical evaluation of epilepsy. *Brain*. 2001; 124:1683–1700.
8. Beleza P. Refractory epilepsy: a clinically oriented review. *Eur Neurol*. 2009;62:65–71.
9. Wiebe S, Blume W, Girvin J, Eliasziw M. A randomized, controlled trial of surgery for temporal-lobe epilepsy. *N Engl J Med*. 2001;345:311–318.
10. Engel Jr J, McDermott M, Wiebe S, et al. Early surgical therapy for drug-resistant temporal lobe epilepsy: a randomized trial. *JAMA*. 2012;307(9):922–930.
11. Schmidt D, Stavem K. Long-term seizure outcome of surgery versus non surgery for drug-resistant partial epilepsy: a review of controlled studies. *Epilepsia*. 2009; 47(suppl 2):28–33.
12. Spencer S, Guimaraes P, Shewmon A. Intracranial electrodes. In: Engle Jr J, Pedley T, eds. *Epilepsy: A Comprehensive Textbook*. New York, NY: Lippincott-Raven.
13. Diehl B, Luders H. Temporal lobe epilepsy: when are invasive recordings needed? *Epilepsia*. 2004;41(suppl 3):S61–S74.
14. Morris III H, Luders H. Electrodes. *Electroencephalogr Clin Neurophysiol*. 1985;37(suppl):3–26.
15. Nair D, Burgess R, McIntyre C, Luders H. Chronic subdural electrodes in the management of epilepsy. *Clin Neurophysiol*. 2008;119:11–28.
16. Ludwig B, Marsan C, Van Buren J. Depth and direct cortical recording in seizure disorders of extratemporal origin. *Neurology*. 1976;26(11):1085–1099.
17. Nunez P. *Electrical Fields of the Brain: The Neurophysics of EEG*. New York, NY: Oxford University Press; 1981.
18. Luders H, Awad I, Burgess R, Wyllie E, van Ness P. Subdural electrodes in the presurgical evaluation for surgery of epilepsy (Review) *Epilepsy Res*. 1992;5(suppl):147–156.
19. Wyllie E, Luders H, Morris III H, et al. Subdural electrodes in the evaluation for epilepsy surgery in children and adults. *Neuropediatrics*. 1988;19(2):80–86.
20. Bingaman W, Bulacio J. Placement of subdural grids in pediatric patients: technique and results. *Childs Nerv Syst*. 2014;30(11):1897–1904.
21. Lesser R, Crone N, Webber W. Subdural electrodes. *Clin Neurophysiol*. 2010;121(9):1376–1392.
22. Voorhies J, Cohen-Gadol A. Techniques for placement of grid and strip electrodes for intracranial epilepsy surgery monitoring: pearls and pitfalls. *Surg Neurol Int*. 2013;4(98).
23. Van Gompel J, Worrell G, Bell M, et al. Intracranial electroencephalography with subdural grid electrodes: techniques, complications, and outcomes. *Neurosurgery*. 2008;63:498–506.
24. WInkler P, Vollmar C, Krishnan K, Pfluger T, Bruckmann H, Noachtar S. Usefulness of 3-D reconstructed images of the human cerebral cortex for localization of subdural electrodes in epilepsy surgery. *Epilepsy Res*. 2000;41:169–178.
25. Arya R, Mangano F, Horn P, Holland K, Rose D, Glauser T. Adverse events related to extraoperative invasive EEG monitoring with subdural grid electrodes: a systematic review and meta-analysis. *Epilepsia*. 2013;54(5):828–839.
26. Hamer H, Morris H, Mascha E, et al. Complications of invasive video-EEG monitoring with subdural grid electrodes. *Neurology*. 2002;58(1):97–103.
27. Schmidt R, Wu C, Lang M, et al. Complications of subdural and depth electrodes in 269 patients undergoing 317 procedures for invasive monitoring in epilepsy. *Epilepsia*. 2016;57(10):1697–1708.
28. Hersh E, Virk M, Shao H, Tsiouris A, Bonci G, Schwartz T. Bone flap explantation, steroid use, and rates of infection in patients with epilepsy undergoing craniotomy for implantation of subdural electrodes. *J Neurosurg*. 2013; 119:48–53.
29. Hedegard E, Bjellvi J, Edelvik A, Rydenhag B, Flink R, Malmgren K. Complications to invasive epilepsy surgery workup with subdural and depth electrodes: a prospective population-based observational study. *Neurol Neurosurg Psychiatry*. 2014;85:716–720.
30. Talairach J, Bancaud J, Bonis A, Szikla G, Tournoux P. Functional stereotaxic exploration of epilepsy. *Confin Neurol*. 1961;22:328–330.

31. Talairach J, Bancaud J. Stereotaxic approach to epilepsy: methodology of anatomofunctional stereotaxic investigations. *Prog Neurol Surg*. 1973;5:297–354.
32. Musolino A, Tournoux P, Missir O, Talairach J. Methodology of "in vivo" anatomical study and stereo-electroencephalograhic exploration in brain surgery for epilepsy. *J Neuroradiol*. 1990;17:67–102.
33. York J, Wharen R, Bloomfield E. Esophageal tear in a patient undergoing stereotactic brain biopsy under general anesthesia. *J Anesth*. 2009;23(3):432–435.
34. Lang M. *Insular Triangulation: A Novel Stereo EEG Technique for Investigation of Insular Lobe Epilepsy*. Chicago, IL; 2016.
35. Wellmer J, von der Groeben F, Klarmann U, et al. Risks and benefits of invasive epilepsy surgery workup with implanted subdural and depth electrodes. *Epilepsia*. 2012;53(8):1322–1332.
36. Mullin J, Shriver M, Alomar S, et al. Is SEEG safe? A systematic review and meta-analysis of stereo-electroencephalography-related complications. *Epilepsia*. 2016;57(3):386–401.
37. Gonzalez-Martinez J, Bulacio J, Thompson S, et al. Technique, results, and complications related to robot-assisted stereoelectroencephalography. *Neurosurgery*. 2016;78:169–180.
38. Safaee M, Burke J, McDermott M. Techniques for the application of stereotactic head frames based on a 25-year experience. *Cureus*. 2016;8(3).
39. Podkorytova I, Hoes K, Lega B. Stereo-encephalography versus subdural electrodes for seizure localization. *Neurosurg Clin N Am*. 2016;27:97–109.
40. Kovac S, Vakharia V, Scott C, Diehl B. Invasive epilepsy surgery evaluation. *Seizure*. 2017;44:125–136.
41. Carpenter M. *Core Text of Neuroanatomy*. 4th ed. Baltimore: Lippincott, Williams & Wilkins; 1991.
42. Kim H, Lee C, Knowlton R, Rozzelle C, Blount J. Safety and utility of supplemental depth electrodes for localizing the ictal onset zone in pediatric neocortical epilepsy. *J Neurosurg Pediatr*. 2011;8:49–56.
43. Serletis D, Bulacio J, Bingaman W, Najm I, Gonzalez-Martinez J. The stereotactic approach for mapping epileptic networks: a prospective study of 200 patients. *J Neurosurg*. 2014;121:1239–1246.
44. Cardinale F, Massimo C, Castana L, et al. Stereoelectroencephalography: surgical methodology, safety, and stereotactic application accuracy in 500 patients. *Neurosurgery*. 2013;72(3):353–366.
45. Unnwongse K, Jehi L, Bulacio J, Gonzalez-Martinez J, Najm I. Contralateral insular involvement producing false lateralizing signs in bitemporal epilepsy: a stereo-encephalography case report. *Seizure*. 2012;21:816–819.
46. Guenot M, Isnard J, Ryvlin P, et al. Neurophysiological monitoring for epilepsy surgery: the Talairach SEEG method. Indications, results, complications and therapeutic applications in a series of 100 consecutive cases. *Ster Funct Neurosurg*. 2001;77(1–4):29–32.
47. Vadera S, Mullin J, Bulacio J, Najm I, Bingaman W, Gonzalez-Martinez J. Stereoelectroencephalography following subdural grid placement for difficult to localize epilepsy. *Neurosurgery*. 2013;72:723–729.
48. Munari C, Hoffmann D, Francione S, et al. Stereo-electroencephalography methodology: advantages and limits. *Acta Neurol Scand Suppl*. 1994;152:52–67.
49. Gonzalez-Martinez J, Bulacio J, Alexopoulos A, Jehi L, Bingaman W, Najm I. Stereoelectroencephalography in the "difficult to localize" refractory focal epilepsy: early experience from a North American epilepsy center. *Epilepsia*. 2013;54:323–330.
50. Cossu M, Cardinale F, Castana L, et al. Stereoelectroencephalography in the presurgical evaluation of focal epilepsy: a retrospective analysis of 215 procedures. *Neurosurgery*. 2005;57:706–718.
51. Alonso F, Sweet J, Miller J. Speech mapping using depth electrodes: the "electric Wada". *Clin Neurol Neurosurg*. 2016;144:88–90.
52. Villanueva V, Giron J, Martin J, et al. Quality of life and economic impact of refractory epilepsy in Spain: the ESPERA study. *Neurologia*. 2013;28(4):195–204.
53. Begley C, Durgin T. The direct cost of epilepsy in the United States: a systematic review of estimates. *Epilepsia*. 2015;56(9):1376–1387.
54. Schiltz N, Kaiboriboon K, Koroukian S, Singer M, Love T. Long-term reduction of health care costs and utilization after epilepsy surgery. *Epilepsia*. 2016;57(2):316–324.
55. Allers K, Essue B, Hackett M, et al. The economic impact of epilepsy: a systematic review. *BMC Neurol*. 2015;15:1–16.

CHAPTER 17

Transcortical Selective Microsurgical Amygdalohippocampectomy for Medically Intractable Seizures Originating in the Mesial Temporal Lobe

KIM J. BURCHIEL, MD, FACS • DAVID C. SPENCER, MD

BACKGROUND

Epilepsy is a common condition that affects nearly 1% of the world's population. Although about two-thirds of patients with epilepsy achieve good seizure control with antiepileptic medications, the remaining one-third have seizures that are resistant to medications and therefore may be considered as candidates for epilepsy surgery. In suitable candidates, surgical therapy is clearly superior to the best medical therapy.[1] Surgery is most often considered and most frequently successful in patients with temporal lobe epilepsy (TLE). Most patients with TLE have seizures that originate from the mesial-basal temporal lobe structures (hippocampus, amygdala, parahippocampal gyrus). Traditionally, the standard surgical treatment has been an en bloc anterior temporal lobectomy (ATL).

This article discusses the indications for a more restrained approach to the surgical management of seizures of temporal lobe origin: the selective microsurgical amygdalohippocampectomy (SMAH) and the techniques used to perform it.

ATL involves resection of approximately 3–6 cm of anterior temporal neocortex (depending on language dominance), which permits the surgeon to access and resect mesial structures, including the amygdala and the hippocampus. A modification popularized by the Yale group limits neocortical resection to 3.5 cm from the temporal pole and spares the superior temporal gyrus, obviating the need for language mapping in most cases.[2,3]

The primary advantages of ATL are the relatively low morbidity and the good surgical exposure that allows complete resection of mesial structures; this procedure also permits pathologic examination of en bloc specimens.

Data from animal models and pathologic, electrophysiologic, and structural and functional imaging studies support the contention that most TLE arises from mesial temporal structures. This suggests the possibility that more targeted mesial temporal resections that spare temporal neocortex (e.g., SMAH) might provide equally good seizure control and result in fewer neuropsychologic sequelae than ATL (Fig. 17.1).

TRANSCORTICAL APPROACH TO SELECTIVE MICROSURGICAL AMYGDALOHIPPOCAMPECTOMY

In 1958, Niemeyer reported such a procedure, using a small incision in the middle temporal gyrus, to access the temporal horn and selectively resect mesial temporal structures.[4] Subsequently, Wieser and Yasargil popularized a transsylvian approach and reported outcomes of large numbers of patients who underwent this procedure.[5,6] Other techniques, including the subtemporal approach[7] and variants of the transcortical approach, have been described.[8] Transsylvian and subtemporal approaches will be briefly discussed below, and the remainder of this chapter will be devoted to the transcortical approach.

Many individual studies suggest that for patients with well-defined mesial temporal onset seizures, particularly those with the syndrome of hippocampal sclerosis, seizure-free outcomes after SMAH are equivalent to outcomes after procedures that involve more

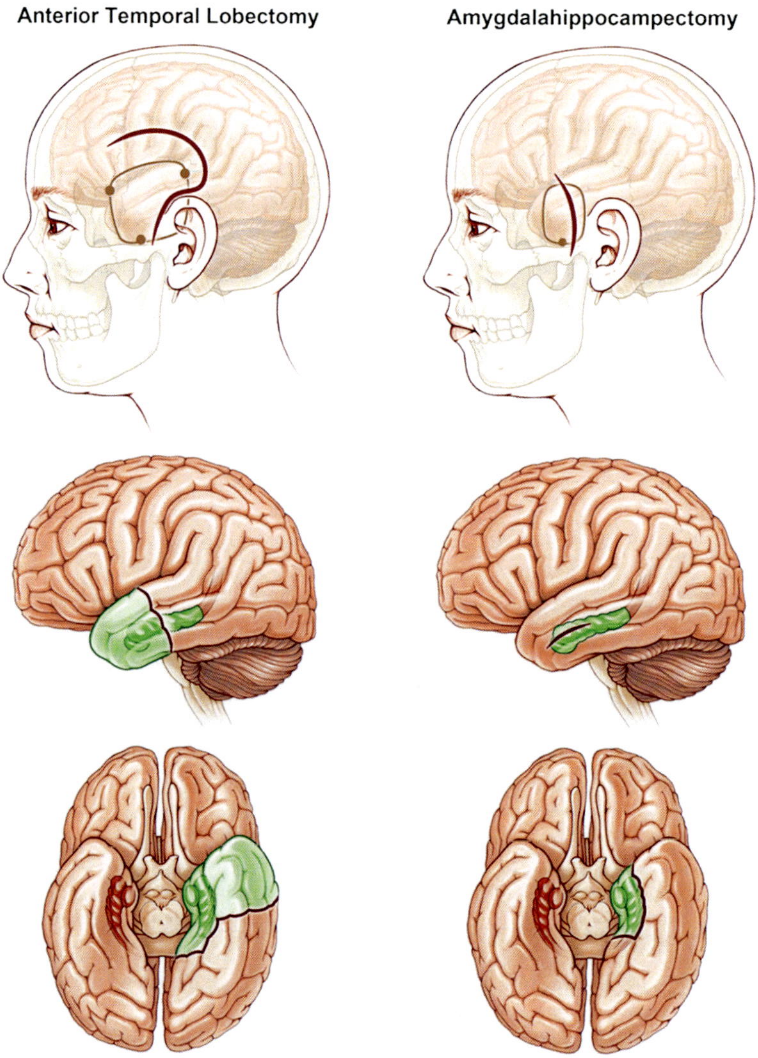

FIG. 17.1 Comparison of anterior temporal lobectomy and selective amygdalohippocampectomy.

extensive temporal neocortical resections.[9–14] A systematic review and metaanalysis suggested a slight advantage in seizure-free rates in patients who underwent ATL; however, methodological concerns from combining potentially biased studies have strengthened the call for a randomized controlled trial of SMAH versus ATL for treatment of mesial TLE.[15,16]

Presuming near equivalence in seizure-free outcomes, SMAH would be preferred over ATL if it could be clearly demonstrated that the more selective procedure would result in superior postoperative neuropsychologic outcomes. Here, the results have been mixed. Although many studies suggest that SAH can spare some aspects of cognitive function as compared with ATL,[5,10,11,17–23] others have reported mixed findings and have not shown the more selective procedure to provide a clear benefit.[24–27] In some of these studies, failure to demonstrate differences in cognitive outcomes may reflect shortcomings in the neuropsychologic batteries administered rather than a lack of difference in cognitive outcomes. Nonetheless, it is clear that SMAH can still cause significant verbal memory impairment in some cases of dominant temporal lobe resection, and it does not eliminate the need for careful preoperative evaluation (including assessment of risk to memory function).

Indications

Most commonly, suitable candidates for SMAH are selected on the basis of the convergence of several lines of evidence implicating unilateral mesial temporal structures as the epileptogenic region. These lines of evidence include (1) a compatible ictal semiology and neurologic history, (2) MRI showing abnormality suggestive of mesial temporal sclerosis (most commonly, hippocampal atrophy and/or mesial temporal signal change on T2-weighted/fluid-attenuated inversion recovery sequences) or exclusively mesial temporal lesions (e.g., low-grade tumor or neurodevelopmental abnormalities), (3) video electroencephalography (EEG) documenting compatible ictal semiology and stereotyped ictal onset on scalp EEG consistent with mesial temporal origin. In these cases, an interictal EEG may reveal concordant unilateral or bilateral (usually predominantly ipsilateral) epileptiform discharges.

For patients in whom these lines of evidence do not converge, or for whom some data points are lacking (e.g., those with no MRI lesion or with poorly localized ictal onsets on EEG), adjunctive studies may be required, such as (1) positron emission tomography, (2) magnetoencephalography, or (3) ictal single-photon emission computed tomography.

Particularly in nonlesional cases, if standard evaluation, supplemented by specialized imaging studies, defines a unilateral temporal lobe onset, intracranial EEG monitoring may be required to distinguish mesial and temporal neocortical onset to determine whether SAH is indicated.

Contraindications

Although ATL or SMAH offer an effective surgical alternative to patients with medically intractable seizures of mesial temporal origin, certain aspects of the seizures would typically exclude patients from consideration of this approach, such as (1) nonepileptic events, (2) idiopathic (primary) generalized epilepsies, (3) extratemporal focal epilepsy, (4) independent bitemporal onset seizures (in most cases), (5) severe impairment of verbal and visuospatial memory (as demonstrated by neuropsychologic testing and intracarotid amytal testing), (6) temporal neocortical epilepsy, and (7) TLE without clear localization to mesial temporal structures.

Surgical Considerations

Routine general anesthesia with endotracheal intubation is indicated. Antibiotics are administered. To minimize intraoperative brain shift, mannitol is avoided. The patient is placed in the supine position, with the head rotated 90 degrees to the opposite side and parallel to the floor. The head is held in position in a three-pin fixateur. Various approaches to SMAH have been developed. Of these, the transcortical approach will be described in some detail.

ATL and SMAH are both performed through a temporal craniotomy, the size of which is dictated by the necessary exposure. Typically, ATL will require a 5- to 6-cm craniotomy, whereas SMAH requires a 3- to 4-cm opening. This more limited exposure, particularly when first undertaken, can lead to disorientation. For this reason, it is highly recommended that neuronavigational guidance is used frequently, particularly during the early learning curve. The surgeon should proceed from safe zone to safe zone and establish routine waypoints for surgical image-guided navigation.

Facial contouring and scalp contouring are used to register the patient's anatomy in the image-guidance system, and the planned entry point is marked on the scalp, along with planned bone flap and scalp incisions. The scalp is prepared, draped, and infiltrated with lidocaine 1%, bupivacaine 0.25%, and epinephrine. A linear scalp incision is performed (Fig. 17.2). The temporalis fascia is incised, separated from the periosteum, and retracted laterally. The neuronavigation system is used to determine the location of the temporal craniotomy. The dura is opened and flapped inferiorly.

The neuronavigation system is used to estimate the distance from the temporal pole and then to plan an entry point in the middle temporal gyrus in a section that is free of cortical vessels. The entry point should be no greater than 3.5 cm from temporal pole (dominant temporal lobe). A 1.5- to 2.0-cm cortical incision is planned. The cortical surface is opened with a bipolar cautery (see Fig. 17.3). Using serial navigation, and two small opposing square self-retaining retractors, the dissection is carried down to the temporal horn, whereupon the ventricle is entered. The amygdala is then partially resected in a direction that is aimed inferiorly and anteriorly so that the pia overlying the most medial middle fossa floor is encountered first.

At this point the surgeon works posteriorly to identify the tentorial incisura, then from anterior to the posterior the uncus is removed (Fig. 17.3), carefully preserving the medial pia along the carotid and suprasellar cisterns. The carotid artery and third nerve are usually visualized during this stage of the resection. Neuronavigational confirmation is obtained frequently at this stage. To avoid injuring the posterior cerebral artery, third cranial nerve, or cerebral peduncle, the mesial pial border must be strictly preserved.

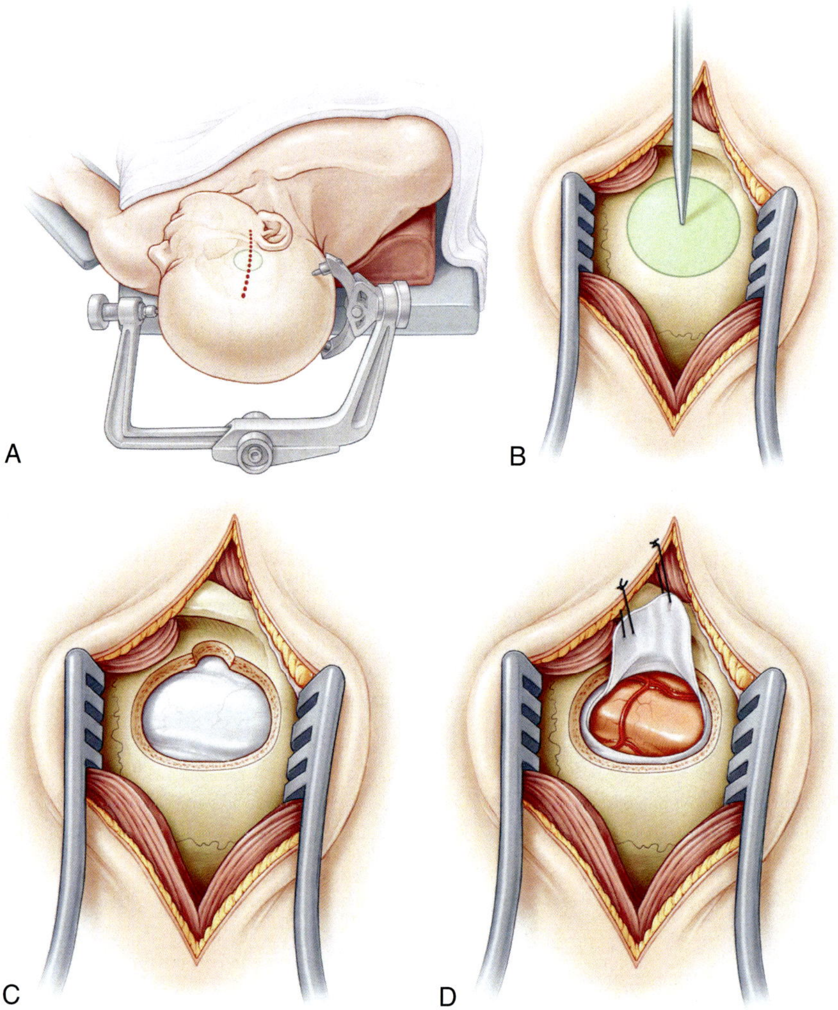

FIG. 17.2 The craniotomy. **(A)** The head is positioned for the procedure, and the incision and craniotomy are planned, **(B)** the planned entry point is marked on the temporal bone, **(C)** a 3- to 4-cm craniotomy is fashioned, and **(D)** the dura is opened.

Once the most medial portion of the uncus is removed, the dissection is then carried back within the temporal horn, to expose the anterior extent of the choroidal fissure. Dissection should never extend superior to the choroidal fissure to prevent inadvertent injury to the optic tract and cerebral peduncle. To prevent this, the white matter superior to the choroidal fissure is effectively "boxed out" by placing a square self-retaining retractor over the choroid plexus with gentle retraction to expose the choroidal fissure. A small square retractor is then placed into the ventricle retracting posteriorly to expose the pes hippocampus. The surgeon then works posteriorly to easily mobilize the hippocampus from the fissure with mobilization of the fimbria and then divides the pes hippocampus posteriorly to coincide with the anteroposterior location of the collicular plate on axial guidance MRI. Neuronavigation is used to confirm the completeness of the resection, usually 2.5 cm of hippocampus proper.

The dissection is then carried out within the parahippocampal gyrus from posterior to anterior to liberate the pes. The liberated pes hippocampus is now free

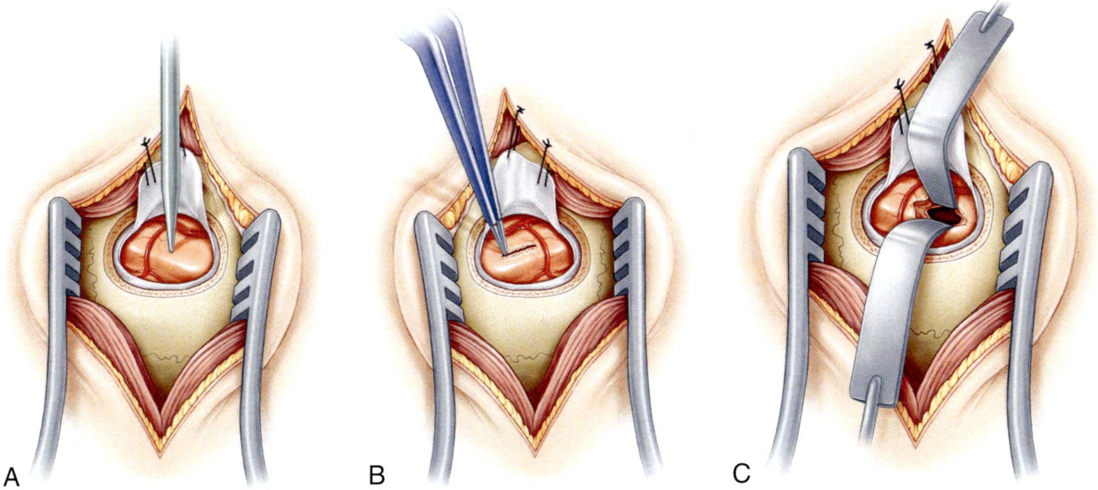

FIG. 17.3 The transcortical approach. **(A)** The entry point on the crest of the midtemporal gyrus is indicated, not more than 3.5 cm posterior to the temporal tip by image guidance, **(B)** a 1.5- to 2.0-cm incision is made in T2, and **(C)** two opposing small square self-retaining retractors are used, with frequent image guidance to locate and enter the temporal horn of the ventricle.

except for the hippocampal fissure (Fig. 17.4). The hippocampus attached to the pia of the hippocampal sulcus is then resected on both sides of the hippocampal fissure, taking care to avoid injury to the anterior choroidal artery or one of its *en passant* branches (Fig. 17.5). This resection incorporates the dentate gyrus, CA4, CA3, CA2, CA1; the entorhinal cortex; and a portion of the parahippocampal gyrus.

Absolute hemostasis is acquired, the medial pial boundary of the resection is lined with thrombin-soaked gelatin sponge (e.g., Gelfoam), and oxidized cellulose fabric is used to line the resection bed proper. The resection cavity is inspected, brain retractors are removed, and the dura is closed. The bone flap is plated, the temporalis muscle is reapproximated, and the scalp is closed in layers to the skin with reabsorbable sutures.

After completion of anesthesia, a neurologic examination is performed. A postoperative computed tomography scan of the head is obtained. Antiepileptic medications are continued. The patient is monitored overnight in a neurologic intensive care unit. The postoperative hospital stay is generally 3–4 days.

Complications

Intraoperative complications can be minimized by strict adherence to timeout procedures, careful patient positioning, and careful visual identification of landmarks coupled with repeated reconfirmation of stereotactic findings. Attention to careful patient selection and preoperative testing can minimize the risk to memory and the chances of mood disturbances and can maximize efficacy by excluding inappropriate patients.

A contralateral homonymous quadranopsia can occur postoperatively, although this is usually asymptomatic.[28] A more serious complication can occur when the anterior choroidal artery, or one of its penetrating branches, is compromised during the procedure. This can result in hemiparesis/hemiplegia and contralateral homonymous hemianopsia due to infarction involving the internal capsule and/or optic tract.

Failure of the neuronavigational system can lead to an inaccurate or incomplete resection. Infections and postoperative hemorrhages are uncommon. Memory impairment,[27] transient dysnomia, and mood changes can also result from this procedure.

OTHER APPROACHES TO SELECTIVE MICROSURGICAL AMYGDALOHIPPOCAMPECTOMY

Transsylvian Approach

The transsylvian approach to SMAH was popularized by Wieser and Yasargil.[6,29] Its advantages were felt to be that it avoided injury to temporal neocortex and underlying white matter, which are traversed in the transcortical procedure, and that it permitted en bloc resections. However, technically, this is a more difficult approach; it affords only limited exposure of the medial temporal

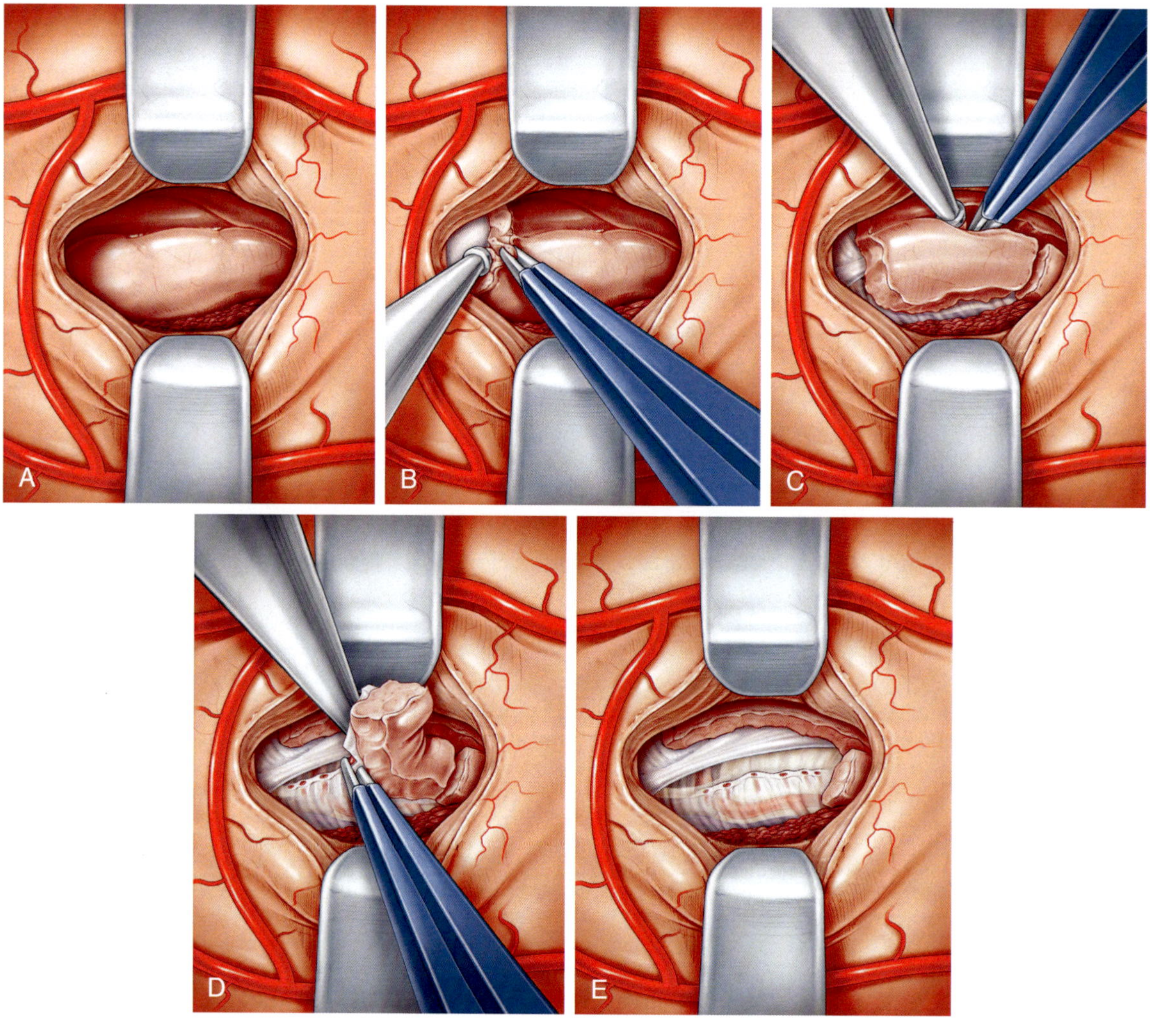

FIG. 17.4 Intraventricular microdissection. **(A)** The amygdala and hippocampus are identified, **(B)** dissection is carried out anterior to the medial pial boundary at the anterior uncus, **(C)** the incisural edge is identified and dissection is carried out posteriorly to encompass the uncus, taking care to preserve the medial pial boundary, and the hippocampal profile is visualized, **(D)** the hippocampus is freed from the choroidal fissure by microdissection of the fimbria, and then at a point which is aligned with the collicular plate on axial image guidance (approximately 2.5 cm of hippocampus), the hippocampus is divided, and the dissection is then carried anteriorly along the margin of the parahippocampal gyrus incorporating in the resection the entorhinal cortex and hippocampus, and the hippocampus is liberated anteriorly taking care to avoid damage to or traction on vessels within the hippocampal sulcus, and **(E)** the hippocampus is dissected free of the pia and vessels on both sides of the hippocampal sulcus and then removed.

lobe, and it transects the temporal stem. Furthermore, exposure of the sylvian vessels poses a risk of vascular injury or vasospasm.[30]

Subtemporal Approach

The advantages of the subtemporal approach[7] to SMAH include the avoidance of injury to the Meyer's loop (visual field defect) and the potential for fewer neuropsychologic sequelae.[20,31] The available data are insufficient to establish whether this is so. The disadvantages are that it may necessitate excessive retraction of the temporal lobe, result in injury to the vein of Labbe, and necessitate removal of the zygomatic process.

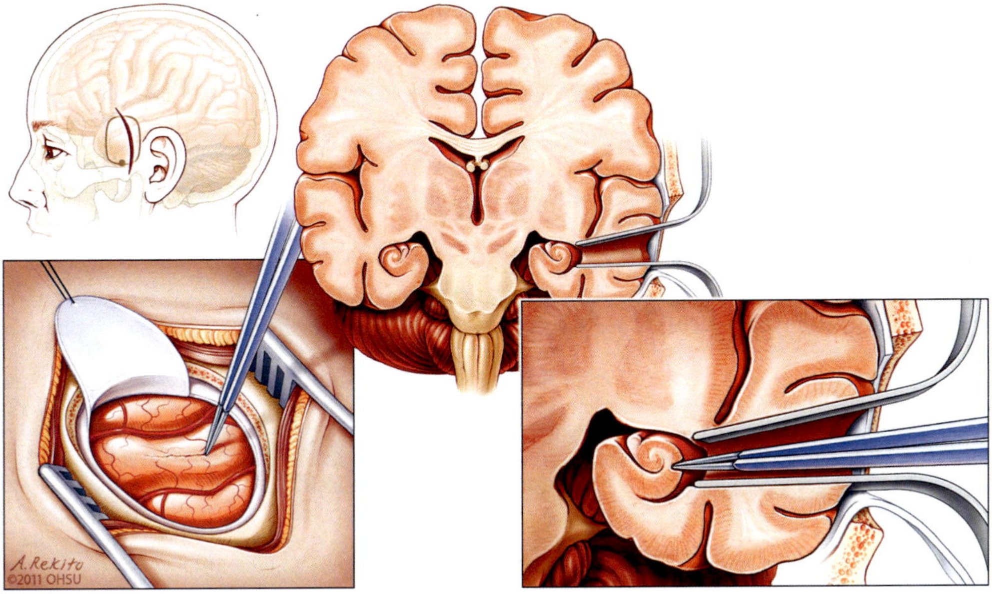

FIG. 17.5 Montage of the transcortical selective microsurgical amygdalohippocampectomy.

CONCLUSIONS

SMAH seizure-free outcomes appear to be comparable with those of a more conventional partial temporal lobectomy or a more limited lobectomy, the ATL. The evidence that this more limited procedure produces superior neuropsychologic outcomes is mixed. Likewise, proof that differences exist between various approaches to SMAH is compromised by small single-center studies with the potential for bias. No truly statistically valid comparative trials of different approaches to SMAH have been published. Currently the choice of procedures is largely determined by the experience of each center. We favor the transcortical approach because it is relatively straightforward and can be accomplished with what has now become routine image-guided surgical technique.

Surgery for epilepsy, particularly resection of the mesial temporal lobe structures in patients with mesial temporal sclerosis, and other pathologies in this area, remains one of the most effective and *underused* surgical procedures in all subspecialties of surgery. As new and increasingly complex, technologically sophisticated, and expensive methods of seizure control emerge, it is wise to remember that in well-selected patients, few surgical procedures rival amygdalohippocampectomy for effectiveness and life-changing potential.

REFERENCES

1. Wiebe S, Blume WT, Girvin JP, Eliasziw M. A randomized, controlled trial of surgery for temporal-lobe epilepsy. *N Engl J Med*. 2001;345(5):311–318.
2. Spencer DD, Spencer SS, Mattson RH, Williamson PD, Novelly RA. Access to the posterior medial temporal lobe structures in the surgical treatment of temporal lobe epilepsy. *Neurosurgery*. 1984;15(5):667–671.
3. Spencer DD. Temporal lobectomy. In: Luders H, ed. *Epilepsy Surgery*. New York, NY: Raven Press; 1991:533–545.
4. Niemeyer P. The transventricular amygdalahippocampectomy in temporal lobe epilepsy. In: Baldwin M, Bailey P, eds. *Temporal Lobe Epilepsy*. Springfield, IL: Charles C. Thomas; 1958:461–482.
5. Wieser HG, Yaşargil MG. Selective amygdalohippocampectomy as a surgical treatment of mesiobasal limbic epilepsy. *Surg Neurol*. 1982;17(6):445–457.
6. Yaşargil MG, Wieser HG, Valavanis A, von Ammon K, Roth P. Surgery and results of selective amygdalahippocampectomy in one hundred patients with nonlesional limbic epilepsy. *Neurosurg Clin N Am*. 1993;4(2): 243–261.
7. Park TS, Bourgeois BF, Silbergeld DL, Dodson WE. Subtemporal transparahippocampal amygdalohippocampectomy for surgical treatment of mesial temporal lobe epilepsy. Technical note *J Neurosurg*. 1996;85(6):1172–1176.
8. Little AS, Smith KA, Kirlin K, et al. Modifications to the subtemporal selective amygdalohippocampectomy using a minimal-access technique: seizure and neuropsychological outcomes. *J Neurosurg*. 2009;111(6):1263–1274.

9. Arruda F, Cendes F, Andermann F, et al. Mesial atrophy and outcome after amygdalohippocampectomy or temporal lobe removal. *Ann Neurol.* 1996;40(3):446–450.
10. Clusmann H, Schramm J, Kral T, et al. Prognostic factors and outcome after different types of resection for temporal lobe epilepsy. *J Neurosurg.* 2002;97(5):1131–1141.
11. Paglioli E, Palmini A, Portuguez M, et al. Seizure and memory outcome following temporal lobe surgery: selective compared with nonselective approaches for hippocampal sclerosis. *J Neurosurg.* 2006;104(1):70–78.
12. Acar G, Acar F, Miller J, Spencer DC, Burchiel KJ. Seizure outcome following transcortical selective amygdalohippocampectomy in mesial temporal lobe epilepsy. *Stereotact Funct Neurosurg.* 2008;86(5):314–319.
13. Tanriverdi T, Olivier A, Poulin N, Andermann F, Dubeau F. Long-term seizure outcome after mesial temporal lobe epilepsy surgery: corticalamygdalohippocampectomy versus selective amygdalohippocampectomy. *J Neurosurg.* 2008;108(3):517–524.
14. Schramm J, Lehmann TN, Zentner J, et al. Randomized controlled trial of 2.5-cm versus 3.5-cm mesial temporal resection—Part 2: volumetric resection extent and subgroup analyses. *Acta Neurochir (Wien).* 2011;153(2): 221–228.
15. Josephson CB, Dykeman J, Fiest KM, et al. Systematic review and meta-analysis of standard vs selective temporal lobe epilepsy surgery. *Neurology.* 2013;80(18): 1669–1676.
16. Mathern GW, Miller JW. Outcomes for temporal lobe epilepsy operations may not be equal: a call for an RCT of ATL vs SAH. *Neurology.* 2013;80(18):1630–1631.
17. Pauli E, Pickel S, Schulemann H, Buchfelder M, Stefan H. Neuropsychologic findings depending on the type of the resection in temporal lobe epilepsy. *Adv Neurol.* 1999;81: 371–377.
18. Gleissner U, Helmstaedter C, Schramm J, Elger CE. Memory outcome after selective amygdalohippocampectomy: a study in 140 patients with temporal lobe epilepsy. *Epilepsia.* 2002;43(1):87–95.
19. Helmstaedter C, Reuber M, Elger CC. Interaction of cognitive aging and memory deficits related to epilepsy surgery. *Ann Neurol.* 2002;52(1):89–94.
20. Hori T, Yamane F, Ochiai T, Hayashi M, Taira T. Subtemporal amygdalohippocampectomy prevents verbal memory impairment in the language-dominant hemisphere. *Stereotact Funct Neurosurg.* 2003;80(1–4):18–21.
21. Gleissner U, Helmstaedter C, Schramm J, Elger CE. Memory outcome after selective amygdalohippocampectomy in patients with temporal lobe epilepsy: one-year follow-up. *Epilepsia.* 2004;45(8):960–962.
22. Morino M, Uda T, Naito K, et al. Comparison of neuropsychological outcomes after selective amygdalohippocampectomy versus anterior temporal lobectomy. *Epilepsy Behav.* 2006;9(1):95–100.
23. Hori T, Yamane F, Ochiai T, et al. Selective subtemporal amygdalohippocampectomy for refractory temporal lobe epilepsy: operative and neuropsychological outcomes. *J Neurosurg.* 2007;106(1):134–141.
24. Goldstein LH, Polkey CE. Short-term cognitive changes after unilateral temporal lobectomy or unilateral amygdalo-hippocampectomy for the relief of temporal lobe epilepsy. *J Neurol Neurosurg Psychiatry.* 1993;56(2): 135–140.
25. Wolf RL, Ivnik RJ, Hirschorn KA, Sharbrough FW, Cascino GD, Marsh WR. Neurocognitive efficiency following left temporal lobectomy: standard versus limited resection. *J Neurosurg.* 1993;79(1):76–83.
26. Jones-Gotman M, Zatorre RJ, Olivier A, et al. Learning and retention of words and designs following excision from medial or lateral temporal-lobe structures. *Neuropsychologia.* 1997;35(7):963–973.
27. Tanriverdi T, Dudley RW, Hasan A, et al. Memory outcome after temporal lobe epilepsy surgery: corticoamygdalohippocampectomy versus selective amygdalohippocampectomy. *J Neurosurg.* 2010;113(6):1164–1175.
28. Egan RA, Shults WT, So N, Burchiel KJ, Kellogg JX, Salinsky M. Visual field deficits in conventional anterior temporal lobectomy versus amygdalohippocampectomy. *Neurology.* 2000;55:1818–1822.
29. Yaşargil MG, Krayenbühl N, Roth P, Hsu SP, Yaşargil DC. The selective amygdalohippocampectomy for intractable temporal limbic seizures. *J Neurosurg.* 2010;112(1): 168–185 (ISSN: 1933–0693).
30. Schaller C, Jung A, Clusmann H, Schramm J, Meyer B. Rate of vasospasm following the transsylvian versus transcortical approach for selective amygdalohippocampectomy. *Neurol Res.* 2004;26(6):666–670.
31. Takaya S, Mikuni N, Mitsueda T, et al. Improved cerebral function in mesial temporal lobe epilepsy after subtemporal amygdalohippocampectomy. *Brain.* 2009;132(Pt 1): 185–194.

CHAPTER 18

Cortical Dysplasia and Extratemporal Resections in Epilepsy

KUNAL GUPTA, MBBChir (Cantab), PHD • NATHAN R. SELDEN, MD, PHD (Cantab)

INTRODUCTION

Focal cortical dysplasias (FCDs) are discrete regions of malformed cerebral cortex, strongly associated with clinical epilepsy in both adults and children. Cortical dysplasias occur primarily or in association with a range of developmental disorders such as lissencephaly, schizencephaly, hemimegalencephaly, and tuberous sclerosis. This chapter will focus on primary FCD. FCDs were originally described by Taylor et al. in 1971.[1] The subsequent advent of magnetic resonance imaging (MRI) has lowered detection thresholds, resulting in FCD identification in 8%–12% of adult patients and up to 14% of pediatric patients with medically refractory epilepsy.[2] A significant proportion of FCDs are not detected on MRI and are only confirmed on surgical pathology; therefore the true prevalence is likely higher. FCDs have become the subject of comprehensive clinical evaluation and surgical resection, with the goal of achieving seizure freedom. With evolving imaging and surgical techniques, clinical success rates have increased over time.[3]

FOCAL CORTICAL DYSPLASIA CLASSIFICATION

Taylor and colleagues originally described 10 patients from a series of 300 patients with epilepsy over 20 years of clinical practice, characterized by a distinct structural abnormality in the cerebral cortex.[1] In these patients, the authors described defined regions of cortical thickening, loss of lamination deep to cortical layer 1, and the presence of large abnormal neurons and malformed cells with large or multiple nuclei and opalescent pseudopodic cytoplasm (later named "balloon cells"). Taylor recognized that this phenomenon shared histopathologic features with tuberous sclerosis; however, he noted that patients did not share any clinical stigmata with tuberous sclerosis. Taylor therefore concluded that there was little to no association between these entities. Thereafter, FCDs were described as non–Taylor-type FCD, or Taylor-type FCD with or without balloon cells. Taylor-type FCD represented cytoarchitectural cortical disruption with giant dysmorphic neurons.[4]

FCDs were reclassified by Colombo et al. in 2003 by histology and correlated with MRI findings[5]; these authors described three subtypes: architectural dysplasia,cytoarchitectural dysplasia, and Taylor-type FCD. In architectural dysplasia, FCDs contained heterotopic neurons and deranged lamination without cellular aberration. Cytoarchitectural dysplasia contained cellular aberration due to giant neurons, and Taylor-type FCD contained neuronal dysmorphism with or without balloon cells.

The Palmini classification,[6] published shortly thereafter, superseded the classification by Colombo et al.[5] as the leading FCD classification. Palmini et al. grouped all disorders of cortical dysgenesis under "malformations due to abnormal cortical development" and reserved the term FCD for a subset of disorders characterized by strictly or mostly intracortical abnormalities.[6] Mild malformations of cortical development demonstrated microscopic neuronal heterotopia, without associated MRI findings. FCDs were categorized under similar histologic criteria to those described by Colombo et al.: type 1a demonstrated architectural abnormalities and dyslamination and type 1b demonstrated cytoarchitectural abnormalities with giant or immature neurons without dysmorphism.[5] Type 2 demonstrated dysmorphic neurons, synonymous with Taylor-type FCD, with types 2a and 2b separated by the absence or presence of balloon cells, respectively. Palmini et al. also correlated individual types of FCD with clinical features, suggesting that types 1a and 1b may be asymptomatic or may present with medically refractory epilepsy and in the latter case have a better prognosis for surgical cure than other subtypes of FCD.[6] These authors also suggested that type 2 FCDs commonly present with medically refractory epilepsy because of high intrinsic epileptogenicity and have a worse prognosis after surgery.

More recently, in 2011, the classification of extratemporal FCDs has been superseded by that of Blumcke.[7] These lesions are currently classified by etiology and histologic features into three subtypes and further subclassified therein.[7] Focal cortical dysplasia types 1 and 2 are primary cortical dysplasias, whereas type 3 represents FCD occurring secondary to other structural abnormalities. This classification system is summarized in Table 18.1.

Focal Cortical Dysplasia Type 1

Focal cortical dysplasia type 1 presents with abnormal cortical layering. Type 1a demonstrates abnormal cortical layering owing to compromised radial migration. There is abundant radial microcolumnar organization, with a microcolumn defined as more than eight neurons aligned in a vertical column. Type 1b is characterized by abnormal tangential cortical organization with loss of clear laminar organization of the six-layered neocortex. Typically, layers 1 and 2, or 2 and 3, are blurred; layer 4 can also be lost or obscured. Furthermore, in this subtype, cellular abnormalities can be encountered, with immature small diameter neurons, hypertrophied pyramidal neurons in layer 5, or normal neurons with aberrant dendritic arborization (Table 18.1).

Focal Cortical Dysplasia Type 2

Focal cortical dysplasia type 2 presents with disrupted cortical lamination and is characterized by the presence of dysmorphic neurons. The laminar disorganization differs from type 1 in which individual laminae are affected; in type 2, there is no identifiable cortical lamination apart from layer 1. The nature of the neuronal abnormality defines the subclass; type 2a demonstrates dysmorphic neurons with significant enlargement of the cell body and nucleus, as well as margination of Nissl granules, without balloon cells. Type 2b is characterized by the presence of balloon cells (Fig. 18.1 and Table 18.1). Balloon cells are large and often multinucleated giant cells that are presumed to have an intermediate cell lineage. The majority of balloon cells express vimentin or nestin, intermediate filament proteins, and a small proportion of balloon cells ($<10\%$) express stem cell markers such as CD34, SOX2, and CD133. The coexpression of glial fibrillary acidic protein and medium chain neurofilament with immature cell markers suggests that these cells are of transitional glial and neuronal lineages.[8]

Focal Cortical Dysplasia Type 3

Focal cortical dysplasia type 3 defines abnormalities in cortical lamination or cellular structure (neuronal hypertrophy outside of layer 5) secondary to a primary pathology that is typically adjacent to or afflicts the same cortical area. Type 3a is associated with hippocampal sclerosis. Type 3a lesions were demonstrated to be epileptogenic by depth electrode recording; seizures were found to propagate both from the sclerotic hippocampus to the neocortical dysplasia and vice versa, with more frequent onset in the hippocampus correlating with worse hippocampal sclerosis. Furthermore, similar ictal patterns were found in temporal neocortical focal cortical dysplasia associated with hippocampal sclerosis as in extratemporal focal cortical dysplasia.[9] In temporal neocortical FCD, hypertrophic neurons are typically found in layers 2–4, with layers 2 and 3 often demonstrating severe neuronal loss and laminar gliosis. Although class 3a also includes temporal lobe subcortical heterotopias, which are often smaller than MRI detection thresholds, true mesial temporal sclerosis and other lesions of the temporal lobe are excluded from class 3a and would be termed "dual pathology." Class 3b includes laminar or cellular aberration due to adjacent epileptogenic tumors, such as ganglioglioma or dysembryoplastic neuroepithelial tumor. Class 3c is associated with vascular malformations, including cavernomas, arteriovenous malformations, dural arteriovenous fistulas, or telangiectasias. Class 3d is associated with injurious lesions acquired in early life, such as prenatal or perinatal ischemic injury, inflammation, infection, or traumatic lesions (Table 18.1).

There is significant overlap between these classification schemes, as well as others not mentioned herein. Each is primarily determined by histologic appearance, based on the degree of lamination disturbance, cellular aberration, and the presence of dysmorphic neurons and balloon cells. Blumcke 1a correlates with both Palmini 1a and Colombo's description of architectural abnormalities, based on the presence of dyslamination alone. Blumcke 1b correlates with Palmini 1b and Colombo's description of cytoarchitectural disturbance, based on the presence of giant neurons and cytologic aberration without dysmorphism. Blumcke 2, Palmini 2, and Taylor-type FCD all share the presence of dysmorphic neurons, with 2a and 2b separated by the absence and presence of balloon cells, respectively, across each classification. Therefore, the terminology used herein remains representative of the original sources.

TABLE 18.1
Blumcke et al. Classification System for Focal Cortical Dysplasia

Focal Cortical Dysplasia							
Type 1		**Type 2**		**Type 3**			
1a	**1b**	**2a**	**2b**	**3a**	**3b**	**3c**	**3d**
				Associated with			
• Abundant radial microcolumnar organization	• Abnormal tangential cortical organization	• Dysmorphic neurons	• Dysmorphic neurons	• Hippocampal sclerosis	• Adjacent epileptogenic tumors	• Vascular malformations	• Injurious lesions
• Compromised radial migration	• Loss of laminar organization		• Presence of balloon cells				
• Partially disrupted cortical lamination		• Widely disrupted cortical lamination with preservation of layer 1					
• Abnormal neurons							

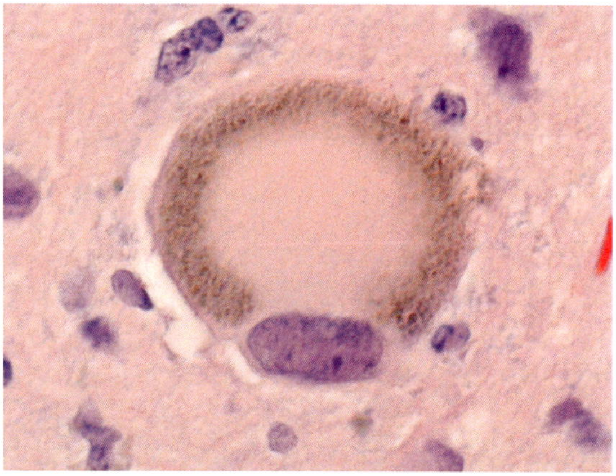

FIG. 18.1 Hematoxylin eosin stain of a balloon cell, demonstrating opalescent cytoplasm and margination of Nissl granules.

CLINICAL PRESENTATION

Focal cortical dysplasias are the most common cause of surgically treatable epilepsy in children and the third most common cause in adults after hippocampal sclerosis and tumors.[3,10] In the pediatric population, patients with FCD develop seizures at younger ages compared with other etiologies (2.6 years vs. 5.1 years), present to surgery at younger ages (7.9 years vs. 10.7 years), and are more likely to have daily seizures (70% vs. 48%).[11] These findings were corroborated in other series.[10] Multifocal lesions are noted in 30% −47% of patients.[11,12] In adults, FCD type 1 typically presents later in life with milder epilepsy, whereas FCD type 2 often presents earlier with a more severe seizure burden. Similarly, patients with multifocal FCD (type 1 or 2) also present earlier with more frequent seizures than patients with isolated focal lesions.[6,10] FCDs are more commonly localized to the lateral hemispheric surfaces rather than medial or basal surfaces, with type 1 lesions often located in the temporal lobe and type 2 lesions often extratemporal in location.[12,13]

PRESURGICAL EVALUATION

Electroencephalogram

Because FCD may present in any cortical lobe, seizure semiology is variable. Scalp electroencephalogram (EEG) also has low diagnostic sensitivity for cortical dysplasia. Interictal EEG abnormalities correspond with the region of cortical dysplasia in between 32% and 62% of cases, whereas ictal EEG corresponds to dysplasia location in 42%–77% of cases.[10,14,15] Furthermore, no specific diagnostic EEG pattern has been identified for cortical dysplasia; however, typical EEG findings may include interictal slowing, spikes, and polyspikes.[10,16] In addition, although some studies have suggested that type 1 FCDs are more likely to present with slowing than type 2,[14] these findings have not be recapitulated in other studies.[10] Therefore, although scalp EEG may provide localization information in up to two-thirds of patients, it does not provide diagnostic information nor does it distinguish between mild and severe FCD.

Imaging

When positive, structural MRI findings are highly predictive for diagnosing FCD. Numerous MRI features have been described in cortical dysplasia, including thickened cortical gray matter, abnormal gyral configuration, blurred gray-white matter junction, white and gray matter T2 signal hyperintensity, focal hypoplasia, white matter atrophy, and transmantle dysplasia.[5,10,17] However, MR images are often normal in patients harboring cortical dysplasia. Patients with FCD type 1 are more likely to present with normal MRI than those with FCD type 2; MRI is normal in approximately 40% of type 1 FCD cases and approximately 15% of type 2 FCD cases.[10]

Colombo et al. attempted to correlate the appearance of FCD on MRI with subtype to guide preoperative diagnosis.[5] Architectural FCD is characterized by lobar or subcortical hypoplasia, atrophy of the underlying white matter, enlargement of the associated subarachnoid space, and blurring of the gray-white matter junction. Cytoarchitectural FCD demonstrates similar MRI findings to Taylor-type FCD, with focal cortical thickening, gray-white matter junction blurring, and white matter T2 hyperintensity and T1 hypointensity. Taylor-type FCD is characterized by focal cortical thickening, blurring of the gray-white matter junction, increased T2 hyperintensity and reduced T1 signal intensity of the subcortical white matter, and white matter tracts leading radially from the FCD to the ventricular surface, also known as transmantle dysplasia (Fig. 18.2).[4–6,17]

The diagnostic value of MRI is variable according to the underlying histologic subtype. MRI findings are diagnostic for Taylor-type/type 2 FCD in 66%–100% of cases.[5,18,19] In cytoarchitectural dysplasia, 50% of cases can be diagnosed by MRI; however, there is significant overlap with findings associated with Taylor-type FCD. In architectural dysplasia, 61% of cases demonstrate diagnostic MRI findings.[5,19] Transmantle dysplasia describes the presence of radial cortical abnormalities between the ventricular surface and the region of cortical dysplasia. This structural abnormality has been described uniquely in FCD type 2 and is present on MRI in 37.5% of cases.[10,14]

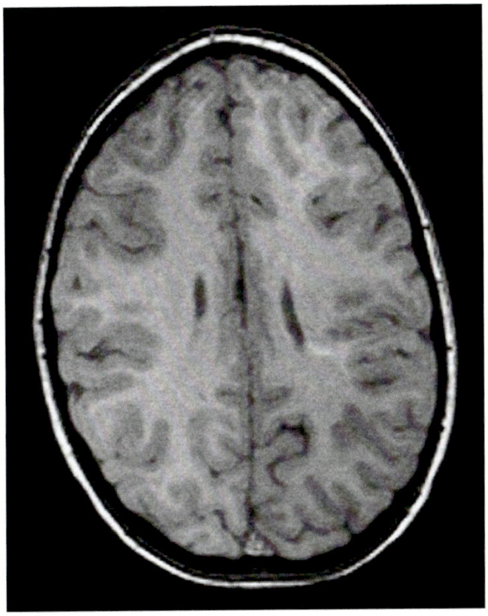

FIG. 18.2 High-resolution axial magnetic resonance imaging T1 weighted image of a patient with type 2 focal cortical dysplasia, demonstrating left frontal transmantle dysplasia.

Hypometabolism on interictal fluorine-18 fluorodeoxyglucose positron emission tomography (18FDG-PET) can be used in correlation with structural MRI to increase the sensitivity of FCD identification. Interictal PET correlates with positive structural MRI findings in 60%–75% of patients with FCD types 1 and 2.[10,14] In the setting of negative MRI findings, FDG-PET has been shown to improve localization in 33%–64% of cases, with particular benefit in FCD type 1 because of its higher association with negative MRI findings.[10,19]

Intracranial Electrode Placement

Intracranial electrode placement can be performed for increased resolution in detection of the epileptogenic zone. Grids may also be used for extraoperative simulation mapping of eloquent cortical function, greatly increasing their use for epilepsy resection evaluation and planning (Fig. 18.3). Published rates for intracranial electrode utilization in cortical dysplasia range widely from 6% to 68% with no significant difference noted between utilization rates for FCD types 1 and 2.[10,14,20] Patients are often selected for intracranial electrode placement because of difficulty in noninvasive seizure localization or proximity to eloquent cortex, and as a result, electrode placement may be associated with poorer postoperative outcomes.[21] Widdes et al. reported on the use of subdural grids to evaluate a series of 48 patients with FCD. The authors reported diffuse ictal onsets in 35% of cases, and in 49% of cases the onset was noted to be at the edge of the grid region. Ictal onset at the edge of the grid was the strongest independent predictor for seizure recurrence and may suggest that the grids need to be relocated or that epilepsy surgery may be a poor option for these patients.[22]

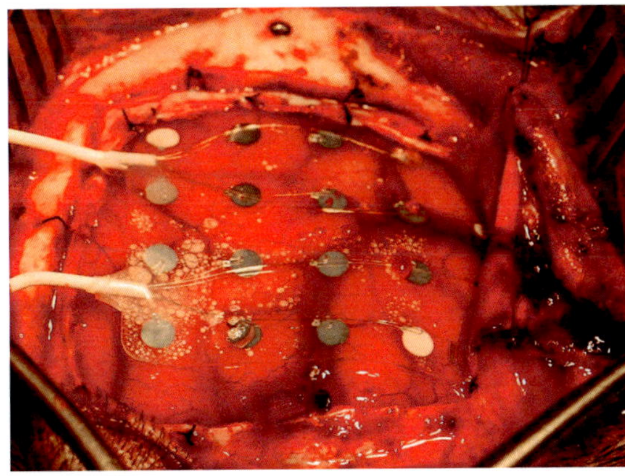

FIG. 18.3 Intraoperative photograph, demonstrating placement of subdural grid for invasive electrocorticography.

Surgical Technique

Surgical treatment for FCD is primarily focused on maximal safe resection. Cortical resection is limited by the involvement of eloquent areas, including primary motor, sensory, visual, and language cortex. The use of image guidance during cortical resection improves the ability to target radiographically apparent lesions and can be used in conjunction with intracranial electrode monitoring to target the neurophysiologic substrate for seizure generation. Surgical techniques using intraoperative pathology to obtain clear margins show increased seizure freedom when clear margins are obtained[20] but remain limited by eloquent cortex. In cases where seizure foci extend into eloquent cortex, multiple subpial transections may limit seizure propagation.[23]

Alternatively, neurostimulation using vagal nerve stimulation (VNS), transcranial magnetic stimulation (TMS), or deep brain stimulation (DBS) has been reported to enhance seizure control with variable efficacy and therefore may present as options for patients with FCDs in eloquent cortex. VNS has been demonstrated in adults to have a low rate of seizure of freedom (7%–30% of patients) and improvement in seizure burden in up to 60% of patients. Earlier implantation, unilateral seizure activity by EEG, and the presence of focal cortical dysplasia predict better seizure control with VNS.[24,25] In the pediatric population, VNS therapy can provide long-term seizure reduction in 60% of patients by a median of 60% at up to 3 years after implantation; 43% had over 75% reduction in seizure burden and 10% were seizure-free.[26] We obtained similar results at our institution, evaluating outcomes after VNS placement in 146 patients over a 10-year period; seizure frequency was reduced in 91% of patients, seizure duration was reduced in 50%, postictal period was reduced in 49%, and medication use was reduced in 75%; no difference was noted between patients with generalized and partial epilepsy.[27] TMS has been trialed in adult patients with FCD who were not surgical candidates, with up to 50% seizure reduction sustained at 8 weeks after treatment compared with control.[28] However, studies are currently limited to small groups and case reports.[28–31] DBS has been trialed, with multiple targets including the anterior nucleus of the thalamus and subthalamic nucleus in cryptogenic refractory epilepsy[32,33] with similar results (approximately 54% of patients having at least 50% seizure reduction at 2 years). More extensive discussion on DBS for epilepsy can be found in reviews by Laxpati et al. and Tykocki et al.[34,35] The gold standard surgical intervention for focal cortical dysplasia remains cortical resection.[36]

Surgical Outcomes

Many groups have reported on seizure freedom after surgical resection since Taylor's original description in 1971.[1] Outcomes are generally favorable with approximately two-thirds of patients achieving seizure freedom. Seizure freedom after surgery is more likely with more severe pathology associated with type 2 FCD (61%–67% in 2a, and 75%–88% in 2b), as opposed to milder pathology associated with type 1 FCD (49%–52% in 1a, and 45%–61% in 1b).[37,38] The variable most associated with seizure freedom is extent of resection; incomplete resection as confirmed by MRI or intracranial EEG is strongly associated with seizure recurrence.[14,20,22,38] Complete resection results in seizure freedom in up to 80%–92% of cases.[20,39,40] Complete resections are achieved in 60%–70% of cases.[20,38]

In the remaining cases, incomplete resection is typically attributed to the presence of eloquent cortex, multifocal or widespread regions of seizure onset, or cryptogenic localization on preoperative studies. Seizure freedom after incomplete resection is reported to be as low as 30%–40%.[20,38] Although use of intracranial EEG is associated with reduced postoperative seizure control,[21] this is likely due to the confounding factor of increased use of intracranial EEG near eloquent cortex. Proximity to eloquent cortex has been cited as the principal reason for incomplete resection.[38,41] Interestingly, in a study of FCDs affecting eloquent cortex, balloon cells were found exclusively in nonfunctional areas that also demonstrated fluid-attenuated inversion recovery hyperintensity on MRI and were absent in functional perirolandic areas. These latter functional regions demonstrated pathology consistent with FCD type 1.[41] Therefore it is possible that the extent of pathologic aberration has an effect on retention of cortical function; regions with milder pathologic changes may be associated with higher retention of cortical function, and regions demonstrating severe pathologic changes may be more likely to be nonfunctional and amenable to resection.

CONCLUSION

In conclusion, FCD is a relatively common cause of epilepsy in both children and adults. Since its original description in 1971, characterization of FCD has undergone extensive evolution based on the observed underlying cortical and cellular aberrations and associated structural abnormalities. Clinical investigation for FCD can be challenging in certain cases owing to poorly localizing EEG and MRI. Despite these limitations, outcomes after targeted surgical resection are typically favorable, with two-thirds of patients becoming seizure-free. Complete surgical resection can be hampered by poor preoperative localization and involvement of eloquent cortex; in these cases, palliative therapies such as neurostimulation by VNS, DBS, or TMS remain viable alternative surgical therapies.

REFERENCES

1. Taylor DC, Falconer MA, Bruton CJ, Corsellis JAN. Focal dysplasia of the cerebral cortex in epilepsy. *J Neurol Neurosurg Psychiatry*. 1971;34(4):369–387.
2. Sisodiya SM. Surgery for malformations of cortical development causing epilepsy. *Brain*. 2000;123(Pt 6):1075–1091.
3. Hauptman JS, Mathern GW. Surgical treatment of epilepsy associated with cortical dysplasia: 2012 update. *Epilepsia*. 2012;53(suppl 4):98–104.
4. Bronen RA, Vives KP, Kim JH, Fulbright RK, Spencer SS, Spencer DD. Focal cortical dysplasia of Taylor, balloon cell subtype: MR differentiation from low-grade tumors. *Am J Neuroradiol*. 1997;18(6):1141–1151.
5. Colombo N, Tassi L, Galli C, et al. Focal cortical dysplasias: MR imaging, histopathologic, and clinical correlations in surgically treated patients with epilepsy. *Am J Neuroradiol*. 2003;24(4):724–733.
6. Palmini A, Najm I, Avanzini G, et al. Terminology and classification of the cortical dysplasias. *Neurology*. 2004; 62(6 suppl 3):S2–S8.

7. Blumcke I, Thom M, Aronica E, et al. The clinicopathologic spectrum of focal cortical dysplasias: a consensus classification proposed by an ad hoc Task Force of the ILAE Diagnostic Methods Commission. *Epilepsia*. 2011;52(1):158–174.
8. Oh HS, Lee MC, Kim HS, et al. Pathophysiologic characteristics of balloon cells in cortical dysplasia. *Childs Nerv Syst*. 2008;24(2):175–183.
9. Fauser S, Schulze-Bonhage A. Epileptogenicity of cortical dysplasia in temporal lobe dual pathology: an electrophysiological study with invasive recordings. *Brain*. 2006;129(Pt 1):82–95.
10. Lerner JT, Salamon N, Hauptman JS, et al. Assessment and surgical outcomes for mild type I and severe type II cortical dysplasia: a critical review and the UCLA experience. *Epilepsia*. 2009;50(6):1310–1335.
11. Harvey AS, Cross JH, Shinnar S, Mathern GW. Defining the spectrum of international practice in pediatric epilepsy surgery patients. *Epilepsia*. 2008;49(1):146–155.
12. Leventer RJ, Phelan EM, Coleman LT, Kean MJ, Jackson GD, Harvey AS. Clinical and imaging features of cortical malformations in childhood. *Neurology*. 1999;53(4):715–722.
13. Fauser S, Sisodiya SM, Martinian L, et al. Multi-focal occurrence of cortical dysplasia in epilepsy patients. *Brain*. 2009;132(Pt 8):2079–2090.
14. Krsek P, Pieper T, Karlmeier A, et al. Different presurgical characteristics and seizure outcomes in children with focal cortical dysplasia type I or II. *Epilepsia*. 2009;50(1):125–137.
15. Siegel AM, Cascino GD, Meyer FB, Marsh WR, Scheithauer BW, Sharbrough FW. Surgical outcome and predictive factors in adult patients with intractable epilepsy and focal cortical dysplasia. *Acta Neurol Scand*. 2006;113(2):65–71.
16. Noachtar S, Bilgin O, Remi J, et al. Interictal regional polyspikes in noninvasive EEG suggest cortical dysplasia as etiology of focal epilepsies. *Epilepsia*. 2008;49(6):1011–1017.
17. Barkovich AJ, Kuzniecky RI, Bollen AW, Grant PE. Focal transmantle dysplasia: a specific malformation of cortical development. *Neurology*. 1997;49(4):1148–1152.
18. Kral T, von Lehe M, Podlogar M, et al. Focal cortical dysplasia: long term seizure outcome after surgical treatment. *J Neurol Neurosurg Psychiatry*. 2007;78(8):853–856.
19. Salamon N, Kung J, Shaw SJ, et al. FDG-PET/MRI coregistration improves detection of cortical dysplasia in patients with epilepsy. *Neurology*. 2008;71(20):1594–1601.
20. Cohen-Gadol AA, Ozduman K, Bronen RA, Kim JH, Spencer DD. Long-term outcome after epilepsy surgery for focal cortical dysplasia. *J Neurosurg*. 2004;101(1):55–65.
21. Widdess-Walsh P, Kellinghaus C, Jeha L, et al. Electro-clinical and imaging characteristics of focal cortical dysplasia: correlation with pathological subtypes. *Epilepsy Res*. 2005;67(1–2):25–33.
22. Widdess-Walsh P, Jeha L, Nair D, Kotagal P, Bingaman W, Najm I. Subdural electrode analysis in focal cortical dysplasia: predictors of surgical outcome. *Neurology*. 2007;69(7):660–667.
23. Sawhney IM, Robertson IJ, Polkey CE, Binnie CD, Elwes RD. Multiple subpial transection: a review of 21 cases. *J Neurol Neurosurg Psychiatry*. 1995;58(3):344–349.
24. Ghaemi K, Elsharkawy AE, Schulz R, et al. Vagus nerve stimulation: outcome and predictors of seizure freedom in long-term follow-up. *Seizure*. 2010;19(5):264–268.
25. Janszky J, Hoppe M, Behne F, Tuxhorn I, Pannek HW, Ebner A. Vagus nerve stimulation: predictors of seizure freedom. *J Neurol Neurosurg Psychiatry*. 2005;76(3):384–389.
26. Alexopoulos AV, Kotagal P, Loddenkemper T, Hammel J, Bingaman WE. Long-term results with vagus nerve stimulation in children with pharmacoresistant epilepsy. *Seizure*. 2006;15(7):491–503.
27. Thompson EM, Wozniak SE, Roberts CM, Kao A, Anderson VC, Selden NR. Vagus nerve stimulation for partial and generalized epilepsy from infancy to adolescence. *J Neurosurg Pediatr*. 2012;10(3):200–205.
28. Fregni F, Otachi PT, Do Valle A, et al. A randomized clinical trial of repetitive transcranial magnetic stimulation in patients with refractory epilepsy. *Ann Neurol*. 2006;60(4):447–455.
29. Menkes DL, Gruenthal M. Slow-frequency repetitive transcranial magnetic stimulation in a patient with focal cortical dysplasia. *Epilepsia*. 2000;41(2):240–242.
30. Misawa S, Kuwabara S, Shibuya K, Mamada K, Hattori T. Low-frequency transcranial magnetic stimulation for epilepsia partialis continua due to cortical dysplasia. *J Neurol Sci*. 2005;234(1–2):37–39.
31. Santiago-Rodriguez E, Cardenas-Morales L, Harmony T, Fernandez-Bouzas A, Porras-Kattz E, Hernandez A. Repetitive transcranial magnetic stimulation decreases the number of seizures in patients with focal neocortical epilepsy. *Seizure*. 2008;17(8):677–683.
32. Benabid AL, Minotti L, Koudsie A, de Saint Martin A, Hirsch E. Antiepileptic effect of high-frequency stimulation of the subthalamic nucleus (corpus luysi) in a case of medically intractable epilepsy caused by focal dysplasia: a 30-month follow-up: technical case report. *Neurosurgery*. 2002;50(6):1385–1391; discussion 1391–1392.
33. Fisher R, Salanova V, Witt T, et al. Electrical stimulation of the anterior nucleus of thalamus for treatment of refractory epilepsy. *Epilepsia*. 2010;51(5):899–908.
34. Laxpati NG, Kasoff WS, Gross RE. Deep brain stimulation for the treatment of epilepsy: circuits, targets, and trials. *Neurotherapeutics*. 2014;11(3):508–526.
35. Tykocki T, Mandat T, Kornakiewicz A, Koziara H, Nauman P. Deep brain stimulation for refractory epilepsy. *Arch Med Sci*. 2012;8(5):805–816.
36. Guerrini R, Duchowny M, Jayakar P, et al. Diagnostic methods and treatment options for focal cortical dysplasia. *Epilepsia*. 2015;56(11):1669–1686.
37. Krsek P, Maton B, Korman B, et al. Different features of histopathological subtypes of pediatric focal cortical dysplasia. *Ann Neurol*. 2008;63(6):758–769.
38. Kim DW, Lee SK, Chu K, et al. Predictors of surgical outcome and pathologic considerations in focal cortical dysplasia. *Neurology*. 2009;72(3):211–216.

39. Alexandre Jr V, Walz R, Bianchin MM, et al. Seizure outcome after surgery for epilepsy due to focal cortical dysplastic lesions. *Seizure.* 2006;15(6):420–427.
40. Kloss S, Pieper T, Pannek H, Holthausen H, Tuxhorn I. Epilepsy surgery in children with focal cortical dysplasia (FCD): results of long-term seizure outcome. *Neuropediatrics.* 2002;33(1):21–26.
41. Marusic P, Najm IM, Ying Z, et al. Focal cortical dysplasias in eloquent cortex: functional characteristics and correlation with MRI and histopathologic changes. *Epilepsia.* 2002;43(1):27–32.

CHAPTER 19

Responsive Neurostimulation

LIA DE LEON ERNST, MD

INTRODUCTION

Approximately, 30% of patients with epilepsy fail to achieve seizure remission with appropriate antiepileptic medication trials. Patients falling into this medically refractory epilepsy group may be evaluated for potential surgical options to treat their epilepsy. Neurostimulation is a rapidly evolving treatment modality for medically refractory epilepsy, offering a palliative and therapeutic option for patients who have been determined to be poor candidates for resective surgery. Therapeutic stimulation can occur directly via subdural electrodes or deep brain stimulation (DBS), or indirectly via stimulation of peripheral nerves. Multiple targets for neurostimulation have been explored, but currently, three modalities of stimulation now have Class I evidence supporting their use: vagal nerve stimulation (VNS), DBS of the anterior nucleus of the thalamus (ANT), and responsive neurostimulation (the RNS System).[1] Only two of these modalities are approved by the FDA for use in the United States—VNS and the RNS System.

The RNS System is a new, cranially implanted medical device that was FDA approved for treatment of medically refractory focal epilepsy in 2013. It is the first neurostimulation treatment modality that involves closed-loop stimulation in response to epileptiform activity detected via electrocorticography.[2,3] A programmable neurostimulator, which is a battery-powered microprocessor embedded in a full-thickness craniectomy, is connected to depth and/or subdural cortical strip leads with four electrodes on each lead (see Fig. 19.1). Leads are surgically placed at one or two predetermined foci that are specifically targeted as seizure onset locations. Up to four leads can be placed, but currently, only two leads can be connected at a given time to the neurostimulator. The electrodes on the leads continuously detect electrocorticographic (ECoG) activity and can be used to both detect abnormal electric activity and provide stimulation in response to epileptiform activity or seizures, according to programmable parameters. The ECoG data can be uploaded to a central database by patients using a specialized wireless telemetry wand and a laptop that functions as a data transmitter, which can later be reviewed by physicians to plan for adjustments in detection and stimulation parameters to optimize control of seizures (see Fig. 19.2).[4]

The neurostimulator is held in place by a tray known as ferrule, which is placed in a full-thickness craniectomy so that it rests flush with the skull surface and is affixed to the skull using bone screws. The neurostimulator battery lasts an average of 4 years with medium settings and requires replacement via scalp incision. The neurostimulator is typically situated over the parietal region of the skull.[5]

RNS SYSTEM FUNCTIONALITY

The main functions of RNS are detection, storage, and stimulation. Several detection methods or tools are used to detect epileptiform activity. The two most commonly used tools are the line length and bandpass tools. The line length tool is designed to detect large increases in amplitude and/or frequency and is typically used in initial programming of the device to have high sensitivity for a wide range of frequencies and amplitudes that may indicate the presence of epileptiform activity. The bandpass tool can be fine-tuned to detect particular ranges of frequency and amplitude specific to the patient's electric patterns of interest, namely, seizures and epileptiform activity. Detection algorithms are adjusted over time to maximize sensitivity and specificity for each individual patient's electric patterns.[2]

Although the neurostimulator continuously monitors cerebral electrographic activity via implanted electrodes, the capacity for stored ECoG segments is limited to 6 min of data. Typically, the device is programmed to store four individual ECoG segments of 90 sec each and can be triggered to store an electrocorticogram based on multiple criteria. When detections

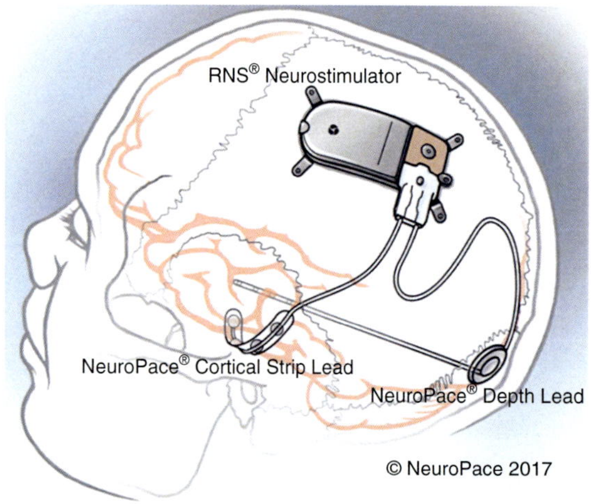

FIG. 19.1 Implanted RNS System neurostimulator, with subdural cortical strip and depth leads. (Copyright 2017, NeuroPace, Inc; image used with permission from NeuroPace, Inc.)

are triggered over a preset duration of time, the event is considered a "long episode," which can trigger storage. Data storage can also be triggered by scheduled times of day or by an external magnet swipe across the scalp over the neurostimulator, which the patient can use to indicate a clinical event.[2] Although storage capacity is limited to 6 min of electrocorticography, data are collected in other ways, including number and timing of detections, long episodes, magnet swipes, and other data points, which can be used with the clinical history to augment the physician's understanding of the patient's seizure burden and frequency. Data can be accessed in graphic format, which may reveal circadian, ultradian, or catamenial patterns to seizures. In patients with bilateral temporal epilepsy, the data can help physicians appreciate the lateralization ratio of seizures in a more natural, long-term ambulatory setting than can be observed during discrete periods of electroencephalogram (EEG) monitoring in the inpatient setting.[6]

The neurostimulator is programmed to deliver charge-balanced biphasic pulses, with bursts durations ranging from 10 to 5000 ms, frequencies ranging from 1 to 333 Hz, current amplitudes ranging from 1 to 12 mA, and pulse widths ranging from 40 to 1000 μs. The stimulation configuration can be arranged to deliver current between any combination of electrodes and the neurostimulator case itself, which results in being able to change the charge density and the area of current field, taking into account the area of the presumed brain region comprising the epileptogenic zone. Typically, electrodes are configured to either deliver stimulation in a bipolar fashion across electrode pairs (often used in patients with mesial temporal seizure onsets) or across all eight electrodes to the neurostimulator case (often used in patients with broader neocortical seizure onsets). Although a wide range of frequencies, current amplitudes, and pulse widths can be programmed, the settings typically programmed are based on settings commonly used in a randomized controlled trial: 1.5–3 mA for current, 160 μs for pulse width, 100–200 ms for burst duration, and 100–200 Hz for frequency.[2,7] Some unofficial guidelines for stimulation programming have been established among epileptologists and by the company NeuroPace that manufactures the device, but there remains much to be learned about the optimal settings for individual cases.

EVIDENCE FOR SAFETY AND EFFICACY

Evidence supporting safety and efficacy of the RNS System began with a "Feasibility Trial," during which 65 patients were implanted with the system and were monitored for adverse events, followed by the randomized controlled "Pivotal Trial," which examined safety and efficacy of the device. In the Pivotal Trial, 191 patients were implanted with the RNS System, and 2 months after surgery (and after optimizing seizure detection parameters), they were randomized to receive responsive stimulation or sham stimulation with only detection settings enabled. Both groups were followed for 12 weeks during this blinded period. Inclusion criteria include an age of 18–70 years, focal seizures, medically refractory epilepsy (failure of $\geq$ 2 AEDs), an average of three or more disabling seizures per month, and EEG evidence of one to two epileptogenic foci. Immediately after implantation, both groups reported a decrease in seizure frequency, reflective of a temporary postsurgery improvement known as "the implantation effect." Over the 3-month follow-up period, stimulated patients reported an average decrease in seizure frequency of 37.9% versus 17.3% in the sham treatment group. During a subsequent open-label period during which all enrolled patients received responsive neurostimulation; the benefit continued to improve in the treatment group, and seizure frequency improved in a similar manner in the group that originally received sham stimulation. Long-term monitoring of implanted patients after the blinded phase showed continued and increased benefit from the device over time, with 43% and 46% of patients achieving a >50% reduction in seizure frequency after 1 and 2 years, respectively. The median percent reduction in seizure frequency was 44% after 1 year and 53% after 2 years.[8]

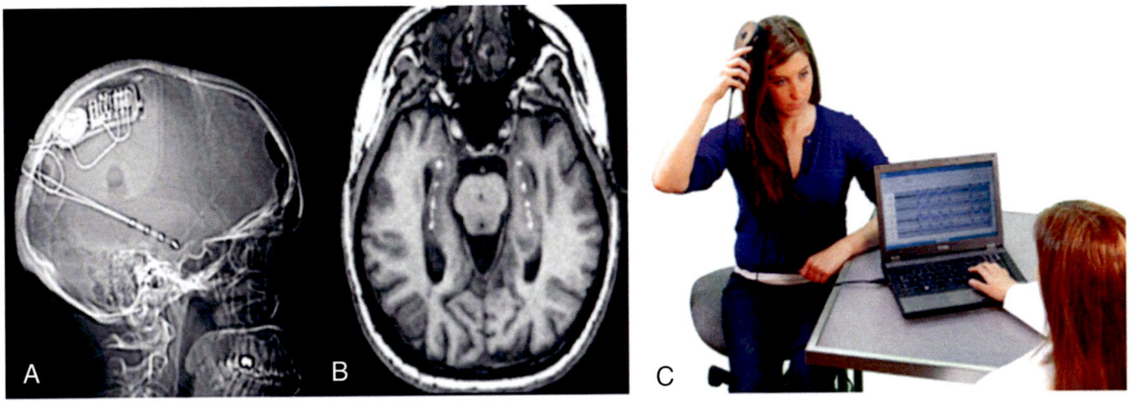

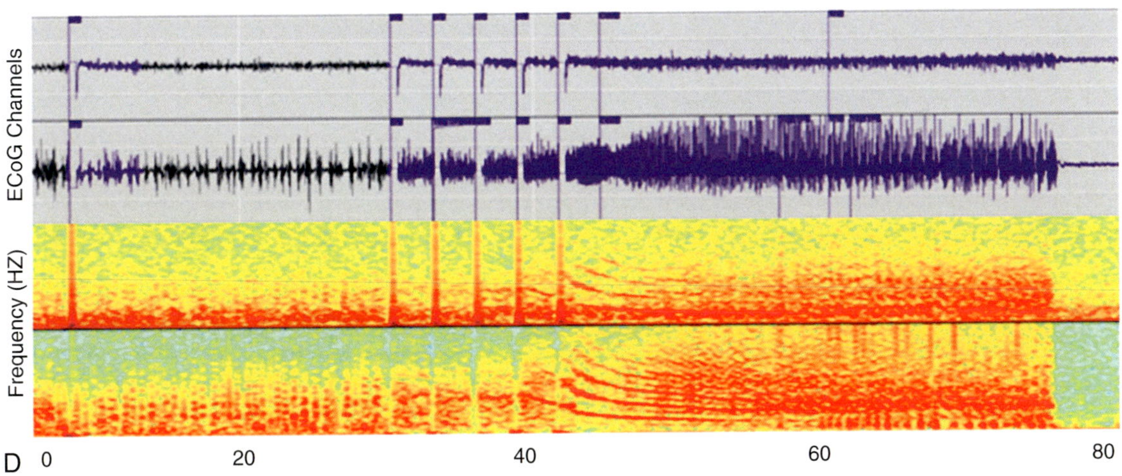

FIG. 19.2 **(A)** Implanted neurostimulator seen on skull X-ray. **(B)** Axial MRI sequence showing placement of bilateral hippocampal depth leads. **(C)** Interrogation of the neurostimulator using the wireless wand and programmer. **(D)** Electrocorticography recorded by a neurostimulator with time-frequency analysis (FFT) showing detection of epileptiform activity and responsive stimulation (*vertical lines*). (Copyright 2017, Neuropace, Inc; image used with permission from NeuroPace, Inc.)

After the conclusion of the Pivotal Trial, patients who were previously enrolled in both the Feasibility and Pivotal Trials were followed in an open-label, long-term trial. Flow chart showing participant accountability with withdrawals is displayed in Fig. 19.3. Median percent seizure reduction in the long-term trial was 60% at 3 years and 65% at 5 years, and most recent data presented at the 2016 American Epilepsy Society Meeting shows a 72% reduction at 7 years postimplantation.[9] Secondary endpoints reported in the long-term trial included adverse events and quality-of-life assessments, as measured by the Quality of Life in Epilepsy Inventory or QOLIE-89.[10] The most common serious adverse event reported was soft tissue infection at the implant site, which occurred in 9% of patients over a mean follow-up time of 5.4 years, either after initial implantation, seizure-related head trauma, or neurostimulator replacement. There was a 3.7% infection rate per neurostimulator procedures. All infections except one were superficial soft tissue infections. dThere were no long-lasting neurologic sequelae related to these infections, but a total of 14 patients had their neurostimulators explanted as a result of site infection and 2 patients were reimplanted.[10a] Mean quality-of-life inventory scores significantly improved at 1 year postimplantation, and improvements were maintained through 5 years.[11]

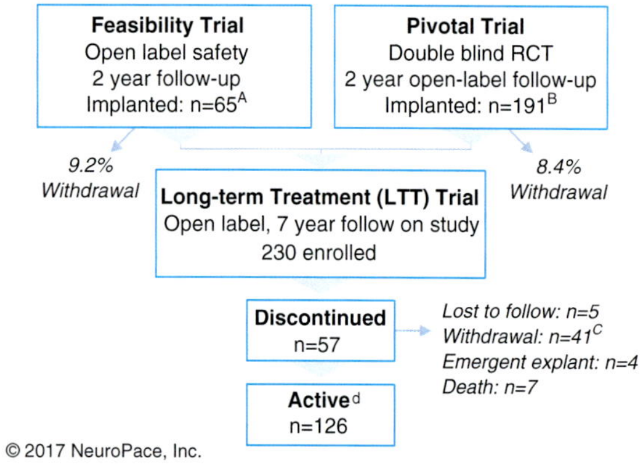

FIG. 19.3 RNS System Clinical Trials Participant Accountability. **(A)** Six patients discontinued before trial completion; two patients completed the trial but elected not to enroll in the long term treatment trial (LTT). **(B)** Fourteen patients discontinued before trial completion; four patients completed the trial, but elected not to enroll in the LTT. **(C)** Discontinuation reasons: to pursue other treatments[9]; insufficient efficacy[7]; participant chose not to replace neurostimulator after expected battery depletion[8] or after resolution of infection[9]; noncompliance[4]; elective explant[1]; ongoing suicidality/noncompliance[1] **(D)** Study ongoing; data as of November 1, 2015. (Copyright 2017, Neuropace, Inc; image used with permission from NeuroPace, Inc.)

EFFECTS OF RNS SYSTEM ON MOOD AND COGNITION

As part of the Pivotal Trial, neuropsychologic data were collected at baseline before implantation and then at 1 and 2 years after starting RNS treatment. Primary cognitive outcomes were scores on the Boston Naming Test and Rey Auditory Verbal Learning Test. There were no significant cognitive declines observed over the 2-year period, and there were small improvements in subcategories of cognitive functioning depending on the patients' region of seizure onset. Patients with neocortical seizure onsets showed significant improvement in naming, whereas patients with mesial temporal seizure onsets showed significant improvement in verbal learning.[12] Mood was also measured during the Pivotal Trial at baseline, 1 year, and 2 year stages via three validated mood inventories, and there was no significant worsening in any score over the course of the blinded period and open-label period of the trial.[8]

SAFETY CONSIDERATIONS

According to Pivotal Trial data, the rate of soft-tissue infection at the surgical site was 3.7% and risk of implant-related hemorrhage was 2.7%. These rates of adverse events are comparable with those associated with intracranial EEG monitoring or DBS. No chronic stimulation side effects were identified.[7] The rate of deaths from sudden unexplained death in epilepsy (SUDEP) in patients with RNS has been calculated to be 2.0 per 1000 stimulation years, based on a total of 707 patients from the long-term treatment study combined with poststudy commercial patients.[13] This rate is comparable and possibly lower than expected for this vulnerable patient population. Previous studies have estimated SUDEP rates at 5.9 per 1000 patient years among patients with medically intractable epilepsy and 9.3 per 1000 patient years among patients being considered for epilepsy surgery.[14,15]

PATIENT SELECTION

RNS is indicated for patients with medically refractory focal epilepsy, who have undergone a presurgical evaluation during which one or two seizure foci have been identified. Based on inclusion criteria used in the Pivotal Trial, patients to be considered for RNS implantation should be adults aged 18 years and above, who experience at least three disabling seizures per month and have failed trials of at least two antiepileptic medications. A neurologist's role, in cooperation with the neurosurgery team and consultation from neuropsychologists and neuroradiologists, is to determine appropriate candidates for RNS implantation. Patients with medically refractory epilepsy should be referred to comprehensive epilepsy centers for presurgical evaluation.[7] Depending on the clinical situation, the patient may be considered for traditional resective epilepsy surgery, laser ablation, or neurostimulation, via either VNS or RNS. Patients with one or two localizable seizure foci, who are deemed to be poor candidates for resective surgery because of having involvement of eloquent cortex in the epileptogenic zone or who may be harmed by removal or destruction of functional tissue, may be considered for RNS implantation. Potential suitable candidates include patients with two seizure foci (most commonly, bilateral temporal foci of either neocortical or mesial origin); seizures that are localized to eloquent cortex such as primary motor, sensory, language, or visual cortex; recurrence of seizures following resective surgery; periventricular nodular heterotopia; or dominant hemisphere hippocampal localization who do not want to risk cognitive decline. Accumulating clinical experience will continue to refine our understanding of the types of patients most likely to benefit from responsive neurostimulation.[3]

CONTRAINDICATIONS

RNS implantation is contraindicated in patients who are at high risk for surgical complications, including patients with active systemic infection and coagulation disorders or patients who are considered high risk for surgery in general. At this time, RNS is not approved for patients who are under 18 years. The medical procedures that are contraindicated for patients with an implanted RNS device include magnetic resonance imaging (MRI), diathermy procedures, electroconvulsive therapy, transcranial magnetic stimulation, and other implanted stimulation devices that deliver electric energy to the brain. MRI is perhaps the most troublesome contraindication because epilepsy patients may encounter situations in which an MRI is desired. At this time, testing has not been performed to ensure safety of RNS in an MRI environment. This fact should be considered when considering candidacy of patients for the device. Thus, patients who are likely to require recurrent MRI, such as patients with brain tumors, are likely poor candidates for RNS. VNS is not a contraindication to receiving RNS, but the use of both neurostimulation devices simultaneously has never been evaluated directly in previous studies.[7]

CONCLUSIONS

The safety and efficacy of responsive neurostimulation has been established, but much remains to be learned about the optimal use of the device. The closed-loop nature of the device was designed with intent to respond directly to epileptiform activity and seizures, thereby preventing or stopping seizures directly, but the actual mechanism of action is likely much more complex. The observation that seizure frequency continues to improve over time suggests that there may be neuromodulatory effects that occur over time and are not yet understood. Drawing from research on rats using DBS, there is evidence that DBS modulates gene expression, both locally and in regions receiving projections from the target being stimulated.[16,17] A similar neuromodulatory process may be occurring with RNS, in addition to immediate benefits associated with direct responsive neurostimulation.

It is poorly understood why some epilepsy patients are refractory to medical treatment in the first place and some are responsive. Among medically refractory patients who receive RNS therapy, there are also responders and nonresponders. One of the goals of future research in responsive neurostimulation will be to determine the ideal stimulation parameters for individual patients, which might be based on specific clinical presentations, anatomic pathology, genetics, or biochemistry. One of the benefits of RNS is the presence of copious data from continuous ambulatory monitoring of electrocorticography. There is enormous potential for future research to help guide future treatment paradigms.

REFERENCES

1. Rolston JD, Englot DJ, Wang DD, Shih T, Chang EF. Comparison of seizure control outcomes and the safety of vagus nerve, thalamic deep brain, and responsive neurostimulation: evidence from randomized controlled trials. *Neurosurg Focus*. 2012;32:E14.
2. Sun FT, Morrell MJ, Wharen RE. Responsive cortical stimulation for the treatment of epilepsy. *Neurotherapeutics*. 2008;5:68–74.
3. Jehi L. Responsive neurostimulation: the hope and the challenges. *Epilepsy Curr*. 2014;14:270–271.
4. Morrell MJ. Responsive cortical stimulation for the treatment of medically intractable partial epilepsy. *Neurology*. 2011;77:1295–1304.
5. RNS® System User Manual. © 2016 NeuroPace, Inc. Available at: http://www.neuropace.com/manuals/RNS_System_User_Manual.pdf.
6. King-Stephens D, Mirro E, Weber PB, et al. Lateralization of mesial temporal lobe epilepsy with chronic ambulatory electrocorticography. *Epilepsia*. 2015;56:959–967.
7. RNS® System, Summary of Safety and Effectiveness, P100026. US Department of Health and Human Services, Food and Drug Administration. Available at: www.accessdata.fda.gov/cdrh_docs/pdf10/p100026b.pdf.
8. Heck CN, King-Stephens D, Massey AD, et al. Two-year seizure reduction in adults with medically intractable partial onset epilepsy treated with responsive neurostimulation: final results of the RNS System Pivotal trial. *Epilepsia*. 2014;55(3):432–441.
9. Weber, et al. *American Epilepsy Society Annual Meeting*. December 2016 (Houston, TX).
10. Devinsky O, Vickrey BG, Cramer J, et al. Development of the quality of life in epilepsy inventory. *Epilepsia*. 1995; 36(11):1089–1104.

10a. Weber PB, Kapur R, Gwinn RP, Zimmerman RS, Courtney TA, Morrell MJ. Infection and erosion in trials of a cranially implanted neurostimulator do not increase with subsequent neurostimulator placements. *Sterotact Funct Neurosurg*. 2017;95(5):325–329. https://www.ncbi.nlm.nih.gov/pmc/articles/PMC5804848.

11. Bergey GK, Morrell MJ, Mizrahi EM, et al. Long-term treatment with responsive brain stimulation in adults with refractory partial seizures. *Neurology*. 2015;84(8): 810–817.
12. Loring DW, Kapur R, Meador KJ, Morrell MJ. Differential neuropsychological outcomes following targeted responsive neurostimulation for partial-onset epilepsy. *Epilepsia*. 2015;56(11):1836–1844.
13. Devinsky Kapur, et al. *American Epilepsy Society Annual Meeting*. December 2016 (Houston, TX).

14. Nashef L, Fish DR, Sander JW, Shorvon SD. Incidence of sudden unexpected death in an adult outpatient cohort with epilepsy at a tertiary referral centre. *J Neurol Neurosurg Psychiatry*. 1995;58:462–464.
15. Dasheiff RM. Sudden unexpected death in epilepsy: a series from an epilepsy surgery program and speculation on the relationship to sudden cardiac death. *J Clin Neurophysiol*. 1991;8:216–222.
16. Thomas GP, Jobst BC. Critical review of the responsive neurostimulator system for epilepsy. *Med Devices (Auckl NZ)*. 2015;8:405.
17. Ewing SG, Porr B, Pratt JA. Deep brain stimulation of the mediodorsal thalamic nucleus yields increases in the expression of zif-268 but not c-fos in the frontal cortex. *J Chem Neuroanat*. 2013;52:20–24.

CHAPTER 20

Brain-Computer Interface (BCI)

ISAAC JOSH ABECASSIS, MD • ANDREW L. KO, MD

INTRODUCTION

Brain-computer (BCI) or brain-machine interfaces, refer to a real-time technology system capable of capturing neural activity (e.g., electrical, chemical, or magnetic) via a recording array and converting this information using mathematical algorithms into a functional output, usually with the governing effects of a behavioral or physiologic conditional signal. At its crux, BCI thereby enables the ability to amplify, modulate, and selectively filter cortical signals in neurologic disease states where the final output signal is diminished or absent, including stroke, spinal cord injury, and neurodegeneration. Accordingly, there is a broad array of various control signals that can be captured and used for BCI. Most efforts have been aimed at improving motor function and thereby overall quality of life, and thus this—and neuromotor prostheses (NMP)—will be the predominant focus of this report; however, cognitive, behavioral, and psychologic circuits are also under investigation with clinical trials underway investigating the use of BCI in attention deficit hyperactivity disorder,[1] depression, chronic pain, Alzheimer dementia, and autism. Regardless of the substrate, it has been very well demonstrated that region- and pathway-specific corticostriatal plasticity plays an important role in learning both physical[2] and abstract[3] skill sets and that BCI should be thought of as a bidirectional interaction. Ultimately, the usefulness of BCI therefore hinges on not only the recording, processing and translation of neural signals into functional output but also the chronic, effects of BCI on the brain itself.

BACKGROUND

Over the past three decades, there has been an evolution of neural recording technologies and modalities, each with its own unique characteristics. In general, the use of any particular approach to deciphering brain activity carries trade-offs with respect to signal fidelity, spatial and temporal resolution, and information content. Broadly speaking, electrophysiologic data can be gathered from single cells, or varying sizes of populations of cells, whose activity is reflected in voltage changes measured over time. BCI relies on detectable changes in these signals to affect a functional output. The most commonly used modalities to gather this signal involve penetrating electrodes for single-cell recordings, subdural electrodes for electrocorticography (ECoG), and scalp electroencephalography (EEG).

Development of novel signal processing techniques, with concomitant improvements in computing capabilities, has resulted in many available strategies for the extraction, processing, and labeling of electrical brain activity for use in BCI. A full discussion of such techniques is beyond the scope of this chapter. Suffice it to say that there are several canonical signals used for control of a BCI system:

1. Single-unit activity is generally reflected as changes in firing rate of individual neurons and is usually derived from voltage changes measured from microelectrodes at very high frequencies (>400 Hz).[4]
2. Measures of neuronal population activity such as local field potentials (LFPs) are derived from voltage changes at less than 300 Hz. Changes in voltage related to activity, such as event-related potentials (ERPs), can be seen in the raw signal or by averaging multiple trials. More information can often be derived from varying frequency components within this signal. Traditional frequency bands that have historically been linked to functional activity include the delta (1–4 Hz), theta (4–7 Hz), alpha (7–12 Hz), and beta (13–30 Hz) bands. These signals are usually measured with subdural or scalp electrodes, with signal processing techniques such as the fast Fourier Transform or other time-frequency analyses used to quantify changes in signal components over time.[5]

Single-unit neuronal activity can be recorded with implantation of approximately 20-μm-diameter electrodes implanted into the cortex, typically with the goal of recording from layer 5 pyramidal cells in the motor cortex. These microelectrodes are either implanted and fixed at the skull or designed to float freely above the surface of cortex to accommodate motion.[6]

Kennedy and Bakay first reported successful implantation of cone-shaped electrodes in human motor cortex, coated with "proprietary neurotrophic factors" aimed at promoting neuronal ingrowth, with successful recording of action potentials (APs) in a patient with amyotrophic lateral sclerosis (ALS)[7] (Fig. 20.1). The same group went on to describe implantation in human patients with brainstem stroke[8] and mitochondrial myopathy[9] with recordings of both fast transients (i.e., APs) and LFPs. This latter recording derives from voltage changes measured at electrodes placed sufficiently far from one particular cell, to capture the "synchronized input" of an extracellular cortical area, with a low pass filter to remove high-frequency fluctuations and individual spikes. Subsequent efforts were aimed at harnessing the tenets of the "population vector" method[10]—whereby individual cells are represented as vectors with weighted contributions along the axis of a preferred direction—for precise three-dimensional motor control.

Although efforts to use neuronal activity as a control signal for BCI have been successful in the acute setting, single-unit recording microelectrodes are prone to high-impedance, gliotic sheath formation in chronic models owing to micromotion,[11] resulting in degradation of this control signal. As a result, investigators have looked at alternative markers for brain activity.

Local field potential recordings have emerged as a major tool for driving long-term, chronically implanted BCI. Voltage changes occurring at lower frequencies (70–300 Hz) than single-unit APs—a range termed the "high γ band" (HGB)—have been demonstrated to correlate to single-unit activity recorded from penetrating electrodes.[6,12] Such signals can be obtained using subdural ECoG,[6,13] which offers a less invasive (nonpenetrating) form of recording that is already widely used in surgical epilepsy practices. Epidural ECoG has been reported in nonhuman primates[14] and subgaleal ECoG in pediatric subjects,[15] both of which associated with an inherent decrease in risk of meningitis and cortical irritation and with similar cortical recording qualities. Moreover, the cortical signals obtained via ECoG have been demonstrated to be stable over time, with reliable indicators of sensorimotor activity unchanged over many months.[16]

Rather than detecting single-cell firing rates as with single-unit BCI systems, ECoG-based BCI, by and large, relies on changes in firing rates of populations of cells being recorded or shifts toward more synchronous activity, which can be easily and reliably detected.[17] For example, changes in HGB power have been shown to correlate with spatially and temporally specific local cortical activity involved in the sensorimotor system,[5,18] as well as activity in other cognitive domains. ECoG electrodes, like microelectrodes, require surgical implantation and are thus invasive. Spatial coverage with these electrodes is also necessarily limited.

EEG, on the other hand, does not necessarily involve surgery. Electrodes are affixed to the scalp and record

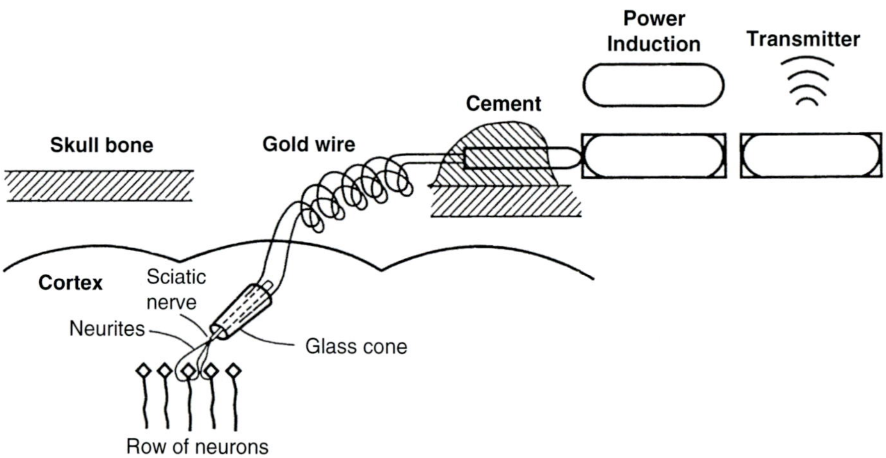

FIG. 20.1 Schematic of the glass conical electrode implanted, and design for collecting signals. (From Kennedy PR, Bakay RA. Restoration of neural output from a paralyzed patient by a direct brain connection. *Neuroreport*. 1998;9(8):1707–1711, with permission.)

signals reflecting the activity of large volumes of brain. This approach allows, in principle, recording voltage changes across the entire supratentorial cortex. Electrical activity has historically been examined in certain low-frequency bands, which are thought to have functional significance: delta (1–4 Hz), theta (4–7 Hz), alpha (7–12 Hz), and beta (13–30 Hz) bands. Importantly, scalp EEG recordings fail to capture HGB activity because of the high resistance and capacitance in the scalp and soft tissues,[19] which filter the higher frequencies generated by smaller neuronal populations and compromising the degree of spatial resolution.[20,21] Moreover, artifacts from muscle activity can often make signal processing challenging. The noninvasive nature of EEG, however, remains a benefit with respect to study recruitment, risks to experimental subjects, and the ability to repeat experiments over time.

In short, each of these approaches has its advantages and disadvantages. Microelectrode-based techniques have high temporal and spatial specificity, and individual cell activity can provide a great deal of information at the cost of being potentially damaging to cortex, with decreasing signal fidelity over time. Widespread spatial coverage of disparate cortical regions may also be impractical. ECoG can cover greater cortical regions, but with loss of spatial resolution, but may be more durable and less invasive. EEG offers wider coverage still and does not require surgical implantation; however, this modality does not offer the spatial or frequency resolution of more invasive techniques.

Overall, two distinct strategies have emerged for how the BCI process implements its functional output. The first aims to complete substitution of lost motor function via "bypassing" the corticospinal tract (assistive BCI, including both noninvasive and invasive technologies); the second approach uses BCI to identify and augment intrinsic neuroplasticity using biofeedback (rehabilitative or restorative BCI), which can sometimes involve brain-computer-brain interfaces (BCBIs).[22]

ASSISTIVE BRAIN-COMPUTER INTERFACE

Noninvasive: Beta and Mu Waves, Beta-Band Desynchronization, Slow Cortical Potentials, and Evoked Response Potentials

Assistive BCI devices rely on an elegant neuroprosthetic design that can seamlessly incorporate into various activities of daily living. Noninvasive modalities for capturing neural recordings largely depend on capturing various segments or frequencies from EEG recordings. At rest, idle cortical activity is conveyed via spontaneous EEG activity with spatiotemporal patterns of "event-related synchronization". Motor, sensory, or cognitive-related cortical activity by both imagery and/or execution creates a local power attenuation in EEG signal termed "event-related desynchronization" (ERD).[23] Sensorimotor EEG activity consists of mu waves at rest (8–13 Hz, in the same frequency range as alpha waves; however, they will not be eliminated with eye opening like posterior dominant occipital alpha waves will) and beta (beta-2 or middle level beta, 15–25 Hz) frequency bands.[24] Each sensorimotor area and supplementary motor area, thus, has a unique intrinsic beta rhythm that undergoes desynchronization with activation, whereby mu activity is suppressed with intended or executed action.[25] Moreover, the amplitude and specific characteristics of beta-band ERD vary during action planning based on the category of action sequences and time course of the actions that are intended.[26] McFarland et al. reported effective movement of a computer cursor in one or two dimensions using mu- and beta-rhythm control.[27,28]

Birbaumer et al. reported the use of BCI in two patients with advanced ALS and a clinically "locked-in syndrome" (similar to the efforts of Kennedy and Bakay), with total loss of motor function/expression and artificial ventilator and feeding support.[29] Slow cortical potentials (SCPs, also called infra-low waves, < 0.5 Hz) were recorded from electroencephalogram (EEG) as well as eye movements, and the subjects were trained to control SCPs based on replicating the visual (upper vs. lower half of the screen) and audiometric (specific tones) features of a signal on a monitor in front of them. SCPs are an event-related (e.g., based on response to a visual or auditory cue), general electrical activity amplitude metric that occurs over 300 ms to multiple seconds (relatively slow for EEG). Increased SCPs negativity reflects greater cell depolarization, a lower threshold for excitement, and hence it is thought to reflect increased neuronal activity.

Initial training in this study advanced to the ability to copy letters and words and ultimately into free spelling. Other efforts capturing "gaze patterns"[30] enabled some function for cursor manipulation as well, however, with the obvious limitation of obstructing natural function (i.e., obstructing gaze). Nonetheless, the fastest speeds of spelling and communication have been demonstrated with the addition of visual evoked potentials (VEPs)[31] and steady-state VEPs,[32] ranging from 20 to 60 characters per minute, respectively. Event-related potentials (ERPs), or the P300 wave as recorded on EEG, are positive deflections in voltage associated with typically audio or visual stimuli. There are two subcomponents including a "P3a" peak (with maximum amplitude over the frontal region and associated with stimulus-driven attention during a task) and a "P3b" peak (with maximum amplitude over the parietal region, however, to be related to improbable events and memory processing).[33] P300-based BCI has been demonstrated with auditory or visual stimuli.[34,35] Sophisticated combinations of technologies have incorporated audiometric feedback (via auditory evoked potentials) into an spinal cord injury (SCI) prosthetic; however, the concept remains to be validated in a disease state.[36] Finally, some groups have attempted to bridge various EEG input BCI techniques to a virtual reality interface.[37]

Invasive—Electrocorticography and Gamma Band Activity

ECoG was first used to capture high gamma range frequencies (40–180 Hz) from sensorimotor and speech cortical areas to direct two-dimensional cursor movement[38] (note that this was performed in patients who were implanted with subdural electrode arrays for epilepsy monitoring, a common trend in ECoG data) (Fig. 20.2). This immediately revealed a shorter training period (3–24 minutes) than had been previously observed in EEG-based BCI. The group later used both LFPs and high gamma (70–200 Hz) from the hand motor cortex to decode the time course of individual finger flexion activity.[39] Indeed, sensory feedback has been incorporated into ECoG-based prostheses, with feedback sensors in the prosthetic translating to direct cortical stimulation of hand somatosensory cortex and creation of a sensorimotor closed-loop system.[40] Interestingly, combining natural visual input and direct

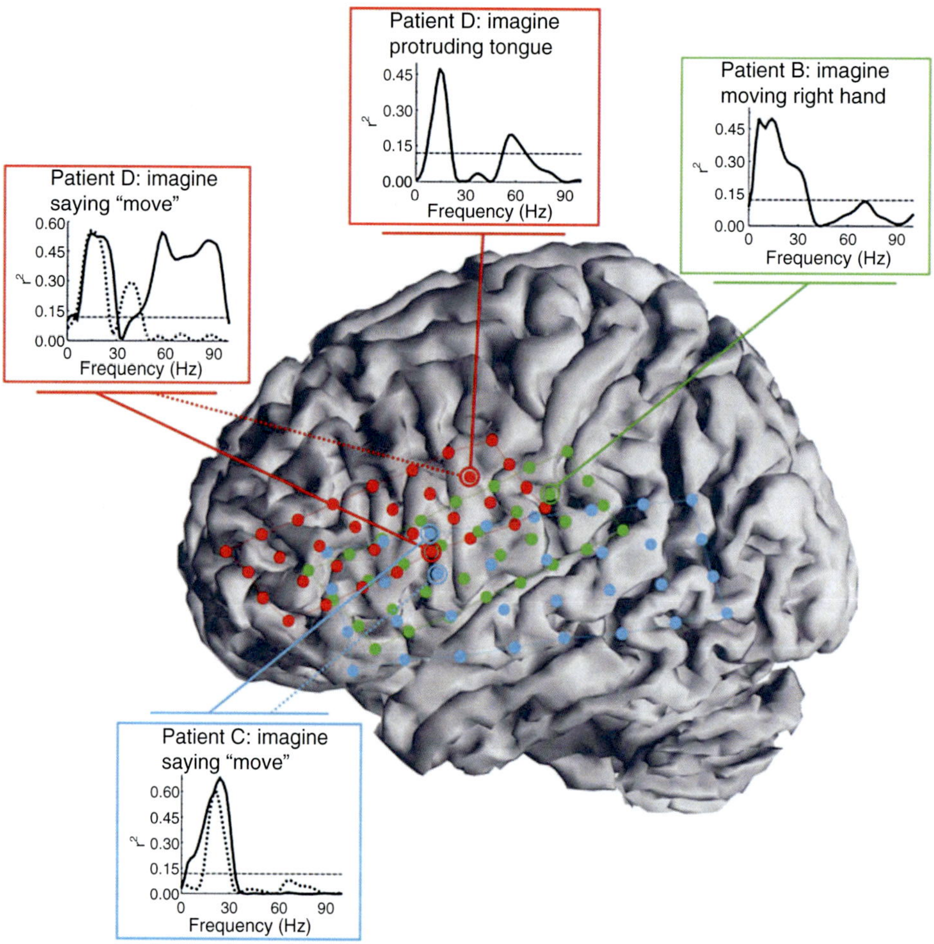

FIG. 20.2 Example of electrocorticography activity collected from three different patients (red, blue, and green) with various imagery tasks indicated. (From Leuthardt EC, Schalk G, Wolpaw JR, Ojemann JG, Moran DW. A brain-computer interface using electrocorticographic signals in humans. *J Neural Eng*. 2004;1(2): 63–71, with permission.)

cortical stimulation over somatosensory cortex in a spatially and temporally congruent manner can induce a feeling of ownership of a "rubber hand," whereas asynchronous stimulation does not .[41] Such experiments show that the brain is capable of integrating visual input with direct somatosensory stimulation to create multisensory perceptions, a bidirectional interface that has the potential to bypass peripheral sensory input, and may be of particularly importance in patients who lack such input owing to spinal cord or other CNS lesions.

Invasive—Single-Unit Recording

Translation from a computer cursor to actual motor function was first modulated in nonhuman primate studies. Moritz et al. captured cortical recordings of the hand and wrist motor areas in monkeys and converted these neural signals into proportional stimuli that were delivered to the actual muscles of the arm and hand—termed "functional electrical stimulation"—after selectively implanting catheters into the radial, ulnar, and median nerves and injecting anesthetic for temporary paralysis.[42] Monkeys were rewarded for displaying smooth control of the limb and accordingly were able to train single neuron discharge patterns from the wrist and hand motor cortex, a concept termed "operant conditioning," which had been reported much earlier by Fetz and Finnochio.[43] These efforts were expanded by Pohlmeyer et al.[44] to include more expansive cortical recording and four rather than two forearm muscles, thus enabling more elaborate upper extremity function. Ultimately, other nonhuman primate studies[45] paved the way for a human-compatible design to record from groups of cells.

With critical financial support by the Defense Advanced Research Projects Agency (DARPA), Hochberg et al.[46] reported the first use of the BrainGate (Cyberkinetics, Inc.) NMP, a 10 × 10 96-channel array of microelectrodes 1 mm in depth with a 4 × 4 mm base, implanted into the hand motor cortex of a quadriplegic spinal cord injury patient, fixed at the skull, with a bundle of cables that are connected externally to a computer system to filter the signal into a cursor that the patient could directly manipulate and direct. AP spikes were recorded from both single and groups of motor neurons, with simultaneous recording of the LFPs (Fig. 20.3). Three populations of neurons emerged including (1) a nonspecific group, (2) a group specific to "imagined" motor movement, and (3) a group correlated to actual (proximal shoulder) muscle activity. This allowed the group to construct a novel linear filter to decode neural activity and highlight "intended action" to be used as a filter. A few years later, the same group reported on additional testing in two patients with ALS and brainstem stroke, whereby they validated a method for decoding kinematics (velocity) with a Kalman filter (a recursive, Bayesian inference algorithm) as an improved conversion tool than the previously described linear filter for position of the cursor (i.e., participants achieved better cursor control at a faster rate in a closed-loop system)[47] (Fig. 20.4). Ultimately, the group reported quite sophisticated motor function in an upper-extremity NMP, including three-dimensional reach and grasp tasks and drinking coffee from a bottle (through a straw).[48] More recently, Collinger et al. implanted two arrays in a tetraplegic patient with spinocerebellar degeneration and successfully reported seven-dimensional control (including three-dimensional orientation, three-dimensional translation, and one-dimensional grasping) using a novel prosthetic device after 13 weeks of training.[49]

REHABILITATIVE BRAIN-COMPUTER INTERFACE

Closed-Loop Systems: Brain-Computer-Brain Interfaces

The governing principles underlying rehabilitative BCI are similar to those underlying basic neurorehabilitation, in which there is a dependence on coordinating novel neuronal ensembles pathways, with adequate rewards to engender a Hebbian plasticity or learning process.[22,50] In other words, rather than using a prosthetic limb to execute endogenous neural activity (albeit with a training process and mathematical algorithm for translation), neural activity is recorded and streamlined through a new conduit within the body so as to harness a "brain-computer-brain" or "brain-spine" circuit. Canadian psychologist Donald Hebb is credited with first developing the underlying concepts that eventually precipitated the field of "Hebbian Plasticity," whereby repetitive assistance with electrical firing of one neuron by another leads to the creation of new interneuron connections. More recent advances in BCI have yielded neuroprosthetic designs that capture a signal from one population of neurons and use this as an input to regulate stimulation of a distinctly separate population of neurons. For example, Guggenmos et al.[51] in a rodent TBI model recruited an adjacent population of neurons through "paired-associated stimulation" (i.e., cortical stimulation of a nearby population of cells during detected premotor action intention) and augmented motor recovery response. Other efforts have focused on a closed-loop circuit involving detection of cortical signals, bypassing an injury, and stimulation of the spinal cord. Jackson et al. first reported the use of a novel battery-powered,

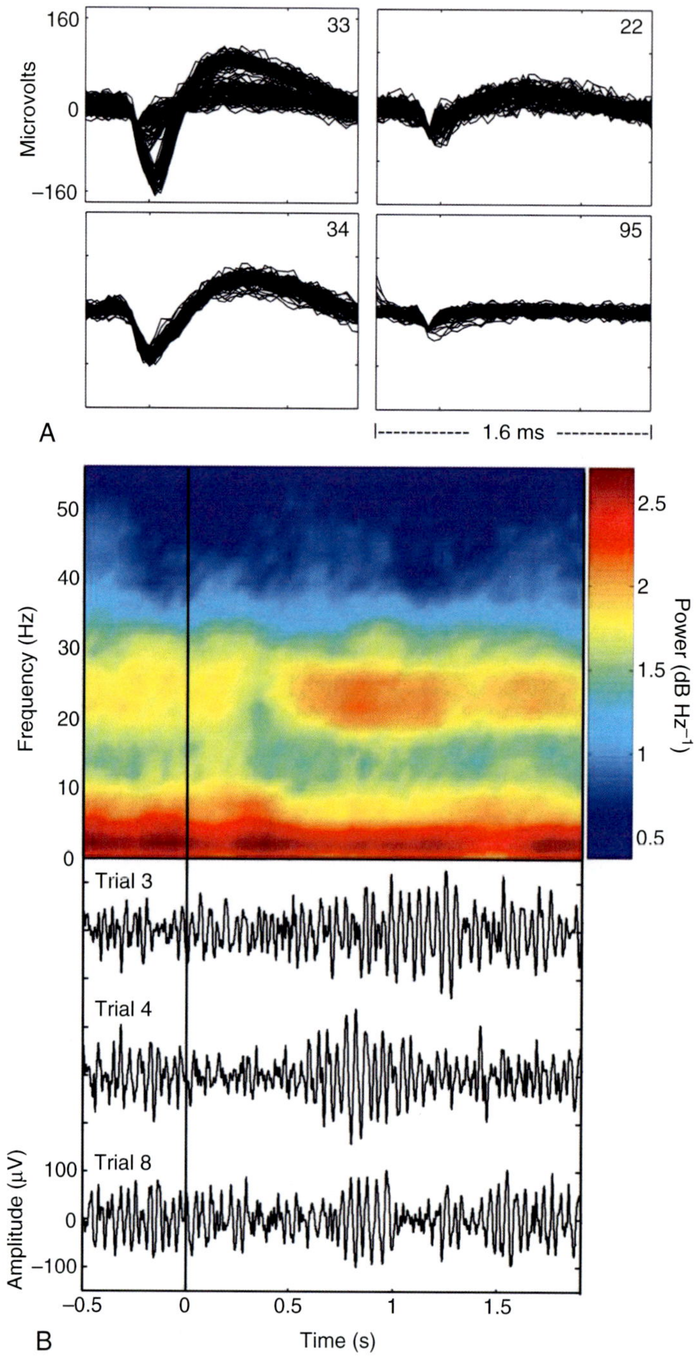

FIG. 20.3 Electrical recordings from four sample electrodes. **(A)** Summation of action potentials in two neuronal units (33), a single unit (34), a low-amplitude signal (22), and triggered noise (95). **(B)** Local field potential recordings from one electrode at three positions (bottom panel) before and after a subject is instructed to move a computer cursor into a part of the screen. The top panel is a pseudocolor power spectral density plot constructed by performing a time-frequency analysis. (From Hochberg LR, Serruya MD, Friehs GM, et al. Neuronal ensemble control of prosthetic devices by a human with tetraplegia. *Nature.* 2006; 442(7099):164–171, with permission.)

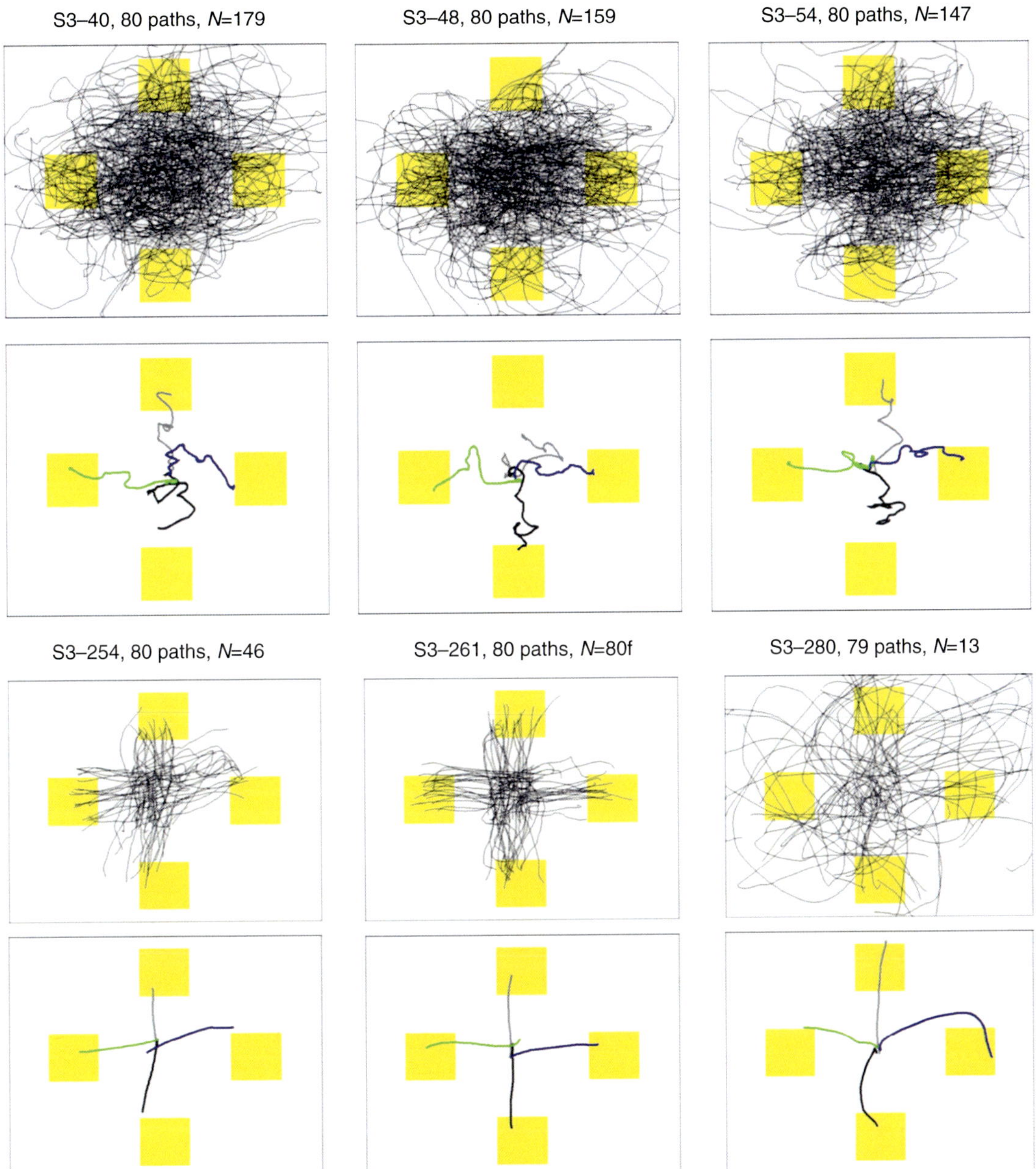

FIG. 20.4 Neural cursor movement with different filtering techniques. *Yellow boxes* approximate target goals. N denotes number of recorded units. Each path (gray, blue, black, and green) comprised 80 neural cursor movements. **(A)** Position-based linear filter in three recording sessions, raw data on the top and filtered data on the bottom. **(B)** Velocity-based Kalman filter in three recording sessions, raw data on the top and filtered data on the bottom. (From Kim SP, Simeral JD, Hochberg LR, Donoghue JP, Black MJ. Neural control of computer cursor velocity by decoding motor cortical spiking activity in humans with tetraplegia. *J Neural Eng.* 2008;5(4): 455–476, with permission.)

"Neurochip" BCI attached to a macaque monkey skull.[52] The device comprises two separate Programmable System-on-Chips (PSoCs) (Cypress Semiconductor Corporation) in parallel, each an 8-bit microprocessor core with the abilities to detect, record, and process APs. One is dedicated to recording cortical data from primary motor cortex (where there are 12 microwires, each 50 μm in diameter) and transmitting the collective data via infrared for external storage/analysis, and the other is responsible for sampling EMG activity from forearm muscles. The two PSoCs communicate, synchronize, rectify (for EMG), filter, and amplify the input signals, with an output electrode capable of microstimulation placed into the cervical spinal cord. Since its inception, intraspinal microstimulation (ISMS) has shown promise in rodent models of cervical contusion SCI.[53,54] Similarly, other groups have validated ISMS in the lumbar spine for locomotion in a rodent model.[55] Closed-loop neuromodulation systems of cortical recording and ISMS have been shown to be efficacious in SCI in both rodent[56] and nonhuman primate models (Fig. 20.5).[57]

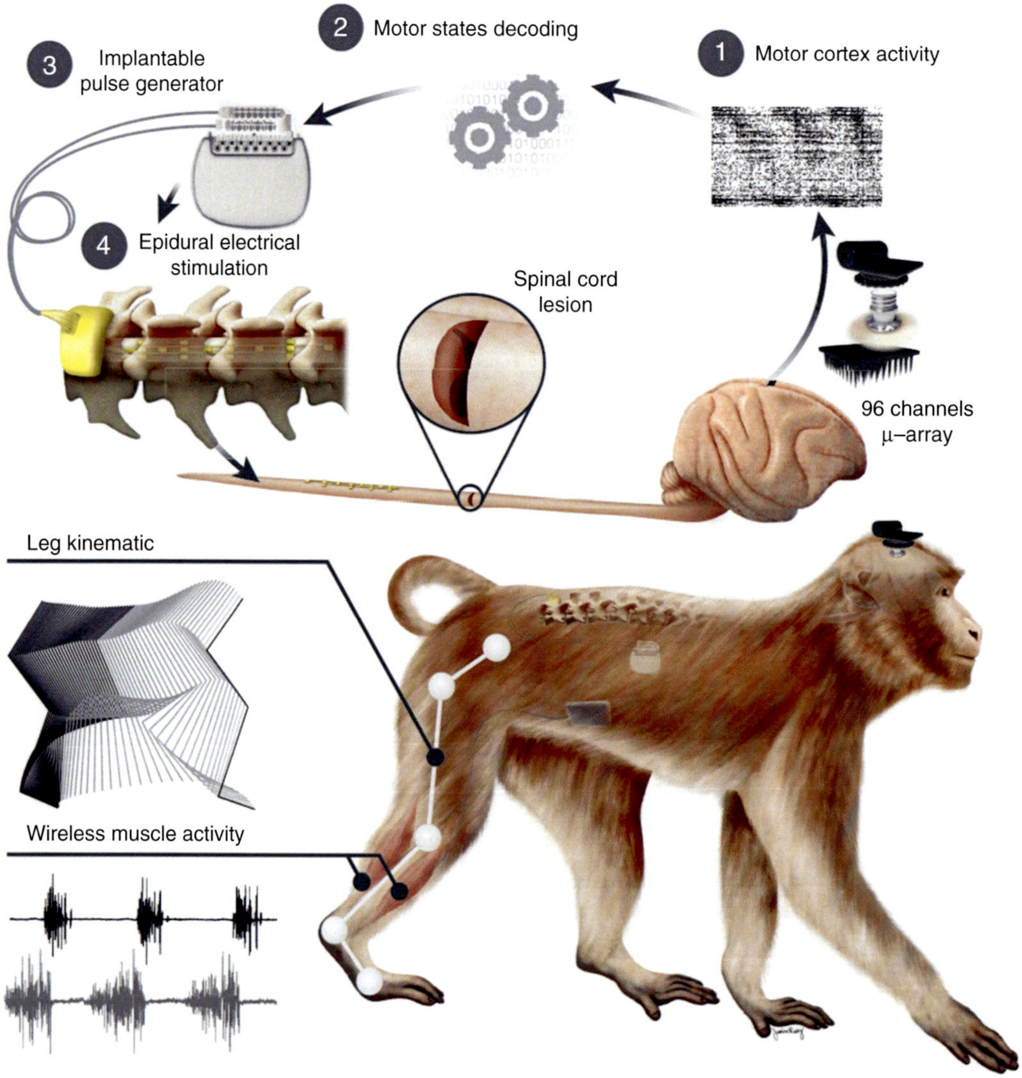

FIG. 20.5 Schematic for brain-computer-spine interface, whereby neural signals are recorded in nonhuman primate motor cortex, modulated, and transmitted to an epidural site for electrical stimulation. This is "closed-loop" type system. (From Capogrosso M, Milekovic T, Borton D, et al. A brain-spine interface alleviating gait deficits after spinal cord injury in primates. *Nature.* 2016;539(7628):284–288, with permission.)

CONCLUSION

In summary, BCI techniques include both noninvasive (EEG) and invasive modalities (ECoG and microelectrode placement) for recording neural signals, within either an assistive (external NMP) or rehabilitative (BCBI, native reanimation) design. Critical to effective performance is an intelligent interpretation, translation, and modulation of raw neural signal into meaningful output. The modalities used to gather this signal often trade spatial and functional resolution for invasiveness and durability of signal; microelectrode arrays have great potential for information bandwidth and dimensionality but are invasive and subject to signal degradation over time. Increasing attention is being paid to bidirectional BCI, where output is directed not only toward an external functional effector but also back to the brain itself, through efforts to provide sensory or multisensory feedback. Although most current efforts have been geared toward sensorimotor restoration, future work aims to build on specific cognitive domains as well.

REFERENCES

1. Ali A, Puthusserypady SA. 3D learning playground for potential attention training in ADHD: a brain computer interface approach. *Conf Proc IEEE Eng Med Biol Soc.* 2015;2015:67–70.
2. Yin HH, Mulcare SP, Hilario MR, et al. Dynamic reorganization of striatal circuits during the acquisition and consolidation of a skill. *Nat Neurosci.* 2009;12(3):333–341.
3. Koralek AC, Jin X, Long JD, Costa RM, Carmena JM. Corticostriatal plasticity is necessary for learning intentional neuroprosthetic skills. *Nature.* 2012;483(7389):331–335.
4. Moritz CT, Fetz EE. Volitional control of single cortical neurons in a brain-machine interface. *J Neural Eng.* 2011;8(2):025017.
5. Miller KJ, Leuthardt EC, Schalk G, et al. Spectral changes in cortical surface potentials during motor movement. *J Neurosci.* 2007;27(9):2424–2432.
6. Moran D. Evolution of brain-computer interface: action potentials, local field potentials and electrocorticograms. *Curr Opin Neurobiol.* 2010;20(6):741–745.
7. Kennedy PR, Bakay RA. Restoration of neural output from a paralyzed patient by a direct brain connection. *Neuroreport.* 1998;9(8):1707–1711.
8. Kennedy PR, Bakay RA, Moore MM, Adams K, Goldwaithe J. Direct control of a computer from the human central nervous system. *IEEE Trans Rehabil Eng.* 2000;8(2):198–202.
9. Kennedy PR, Kirby MT, Moore MM, King B, Mallory A. Computer control using human intracortical local field potentials. *IEEE Trans Neural Syst Rehabil Eng.* 2004;12(3):339–344.
10. Georgopoulos AP, Schwartz AB, Kettner RE. Neuronal population coding of movement direction. *Science.* 1986;233(4771):1416–1419.
11. Sohal HS, Clowry GJ, Jackson A, O'Neill A, Baker SN. Mechanical flexibility reduces the foreign body response to long-term implanted microelectrodes in rabbit cortex. *PLoS One.* 2016;11(10):e0165606.
12. Heldman DA, Wang W, Chan SS, Moran DW. Local field potential spectral tuning in motor cortex during reaching. *IEEE Trans Neural Syst Rehabil Eng.* 2006;14(2):180–183.
13. Miller KJ. Broadband spectral change: evidence for a macroscale correlate of population firing rate? *J Neurosci.* 2010;30(19):6477–6479.
14. Rouse AG, Moran DW. Neural adaptation of epidural electrocorticographic (EECoG) signals during closed-loop brain computer interface (BCI) tasks. *Conf Proc IEEE Eng Med Biol Soc.* 2009;2009:5514–5517.
15. Olson JD, Wander JD, Johnson L, et al. Comparison of subdural and subgaleal recordings of cortical high-gamma activity in humans. *Clin Neurophysiol.* 2016;127(1):277–284.
16. Herron JA, Thompson MC, Brown T, Chizeck HJ, Ojemann JG, Ko AL. Chronic electrocorticography for sensing movement intention and closed-loop deep brain stimulation with wearable sensors in an essential tremor patient. *J Neurosurg.* 2016:1–8.
17. Ray S, Crone NE, Niebur E, Franaszczuk PJ, Hsiao SS. Neural correlates of high-gamma oscillations (60-200 Hz) in macaque local field potentials and their potential implications in electrocorticography. *J Neurosci.* 2008;28(45):11526–11536.
18. Ray S, Niebur E, Hsiao SS, Sinai A, Crone NE. High-frequency gamma activity (80-150Hz) is increased in human cortex during selective attention. *Clin Neurophysiol.* 2008;119(1):116–133.
19. Pfurtscheller G, Cooper R. Frequency dependence of the transmission of the EEG from cortex to scalp. *Electroencephalogr Clin Neurophysiol.* 1975;38(1):93–96.
20. Freeman WJ, Holmes MD, Burke BC, Vanhatalo S. Spatial spectra of scalp EEG and EMG from awake humans. *Clin Neurophysiol.* 2003;114(6):1053–1068.
21. Srinivasan R, Nunez PL, Silberstein RB. Spatial filtering and neocortical dynamics: estimates of EEG coherence. *IEEE Trans Biomed Eng.* 1998;45(7):814–826.
22. Soekadar SR, Birbaumer N, Slutzky MW, Cohen LG. Brain-machine interfaces in neurorehabilitation of stroke. *Neurobiol Dis.* 2015;83:172–179.
23. Meirovitch Y, Harris H, Dayan E, Arieli A, Flash T. Alpha and beta band event-related desynchronization reflects kinematic regularities. *J Neurosci.* 2015;35(4):1627–1637.
24. Pfurtscheller G, Brunner C, Schlogl A, Lopes da Silva FH. Mu rhythm (de)synchronization and EEG single-trial classification of different motor imagery tasks. *Neuroimage.* 2006;31(1):153–159.
25. Pfurtscheller G, Neuper C, Andrew C, Edlinger G. Foot and hand area mu rhythms. *Int J Psychophysiol.* 1997;26(1–3):121–135.
26. Park H, Kim JS, Chung CK. Differential beta-band event-related desynchronization during categorical action sequence planning. *PLoS One.* 2013;8(3):e59544.

27. Wolpaw JR, McFarland DJ, Vaughan TM, Schalk G. The Wadsworth Center brain-computer interface (BCI) research and development program. *IEEE Trans Neural Syst Rehabil Eng.* 2003;11(2):204–207.
28. McFarland DJ, Kruslenski DJ, Wolpaw JR. Brain-computer interface signal processing at the Wadsworth Center: mu and sensorimotor beta rhythms. *Prog Brain Res.* 2006; 159:411–419.
29. Birbaumer N, Ghanayim N, Hinterberger T, et al. A spelling device for the paralysed. *Nature.* 1999; 398(6725):297–298.
30. Thoumie P, Charlier JR, Alecki M, et al. Clinical and functional evaluation of a gaze controlled system for the severely handicapped. *Spinal Cord.* 1998;36(2):104–109.
31. Spuler M, Rosenstiel W, Bogdan M. Online adaptation of a c-VEP Brain-computer Interface (BCI) based on error-related potentials and unsupervised learning. *PLoS One.* 2012;7(12):e51077.
32. Chen X, Wang Y, Nakanishi M, Gao X, Jung TP, Gao S. High-speed spelling with a noninvasive brain-computer interface. *Proc Natl Acad Sci USA.* 2015;112(44): E6058–E6067.
33. Polich J. Updating P300: an integrative theory of P3a and P3b. *Clin Neurophysiol.* 2007;118(10):2128–2148.
34. Piccione F, Giorgi F, Tonin P, et al. P300-based brain computer interface: reliability and performance in healthy and paralysed participants. *Clin Neurophysiol.* 2006;117(3): 531–537.
35. Sellers EW, Donchin E. A P300-based brain-computer interface: initial tests by ALS patients. *Clin Neurophysiol.* 2006;117(3):538–548.
36. Tidoni E, Gergondet P, Fusco G, Kheddar A, Aglioti S. The role of audio-visual feedback in a thought-based control of a humanoid robot: a BCI study in healthy and spinal cord injured people. *IEEE Trans Neural Syst Rehabil Eng.* 2016; 25(6):772–781.
37. Rutkowski TM. Robotic and virtual reality BCIs using spatial tactile and auditory oddball paradigms. *Front Neurorobot.* 2016;10:20.
38. Leuthardt EC, Schalk G, Wolpaw JR, Ojemann JG, Moran DW. A brain-computer interface using electrocorticographic signals in humans. *J Neural Eng.* 2004;1(2): 63–71.
39. Kubanek J, Miller KJ, Ojemann JG, Wolpaw JR, Schalk G. Decoding flexion of individual fingers using electrocorticographic signals in humans. *J Neural Eng.* 2009;6(6): 066001.
40. Cronin JA, Wu J, Collins KL, et al. Task-specific somatosensory feedback via cortical stimulation in humans. *IEEE Trans Haptics.* 2016;9(4):515–522.
41. Collins KL, Guterstam A, Cronin J, Olson JD, Ehrsson HH, Ojemann JG. Ownership of an artificial limb induced by electrical brain stimulation. *Proc Natl Acad Sci USA.* 2017;114(1):166–171.
42. Moritz CT, Perlmutter SI, Fetz EE. Direct control of paralysed muscles by cortical neurons. *Nature.* 2008; 456(7222):639–642.
43. Fetz EE, Finocchio DV. Operant conditioning of specific patterns of neural and muscular activity. *Science.* 1971; 174(4007):431–435.
44. Pohlmeyer EA, Oby ER, Perreault EJ, et al. Toward the restoration of hand use to a paralyzed monkey: brain-controlled functional electrical stimulation of forearm muscles. *PLoS One.* 2009;4(6):e5924.
45. Serruya MD, Hatsopoulos NG, Paninski L, Fellows MR, Donoghue JP. Instant neural control of a movement signal. *Nature.* 2002;416(6877):141–142.
46. Hochberg LR, Serruya MD, Friehs GM, et al. Neuronal ensemble control of prosthetic devices by a human with tetraplegia. *Nature.* 2006;442(7099):164–171.
47. Kim SP, Simeral JD, Hochberg LR, Donoghue JP, Black MJ. Neural control of computer cursor velocity by decoding motor cortical spiking activity in humans with tetraplegia. *J Neural Eng.* 2008;5(4):455–476.
48. Hochberg LR, Bacher D, Jarosiewicz B, et al. Reach and grasp by people with tetraplegia using a neurally controlled robotic arm. *Nature.* 2012;485(7398):372–375.
49. Collinger JL, Wodlinger B, Downey JE, et al. High-performance neuroprosthetic control by an individual with tetraplegia. *Lancet.* 2013;381(9866):557–564.
50. Dobkin BH. Brain-computer interface technology as a tool to augment plasticity and outcomes for neurological rehabilitation. *J Physiol.* 2007;579(Pt 3):637–642.
51. Guggenmos DJ, Azin M, Barbay S, et al. Restoration of function after brain damage using a neural prosthesis. *Proc Natl Acad Sci USA.* 2013;110(52):21177–21182.
52. Jackson A, Moritz CT, Mavoori J, Lucas TH, Fetz EE. The Neurochip BCI: towards a neural prosthesis for upper limb function. *IEEE Trans Neural Syst Rehabil Eng.* 2006; 14(2):187–190.
53. Sunshine MD, Cho FS, Lockwood DR, Fechko AS, Kasten MR, Moritz CT. Cervical intraspinal microstimulation evokes robust forelimb movements before and after injury. *J Neural Eng.* 2013;10(3):036001.
54. Kasten MR, Sunshine MD, Secrist ES, Horner PJ, Moritz CT. Therapeutic intraspinal microstimulation improves forelimb function after cervical contusion injury. *J Neural Eng.* 2013;10(4):044001.
55. Grahn PJ, Lee KH, Kasasbeh A, et al. Wireless control of intraspinal microstimulation in a rodent model of paralysis. *J Neurosurg.* 2015;123(1):232–242.
56. Wenger N, Moraud EM, Gandar J, et al. Spatiotemporal neuromodulation therapies engaging muscle synergies improve motor control after spinal cord injury. *Nat Med.* 2016;22(2):138–145.
57. Capogrosso M, Milekovic T, Borton D, et al. A brain-spine interface alleviating gait deficits after spinal cord injury in primates. *Nature.* 2016;539(7628):284–288.

CHAPTER 21

Laser Interstitial Thermal Therapy

PURVEE PATEL, MD • NITESH V. PATEL, MD • SHABBAR F. DANISH, MD, FAANS

INTRODUCTION

Laser-induced thermal therapy (LITT) is a relatively novel technique that has revolutionized the use of minimally invasive techniques to treat intracranial diseases in the past few decades. It allows treatment of lesions that were otherwise deemed inoperable and terminal. In the midst of centuries-old traditional surgical interventions, LITT was met with some initial resistance in the neurosurgical field. However, as its popularity grew and institutions presented their experiences with the procedure, it has established itself as a first-line consideration for a variety of intracranial pathologies. We review the historical developments that led to current LITT technology, techniques and indications practiced in institutions throughout the world, and the outcomes and complications that have resulted, as well as future advances of LITT, further establishing itself as a significant tool in the neurosurgeon's armamentarium.

HISTORY

Laser Development and Early Uses

The major events in the history of lasers in neurosurgery are summarized in Fig. 21.1. The idea of a laser was first conceptualized by Albert Einstein back in 1917, as he described the theories of spontaneous and stimulated emission and absorption in his book "Zur Quantum Theorie der Strahlung" (*The Quantum Theory of Radiation*).[1] The first laser was operated in 1960, when Maiman produced a laser pulse with a 694-nm wavelength, using ruby as the active medium.[2] Other lasers using different solid- and gas-state mediums and of various wavelengths were created shortly thereafter. The Nd-in-glass laser was developed 1 year later in 1961 and it, too, emitted in pulses, like the ruby laser.[3]

The initial uses of the laser were in the industrial and military fields.[2,4] The medical community began to explore the applications of the laser soon after. Some of the first biomedical uses of laser were in general surgery for the excision of tumors. Starting as early as 1962, the laser was used in ophthalmic surgery to operate on detached retinas.[3] However, the initial lasers were limited in their application owing to the wavelength in which they are operated and pulselike nature of their emissions. They were only effective and safe when used in the treatment of retinas but could be fatal to small animals when used at higher powers.[3]

Animal Models in Neurosurgery

The early lasers were tested in experiments using animal models. In 1965, Earle and Fine first demonstrated use of ruby laser in mice models, showing that the laser caused rapid expansion of mice brain and cerebral herniation, leading to instant death.[2,5] Fox et al. conducted similar studies in guinea pigs and concluded the cause of death to be apnea secondary to brainstem compression.[5] Subsequent studies using lasers in animal models that were craniectomized resulted in survival. With this newfound knowledge, studies could be conducted in craniectomized animals and effects of laser could be studied in these surviving animals.[2,5]

Human pathologies were introduced into animal models to understand the tissue interactions and outcomes after laser radiation. McGuff et al. applied the ruby laser to human-origin malignant melanomas and adenocarcinomas that were implanted into hamsters.[6] They found that all animals that completed laser treatment had complete resolution of the tumor, confirmed grossly and histologically. They also concluded that for effective laser therapy, the tumors must be exposed to allow for direct treatment. Similar outcomes were found in mice with implanted melanomas of human origin.[7] Minton et al. applied radiation via the ruby laser and found that the melanomas were destroyed.

Introduction of the CO_2 Laser

A major milestone came in 1964, when Patel introduced the first molecular laser using CO_2.[2] This laser radiated continuously at a long wavelength of 10.6 μm, with high absorption in all soft tissue and

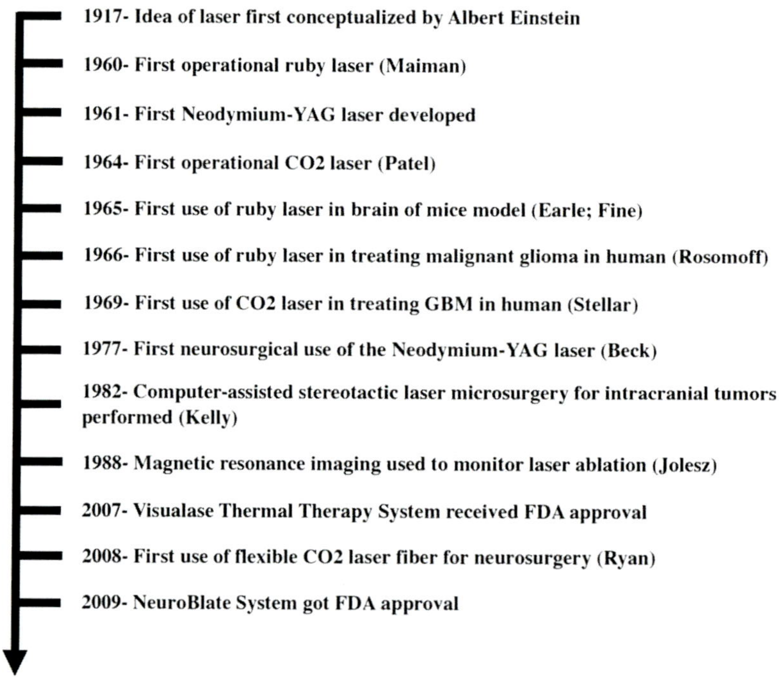
1917- Idea of laser first conceptualized by Albert Einstein
1960- First operational ruby laser (Maiman)
1961- First Neodymium-YAG laser developed
1964- First operational CO2 laser (Patel)
1965- First use of ruby laser in brain of mice model (Earle; Fine)
1966- First use of ruby laser in treating malignant glioma in human (Rosomoff)
1969- First use of CO2 laser in treating GBM in human (Stellar)
1977- First neurosurgical use of the Neodymium-YAG laser (Beck)
1982- Computer-assisted stereotactic laser microsurgery for intracranial tumors performed (Kelly)
1988- Magnetic resonance imaging used to monitor laser ablation (Jolesz)
2007- Visualase Thermal Therapy System received FDA approval
2008- First use of flexible CO2 laser fiber for neurosurgery (Ryan)
2009- NeuroBlate System got FDA approval

FIG. 21.1 **Timeline for the History of Lasers in Neurosurgery.** Chronologic events that played a major role in the development and evolution of lasers in the neurosurgical field.

water. The CO_2 laser could allow for rapid conversion of light energy into heat within a small volume of tissue, thereby treating the targeted region with minimal damage to the nearby structures. These properties made the CO_2 laser seem a promising, potential instrument in the surgical field, allowing for precise cutting and vaporizing of tissues.[3,8] In 1970, Stellar et al. were able to use the CO_2 laser to vaporize and resect intracranial tumors in mice.[2]

Transition to Human Use

The first clinical experience in humans was using the ruby laser to treat malignant gliomas, performed by Rosomoff and Carroll in 1966.[2,5,9] To avoid thermal damage to adjacent brain matter, low energy pulses were used and physicians did not try to resect the tumor. However, the laser radiation induced some areas of radiation necrosis.[2] Stellar et al. were the first in the world to use the continuous-wave CO_2 laser to try to resect a recurrent glioblastoma multiforme in a human in 1969.[3] They were able to partially excise the tumor, without causing any damage to the surrounding structures.

Evolution to Laser-Induced Thermal Therapy and Further Advances

After these initial milestones, progress slowed down as physicians were faced with the technical difficulties of operating these lasers and being able to treat tumors that were embedded deeper in the body. Bown introduced the idea of LITT with the concept of laser beams being transmitted through flexible fibers to target areas inside the body and allowing for destruction of large tumors without causing damage to the surrounding areas.[10] The earliest thoughts of thermal therapy date back as early as the 19th century when physicians noted that tumors seemed to regress at times of systemic fever or infection. This introduced the idea of using hyperthermia to treat malignant tumors.[5] A number of experiments conducted in animal models demonstrated changes in brain tissue in response to LITT.[11–15] This gave rise to the development of a number of lasers that could transmit energy through fiber optics.

One such laser was the Nd:YAG laser, which could be conducted through quartz glass fibers.[16] Although the CO_2 laser was able to cut into and vaporize tissues without causing thermal damage to the adjacent tissue, a drawback was its inability to coagulate vessels.[2] The Nd:YAG laser was developed and applied to the neurosurgical field as an instrument useful for coagulation and hemostasis.[17] The initial type of Nd:YAG laser had a wavelength of 1064 nm. It was found to scatter widely throughout biologic tissue, producing a wider area of effect and therefore being able to coagulate vessels. In 1980, Beck et al. demonstrated the efficacy of Nd:YAG laser in neurosurgery, as it created more extensive tissue damage to the desired area, reaching into deeper layers of the brain.[18] However, the wider transition zone of the thermal impact also limited its use near eloquent structures.[2]

The argon laser also could be used for coagulation. It had a shorter wavelength of 488–516 nm, which allowed it to scatter more broadly in tissue, thus having a wider area of heating. At those wavelengths, it was also absorbed by hemoglobin, making it good for coagulation.[2] Boggan et al. conducted a study in 1982 comparing the effects on brain tissue in rats after the CO_2 and argon lasers.[19] There were no significant differences found in the brain matter after exposure with the two lasers. However, the argon laser was better than the CO_2 laser at producing hemostasis. Powers et al. presented their clinical experience with the argon laser in 68 patients.[20] They concluded that although the CO_2 laser was better for debulking larger tumors, the argon laser may be a better option for microsurgical cases. With the advent of fiberoptic delivery systems, the argon laser allowed for easier maneuverability. It could also transmit radiation through aqueous fluids such as cerebrospinal and irritating fluids, making it possible to work in operative fields that may be near or within cerebrospinal fluid–containing spaces.[20]

Further advances led to the development of the 1.32 Nd:YAG, 1.44 Nd:YAG, and high diode lasers, all of which could be applied through fiberoptic delivery systems to induce thermal therapy and treat intracranial lesions.[16,21–23] In 2008, Ryan and colleagues described the first use of the flexible CO_2 laser fiber for neurosurgery.[24] The introduction of LITT was a major milestone in the neurosurgical field.

Introduction of Imaging and Real-Time Monitoring

As LITT and the fiberoptic delivery systems allowed neurosurgeons to treat tumors deeply seated without full exposure, the issue arose of being able to visualize the target lesion and assess accurate placement. This gave rise to computer-assisted stereotactic tumor ablation and resection, first suggested by Kelly in 1982.[25] Using imaging modalities such as CT and MRI, trajectories could be planned and progression and position of the laser along that trajectory would be displayed on a graphics monitor in the operating suite. Kelly reported favorable outcomes in a large series of patients who underwent computer-assisted stereotactic resection of deeply seated intracranial tumors.[26]

Imaging modalities could now be used to assess ideal trajectories and monitor accurate placement of the laser at the treatment site. Jolesz et al. further expanded the use of imaging guidance to allow physicians to monitor the hyperthermia induced at the tumor site.[27] They presented a new application of the MRI to map the spatial and temporal effects of Nd-YAG LITT on tissue, as MR is highly sensitive in detecting the changes in mobility and distribution of tissue water resulting from the deposition of thermal energy. The group was able to use MRI for real-time thermal analysis of the target brain tissue. Image guidance would not only allow for target definition and appropriate placement of the target device but also measure and monitor temperature, establish heat and cold zones, and allow neurosurgeons to have more control over thermal ablation while maintaining a desired temperature.[28] The feasibility of MRI for monitoring interstitial thermal therapy has been demonstrated in a number of experimental animal models.[15,29,30]

PHYSICS AND HARDWARE OF LASER-INDUCED THERMAL THERAPY

Lasers are nonionizing radiation that is delivered through a highly coherent energy beam. They often may travel relatively long distances with high energy fidelity. Lasers in medicine are often used for treatment and frequently as surgical devices. For brain interventions, lasers are highly compact and mobile classified as class IV solid-state diodes with outputs in the 2–40 W range.[31,32] An optimal wavelength is necessary to balance absorption and penetration; this allows for efficient photothermic heating of tissue.

As brain tissue is essentially a turbid, water-dominated medium, wavelengths of light that have a good level of penetration and local absorption are desired. Two groups of factors are important for laser efficacy: optical properties of lasers and thermal properties of tissue. When a single photon encounters tissue, the absorption coefficient determines whether that photon will thermally damage that tissue; however, the scattering coefficient determines whether that tissue will deflect and change the trajectory of that photon. Tissue properties also affect ablation, namely, tissue conductivity, tissue perfusion, and specific heat. As the absorption coefficient is a measure of absorption of light as a function of depth, it is important to consider when determining the ideal wavelength. Wavelengths near the infrared spectrum tend to have a dominance of photon scattering over absorption and therefore lead to rapid photothermal heating of tissue through higher penetration. Within the range near the lower wavelengths of this spectrum, key absorbers are deoxyhemoglobin and oxyhemoglobin; at the higher end, water dominates. The two commonly used wavelengths for LITT are 980 and 1064 nm, corresponding to the two popular LITT systems presently used (Visualase and Monteris, respectively).[33,34] The 980 nm wavelength has a slightly higher absorption coefficient in both water and blood when compared with 1064 nm (Fig. 21.2).[32]

For LITT, laser energy is delivered through long, flexible optical fibers.[31,32] These fibers may be up to 10 m in length, as they have to reach from the LITT console (outside of the MRI) to the patient. Laser therapy is delivered to the target; however, the shape of the fiber tip can affect how this therapy is delivered. A diffusing tip allows for three-dimensional radial delivery while a directional firing tip can be used to better conform more complex lesion geometry.[31,32] The exact nanometer wavelength and tip style are largely dependent on the manufacturer of the LITT system being used. Power in LITT is measured in watts and often exceeding 10 W. To protect the laser fibers from thermal damage, catheters are placed within a cooling sheath, with either flowing water or CO_2 gas.[31,32] Ablation extent is largely a balance between thermal control, local perfusion, cooling, laser power, and laser-on time.

At the basic level, LITT hardware consists of a laser catheter with a diode laser, LITT clinician workstation, and MRI machine. The two commercially available systems at the present time vary in terms of catheter structural design, size, thermal output, cooling mechanism, and software.[34] The Medtronic-Visualase system uses a polymer-sheathed silica catheter, whereas the Monteris system uses a sapphire-sheathed silica catheter. Catheter diameter is 1.65 mm for the Visualase system and 2.2/3.3 mm for Monteris. Thermal delivery is continuous wave for Visualase, whereas it is pulsed for Monteris. Cooling is an important feature for both systems; Visualase uses a saline circulator, whereas Monteris uses a CO_2 cooling mechanism with thermocoupled feedback control. Although the user interface varies, the software for both systems accomplish similar goals in terms of real-time monitoring of thermal damage and laser control.

Monitoring of the laser procedure is performed through the commercially available workstations associated with the common LITT systems (Fig. 21.3). Serial MRI sequences are obtained throughout the duration of the procedure at varying intervals (usually in the range

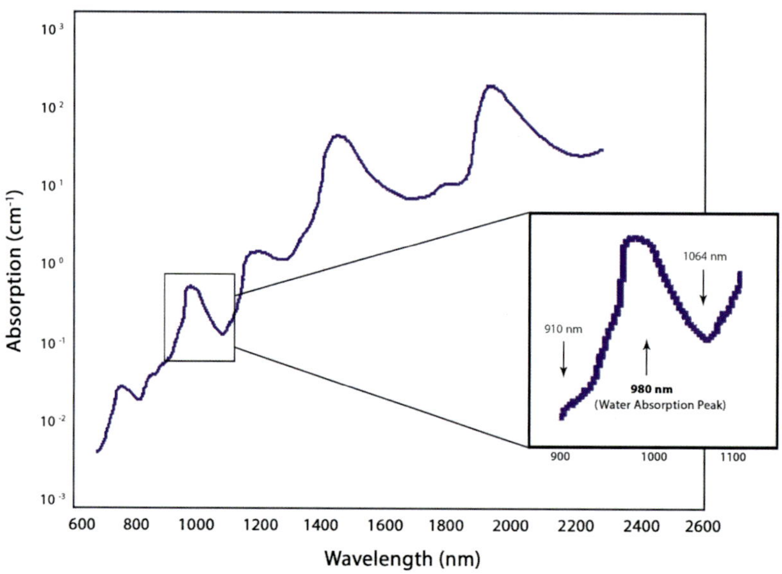

FIG. 21.2 **Laser Wavelengths for Optimal Absorption.** A spectrum of wavelengths is plotted against the absorption coefficients. The two most commonly used wavelengths for laser-induced thermal therapy in the current thermal therapy systems—Monteris and Visualase—are 980 and 1064 nm, respectively.

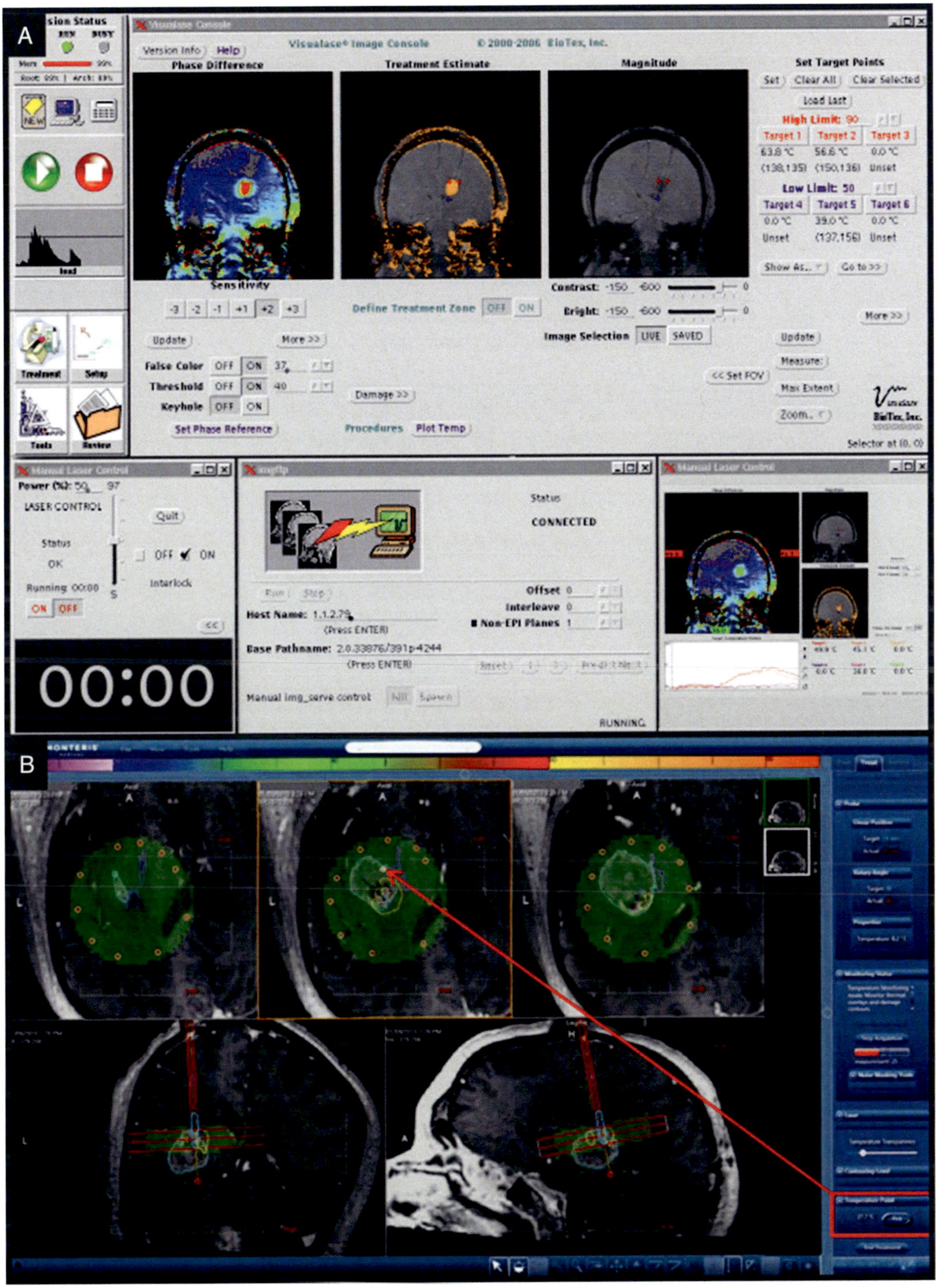

FIG. 21.3 **Visualase and Monteris Workstations.** **(A)** The Visualase and **(B)** Monteris workstations, although with distinct unique features, allow for real-time thermal monitoring of ablation sites using MRI sequences obtained intraoperatively. Both systems highlight the lesion of interest and display real-time temperature changes for neurosurgeons to easily monitor through these workstations.

of seconds). Gradient recalled ECHO image phases are used to estimate temperature change, and the LITT software computes an estimate of the extent of thermal damage based on cumulative heating.[35]

INDICATIONS AND DECISION-MAKING

Despite its promising features and minimal invasiveness, the use of LITT is inherently dependent on operator decision-making. For epilepsy and infield recurrent metastatic lesions, there have been decision-making algorithms reported in the literature (Fig. 21.4).[36,37] Often, operators rely on the case series in the literature and their experience and outcomes. However, LITT is seldom used as the sole initial intervention in a routine or common neurosurgical oncologic case. For other uses, such as chronic pain or epilepsy, LITT may be the initial surgical approach.[38,39] There have been reports of LITT use in spinal cases as well.[40]

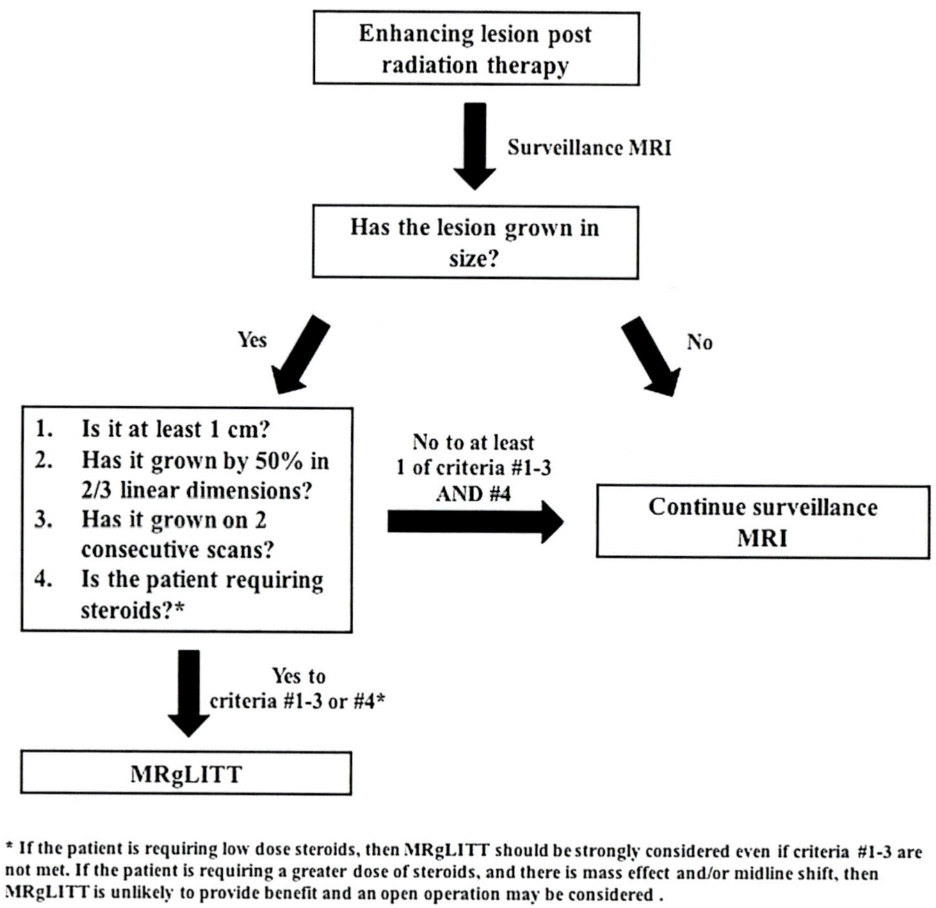

A

FIG. 21.4 **Recurrent Mets and Epilepsy Algorithms.** **(A)** This clinical algorithm presents a number of criteria that can be applied to assess when a progressive infield metastatic recurrence (or radiation necrosis) should be treated with laser-induced thermal therapy (LITT) and when it is sufficient to continue image surveillance. **(B)** A comprehensive clinical algorithm presents diagnostic evaluation of mesial temporal lobe epilepsy to determine when a patient may be a surgical candidate for stereotactic laser amygdalohippocampectomy (SLAH) using LITT. (Reproduced from: Patel PD, Patel NV, Davidson C, Danish SF. The role of MRgLITT in overcoming the challenges in managing infield recurrence after radiation for brain metastasis. *Neurosurgery*. 2016;79(suppl 1):S40–S58; Reproduced from: Gross RE, Willie JT, Drane DL. The role of stereotactic laser amygdalohippocampotomy in mesial temporal lobe epilepsy. *Neurosurg Clin N Am*. 2016;27(1):37–50.)

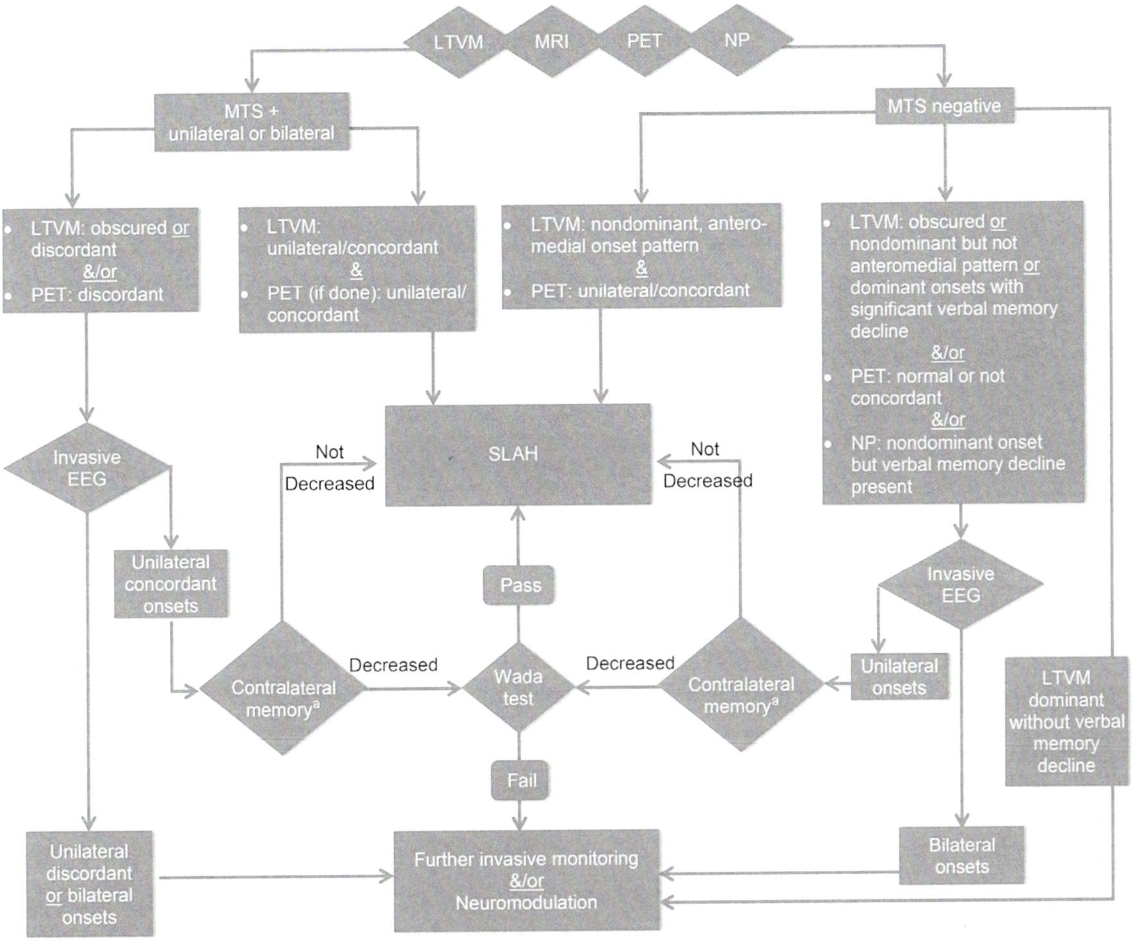

B

FIG. 21.4 cont'd. LTVM = Long term video monitoring; MRI = Magnetic resonance imaging; PET = Positron emission tomography; NP = Neurophysiologic testing; EEG = Electroencephalography; SLAH = Selective laser amygdalohippocampectomy; MTS = Mesial temporal lobe sclerosis.

For intracranial tumors, the typical scenario for LITT use is in the case of recurrence and radiation necrosis, when the patient is a poor surgical candidate, or in cases of unfavorable anatomy.[41] For each of these situations, there is significant operator variability. As LITT is not yet a gold standard approach for any specific indication, there remains significant debate over application. In fact, at the time this chapter was written, the only FDA indication was soft-tissue ablation. The FDA has not approved the specific treatment of a disease or specific histopathology. The first and foremost question in decision-making is lesion size, location, and morphology. For lesions that are wider than 2.0–2.5 cm, are multilobulated, have large cystic components, are near highly eloquent cortex, or are near large fluid bodies, LITT may not be as effective.[42] The laser therapy is delivered in a spherical fashion with the commonly used LITT systems, and therefore larger lesions pose a challenge, although the primary treatment of large tumors with LITT has been reported.[42,43] Complex lesion shapes also lead to similar problems, as spherical energy dispersion may not cover the contours of the target. The type of the tip used is important, as both diffusing and side-firing tips are available. As the laser may be moved back and forth along its implanted trajectory, depending on the tip being used, varying sized ablation columns may be created. Fluid within or outside of the lesion may function as a heat sink and draw heat energy away from the target, leading to an asymmetric ablation outcome. Thermal injury to nearby eloquent cortex is also a concern as is postoperative edema development. Patients with recurrence often have other comorbidities and may not be ideal candidates for open surgery because of invasiveness, inability to tolerate longer general anesthesia times, or risk of wound breakdown. In such patients, LITT may be of use, as it is relatively quick and minimally invasive. Radiation necrosis is a challenging entity, and without pathologic analysis, it is often difficult to confirm. This difficulty stems from variation among institutions in determining what defines radiation necrosis versus infield recurrence and what it means when the pathology falls between the two spectrums.[36] Prior studies have discussed the concept of treating symptomatic radiation necrosis and recurrent metastasis as the same clinical entity from a surgical management standpoint.[36] Although this is a controversial topic, recent work by Patel et al. suggested treating both as the same in terms of LITT applicability as well.[36]

Epileptic foci and chronic pain are two other areas in which LITT has gained use.[38,39] For epilepsy cases, the common goal is to ablate the seizure causing foci in an effort to terminate the seizure source. The use of LITT in epilepsy revolves around the desire to achieve seizure freedom while minimizing collateral damage. The ideal LITT target in epilepsy cases is one that has a relatively well-defined region on preoperative imaging. LITT may be used as an initial treatment option for medically refractory focal epilepsy and has gained enthusiasm for lesional epilepsy syndromes.

Chronic pain is less commonly an indication for LITT. For appropriate chronic pain cases, bilateral cingulotomy can be performed with LITT. Certainly, the image guidance helps to visualize the ablation. Whether this in fact leads to an outcome that is different from radiofrequency ablation is debatable (Fig. 21.5).[39]

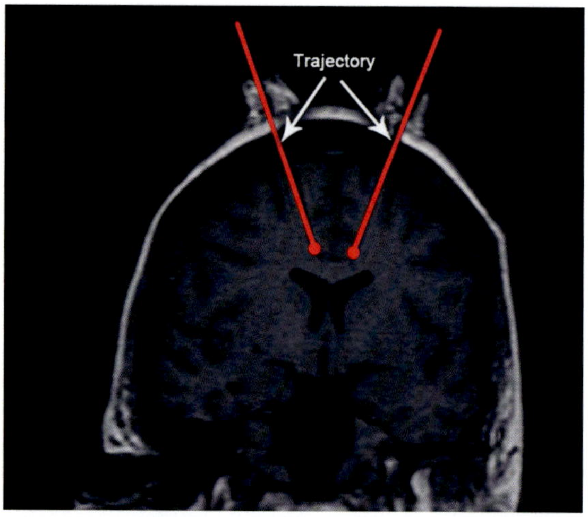

FIG. 21.5 Cingulotomy for Chronic Pain. Preoperatively, two individual trajectories (shown in red) are planned for laser ablation to the bilateral cingulate gyri for the treatment of chronic pain. (Reproduced from: Patel NV, Agarwal N, Mammis A, Danish SF. Frameless stereotactic magnetic resonance imaging-guided laser interstitial thermal therapy to perform bilateral anterior cingulotomy for intractable pain: feasibility, technical aspects, and initial experience in 3 patients. *Neurosurgery*. 2015;11(suppl 2):17–25; Discussion 25.)

SURGICAL PROCEDURE

Preoperative planning is critical for maximal ablation results. Although more than one commercially available system exists, the general steps for laser catheter placement and securement are similar. Stereotactic planning is used for entry point, target, and trajectory identification; this is followed by burr hole creation, catheter insertion, and laser ablation. The general steps are identified below, adapted from Patel et al. (Fig. 21.6).[31]

1. Stereotactic registration with burr hole creation—Before burr hole creation, an entry point and target point are identified and this guides trajectory planning. Stereotactic registration may be performed as frameless, trajectory-guided platform, and traditional stereotactic frame based and with robotic assistance. Frameless approaches use either anatomic landmarks, gadolinium fiducials, or implanted skull fiducials. Trajectory-guided platforms use a small platform that is fixed to the skull and used as a reference for the stereotactic software and can be performed completely in the MRI suite with the ClearPoint system (MRI Innovations, Irvine, CA) without the need for an operating room placement. Traditional stereotactic frames are used for LITT, and planning is similar to that for a stereotactic biopsy. Once the trajectory is identified, a burr hole is created at the entry point. A small bone anchor is placed, which holds the laser catheter in place.
2. Laser catheter placement—After the skull and dural opening are created, and the bone anchor is in place, the laser catheter is marked to the appropriate trajectory and inserted until the target is reached. The Visualase system typically requires that the laser is placed in the operating room, whereas the laser is inserted in MRI suite when using the Monteris NeuroBlate system. Once at target, the bone anchor is locked and the laser catheter and wiring are secured. Of note, it is important to factor in the length of the bone anchor and any stylets or cannulas used to mark the appropriate trajectory length.

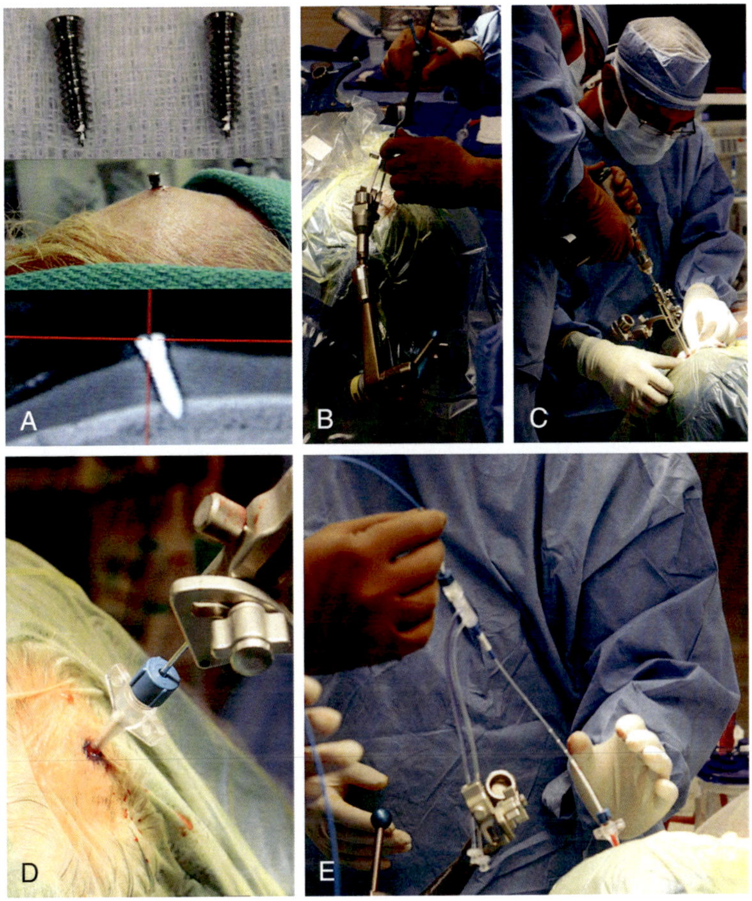

FIG. 21.6 **LITT (Visualase) Surgical Steps.** **(A)** Skull pins are implanted for the frameless stereotactic approach. **(B)** Stereotactic registration is performed using the Medtronic StealthStation S7 and preoperative MRI sequences that were uploaded and fused onto this software. Neurosurgeons can use this to plan a trajectory for the laser. **(C)** Based on the planned trajectory, a burr hole is created at the entry point. **(D)** A small bone anchor is placed to secure the laser catheter at this position. **(E)** The laser catheter is then marked to the appropriate trajectory and inserted until it reaches the target lesion. (Reproduced from: Patel NV, Mian M, Stafford RJ, et al. Laser interstitial thermal therapy technology, physics of magnetic resonance imaging thermometry, and technical considerations for proper catheter placement during magnetic resonance imaging-guided laser interstitial thermal therapy. *Neurosurgery*. 2016;79(suppl 1):S8-S16.)

3. Laser ablation—The laser and its cooling line are linked to the workstation in the MRI control room. Next a series of MR images are obtained to confirm catheter placement and identify appropriate treatment planes. The goal is to find a plane in which the entire length of the intralesional catheter is visualized along with relevant and critical surrounding anatomy. A secondary plane is also obtained, ideally orthogonal to the first. The Monteris system allows for a tertiary plane in addition to an above and below plane relative to the lesion. A test dose is delivered to assure appropriate heat delivery. The procedure is then performed and monitored. The Visualase console allows for setting of thermal boundaries. As temperature exceeds a defined degree at the chosen boundary, the system will stop the ablation. The thermal damage is shown as a single colored overlay on the target lesion. A temperature map may also be overlain showing the extent of heating across the lesion. The Monteris system uses thermal boundary control system as well; however, it consists of thermal dose threshold lines predicting areas of irreversible damage and those of recoverable tissue.

4. Postprocedure—After completion of the procedure, the laser catheter and bone anchor are removed. The entry site is closed with a single absorbable suture, and the patient is recovered. Post-LITT MRI with and without contrast is obtained immediately after the procedure and sometimes 24 h after the procedure. Typically, patients spend 24–48 h in the hospital post-LITT and are discharged home.

CURRENT USES

In the recent years, LITT has progressed to become a minimally invasive alternative to conventional surgical techniques for the treatment of a wide variety of neurosurgical and nonneurosurgical pathologies. Some of the most common intracranial pathologies include malignant gliomas, cerebral metastases, radiation necrosis, epilepsy, and chronic pain syndrome. The technique has also been used successfully for the treatment of pediatric neurosurgical conditions.

Malignant Gliomas

Among neurosurgical conditions, the one for which LITT has been used and studied most extensively is malignant gliomas (Fig. 21.7). Gliomas are the most common primary intracranial tumor, representing as high as 81% of all malignant intracranial tumors.[44] One of the most significant prognostic factors in these patients is the extent of tumor resection, with gross total resection being associated with longer survival and improved quality of life.[44,45] However, there is a delicate balance of obtaining complete tumor resection and avoiding surgically acquired neurologic deficits.[46] Considering the functional impairments that may be associated with open surgery especially for surgically inaccessible tumors, LITT is emerging as an important surgical tool that allows for an improved balance of tumor resection and preservation of brain function.[47]

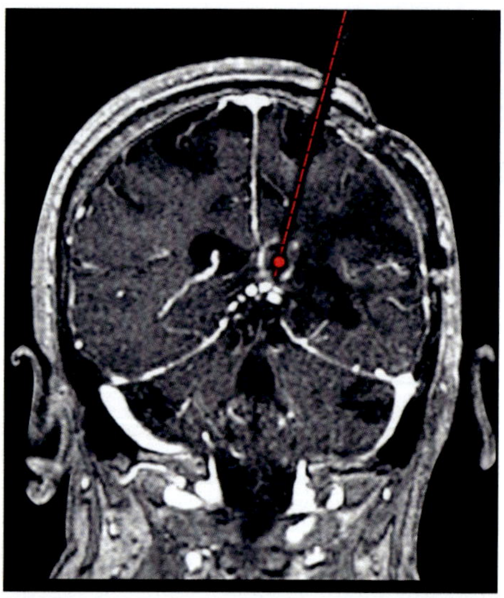

FIG. 21.7 Glioma Case Treated With Laser-Induced Thermal Therapy (LITT). A 58-year-old woman presented with a left deep parietal region ependymoma, which was treated with LITT. The trajectory to this tumor is highlighted in red. (Reproduced from: Purvee P, Patel NV, Shabbar DF. Intracranial MR-guided laser-induced thermal therapy: single-center experience with the Visualase thermal therapy system. *J Neurosurg*. 2016;125:853–860.)

The initial reports of LITT for gliomas date back to the early 1990s when several groups reported their clinical outcomes after treatment. Ascher and colleagues had started using interstitial thermotherapy with the laser and real-time MRI monitoring in 1984.[48] They concluded that this novel treatment option could be used palliatively for malignant tumors and possibly as a cure for benign pathologies. It also seemed promising for the treatment of all types of tumors without high risk to the patient's neurologic function and life. Sugiyama et al. treated five patients using computed tomography stereotactic laser hyperthermia and found all the lesions to have disappeared after the procedure.[49] In 1998, Reimer et al. presented their experience with the MRgLITT as a palliative treatment option in four patients with high-grade gliomas.[50] They reported local tumor control and clinically stable conditions for more than 6 months after the procedure and no permanent neurologic deficits or infections. In addition, compared with palliative surgery, the length of hospital stay, risk of infections, cost, and chance of patients being psychologically affected were all reduced with LITT. Other groups also reported their experience with this new, emerging technique.[51,52]

Many of the earlier studies were limited to a small number of cases. Over time, as the use of image-guided LITT grew, larger series were presented to assess safety and efficacy and compare with the traditional treatment options. Schwarzmaier et al.[53] treated 16 patients with recurrent glioblastoma multiforme using LITT. They found the median survival after LITT to be 6.9 months, which increased to 11.2 months after the learning curve was overcome. This was longer than the survival rates that had been reported for natural history (<5 month) and after chemotherapy treatment with temozolomide (5.4–7.1 months). Overall, the group demonstrated a relatively longer survival after local LITT for recurrent (Glioblastoma Multiforme) GBM. No permanent neurologic deficits or mortality were reported in this series. Hawasli and colleagues[54] reported their experience using LITT for the treatment of 11 gliomas (and 5 metastatic lesions and 1 epileptogenic focus). Most complications were transient, and there were relatively short ICU and hospital stays. The technique resulted in an overall 93% tumor ablation. The study proposed LITT as a potential treatment option for deep-seated recurrent gliomas that were deemed inoperable.

Institutions also reported their individual experiences with the two commercially available operating systems—Visualase, which received FDA approval in 2007, and NeuroBlate, which was approved in 2009.[55] Carpentier and colleagues[56] presented one of the first studies using the Visualase thermal therapy system for the treatment of four recurrent glioblastomas. The real-time guidance offered by the system was of great significance at controlling the extent of ablation (EOA) without complications and ensuring that the entire target tumor was treated. It was a safe procedure with no neurologic deterioration or permanent complications and with a decrease in size of treated tumor postoperatively. Jethwa et al.[35] presented their initial experience using the same system for treating 20 intracranial lesions, mostly gliomas and metastatic tumors. Major complications were relatively low, occurring in four patients, and further decreased as the physicians gained more experience in the procedure and patient selection. The Visualase thermal therapy system used a 980-nm diode laser, a more efficient laser in comparison with other diode and Nd:YAG lasers. In addition to the laser type, the diffusing tipped laser fiber, cooling system, and continuous MR thermal monitoring all collectively made this thermal therapy system efficient and promising for the treatment of intracranial lesions.

The largest series till date has been reported by Patel and colleagues,[57] who described their results in 102 patients treated the Visualase thermal therapy system, 50 of which had primary brain tumors. There were a total of 27 complications that arose, all in patients who underwent the procedure for primary or metastatic brain tumors. However, the majority of these complications also resolved with therapy, and overall, the procedure was found to have a relatively low complication rate. It is important to note that the baseline health of patients with intracranial lesions is often compromised relative to patients who undergo the procedure for primary diagnosis of epilepsy or pain, who experienced no complications in this series. Therefore, patient selection and comorbidities are important to consider when offering LITT.

The NeuroBlate system uses a 1064-nm Nd:YAG laser with the option for both side-firing and diffuse-tip probes.[58] Sloan and colleagues[34] presented outcomes of the first-in-humans phase I clinical trial of the system for treatment of recurrent glioblastomas. The median survival time was 316 days in this series compared with 90–150 days typically seen with recurrent glioblastomas. There were two significant neurologic complications that arose secondary to the procedure; however, both were successfully managed with overall improvement. The group concluded the NeuroBlate system was a safe and well-tolerated procedure based on their experience. Another group presented their experience with the NeuroBlate in 34 patients treated for high-grade, difficult-to-access gliomas.[43] The median progression free survival (PRS) was 5.1 months, and the estimated 1-year overall survival was 68 ± 9%. After being heated at 43°C for 10 min, the median tumor ablation coverage was 98% and it was suggested that greater EOA or tumor coverage correlated with longer PRS.

In the recent years, many institutions have heavily adapted LITT and were able to draw conclusions on its efficacy and safety. Furthermore, the technique was compared with the conventional craniotomy for resection of high-grade gliomas.[59] In a metaanalysis undertaken to answer such questions, the EOA or extent of resection was found to be significantly higher with LITT (85.4%) than with craniotomy (77.0%). In addition, craniotomies were associated with significantly more complications (13.8%) compared with LITT (5.7%). The goal of surgery in such cases is maximal resection of the tumor while maintaining neurocognitive function with minimal complications, and LITT may be able to achieve these goals better than conventional open surgery.

Another important advantage of LITT for the treatment of malignant gliomas is its potential role in disruption of the blood-brain barrier (BBB). A major limiting factor in central nervous system delivery of therapeutic drugs for the treatment of brain tumors has been the BBB.[60] The hyperthermia induced by LITT results in a transient disruption of the BBB, which allows for greater delivery of chemotherapeutic drugs to the cancerous cells of the tumor.[61] Leuthardt and colleagues[60] demonstrated that there was a break in the BBB with the highest permeability being within 1–2 weeks after ablation and gradually decreasing by 6 weeks. This proposed an optimal window for treatment with therapeutic agents to be administered for greater delivery to the tumor cells. In addition, because of the minimally invasive nature of LITT, patients can start their chemotherapy regimen sooner postoperatively than if they have undergone an open craniotomy for resection.[62]

Overall, LITT has been proving to be a promising, safe, and effective treatment for gliomas. It has the benefits of causing maximal tissue ablation with relatively fewer complications when compared with open surgery, while also enhancing the delivery and effectiveness of adjuvant chemotherapeutic agents. Complications do still arise and are discussed in more detail in later sections, but many institutions have been able to overcome them with experience in the procedure and patient selection. In addition to treating gliomas that are deeply seated and deemed unresectable, LITT also offers treatment to patients with significant comorbidities who may not be candidates for open surgery.[62] This is beneficial considering that as the population is aging, there will be an increase in the number of older patients diagnosed with gliomas.[63] Lastly, LITT with MR guidance not only improves overall survival in patients treated for high-grade gliomas compared with open resection but also does so at a cost significantly less than the international and US thresholds for good value.[64]

Cerebral Metastases and Radiation Necrosis

After gliomas, the second most studied lesions using LITT are intracranial metastatic tumors. Brain metastases are the most common type of brain tumor in adults, with the incidence being approximately 10 times more than primary intracranial tumors.[42,65] The standard treatment for localized metastatic lesions has been surgical resection with adjuvant stereotactic radiosurgery (SRS) and/or whole brain radiation therapy (WBRT), whereas for multiple lesions, radiation therapy (SRS and/or WBRT) is preferred mainstay treatment.[36] Unfortunately, following radiation therapy, tumor recurrence or progression can occur, with incidences up to 31% when only SRS and 19% when both SRS and WBRT were administered.[66,67] Multiple studies have demonstrated the efficacy of LITT in successfully treating metastatic tumors resistant to a range of treatment, including chemotherapy, WBRT, and SRS.

Carpentier and colleagues[42] presented their results of a pilot clinical trial treating treatment-resistant metastatic brain tumors with MRgLITT using the Visualase thermal therapy system. Six lesions were treated in four patients. The procedure was well tolerated with no periprocedural complications, and there were no tumor recurrences within the thermal ablation zone. The group later reported follow-up results of the trial with a total of 15 metastatic tumors in seven patients.[68] There were still no tumor recurrences within the ablation region, and most patients were discharged within 24 h. The median survival was 19.8 months, and there were no permanent complications. Radiologically, it was noted that postoperatively there was an acute increase in the lesion size owing to edema, which then gradually decreased. Hawasli et al.[54] presented their experience using the NeuroBlate LITT for the treatment of five metastatic tumors. They reported the median recurrence-free survival and overall survival after LITT to be 5.8 months for each. Several case reports also demonstrate the use of LITT for treating enhancing lesions postradiation for metastatic tumors.[69,70]

Although LITT has initially shown success in the treatment of metastatic intracranial tumors, a study conducted by Fabiano et al.[71] demonstrated delayed failure and tumor recurrence in two cases 6 and 11 months after the LITT procedure. In both of their cases, pathology confirmed the enhancing lesions to be entirely tumor recurrence and not radiation necrosis.

LITT can also be used for the treatment of radiation necrosis, which is a common sequela of radiation therapy that can illicit clinical symptoms. The incidence ranges from 5% to 50%.[72] The first case report of using LITT to treat radiation necrosis was presented in 2012.[73] The patient had been previously treated for a metastatic brain tumor with SRS and presented with a focal lesion at the site at follow-up, consistent with radiation necrosis. The patient was treated with LITT, which was well tolerated and had near-total resolution of symptoms. Torres-Reveron and colleagues[74] reported their experience with six cases of biopsy-confirmed radiation necrosis that underwent MRgLITT. The patients tolerated the procedure well, and there were no complications directly secondary to the procedure. Four of the six patients had improvement in neurologic symptoms. In the largest series to date, Smith et al.[75] presented 25 cases of biopsy-proven radiation necrosis who were treated with MRgLITT. The overall survival after LITT for radiation necrosis with prior treatment for grade 3 and grade 4 primary brain tumor and metastatic tumor were 12.2, 13.1, and 19.2 months, respectively. The PRSs were 8.5, 9.1, and 11.4 months, respectively. When monitoring radiologic volumetric trends, the authors found results similar to prior reports—the lesions initially increased in size following ablation, with subsequent gradual decrease.

Both recurrent metastatic tumors and radiation necrosis appear as enhancing lesions that progress after SRS and are often difficult to distinguish from one another (Fig. 21.8).[76] Fig. 21.8 shows similarities in the MR images of the two entities. Kano et al.[77] demonstrated use of T1 and T2 MRI sequences to distinguish between the two. They found that T1/T2 match between the sequences was associated with recurrent tumors,

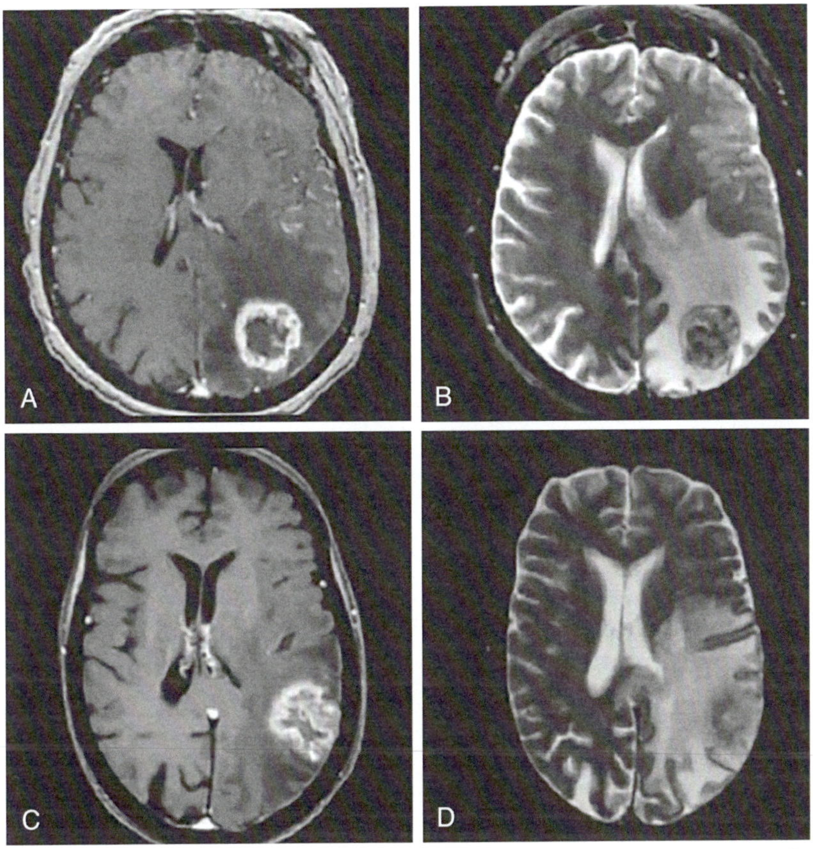

FIG. 21.8 **Recurrent Metastatic Tumor and Radiation Necrosis on MRI After Stereotactic Radiosurgery.** **(A and B)** T1- and T2-weighted images from a patient with colon cancer and brain metastasis. There is a T1/T2 mismatch. This is biopsy-confirmed recurrent tumor. **(C and D)** T1- and T2-weighted images from a patient with non–small cell lung cancer and brain metastasis. There is a T1/T2 mismatch. This is biopsy-confirmed radiation necrosis. (Reproduced from: Kano H, Kondziolka D, Lobato-Polo J, Zorro O, Flickinger JC, Lunsford LD. T1/T2 matching to differentiate tumor growth from radiation effects after stereotactic radiosurgery. *Neurosurgery*. 2010;66(3):486–491; Discussion 491-482.)

and T1/T2 mismatch, with radiation necrosis. Two case examples in Fig. 21.8 emphasize these associations. However, despite such diagnostic methods, there remains a major dilemma in the neurooncology field to accurately differentiate between the two entities.[36] LITT can potentially overcome this issue, as it can successfully treat both, eliminating the need to diagnose individually.[36] Patel and colleagues[36] proposed that the two diagnoses be grouped together as a single entity termed progressive infield recurrence. Many institutions have been using LITT to treat both diagnoses and have had favorable outcomes. Rao and colleagues[76] performed 15 LITT ablations on 14 patients with postradiosurgery recurrence and/or radiation necrosis. Local control for the cohort was 75.8%, median PRS was 37 weeks, and overall survival was 57%. Patel and colleagues[57] used MRgLITT to treat a total of 37 cases grouped as metastatic tumor recurrence or radiation necrosis. Our internal data has shown a nearly 80% control rate across 43 selected cases (unpublished data).[78]

LITT offers a minimally invasive alternative to treating progression of treatment-resistant metastatic lesions, as well as radiation necrosis. Although the neurosurgical community has faced dilemmas in distinguishing between these two entities, LITT has an additional advantage in successfully treating both pathologies and, therefore, eliminating the need to make a definite diagnosis. This theoretically eliminates costs and diagnostic steps in the medical management of these patients, thereby providing a sooner treatment. As of now, the application of LITT is limited to treating metastatic lesions that progress after other treatments were offered and exhausted.

Epilepsy

Epilepsy, characterized by recurrent seizures, has an estimated prevalence of 3%.[79] As many as one-third of cases are resistant to anticonvulsant drugs, which is the first-line treatment. For such cases, the mainstay treatment is often open resection surgery such as anterior temporal lobectomy (ATL) and selective amygdalohippocampectomy (SAH). For many years, there have been efforts to find less invasive methods of treatments, and most recently, MRgLITT has shown promising results (Fig. 21.9). Curry et al.[38] presented the first study using LITT for the treatment of epilepsy in five pediatric patients. At the latest follow-up, all the patients in the series were seizure free and had no complications. Since this initial study, further research has been performed looking at various underlying etiologies causing epilepsy, including hypothalamic hamartomas, mesial temporal lobe epilepsy (MTLE), periventricular nodular heterotopia (PVNH), focal cortical dysplasias (FCDs), tuberous sclerosis complex (TSC), and cavernous malformations.

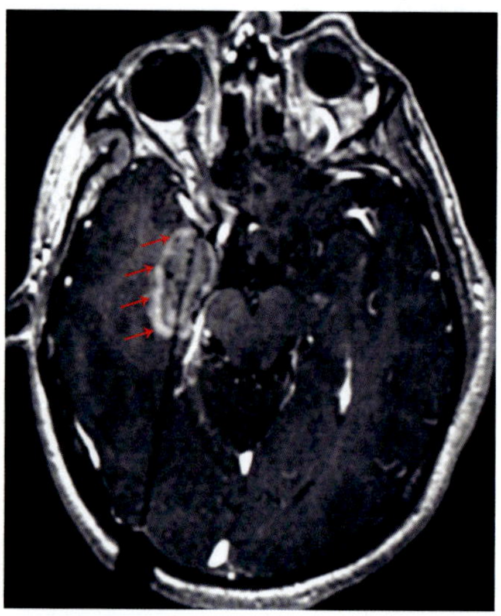

FIG. 21.9 Epilepsy Case Treated With Laser-Induced Thermal Therapy (LITT). Postablation changes are seen after patient underwent LITT to the right anterior temporal lobe for treatment of mesial temporal lobe epilepsy. The laser applicator can also be seen along a preplanned trajectory to the target epileptogenic foci. The *red arrows* show the lateral boundary of ablation.

Hypothalamic hamartomas are nonneoplastic, developmental lesions that cause gelastic, drug-resistant seizures starting in infancy with associated behavioral and developmental decline.[80] Wilfong and colleagues[80] reported on their series of 14 patients with hypothalamic hamartomas who were treated with LITT using the Visualase thermal therapy system. Seizure freedom was achieved in 86% of all patients at a mean follow-up of 9 months. There were no permanent perioperative complications, neurologic deficits, or neuroendocrine changes as a result of the procedure, and the majority of patients were discharged within 1 day after LITT. A case report was presented of a 3-year-old treated for a hypothalamic hamartoma using LITT.[81] Postoperatively, the child had significant improvement in behavior and presenting symptoms and remained seizure-free at the latest follow-up at 6 months.

MTLE is the most common epileptic disorder in adults.[82,83] Willie and colleagues[84] presented the first series in which they treated 13 adult patients with intractable mesial temporal lobe epilepsy with and without mesial temporal sclerosis (MTS) using MRgLITT. 77% of patients had significant reduction of seizures, and 67% of MTS patients had seizure freedom postoperatively. There was a visual field defect and a small acute subdural hemorrhage that occurred during stereotactic insertion. Another study compared outcomes in seven patients with MTLE who underwent MRgLITT with those in seven patients who underwent resection of the anterior medial temporal lobe (AMTL).[85] The seizure freedom rate was comparable—80% in MRgLITT versus 100% of AMTL resection. The length of stay was significantly shorter for patients who underwent MRgLITT, and the neuropsychologic outcomes were comparable between the two. Kang and colleagues[86] presented a larger series of 20 patients with intractable MTLE who underwent LITT. When compared with ATL, patients who underwent LITT had minimal postoperative pain, shorter hospital stay, and shorter recovery period. However, it was concluded that the chances of achieving seizure freedom are lower after LITT versus ATL. Seizure freedom after LITT treatment ranges from 40% to 60%, whereas they range from 60% to 80% after ATL.[87]

PVNH is a neuronal migration disorder that leads to malformation of cortical development and can result in severe focal epilepsy.[88] A few cases of PVNH treated with LITT have been reported.[89–91] Esquenazi and colleagues[89] discussed the outcomes of using laser ablation for the treatment of PVNH in two patients. One patient remained seizure-free for 1 month and then was placed on anticonvulsant medications that led to seizure freedom. The second patient remained seizure-free for

12 weeks and then had follow-up ATL and amygdalohippocampectomy that resulted in seizure freedom. Another case report[90] presented a young patient with bilateral involvement. The patient underwent laser ablation bilaterally and remained seizure-free 8 months postoperatively. Although there are not too many patients with PVNH reported being treated with LITT, this novel technique still may be a promising alternative treatment, as PVNHs are often difficult to access surgically.[79]

Focal cortical dysplasia is the most common structural brain lesion in the pediatric population.[92,93] Bandt and colleagues[94] described a case of a patient with a right temporal cortical malformation that led to treatment refractory epilepsy. After undergoing LITT, the patient achieved seizure freedom for 18 months postoperatively. In a larger series of 17 pediatric patients undergoing LITT to ablate epileptogenic foci, 11 patients had evidence of FCD.[95] The procedure was found to significantly reduce the postoperative hospital stay compared with surgery. However, the authors found that LITT was less effective in achieving seizure freedom compared with conventional surgery.

In the same study, 5 of the 17 patients were found to have evidence of TSC.[95] TSC is a genetic disorder affecting multiple systems in affected persons, with epilepsy being the most common neurologic symptom.[96,97] Unfortunately, there is limited literature and results describing treatment of TSC by LITT. Another epileptic etiology is cerebral cavernous malformations. These lesions consist of a network of intertwined vascular sinusoids that are lined by endothelial cells without intervening parenchyma, and they can lead to seizures in up 70% of patients.[98] McCracken and colleagues[98] reported their experience treating five patients with cavernous malformations using LITT (Fig. 21.10). The authors reported no complications or neurologic deficits and seizure freedom was achieved in 80% of patients. Other less frequently reported causes of epilepsy treated with LITT include encephalocele and poststroke insular epilepsy.[94]

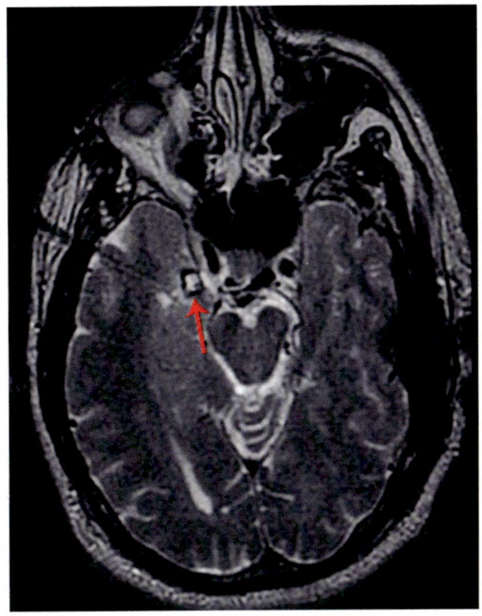

FIG. 21.10 Cavernous Malformation Treated With Laser-Induced Thermal Therapy (LITT). Note the right side medial temporal lesion. This patient had seizures localized to this region, and it was thought that the lesion was the cause of the seizures. LITT was performed and the patient tolerated the procedure well. He was seizure-free thereafter. (Reproduced from: Patel P, Patel NV, Danish SF. Intracranial MR-guided laser-induced thermal therapy: single-center experience with the Visualase thermal therapy system. *J Neurosurg*. 2016:1–8.)

Chronic Pain

As many as 9 million people suffer from intractable cancer-associated pain annually.[99] In hopes of finding more long-term alleviation of the pain, MRgLITT has been investigated as an alternative to radiofrequency for anterior cingulotomy. Patel and colleagues[39] reported their outcomes in three patients who underwent bilateral anterior cingulotomy using MRgLITT (Fig. 21.11). There was significant alleviation of pain in all patients (one required two MRgLITT procedures). There were

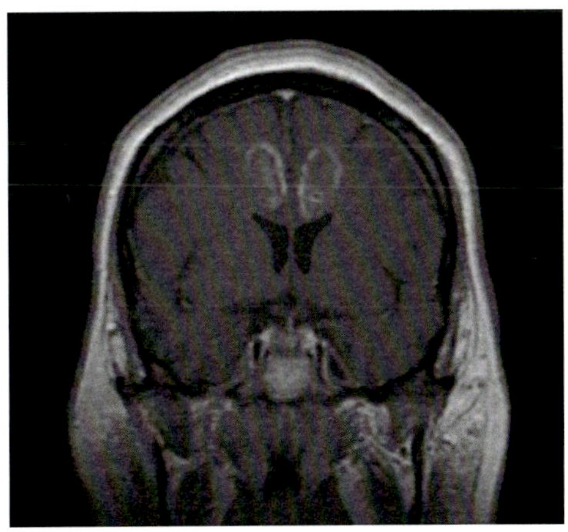

FIG. 21.11 Bilateral Cingulotomy Case Treated With Laser-Induced Thermal Therapy. Postoperative changes are seen after laser ablation to bilateral cingulate gyrus for the treatment of chronic pain. (Reproduced from: Patel NV, Agarwal N, Mammis A, Danish SF. Frameless stereotactic magnetic resonance imaging-guided laser interstitial thermal therapy to perform bilateral anterior cingulotomy for intractable pain: feasibility, technical aspects, and initial experience in 3 patients. *Neurosurgery*. 2015;11(suppl 2):17–25; discussion 25.)

no complications reported. Other studies also confirmed successful treatment of chronic cancer pain using LITT.[57,100] Stereotactic cingulotomies have been performed since the 1970s with most procedures using radiofrequency ablation.[39] However, there have been mixed outcomes in terms of the longevity of pain relief. Whether there is real value in using MRgLITT over radiofrequency in this procedure remains to be seen.

Pediatric Neurooncology and Epilepsy

The earliest use of LITT in the pediatric population was limited to deep-seated brain tumors.[101] In fact, two of the first case reports using MRgLITT were for pediatric cases of thalamic and hypothalamic tumors. Jethwa and colleagues presented the first case report of a child with a thalamic supratentorial primitive neuroectodermal tumor.[102] The patient tolerated the procedure well with almost complete resolution of preoperative neurologic deficits at 6 months' follow-up. As was previously described (in the Epilepsy section), another case report described favorable outcomes of treating a hypothalamic hamartoma in a 3-year-old child.[81]

As more studies were conducted and literature reported, the evidence for the safety and efficacy of LITT expanded its indications to include various tumor types located more superficially as well. In the first series looking at pediatric brain tumors treated with LITT, Tovar-Spinoza and colleagues presented a wide range of etiologies including pilocytic astrocytoma, ependymoma (see Fig. 21.12), medulloblastoma, choroid plexus xanthogranuloma, subependymal giant cell astrocytoma, and ganglioglioma.[103] The tumors included deep-seated lesions, recurrent tumors that were resistant to adjuvant therapies, and tumors that could be difficult to identify intraoperatively, further emphasizing the range of the tumor types that can be offered LITT. Of the 11 patients in this series, 2 patients experienced postoperative complications but both had improvement over time with rehabilitation. The same group presented a case report of a 19-month-old male child with a ganglioglioma.[104] The child underwent ablation with the LITT and was discharged the following day without operative or perioperative complications. Follow-up visits confirmed significant reduction of tumor volume. Numerous other studies have also demonstrated the use of LITT in pediatric intracranial diagnoses.[38,95,105]

In general, LITT has many advantages over conventional surgery, which are even more relevant when considering the pediatric population. This novel procedure can be used in all age groups and can be repeated multiple times without any adverse side effects.[103] LITT is also associated with shorter operative times and hospital stays, allowing for shorter time to return to normal life for children. For low-grade gliomas, the treatments of choice are usually total resection accompanied by adjuvant chemotherapy and radiotherapy. However, radiation and chemotherapy can lead to developmental problems and cognitive deficits in young children.[104] In such cases, MRgLITT would be a safer alternative to offer to pediatric patients. Lastly, this technique allows for cosmetically more appealing results and is thus a less traumatic experience for a child.

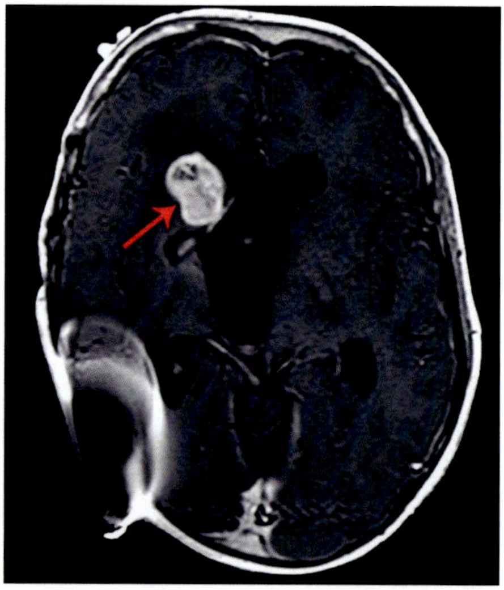

FIG. 21.12 Pediatric Ependymoma Case Treated With Laser-Induced Thermal Therapy (LITT). A 13-year-old pediatric patient presented with a right frontal ventricular ependymoma. This preoperative MRI shows the tumor of interest, which was then treated with LITT. (Reproduced from: Patel NV, Jethwa PR, Shetty A, Danish SF. Does the real-time thermal damage estimate allow for estimation of tumor control after MRI-guided laser-induced thermal therapy? Initial experience with recurrent intracranial ependymomas. *J Neurosurg Pediatr*. 2015;15(4):363–371.)

REPORTED COMPLICATIONS

Although long-term studies are still warranted to determine long-term benefits and clinical outcomes for many of the intracranial pathologies, a lot is already known about the safety profile of this procedure. Many of the studies documented complications that arose in the perioperative and postoperative periods. These include neurologic deficits, hemorrhage, infection, thermal injury, refractory edema, and technical issues.

Neurologic Deficits

According to Medvid et al.[55] who analyzed a large number of LITT studies with reported complications, transient neurologic deficits are the most commonly reported complications, with an overall incidence of about 13%. These resolved either spontaneously or following steroid administration and included symptoms such as dysphagia, weakness, hemianopsia, and seizures. New progressive or permanent neurologic deficits occur in about 3% of patients undergoing MRgLITT.[55]

The largest series of patients to undergo LITT using the Visualase thermal therapy system was presented by Patel and colleagues.[57] They reported outcomes in 102 patients who were treated for a variety of pathologies including primary intracranial tumors, metastatic tumors/radiation necrosis, epilepsy, and chronic pain syndrome. In their series, neurologic deficits were also the most frequent complication to arise, accounting for 13.7%. This included mostly motor deficits and also cognitive decline and visual changes. Of these deficits, 64.3% had complete resolution within 1 month and 7.1% had partial resolution. Permanent deficits were seen in 14.3% of the total deficits and another 14.3% died before resolution.

Patel et al. believed that the deficits that were transient were secondary to postoperative edema in the ablation bed, and as the edema resolved, the deficits also resolved over time.[57] In the cases of permanent deficits, there was potentially permanent thermal injury to the motor tract, which led to motor deficits in those patients. Sharma and colleagues[106] found that permanent neurologic deficits occurred in patients who had larger overlapping volumes and areas between CSTs and hyperthermic fields. Pruitt and colleagues[107] described alterations they made after experiencing three cases of permanent neurologic deficits secondary to thermal injury in their series of 49 LITT procedures. The authors used a smaller, 3-mm diffusing tip and modified thermal energy doses to ensure more controlled ablation, especially for lesions in close vicinity to critical structures such as the brainstem, spinal cord, or eloquent cortex.

Sloan and colleagues[34] conducted the first clinical trial using the NeuroBlate Thermal Therapy system. Of the 10 patients in their series, 2 (20%) patients experienced temporary neurologic deficits, which resolved after steroid treatment. Another group presented 34 patients who underwent LITT using the NeuroBlate System.[43] They found neurologic deficits in seven patients (20%), of which five (14%) were transient and resolved within a few days, whereas the other two (6%) were permanent deficits.

Hemorrhage

Hemorrhage is a potential complication in any procedure that involves intracranial catheter insertion.[57] In the series presented by Patel and colleagues,[57] three patients (2.9%) experienced hemorrhages, which required conversion to open surgery to evacuate the hemorrhage (see Fig. 21.13). It was determined that vessels could have been damaged when the catheter was placed, despite careful trajectory planning. Pruitt and colleagues[107] reported three (6.1%) incidences of hemorrhage in their series of 49 patients who underwent LITT. The authors described each case and made alterations in their procedure and management to avoid such future complications. Various events were hypothesized to have led to the hemorrhages including vascular injury during insertion of the device, inadequate puncture of the dura, improper catheter removal, and use of multiple devices. In response, the group adopted a sharper tool to adequately open dura, fused computed tomographic angiography (CTA) and MRI for better anatomic accuracy, and trajectory planning in relation to vasculature and aimed to limit the number of devices and reduce device malfunction.

Infection

The overall incidence of infections is approximately 2.5%.[55] These infections can be superficial at the incision site or more severe such as ventriculitis and

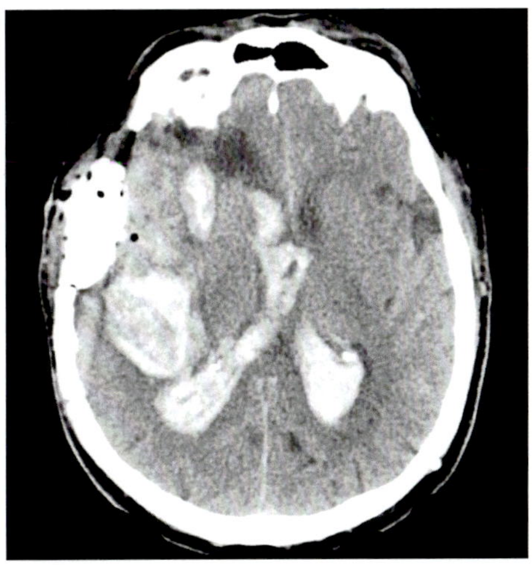

FIG. 21.13 **Hemorrhage From Laser-Induced Thermal Therapy (LITT) Image.** An example of a significant LITT-related complication. A large hemorrhage noted secondary to vascular injury during an LITT procedure. (Reproduced from: Patel P, Patel NV, Danish SF. Intracranial MR-guided laser-induced thermal therapy: single-center experience with the Visualase thermal therapy system. *J Neurosurg*. 2016:1–8.)

meningitis. Several studies showed similar rates. Patel et al.[57] reported two (2.0%) cases of superficial wound infections at the insertion site in their series. Mohammadi and colleagues[43] had an infection rate of 6%, of which one case was superficial and the other was ventriculitis. Lastly, Hawasli et al.[54] reported a case of fatal meningitis.

Refractory Edema

Refractory edema can be defined as edema that is persistent, symptomatic, and unresponsive to conservative treatment methods.[57] The peak of postablation edema is usually around 3–4 days postoperatively that can then be managed sufficiently with steroid tapers (see Fig. 21.14).[35] In the study by Patel and colleagues,[57] there were five complications attributed to refractory edema, two of which led to perioperative deaths. Of the perioperative deaths, one of the lesions had a large volume and the other lesion was located near the midbrain and pons. Rapid progression of malignant edema in these two lesions led to global neurologic decline and the demise of the patients. Measures taken to reduce such complications are discussed in further detail in a later section.

Inaccurate Laser Placement

Complications can also arise from device malposition such as subdural hematoma, subarachnoid hemorrhage, other arterial injuries, and even seeding of neoplastic cells along catheter trajectory.[107] In one study, two cases of laser misplacement led to abortion of the LITT procedure (Fig. 21.15).[57] Therefore, accurate and proper placement is important for efficiency of the procedure and reduction of postoperative complications. Methods to avoid catheter and laser malposition are discussed in the next section.

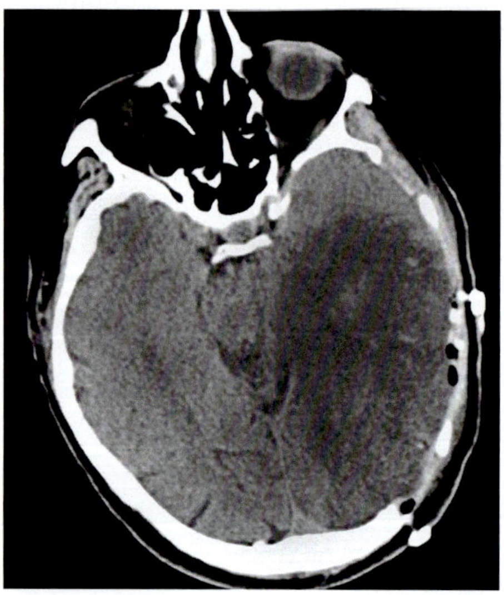

FIG. 21.14 Post–Laser-Induced Thermal Therapy Refractory Edema. This image shows extensive left-sided edema, marked by hypodense region on this CT image, after patient underwent laser ablation for tumor. The patient is postdecompressive craniectomy.

Complication Avoidance

Multiple techniques and changes have been adopted to try to reduce the number of complications associated with LITT. The use of intraoperative image guidance, computer assistance, and frameless surgical navigation systems has revolutionized and advanced treatment of many intracranial pathologies and has been associated with lower complication rates.[108,109] In addition to the preoperative CT/MR images that are taken for trajectory planning, it has been suggested to also include magnetic resonance angiography or CTA and diffusion tensor imaging with fiber tracking in preoperative imaging.[34,107] This could improve trajectory planning by avoiding vital structures such as vessels and cerebrospinal fluid (CSF) when navigating the catheter or laser to the target lesion, thus potentially reducing the incidence of hemorrhage and motor deficits.

Precautions can also be taken in an attempt to prevent complications secondary to refractory edema. If there are lesions for which large ablation volumes would be expected or if lesions are in close vicinity to critical structures, high-dose steroid administration preoperatively may assist in decreasing adverse events due to postablation edema.[35] In addition, the procedure should not be offered to patients who required high-dose steroids preoperatively for symptom relief.[57] More aggressive surveillance and treatment before development of edema have also been attempted to prevent postoperative occurrences. Habboub and colleagues presented a novel combination of laser ablation and subsequent minimally invasive debulking for the treatment of large intracranial tumors.[110] As thermal coagulation from the ablation can lead to edema and mass effect, postablation debulking would theoretically aim to control for the swelling and volume expansion and thus lower the risk of developing edema-related complications.

Frame-based techniques such as use of anchoring devices can help reduce complications secondary to device malposition and inaccurate laser placement.[107] A variety of stereotactic techniques have been introduced to further improve laser placement, including traditional frames, robot-assisted systems, optical frameless

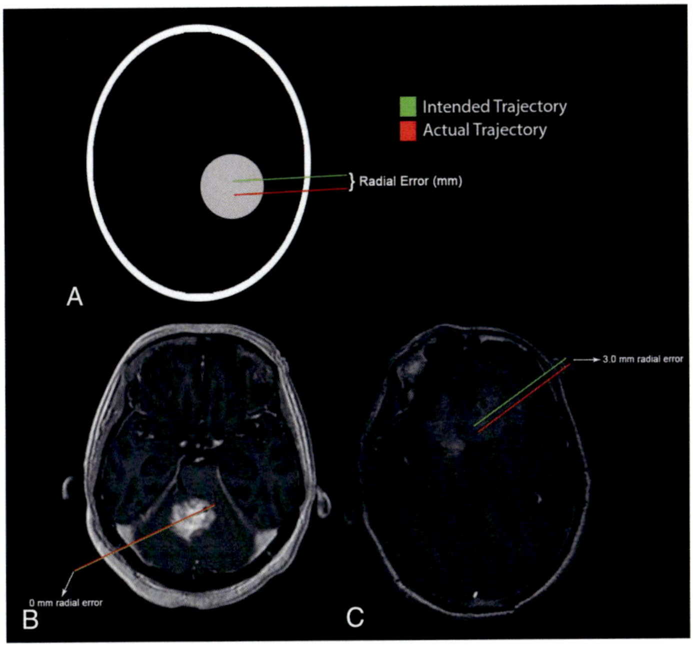

FIG. 21.15 **Inaccurate Laser Insertion.** **(A)** A goal of preoperative stereotactic registration and trajectory planning is to ensure a minimal radial error (mm) between the intended trajectory (in green) and actual trajectory (in red). **(B)** In this case, there is a 0 mm radial error, meaning the actual trajectory was accurate and identical to the intended trajectory that was planned preoperatively. **(C)** In this case, there is a 3.0 mm radial error between the planned trajectory (green) and actual trajectory (red). This can increase the risk of damage to eloquent brain matter and vasculature during laser placement. (Reproduced from: Attaar SJ, Patel NV, Hargreaves E, Keller IA, Danish SF. Accuracy of laser placement with frameless stereotaxy in magnetic resonance-guided laser-induced thermal therapy. *Oper Neurosurg*. 2015;11(4):554–563.)

systems, MRI-assisted techniques, and most recently, custom 3D printed stereotactic frames.[111] Attaar and colleagues reported their consistent accuracy in laser placement and resultant complete ablations when using skull pin–based frameless stereotaxy.[112] Other technical advances such as novel miniframes can permit more trajectory angles and multiple trajectories from a single burr hole.[34] In addition, new MRI coils that would improve access to targets from a range of angles allowing greater coverage of tumor are also under development.

As physicians gain experience with the LITT procedure and patient selection, the efficacy and safety profile are also expected to improve. Several studies have shown that with more experience, they observed increased survival and laser placement accuracy and decreased incidences of major complications.[35,53,57] It is also important to consider patient comorbidities when offering any surgical procedure. Although LITT is minimally invasive relative to open surgery, there are nevertheless complications that can arise, especially in patients in medically more compromised states. Patel and colleagues[57] noted that in their series of 102 patients, all complications occurred in patients who had a primary or metastatic intracranial tumor versus those with epilepsy or chronic pain. These patients were medically more debilitated, which may have also increased their chances of developing complications in the peri- and postoperative periods.

FUTURE DIRECTIONS

Nanotechnology is currently being investigated for its potential in cancer treatment, and LITT may be a vital component to this novel therapy. Gold nanoparticles, in particular, have been able to successfully achieve controlled thermal damage within tumors when used with laser light.[113] Nanoparticles work by increasing absorption in tissues such as cancerous cells, allowing greater degree of heating of those cells.[114] Macrophages can be used as vectors to deliver nanoparticles through the BBB to the target site.[115] Once there, increased accumulation of the particles within the tissue allows the target lesion to be ablated with higher selectivity relative to surrounding areas. LITT can act as the source of laser irradiation to the nanoparticle-filled target tissues. Schwartz and colleagues[116] used MRgLITT for the nanoparticle-directed ablation of canine prostates and concluded that the method allowed for precise tumor ablation while also preventing damage to nearby critical structures. This novel technique has been tested on multiple animal models and on in vitro tumor cell lines, specifically GBM, with promising outcomes.[113,116–120] Further experimentation is required to assess the safety, feasibility, and efficacy in clinical cases. The future direction and association of LITT in nanotechnology may lead to a turning point for cancer therapies.

REFERENCES

1. Takac S, Stojanovic S. Characteristics of laser light. *Med Pregl.* 1999;52(1–2):29–34.
2. Ryan RW, Spetzler RF, Preul MC. Aura of technology and the cutting edge: a history of lasers in neurosurgery. *Neurosurg Focus.* 2009;27(3):E6.
3. Stellar S, Polanyi TG. Lasers in neurosurgery: a historical overview. *J Clin Laser Med Surg.* 1992;10(6):399–411.
4. Jain KK. Lasers in neurosurgery: a review. *Lasers Surg Med.* 1983;2(3):217–230.
5. Krishnamurthy S, Powers SK. Lasers in neurosurgery. *Lasers Surg Med.* 1994;15(2):126–167.
6. McGuff PE, Deterling Jr RA, Gottlieb LS, Fahimi HD, Bushnell D. Surgical applications of laser. *Ann Surg.* 1964;160:765–777.
7. Minton JP, Ketcham AS. The effect of ruby laser radiation on the cloudman S-91 melanoma in the CDBA-2F hybrid mouse. *Cancer.* 1964;17:1305–1309.
8. Ascher PW, Heppner F. CO_2-laser in neurosurgery. *Neurosurg Rev.* 1984;7(2–3):123–133.
9. Rosomoff HL, Carroll F. Reaction of neoplasm and brain to laser. *Arch Neurol.* 1966;14(2):143–148.
10. Bown SG. Phototherapy in tumors. *World J Surg.* 1983; 7(6):700–709.
11. Chen L, Wansapura JP, Heit G, Butts K. Study of laser ablation in the in vivo rabbit brain with MR thermometry. *J Magn Reson Imag.* 2002;16(2):147–152.
12. Cheng MK, McKean J, Boisvert D, Tulip J, Mielke BW. Effects of photoradiation therapy on normal rat brain. *Neurosurgery.* 1984;15(6):804–810.
13. Elias Z, Powers SK, Atstupenas E, Brown JT. Hyperthermia from interstitial laser irradiation in normal rat brain. *Lasers Surg Med.* 1987;7(4):370–375.
14. Tracz RA, Wyman DR, Little PB, et al. Magnetic resonance imaging of interstitial laser photocoagulation in brain. *Lasers Surg Med.* 1992;12(2):165–173.
15. Tracz RA, Wyman DR, Little PB, et al. Comparison of magnetic resonance images and the histopathological findings of lesions induced by interstitial laser photocoagulation in the brain. *Lasers Surg Med.* 1993;13(1): 45–54.
16. Roux FX, Devaux B, Mordon S, Nguyen S, Chodkiewicz JP. The use of 1.32 Nd:YAG laser in neurosurgery: experimental data and clinical experience from 70 patients. *J Clin Laser Med Surg.* 1990;8(4):55–61.
17. Wharen Jr RE, Anderson RE, Scheithauer B, Sundt Jr TM. The Nd:YAG laser in neurosurgery. Part 1. Laboratory investigations: dose-related biological response of neural tissue. *J Neurosurg.* 1984;60(3):531–539.
18. Beck OJ. The use of the Nd-YAG and the CO_2 laser in neurosurgery. *Neurosurg Rev.* 1980;3(4):261–266.
19. Boggan JE, Edwards MS, Davis RL, Bolger CA, Martin N. Comparison of the brain tissue response in rats to injury by argon and carbon dioxide lasers. *Neurosurgery.* 1982; 11(5):609–616.
20. Powers SK, Edwards MS, Boggan JE, et al. Use of the argon surgical laser in neurosurgery. *J Neurosurg.* 1984; 60(3):523–530.
21. Roux FX, Mordon S, Fallet-Bianco C, Merienne L, Devaux BC, Chodkiewicz JP. Effects of 1.32-micron Nd-YAG laser on brain thermal and histological experimental data. *Surg Neurol.* 1990;34(6):402–407.
22. Martiniuk R, Bauer JA, McKean JD, Tulip J, Mielke BW. New long-wavelength Nd:YAG laser at 1.44 micron: effect on brain. *J Neurosurg.* 1989;70(2):249–256.
23. Devaux BC, Roux FX, Nataf F, Turak B, Cioloca C. High-power diode laser in neurosurgery: clinical experience in 30 cases. *Surg Neurol.* 1998;50(1):33–39; discussion 39–40.
24. Ryan RW, Wolf T, Spetzler RF, Coons SW, Fink Y, Preul MC. Application of a flexible CO(2) laser fiber for neurosurgery: laser-tissue interactions. *J Neurosurg.* 2010;112(2):434–443.
25. Kelly PJ, Alker Jr GJ, Goerss S. Computer-assisted stereotactic microsurgery for the treatment of intracranial neoplasms. *Neurosurgery.* 1982;10(3):324–331.
26. Kelly PJ. Future perspectives in stereotactic neurosurgery: stereotactic microsurgical removal of deep brain tumors. *J Neurosurg Sci.* 1989;33(1):149–154.
27. Jolesz FA, Bleier AR, Jakab P, Ruenzel PW, Huttl K, Jako GJ. MR imaging of laser-tissue interactions. *Radiology.* 1988;168(1):249–253.
28. McDannold NJ, Jolesz FA. Magnetic resonance image-guided thermal ablations. *Top Magn Reson Imaging.* 2000;11(3):191–202.
29. Anzai Y, Lufkin RB, Saxton RE, et al. Nd:YAG interstitial laser phototherapy guided by magnetic resonance imaging in an ex vivo model: dosimetry of laser-MR-tissue interaction. *Laryngoscope.* 1991;101(7 Pt 1):755–760.
30. Matsumoto R, Oshio K, Jolesz FA. Monitoring of laser and freezing-induced ablation in the liver with T1-weighted MR imaging. *J Magn Reson Imag.* 1992;2(5):555–562.

31. Patel NV, Mian M, Stafford RJ, et al. Laser interstitial thermal therapy technology, physics of magnetic resonance imaging thermometry, and technical considerations for proper catheter placement during magnetic resonance imaging-guided laser interstitial thermal therapy. *Neurosurgery*. 2016;79(suppl 1):S8–S16.
32. Stafford RJ, Fuentes D, Elliott AA, Weinberg JS, Ahrar K. Laser-induced thermal therapy for tumor ablation. *Crit Rev Biomed Eng*. 2010;38(1):79–100.
33. Lagman C, Chung LK, Pelargos PE, et al. Laser neurosurgery: a systematic analysis of magnetic resonance-guided laser interstitial thermal therapies. *J Clin Neurosci*. 2017;36: 20–26.
34. Sloan AE, Ahluwalia MS, Valerio-Pascua J, et al. Results of the NeuroBlate System first-in-humans Phase I clinical trial for recurrent glioblastoma: clinical article. *J Neurosurg*. 2013;118(6):1202–1219.
35. Jethwa PR, Barrese JC, Gowda A, Shetty A, Danish SF. Magnetic resonance thermometry-guided laser-induced thermal therapy for intracranial neoplasms: initial experience. *Neurosurgery*. 2012;71(1 suppl Operative): 133–144; 144–145.
36. Patel PD, Patel NV, Davidson C, Danish SF. The role of MRgLITT in overcoming the challenges in managing infield recurrence after radiation for brain metastasis. *Neurosurgery*. 2016;79(suppl 1):S40–S58.
37. Gross RE, Willie JT, Drane DL. The role of stereotactic laser amygdalohippocampotomy in mesial temporal lobe epilepsy. *Neurosurg Clin N Am*. 2016;27(1):37–50.
38. Curry DJ, Gowda A, McNichols RJ, Wilfong AA. MR-guided stereotactic laser ablation of epileptogenic foci in children. *Epilepsy Behav*. 2012;24(4):408–414.
39. Patel NV, Agarwal N, Mammis A, Danish SF. Frameless stereotactic magnetic resonance imaging-guided laser interstitial thermal therapy to perform bilateral anterior cingulotomy for intractable pain: feasibility, technical aspects, and initial experience in 3 patients. *Neurosurgery*. 2015;11(suppl 2):17–25; discussion 25.
40. Ahn H, Mousavi P, Chin L, et al. The effect of pre-vertebroplasty tumor ablation using laser-induced thermotherapy on biomechanical stability and cement fill in the metastatic spine. *Eur Spine J*. 2007;16(8):1171–1178.
41. Diaz R, Ivan ME, Hanft S, et al. Laser interstitial thermal therapy: lighting the way to a new treatment option in neurosurgery. *Neurosurgery*. 2016;79(suppl 1):S3–S7.
42. Carpentier A, McNichols RJ, Stafford RJ, et al. Real-time magnetic resonance-guided laser thermal therapy for focal metastatic brain tumors. *Neurosurgery*. 2008; 63(1 suppl 1): ONS21–28; discussion ONS28–29.
43. Mohammadi AM, Hawasli AH, Rodriguez A, et al. The role of laser interstitial thermal therapy in enhancing progression-free survival of difficult-to-access high-grade gliomas: a multicenter study. *Cancer Med*. 2014;3(4): 971–979.
44. Ostrom QT, Bauchet L, Davis FG, et al. The epidemiology of glioma in adults: a "state of the science" review. *Neuro Oncol*. 2014;16(7):896–913.
45. Brown PD, Maurer MJ, Rummans TA, et al. A prospective study of quality of life in adults with newly diagnosed high-grade gliomas: the impact of the extent of resection on quality of life and survival. *Neurosurgery*. 2005;57(3): 495–504; discussion 495–504.
46. Gulati S, Jakola AS, Nerland US, Weber C, Solheim O. The risk of getting worse: surgically acquired deficits, perioperative complications, and functional outcomes after primary resection of glioblastoma. *World Neurosurg*. 2011;76(6):572–579.
47. Hawasli AH, Kim AH, Dunn GP, Tran DD, Leuthardt EC. Stereotactic laser ablation of high-grade gliomas. *Neurosurg Focus*. 2014;37(6):E1.
48. Ascher PW, Justich E, Schrottner O. Interstitial thermotherapy of central brain tumors with the Nd:YAG laser under real-time monitoring by MRI. *J Clin Laser Med Surg*. 1991;9(1):79–83.
49. Sugiyama K, Sakai T, Fujishima I, Ryu H, Uemura K, Yokoyama T. Stereotactic interstitial laser-hyperthermia using Nd-YAG laser. *Stereotact Funct Neurosurg*. 1990; 54–55:501–505.
50. Reimer P, Bremer C, Horch C, Morgenroth C, Allkemper T, Schuierer G. MR-monitored LITT as a palliative concept in patients with high grade gliomas: preliminary clinical experience. *J Magn Reson Imag*. 1998;8(1):240–244.
51. Bettag M, Ulrich F, Schober R, et al. Stereotactic laser therapy in cerebral gliomas. *Acta Neurochir Suppl (Wien)*. 1991;52:81–83.
52. Fan M, Ascher PW, Schrottner O, Ebner F, Germann RH, Kleinert R. Interstitial 1.06 Nd:YAG laser thermotherapy for brain tumors under real-time monitoring of MRI: experimental study and phase I clinical trial. *J Clin Laser Med Surg*. 1992;10(5):355–361.
53. Schwarzmaier HJ, Eickmeyer F, von Tempelhoff W, et al. MR-guided laser-induced interstitial thermotherapy of recurrent glioblastoma multiforme: preliminary results in 16 patients. *Eur J Radiol*. 2006;59(2):208–215.
54. Hawasli AH, Bagade S, Shimony JS, Miller-Thomas M, Leuthardt EC. Magnetic resonance imaging-guided focused laser interstitial thermal therapy for intracranial lesions: single-institution series. *Neurosurgery*. 2013; 73(6):1007–1017.
55. Medvid R, Ruiz A, Komotar RJ, et al. Current applications of MRI-guided laser interstitial thermal therapy in the treatment of brain neoplasms and epilepsy: a radiologic and neurosurgical overview. *Am J Neuroradiol*. 2015; 36(11):1998–2006.
56. Carpentier A, Chauvet D, Reina V, et al. MR-guided laser-induced thermal therapy (LITT) for recurrent glioblastomas. *Lasers Surg Med*. 2012;44(5):361–368.
57. Patel P, Patel NV, Danish SF. Intracranial MR-guided laser-induced thermal therapy: single-center experience with the Visualase thermal therapy system. *J Neurosurg*. 2016:1–8.
58. Missios S, Bekelis K, Barnett GH. Renaissance of laser interstitial thermal ablation. *Neurosurg Focus*. 2015;38(3):E13.

59. Barnett GH, Voigt JD, Alhuwalia MS. A systematic review and meta-analysis of studies examining the use of brain laser interstitial thermal therapy versus craniotomy for the treatment of high-grade tumors in or near areas of eloquence: an examination of the extent of resection and major complication rates associated with each type of surgery. *Stereotact Funct Neurosurg*. 2016;94(3): 164–173.
60. Leuthardt EC, Duan C, Kim MJ, et al. Hyperthermic laser ablation of recurrent glioblastoma leads to temporary disruption of the peritumoral blood brain barrier. *PLoS One*. 2016;11(2):e0148613.
61. Lee I, Kalkanis S, Hadjipanayis CG. Stereotactic laser interstitial thermal therapy for recurrent high-grade gliomas. *Neurosurgery*. 2016;79(suppl 1):S24–S34.
62. Ivan ME, Mohammadi AM, De Deugd N, et al. Laser ablation of newly diagnosed malignant gliomas: a meta-analysis. *Neurosurgery*. 2016;79(suppl 1):S17–S23.
63. Leonardi MA, Lumenta CB. Stereotactic guided laser-induced interstitial thermotherapy (SLITT) in gliomas with intraoperative morphologic monitoring in an open MR: clinical experience. *Minim Invasive Neurosurg*. 2002;45(4):201–207.
64. Voigt JD, Barnett G. The value of using a brain laser interstitial thermal therapy (LITT) system in patients presenting with high grade gliomas where maximal safe resection may not be feasible. *Cost Eff Resour Alloc*. 2016;14:6.
65. Torcuator RG, Hulou MM, Chavakula V, Jolesz FA, Golby AJ. Intraoperative real-time MRI-guided stereotactic biopsy followed by laser thermal ablation for progressive brain metastases after radiosurgery. *J Clin Neurosci*. 2016;24:68–73.
66. Kocher M, Soffietti R, Abacioglu U, et al. Adjuvant whole-brain radiotherapy versus observation after radiosurgery or surgical resection of one to three cerebral metastases: results of the EORTC 22952-26001 study. *J Clin Oncol*. 2011;29(2):134–141.
67. Rajakesari S, Arvold ND, Jimenez RB, et al. Local control after fractionated stereotactic radiation therapy for brain metastases. *J Neurooncol*. 2014;120(2):339–346.
68. Carpentier A, McNichols RJ, Stafford RJ, et al. Laser thermal therapy: real-time MRI-guided and computer-controlled procedures for metastatic brain tumors. *Lasers Surg Med*. 2011;43(10):943–950.
69. Hawasli AH, Ray WZ, Murphy RK, Dacey Jr RG, Leuthardt EC. Magnetic resonance imaging-guided focused laser interstitial thermal therapy for subinsular metastatic adenocarcinoma: technical case report. *Neurosurgery*. 2012;70(2 suppl Operative):332–337; discussion 338.
70. Fabiano AJ, Alberico RA. Laser-interstitial thermal therapy for refractory cerebral edema from post-radiosurgery metastasis. *World Neurosurg*. 2014;81(3–4):652.e651–e654.
71. Fabiano AJ, Qiu J. Delayed failure of laser-induced interstitial thermotherapy for postradiosurgery brain metastases. *World Neurosurg*. 2014;82(3–4):e559–e563.
72. Rahmathulla G, Marko NF, Weil RJ. Cerebral radiation necrosis: a review of the pathobiology, diagnosis and management considerations. *J Clin Neurosci*. 2013; 20(4):485–502.
73. Rahmathulla G, Recinos PF, Valerio JE, Chao S, Barnett GH. Laser interstitial thermal therapy for focal cerebral radiation necrosis: a case report and literature review. *Stereotact Funct Neurosurg*. 2012;90(3):192–200.
74. Torres-Reveron J, Tomasiewicz HC, Shetty A, Amankulor NM, Chiang VL. Stereotactic laser induced thermotherapy (LITT): a novel treatment for brain lesions regrowing after radiosurgery. *J Neurooncol*. 2013;113(3): 495–503.
75. Smith CJ, Myers CS, Chapple KM, Smith KA. Long-term follow-up of 25 cases of biopsy-proven radiation necrosis or post-radiation treatment effect treated with magnetic resonance-guided laser interstitial thermal therapy. *Neurosurgery*. 2016;79(suppl 1):S59–S72.
76. Rao MS, Hargreaves EL, Khan AJ, Haffty BG, Danish SF. Magnetic resonance-guided laser ablation improves local control for postradiosurgery recurrence and/or radiation necrosis. *Neurosurgery*. 2014;74(6):658–667; discussion 667.
77. Kano H, Kondziolka D, Lobato-Polo J, Zorro O, Flickinger JC, Lunsford LD. T1/T2 matching to differentiate tumor growth from radiation effects after stereotactic radiosurgery. *Neurosurgery*. 2010;66(3):486–491; discussion 491–492.
78. Hernandez RN, Patel PD, Iqbal MO, Hargreaves EL, Danish SF. Magnetic resonance-guided laser-induced thermal therapy for infield progression following stereotactic radiosurgery for metastatic brain disease. *J Neuro-Oncology*. 2017. In press.
79. LaRiviere MJ, Gross RE. Stereotactic laser ablation for medically intractable epilepsy: the next generation of minimally invasive epilepsy surgery. *Front Surg*. 2016;3:64.
80. Wilfong AA, Curry DJ. Hypothalamic hamartomas: optimal approach to clinical evaluation and diagnosis. *Epilepsia*. 2013;54(suppl 9):109–114.
81. Tovar-Spinoza Z, Carter D, Ferrone D, Eksioglu Y, Huckins S. The use of MRI-guided laser-induced thermal ablation for epilepsy. *Childs Nerv Syst*. 2013;29(11): 2089–2094.
82. Engel Jr J. Mesial temporal lobe epilepsy: what have we learned? *Neuroscientist*. 2001;7(4):340–352.
83. Sharma AK, Reams RY, Jordan WH, Miller MA, Thacker HL, Snyder PW. Mesial temporal lobe epilepsy: pathogenesis, induced rodent models and lesions. *Toxicol Pathol*. 2007;35(7):984–999.
84. Willie JT, Laxpati NG, Drane DL, et al. Real-time magnetic resonance-guided stereotactic laser amygdalohippocampotomy for mesial temporal lobe epilepsy. *Neurosurgery*. 2014;74(6):569–584; discussion 584–565.
85. Waseem H, Osborn KE, Schoenberg MR, et al. Laser ablation therapy: an alternative treatment for medically resistant mesial temporal lobe epilepsy after age 50. *Epilepsy Behav*. 2015;51:152–157.

86. Kang JY, Wu C, Tracy J, et al. Laser interstitial thermal therapy for medically intractable mesial temporal lobe epilepsy. *Epilepsia*. 2016;57(2):325–334.
87. Kang JY, Sperling MR. Magnetic resonance imaging-guided laser interstitial thermal therapy for treatment of drug-resistant epilepsy. *Neurotherapeutics*. 2017;14(1):176–181.
88. Battaglia G, Chiapparini L, Franceschetti S, et al. Periventricular nodular heterotopia: classification, epileptic history, and genesis of epileptic discharges. *Epilepsia*. 2006; 47(1):86–97.
89. Esquenazi Y, Kalamangalam GP, Slater JD, et al. Stereotactic laser ablation of epileptogenic periventricular nodular heterotopia. *Epilepsy Res*. 2014;108(3):547–554.
90. Clarke DF, Tindall K, Lee M, Patel B. Bilateral occipital dysplasia, seizure identification, and ablation: a novel surgical technique. *Epileptic Disord*. 2014;16(2): 238–243.
91. Gonzalez-Martinez J, Vadera S, Mullin J, et al. Robot-assisted stereotactic laser ablation in medically intractable epilepsy: operative technique. *Neurosurgery*. 2014; 10(suppl 2):167–172; discussion 172–163.
92. Kabat J, Krol P. Focal cortical dysplasia - review. *Pol J Radiol*. 2012;77(2):35–43.
93. Shaker T, Bernier A, Carmant L. Focal cortical dysplasia in childhood epilepsy. *Semin Pediatr Neurol*. 2016;23(2): 108–119.
94. Bandt SK, Leuthardt EC. Minimally invasive neurosurgery for epilepsy using stereotactic MRI guidance. *Neurosurg Clin N Am*. 2016;27(1):51–58.
95. Lewis EC, Weil AG, Duchowny M, Bhatia S, Ragheb J, Miller I. MR-guided laser interstitial thermal therapy for pediatric drug-resistant lesional epilepsy. *Epilepsia*. 2015;56(10):1590–1598.
96. Connolly MB, Hendson G, Steinbok P. Tuberous sclerosis complex: a review of the management of epilepsy with emphasis on surgical aspects. *Childs Nerv Syst*. 2006; 22(8):896–908.
97. Holmes GL, Stafstrom CE, Tuberous Sclerosis Study G. Tuberous sclerosis complex and epilepsy: recent developments and future challenges. *Epilepsia*. 2007;48(4): 617–630.
98. McCracken DJ, Willie JT, Fernald B, et al. Magnetic resonance thermometry-guided stereotactic laser ablation of cavernous malformations in drug-resistant epilepsy: imaging and clinical results. *Oper Neurosurg Hagerst*. 2016; 12(1):39–48.
99. Tiwari P, Danish S, Madabhushi A. Identifying MRI markers to evaluate early treatment related changes post laser ablation for cancer pain management. *Proc SPIE*. 2014;9036:90362L.
100. Sundararajan SH, Belani P, Danish S, Keller I. Early MRI characteristics after MRI-guided laser-assisted cingulotomy for intractable pain control. *Am J Neuroradiol*. 2015;36(7):1283–1287.
101. Riordan M, Tovar-Spinoza Z. Laser induced thermal therapy (LITT) for pediatric brain tumors: case-based review. *Transl Pediatr*. 2014;3(3):229–235.
102. Jethwa PR, Lee JH, Assina R, Keller IA, Danish SF. Treatment of a supratentorial primitive neuroectodermal tumor using magnetic resonance-guided laser-induced thermal therapy. *J Neurosurg Pediatr*. 2011;8(5):468–475.
103. Tovar-Spinoza Z, Choi H. Magnetic resonance-guided laser interstitial thermal therapy: report of a series of pediatric brain tumors. *J Neurosurg Pediatr*. 2016;17(6): 723–733.
104. Tovar-Spinoza Z, Choi H. MRI-guided laser interstitial thermal therapy for the treatment of low-grade gliomas in children: a case-series review, description of the current technologies and perspectives. *Childs Nerv Syst*. 2016; 32(10):1947–1956.
105. Patel NV, Jethwa PR, Shetty A, Danish SF. Does the real-time thermal damage estimate allow for estimation of tumor control after MRI-guided laser-induced thermal therapy? Initial experience with recurrent intracranial ependymomas. *J Neurosurg Pediatr*. 2015;15(4):363–371.
106. Sharma M, Habboub G, Behbahani M, Silva D, Barnett GH, Mohammadi AM. Thermal injury to corticospinal tracts and postoperative motor deficits after laser interstitial thermal therapy. *Neurosurg Focus*. 2016;41(4):E6.
107. Pruitt R, Gamble A, Black K, Schulder M, Mehta AD. Complication avoidance in laser interstitial thermal therapy: lessons learned. *J Neurosurg*. 2016:1–8.
108. Barnett GH. The role of image-guided technology in the surgical planning and resection of gliomas. *J Neurooncol*. 1999;42(3):247–258.
109. Siomin V, Barnett G. Intraoperative imaging in glioblastoma resection. *Cancer J*. 2003;9(2):91–98.
110. Habboub G, Sharma M, Barnett GH, Mohammadi AM. A novel combination of two minimally invasive surgical techniques in the management of refractory radiation necrosis: technical note. *J Clin Neurosci*. 2017;35:117–121.
111. Brandmeir NJ, McInerney J, Zacharia BE. The use of custom 3D printed stereotactic frames for laser interstitial thermal ablation: technical note. *Neurosurg Focus*. 2016; 41(4):E3.
112. Attaar SJ, Patel NV, Hargreaves E, Keller IA, Danish SF. Accuracy of laser placement with frameless stereotaxy in magnetic resonance-guided laser-induced thermal therapy. *Oper Neurosurg*. 2015;11(4):554–563.
113. Fernandez Cabada T, Sanchez Lopez de Pablo C, Martinez Serrano A, del Pozo Guerrero F, Serrano Olmedo JJ, Ramos Gomez M. Induction of cell death in a glioblastoma line by hyperthermic therapy based on gold nanorods. *Int J Nanomedicine*. 2012;7:1511–1523.
114. Norred SE, Johnson JA. Magnetic resonance-guided laser induced thermal therapy for glioblastoma multiforme: a review. *Biomed Res Int*. 2014;2014:761312.
115. Madsen SJ, Baek SK, Makkouk AR, Krasieva T, Hirschberg H. Macrophages as cell-based delivery systems for nanoshells in photothermal therapy. *Ann Biomed Eng*. 2012;40(2):507–515.
116. Schwartz JA, Price RE, Gill-Sharp KL, et al. Selective nanoparticle-directed ablation of the canine prostate. *Lasers Surg Med*. 2011;43(3):213–220.

117. Schwartz JA, Shetty AM, Price RE, et al. Feasibility study of particle-assisted laser ablation of brain tumors in orthotopic canine model. *Cancer Res.* 2009;69(4):1659–1667.
118. Baek SK, Makkouk AR, Krasieva T, Sun CH, Madsen SJ, Hirschberg H. Photothermal treatment of glioma; an in vitro study of macrophage-mediated delivery of gold nanoshells. *J Neurooncol.* 2011;104(2):439–448.
119. Yang TD, Choi W, Yoon TH, et al. In vivo photothermal treatment by the peritumoral injection of macrophages loaded with gold nanoshells. *Biomed Opt Exp.* 2016; 7(1):185–193.
120. Day ES, Thompson PA, Zhang L, et al. Nanoshell-mediated photothermal therapy improves survival in a murine glioma model. *J Neurooncol.* 2011;104(1):55–63.

CHAPTER 22

Microelectrode Recording in Functional Neurosurgery

MICHAEL D. STAUDT, MD, MSc • JONATHAN P. MILLER, MD

INTRODUCTION

Stereotactic neurosurgery has revolutionized the management of movement disorders such as Parkinson disease (PD), essential tremor (ET), and dystonia. Clinical efficacy of stereotactic procedures is critically dependent on accurate intraoperative targeting, but before the advent of modern imaging modalities, only indirect targeting based on ventricular imaging was possible. In an effort to improve localization and adjust for individual anatomic variability, in the 1960s, microelectrode recording (MER) of action potentials from single cells was translated from the laboratory to the clinical setting. MER made it possible not only to distinguish gray from white matter but also to discriminate the borders of different subcortical nuclei by resolving each structure's characteristic neural firing pattern.[1] Subsequently, microelectrode design has been refined to allow precise physiologic localization using electrophysiologic activity, synchrony with movement or tremor activity, relationship to local field potentials, and response to microstimulation.[2–5] Even after the clinical success of levodopa led to a transition away from surgery toward medical management,[6,7] observations made using MER facilitated novel therapeutic applications that led to a continued interest in surgery as an important component of movement disorder management[8] and the delineation of new therapeutic targets such as the subthalamic nucleus (STN).[9] Moreover, the development of deep brain stimulation (DBS) as a reversible and titratable application reinvigorated MER as an important adjunct for target localization when placing DBS electrodes.[10] As imaging and intraoperative techniques have improved, some centers have abandoned MER techniques in favor of direct anatomic targeting, but MER and intraoperative stimulation have an important role and continue to be widely used in functional neurosurgery.

Radiographic and anatomic localization of intracranial targets is the essential first step in planning stereotactic procedures, and modern imaging technologies allow for greater visualization and identification of therapeutic targets than ever before. However, even the most advanced imaging modalities are affected by some degree of distortion and sometimes do not clearly display the target structure. MER offers the potential for accurate target localization based on physiologic criteria, correction for any targeting error, and definition of the physiologic target, which may differ from the anatomic target. Potential disadvantages of MER include increased time, cost, and complexity of the surgical case and an elevated risk of complications (especially hemorrhage) associated with multiple electrode tracts. The aim of this chapter is to describe the use of MER for localization of intracranial targets in stereotactic neurosurgery, outline principles of its use for specific targets, and list the advantages and disadvantages associated with the use of MER.

MICROELECTRODE TECHNOLOGY AND TECHNIQUE

Although use of MER varies widely across different centers, the setup and technical aspects of insertion and recording are relatively uniform. The basic apparatus includes the microelectrode or semimicroelectrode, an amplifier/oscilloscope, and video/audio monitors. A motorized microdriver compatible with the available stereotactic targeting system is sometimes used. Intraoperative stimulation through the high-impedance recording contact (microstimulation) or referential contact (macrostimulation) can be performed using a current-isolation stimulator. Patient medications are often withheld up to 12 h before surgery to induce an "off-medication" state to accentuate the underlying pathologic activity.

The microelectrode usually consists of a platinum-iridium or tungsten bipolar electrode with a glass-insulated tapered tip and a 10- to 15-μm segment for recording. Semimicroelectrodes have a larger tip diameter (approximately 25 μm) with lower impedance and have greater sensitivity to neural activity; however, they are unable to discriminate single cell recordings and therefore provide less specific information.[11] Microelectrode impedance is generally greater than 500 kΩ, as high impedance is needed to isolate single units in regions with a high density of neurons.[12,13] The electrodes are durable to microstimulation; passage of current degrades the glass insulation and lowers the impedance, which decreases noise and also makes it more difficult to isolate single units.

The microelectrode is inserted within a protective stainless steel cannula that allows for retraction of the electrode tip during advancement through brain parenchyma. The MER process starts at a position at some distance above target (typically 15–25 mm), and recording is performed as the electrode is slowly advanced to target and a short distance beyond. As the microelectrode is advanced, the signal is filtered and amplified via isolated preamplifiers and excess noise is eliminated by processing the signal through low- and high-pass filters. This signal is then displayed on an oscilloscope, often enhanced through digital processing, and sound is transmitted through speakers. The signal is heard as multiple discharges, and window discriminators can be used to isolate individual neuronal firing activity.

MER can be used in different ways depending on the implantation philosophy based on how much detail is desired. For example, a single pass along a single trajectory can verify the presence of the target structure and define its depth along that trajectory. Alternatively, multiple parallel passes can be used to produce detailed three-dimensional maps of the borders of multiple subcortical structures. It is possible to insert and record from multiple electrodes simultaneously during a single pass using a multichannel microarray such as the "Ben gun," which has a central channel and four side channels that advance up to five parallel microelectrodes simultaneously.[14] Purported advantages of this technique include the ability to directly compare recordings between electrodes and map a theoretical volume of tissue given the fixed distance between the electrodes.[15]

MER can be used alone or in conjunction with micro- or macrostimulation delivered via an isolated current stimulator. Whereas recordings from MER are accurate to about 0.1 mm, stimulation current spreads over much a wider area of up to a few millimeters, so mapping by stimulation is somewhat less precise. Stimulation is performed using monopolar or bipolar biphasic charge-balanced square wave pulse trains of 0.06–0.3 ms at 130–300 Hz. The clinical response varies depending on the electrode position, and the resultant sensory, pyramidal, or extrapyramidal manifestations assist in physiologic mapping. Skilled interpretation of these manifestations is essential; for example, changes in tremor may be simple to quantify, but tremor arrest may also be seen in areas outside of target, including the zona incerta and corticospinal tract. Furthermore, stimulation tends to be accurate only to approximately 5 mm of targeted tissue, raising the possibility of false negatives.

GLOBUS PALLIDUS

Globus pallidus is divided into a medial internal segment (GPi) and a lateral external segment (GPe). The distribution of pallidal tremor cells appears to be primarily within the ventral portion of GPi,[16] corresponding to the sensorimotor component located laterally, posteriorly, and ventrally.[8] The target location for DBS is approximately 3–5 mm from the pallidocapsular border and 1–2 mm from the external segment of GPe,[17] ideally as far posterior as possible without inducing muscle contractions with stimulation.[18] The GPi is relatively easy to visualize on MRI.

GPi is the preferred target for the treatment of primary dystonia,[19,20] tardive dystonia,[21] and some forms of secondary dystonia.[22] It is also an effective treatment of parkinsonian symptoms.[23] GPi has different firing patterns depending on the movement disorder pathology. In PD patients, dopamine depletion causes a striking increase in the GPi firing rate [24]; these responses to kinesthetic movements are exaggerated and lack specificity with greater spread of response across multiple joints including ipsilateral to recording, and the firing pattern may be synchronous with tremor.[25,26] In patients with dystonia, there is a less pronounced increase in GPi firing compared with GPe,[27] which can make discrimination of the nuclei more problematic. In addition, dystonia is associated with changes in the specificity of receptive fields and an increased tendency for group discharges.[28] Some of these effects may be artifact because many patients with dystonia require anesthesia to facilitate implantation.[29]

Microelectrode Mapping of Globus Pallidus Interna

As the microelectrode passes through the striatum, minimal activity is usually seen, with rare discharges related to injury and occasional tonically active cells at 4–6 Hz.[26] As GPe is entered, large spontaneously active units are encountered with two distinct patterns: (1) intermediate-frequency discharges (60 Hz) with occasional pauses ("pauser" cells) and (2) low-frequency discharges (10–20 Hz) punctuated by rapid bursts ("burster" cells). Once the GPe is exited ventrally, there is an area with minimal activity because of the 1–2 mm band of white matter fibers known as the medial pallidal lamina. "Border cells" are sometimes seen at the border of the nuclei, which are cholinergic cells with diffuse cortical inputs that produce a regular, slow steady tonic discharge (20–40 Hz) of wide action potentials at a nearly constant interspike interval. These cells will occasionally fire in a spontaneous bursting pattern or in response to movement.

When the GPi is encountered, discharges are seen to be more rapid and regular than in GPe, particularly in PD where the frequency can approach 80–90 Hz. Approximately 25% of cells respond to kinesthetic movements, with representation of the face, extraocular muscles, and upper and lower limbs. This response may be an increase, decrease, or reciprocal increase/decrease in the firing rate. The internal and external segments of the GPi are separated by an incomplete pallidal lamina.

Past the target, white matter is encountered where the optic and corticospinal tracts pass. Flashes of light will produce potentials within the optic tract, and microstimulation as low as 1 μA and 300 Hz will cause the patient to perceive phosphenes of light in the contralateral visual field.[30] Entry into the corticospinal tract is associated with lack of action potentials and contralateral muscle tetanus with stimulation. The threshold of muscle contractions in relation to stimulation is an indirect measure of the electrode position relative to the internal capsule, and somatotopy may provide information regarding laterality (face represented most medial, then upper extremities, and then lower extremities).[26]

VENTRAL THALAMUS

DBS of the ventral thalamic nuclei is commonly used to treat movement disorders. There include the ventral oral (Vo) or pallidal relay nucleus, used to treat dystonia or parkinsonism; the ventral intermediate (Vim) or cerebellar relay nucleus, used to treat tremor; and the ventral caudal (Vc) or somatic sensory nucleus, used for localization of Vim and also to treat neuropathic pain.[31,32] Because none of these targets is clearly visualized on MRI, targeting is performed indirectly relative to the anterior and posterior commissures (AC-PC line) and physiologic localization can then be performed with recording and/or stimulation to identify the thalamic nuclei based on their unique electrophysiologic responses.

Kinesthetic cells of the thalamic Vim demonstrate firing synchronous with tremor activity.[33–35] Firing rates are dependent on the disease pathology. Kinesthetic cells fire at a higher frequency in ET compared with PD or pain.[32,36] In comparison, the neuronal firing rate in intention tremor is quite low compared with control patients, suggestive of potential cerebellar deafferentation.[32] It has been proposed that targeting the anterior Vo (Voa) nucleus is superior for rigidity control, whereas the posterior Vo (Vop) is preferred for tremor,[37,38] and MER has demonstrated rhythmic bursting activity at tremor frequencies in Vop.

Microelectrode Mapping of Vc, Vim, and Voa/Vop

Vc is the most easily identifiable of the ventral thalamic nuclei using MER. Cell firing within Vc demonstrates rate changes in response to sensory stimulation in small, well-defined receptive fields with mediolateral somatotopy (orofacial medial, leg lateral).[39] Stimulation of tactile cells in Vc produces paresthesia within the region of the corresponding receptive field. There tends to be a distinct reduction in background noise and unit recordings, as the microelectrode passes through the bottom of the thalamus. Stimulation in this region may continue to produce paresthesias, however, requiring higher thresholds, and muscle contractions may be elicited if the electrode is too close to the internal capsule.

Cells anterior to the cutaneous core in the anterior dorsal cap of Vc and within Vim comprise the kinesthetic region. These cells respond to joint movement, deep pressure, and squeezing of muscles and tendons but not manipulation of skin deformed by these movements. Kinesthetic cells may fire concurrently with tremor if the receptive fields overlap,[40] particularly in PD. Vim has similar somatotopy to Vc, with deep sensory cells of the wrist anterior to the cutaneous representation of digits.[39,41] The border between Vim and Vc is difficult to identify, as macrostimulation produces paresthesias within similar parts of the body, however, usually with higher thresholds of activation.

Spontaneous firing activity is less frequent in Vop and Voa compared with the other targets. Neuronal activity within these areas correlates with movement in response to commands, the active phase of movement, and a state of maximal muscle contraction.[34,42,43] The largest proportion change firing rates in response to active movement (the so-called "voluntary cells"), and tremor cells that fire in synchrony with the patient's tremor may be encountered. Firing is often preferentially related to the execution of particular movements, with a somatotopy parallel to the cutaneous core of Vc.[42] Vim and Vop can readily be identified by the response to stimulation of deep structures (e.g., tendons) or movement of joints and phasic tremor frequency. Certain cells also respond to both active movement and somatosensory stimulation. Vop can also be identified by spindle activity on EEG, which demonstrates a 7–10 Hz rhythm with increases and decreases in amplitude.[32]

SUBTHALAMIC NUCLEUS

The STN plays an important role in movement disorder pathophysiology because of its extensive connectivity and influence within cortical and thalamic loops. It forms an essential component of the "indirect pathway," receiving input from the striatum via the GPe and projecting to GPi and substantia nigra pars reticulata (SNr),[44] and also receives extensive direct excitatory cortical input.[45] Early preclinical studies highlighted its importance in motor circuitry and the pathophysiology of PD: selective lesioning in rhesus monkeys resulted in hemiballismus[46] but also improved parkinsonian symptoms in primate models of PD.[9,47] Thereafter, high-frequency stimulation via DBS was shown to improve tremor, rigidity, and akinesia in primate models[48,49] and humans with PD.[14,50] STN, specifically the dorsolateral motor segment,[51,52] is the most common target for the surgical treatment of PD.

In the context of PD, STN undergoes a change in firing pattern and increase in the firing rate because of nigrostriatal dopamine depletion.[53,54] STN normally fires at 20 Hz but at greater than 40 Hz in PD. Oscillatory activity, normally rare, is found in up to 20% of cells.[55,56] Augmented synchrony is observed with loss of specificity of receptive fields and spread through multiple joints. A loss of center-surround inhibition is observed, resulting in increased bursting activity. Firing is observed with active or passive contralateral joint activation, with ipsilateral response in up to 25% of cells.

Microelectrode Mapping of Subthalamic Nucleus

The striatum is relatively quiet on MER with occasional injury discharges and tonically active cells at 4–6 Hz. Entry into the reticular shell of the thalamus demonstrates relatively slow, regular discharges,[57] followed by the cell-poor zona incerta.

As STN is encountered, there is a sudden increase in cellularity with a dramatic increase in the number of action potentials. These cells primarily demonstrate spikes with a negative wave followed by a smaller and narrower positive deflection. Two different extracellular spike waveforms are encountered demonstrating both monophasic and biphasic behavior: (1) a mixed pattern, defined by tonic activity with an irregular discharge pattern and occasional bursts, and (2) a burst pattern, with periodic oscillatory bursts that are synchronous with the rest tremor, although not as much bursting as seen in the thalamus.[58] Approximately 40%–50% of cells will respond to passive movement. Microelectrode stimulation in these regions aids in localization, as ipsilateral eye deviation may indicate medial proximity to the oculomotor nerve or nucleus and bulbar responses, lateral proximity to the corticobulbar tract.[59]

Past the target (deep to STN), SNr is less rich and sparser than the STN but produces a continuous almost melodic hum of irregular firing. Spikes are symmetrical, biphasic, and of large amplitude, with a rate of approximately 30 Hz and a range of 8–80 Hz,[58] although higher firing rates have been described.[57] Importantly, these cells are always tonic and never burst.

THE CASE FOR (AND AGAINST) MAPPING

Potential Advantages

Even under optimal conditions, stereotaxy is prone to small errors that can add up to several millimeters. Potential causes of error include the spatial inaccuracy and distortion of MRI, brain shift due to intraoperative cerebrospinal fluid loss and pneumocephalus,[60,61] and deflection caused by entry of a stiff cannula or electrode into the soft brain parenchyma. Indirect targeting with the use of routine landmarks can be quite variable because of differences in the location of subcortical nuclei in relation to the AC-PC line.[62,63] Because it indicates what is happening at the electrode tip in real time, MER has the potential to correct for all of these sources of error at a resolution of less than 0.1 mm. When the surgical target is modified based on MER data, it is often observed on postoperative imaging that the electrode is in the originally intended location, suggesting that physiologic data allowed compensation for a targeting error that would otherwise have been unrecognized.

Another advantage of MER is its ability to identify physiologic structures directly. Anatomy and physiology do not always correspond, so there may be a difference between the "selected target" and the "actual target." Spontaneous firing rates, patterns, and responses to movement differ between individual nuclei, and MER can identify these with better spatial accuracy and resolution than many MRI sequences. Despite advances in MRI technology, intracranial targets are not always easy to identify: GPi is best visualized, STN is somewhat less so, and Vim is least because the image borders of individual thalamic nuclei are indistinct at clinical field strength. MER allows for precise mapping in three dimensions, including the contours of the nuclei.[64] Mapping of borders can aid in maximizing the physiologic effects and minimizing side effects or unintended injury.[65,66] There is also the possibility of micro- or macrostimulation alone producing variable or delayed effects, even at target, so localization requires skilled interpretation of MER and neuronal firing patterns.[30,57,67]

Finally, MER also has a valuable role in research by helping to delineate the physiology of deep brain structures, the pathophysiology of movement disorders, the effect of DBS on downstream neurons, and the effect of drugs on these mechanisms. MER has also helped to identify new targets for DBS; for example, the pedunculopontine nucleus contains cells that respond to movement and exhibit β oscillations,[68,69] and firing patterns in the anterior nucleus of the thalamus support its potential as a target for treatment of refractory epilepsy.[70]

Potential Disadvantages

Despite the benefits, there are numerous downsides to the routine use of MER. Recent evidence suggests that exclusively anatomic targeting is associated with excellent results, which suggests that the anatomic target may be the same as the physiologic target. The extremely high degree of accuracy afforded by MER (less than 0.1 mm) may not be necessary, as the area stimulated by the DBS electrode is both large and defined empirically during programming. Before the development of modern imaging techniques, a survey of functional neurosurgeons demonstrated their preferred thalamic surgical target for PD varied widely with nevertheless excellent results.[71] An analysis by Hariz[72] suggested that numerous seminal publications defining the use of MER for ablative target localization actually published MRIs demonstrating many lesion locations to be off-target,[23,73] sometimes widely so,[74,75] and this is also true of studies for MER-guided DBS.[76,77] Two non-MER pallidotomy studies described excellent clinical results with no mortality and low morbidity.[78,79]

As imaging technology has steadily advanced, MRI modalities allow for progressively better preoperative visualization of subcortical targets and white matter tracts,[80] and intraoperative imaging modalities have been developed that allow intraoperative image-guided DBS. Two such technologies, Nexframe (Medtronic, Minneapolis, MN, USA) and ClearPoint (MRI Interventions, Irvine, CA, USA), integrate planning, targeting, and confirmation of DBS lead placement. Numerous studies have now been published, demonstrating safety and efficacy using these technologies (Table 22.1). These studies have reported similar lead placement accuracy to what has been reported using MER,[81–84] excellent clinical results, decreased procedure time, little to no overall complications,[85–87] and lower hemorrhage risk compared with MER.[88,89] In addition, the ability to perform DBS surgeries under general anesthesia has the potential to maintain clinical efficacy while reducing fear, anxiety, and pain associated with awake surgery under local anesthesia[90,91] because even sedation with propofol interferes with MER and the identification of intracranial targets.[92,93] However, the use of dexmedetomidine, a short-acting and easily reversible sedative, has been reported to maintain the rate of STN firing, however, with reduced neuronal variability.[94]

There is evidence that MER is associated with an increased risk of complications, particularly hemorrhage,[95–99] which is correlated with the number of microelectrode passes[100–102] (Table 22.2). When assessing significant literature reviews from 1988 to 2002, Hariz concluded that MER techniques were at least five times as dangerous as macrostimulation techniques, with no indication that outcomes are better when MER is used.[103] However, confirmation that MER is either less safe or more efficacious than other techniques would require a controlled clinical trial, and no such study has ever been performed.

Finally, MER considerably increases the cost and complexity of stereotactic cases. Considerable expertise

TABLE 22.1
Image-Guided DBS Targeting Methods

References	Techniques	Patients	Results
Starr et al.[85]	MRI (NexFrame)	29	Single penetration in 87%; UPDRS decreased 60%; no complications; faster, greater comfort
Larson et al.[81]	MRI (ClearPoint)	18	Error 0.2 ± 0.1 mm, 88 min procedure time
Ostrem et al.[86]	MRI (NexFrame)	17	UPDRS from 44.5 to 22.5 (49.4%), no complications
Burchiel et al.[82]	CT (NexFrame)	60	Mean deviation off trajectory 1.59 ± 1.11 mm, one infection, no hemorrhage, no pneumocephalus
Starr et al.[83]	MRI (ClearPoint)	6	Error 0.6 ± 0.5 mm, BFMDRS decreased 87.6 ± 19.2%, no complications
Jimenez-Shahed et al.[89]	MRI (ClearPoint)	3 MRI, 5 MER (randomized)	MER more likely than MRI to have microlesion (80% vs. 33%), targeting error (0.6 vs. 1.1 mm), and postoperative confusion
Saleh et al.[88]	MRI (ClearPoint)	14 MER, 23 MRI	LEDD decreased 38% for MER, 49% for MRI (NS)
Chen et al.[90]	CT (NexFrame or Leksell)	40 awake, 17 asleep (no MER in either)	No difference in BFTADL (−32.1 awake, −27.0 asleep, NS); error higher in awake patients (1.7 vs. 0.8 mm)
Ostrem et al.[87]	MRI (ClearPoint)	26	Single penetration in all cases, significant improvement in UPDRS (40.75–24.35, $P = .001$) and LEDD, one infection, no hemorrhage or cognitive/mood decline
Mirzadeh et al.[84]	CT (Leksell)	35	Error 0.8 mm, significant improvement in UPDRS (48.4–28.9, $P < .001$), also PDQ-39 and LEDD, no complications
Jacob et al.[91]	CT (NexFrame)	53 awake, 158 asleep	Asleep has less variable costs; overall cost is half national average

BFMDRS, Burke-Fahn-Marsden Dystonia rating scale; *LEDD*, levodopa equivalent dose; *MER*, microelectrode recording; *NS*, not significant; *PDQ-39*, Parkinson's Disease Questionnaire, *UPDRS*, Unified Parkinson's Disease Rating Scale.

is required to interpret the physiologic recordings, and specialized equipment and personnel, as well as additional operating room time, are necessary. The use of MER has been reported to increase operative time for unilateral and bilateral DBS implantation by 3 h and staged bilateral implantation by 6 h, with an associated doubling or tripling of costs related to operating room time, equipment, and personnel.[104] Performing DBS surgeries asleep using image guidance has been reported to lower costs relative to awake surgeries, with the overall cost being less than half of the national average.[91]

TABLE 22.2
Safety of Microelectrode Recording

References	Study Type	With MER	Without MER	Difference in Complications With MER	Difference in Outcomes With MER
Alkhani and Lozano[95]	Metaanalysis, pallidotomy	903	1051	Significantly higher rate of hemorrhage with MER, postoperative weakness/ dysphagia, and overall risk of complication ($P = .003$)	No difference in UPDRS
Palur et al.[96]	Metaanalysis, pallidotomy	302	184	Significantly higher risk of hemorrhage with MER (1.3% vs. 0.25%, $P = .012$)	No difference in UPDRS or dyskinesia
de Bie et al.[97]	Metaanalysis, pallidotomy	198	136	Adverse effects 14.4% higher, stroke 4.9% higher with MER	N/A
Hariz[103]	Metaanalysis, thalamotomy and pallidotomy	N/A	N/A	Fivefold increase in risk of complications	No difference
Higuchi and Iacono[98]	Retrospective single-institution, pallidotomy	73	723	Risk of hemorrhage 3.82× higher with MER, risk of postoperative hemiparesis without hemorrhage 6.1× ($P = .001$)	N/A
Gorgulho et al.[100]	Retrospective single-institution, pallidotomy and DBS	104	144	Hemorrhage increased from 1.4% to 2.9% when MER used, correlated with number of passes	N/A
DBS for PD Study Group[101]	Prospective double-blind study, DBS	134	0	Number of passes strongly correlated with hemorrhage (4.1 passes in patients with hemorrhage vs. 2.9 without)	N/A
Binder et al.[102]	Retrospective single-institution, DBS	280	0	Hemorrhage rate 3.3%; correlated with number of passes and target (GPi worse)	N/A
Zrinzo et al.[99]	Retrospective single-institution, DBS	0	214	Hemorrhage rate 0.9% compared with 5.0% in literature	N/A

DBS, deep brain stimulation; *GPi*, globus pallidus interna; *MER*, microelectrode recording; *PD*, Parkinson disease; *UPDRS*, Unified Parkinson's Disease Rating Scale.

SUMMARY

MER has a long history in the experimental study and clinical treatment of movement disorders, particularly to delineate the anatomic relationships for targeting. MER offers a degree of precision unparalleled by any other implantation technology and can allow for correction of stereotactic targeting error and provide confirmation that the physiologic target has been identified. Improvements in imaging and stereotactic technology have mitigated some of these benefits, and MER may be associated with increased complexity and risk of complications without necessarily improving outcome. Although excellent outcomes have been reported with and without MER, a direct comparison has never been performed. With the advent of new technologies for intraoperative targeting, the role of MER in the stereotactic implantation of DBS electrodes is likely to continue to evolve.

REFERENCES

1. Albe-Fessard D, Arfel G, Guiot G, et al. Identification and precide delimitation of certain subcortical structures in man by electrophysiology. Its importance in stereotaxic surgery of dyskinesia. *C R Hebd Seances Acad Sci.* 1961; 253:2412–2414.
2. Albe-Fessard D, Arfel G, Guiot G, et al. Electrophysiological studies of some deep cerebral structures in man. *J Neurol Sci.* 1966;3:37–51.
3. Albe-Fessard D, Arfel G, Guiot G, Derome P, Guilbaud G. Thalamic unit activity in man. *Electroencephalogr Clin Neurophysiol.* 1967;(suppl 25):132+.
4. Gaze RM, Gillingham FJ, Kalyanaraman S, Porter RW, Donaldson AA, Donaldson IM. Microelectrode recordings from the human thalamus. *Brain.* 1964;87:691–706.
5. Hardy J. Electrophysiological localization and identification of subcortical structures as an aid to stereotaxic surgery: a preliminary report. *Can Med Assoc J.* 1962;86: 498–499.
6. Rascol O, Lozano A, Stern M, Poewe W. Milestones in Parkinson's disease therapeutics. *Mov Disord.* 2011;26: 1072–1082. https://doi.org/10.1002/mds.23714.
7. Tasker RR, Siqueira J, Hawrylyshyn P, Organ LW. What happened to VIM thalamotomy for Parkinson's disease? *Appl Neurophysiol.* 1983;46:68–83.
8. Laitinen LV, Bergenheim AT, Hariz MI. Leksell's posteroventral pallidotomy in the treatment of Parkinson's disease. *J Neurosurg.* 1992;76:53–61. https://doi.org/10.3171/jns.1992.76.1.0053.
9. Bergman H, Wichmann T, DeLong MR. Reversal of experimental parkinsonism by lesions of the subthalamic nucleus. *Science.* 1990;249:1436–1438.
10. Hariz MI, Blomstedt P, Zrinzo L. Deep brain stimulation between 1947 and 1987: the untold story. *Neurosurg Focus.* 2010;29:E1. https://doi.org/10.3171/2010.4.FOCUS10106.
11. Favre J, Taha JM, Nguyen TT, Gildenberg PL, Burchiel KJ. Pallidotomy: a survey of current practice in North America. *Neurosurgery.* 1996;39:883–890; discussion 890–882.
12. Lenz FA, Dostrovsky JO, Kwan HC, Tasker RR, Yamashiro K, Murphy JT. Methods for microstimulation and recording of single neurons and evoked potentials in the human central nervous system. *J Neurosurg.* 1988;68: 630–634. https://doi.org/10.3171/jns.1988.68.4.0630.
13. Bertrand G, Jasper H, Wong A, Mathews G. Microelectrode recording during stereotactic surgery. *Clin Neurosurg.* 1969;16:328–355.
14. Limousin P, Krack P, Pollak P, et al. Electrical stimulation of the subthalamic nucleus in advanced Parkinson's disease. *N Engl J Med.* 1998;339:1105–1111. https://doi.org/10.1056/NEJM199810153391603.
15. Pollak P, Krack P, Fraix V, et al. Intraoperative micro- and macrostimulation of the subthalamic nucleus in Parkinson's disease. *Mov Disord.* 2002;17(suppl 3):S155–S161.
16. Hutchison WD, Lozano AM, Tasker RR, Lang AE, Dostrovsky JO. Identification and characterization of neurons with tremor-frequency activity in human globus pallidus. *Exp Brain Res.* 1997;113:557–563.
17. Starr PA, Turner RS, Rau G, et al. Microelectrode-guided implantation of deep brain stimulators into the globus pallidus internus for dystonia: techniques, electrode locations, and outcomes. *J Neurosurg.* 2006;104:488–501. https://doi.org/10.3171/jns.2006.104.4.488.
18. Tisch S, Zrinzo L, Limousin P, et al. Effect of electrode contact location on clinical efficacy of pallidal deep brain stimulation in primary generalised dystonia. *J Neurol Neurosurg Psychiatry.* 2007;78:1314–1319. https://doi.org/10.1136/jnnp.2006.109694.
19. Kupsch A, Benecke R, Muller J, et al. Pallidal deep-brain stimulation in primary generalized or segmental dystonia. *N Engl J Med.* 2006;355:1978–1990. https://doi.org/10.1056/NEJMoa063618.
20. Vidailhet M, Vercueil L, Houeto JL, et al. Bilateral deep-brain stimulation of the globus pallidus in primary generalized dystonia. *N Engl J Med.* 2005;352:459–467. https://doi.org/10.1056/NEJMoa042187.
21. Trottenberg T, Paul G, Meissner W, Maier-Hauff K, Taschner C, Kupsch A. Pallidal and thalamic neurostimulation in severe tardive dystonia. *J Neurol Neurosurg Psychiatry.* 2001;70:557–559.
22. Vitek JL, Delong MR, Starr PA, Hariz MI, Metman LV. Intraoperative neurophysiology in DBS for dystonia. *Mov Disord.* 2011;26(suppl 1):S31–S36. https://doi.org/10.1002/mds.23619.
23. Gross RE, Lombardi WJ, Lang AE, et al. Relationship of lesion location to clinical outcome following microelectrode-guided pallidotomy for Parkinson's disease. *Brain.* 1999;122(Pt 3):405–416.
24. Hutchinson WD, Levy R, Dostrovsky JO, Lozano AM, Lang AE. Effects of apomorphine on globus pallidus neurons in parkinsonian patients. *Ann Neurol.* 1997;42: 767–775. https://doi.org/10.1002/ana.410420513.

25. Hutchison WD, Lozano AM, Davis KD, Saint-Cyr JA, Lang AE, Dostrovsky JO. Differential neuronal activity in segments of globus pallidus in Parkinson's disease patients. *Neuroreport*. 1994;5:1533–1537.
26. Lozano AM, Hutchison WD. Microelectrode recordings in the pallidum. *Mov Disord*. 2002;17(suppl 3):S150–S154.
27. Vitek JL. Pathophysiology of dystonia: a neuronal model. *Mov Disord*. 2002;17(suppl 3):S49–S62.
28. Vitek JL, Chockkan V, Zhang JY, et al. Neuronal activity in the basal ganglia in patients with generalized dystonia and hemiballismus. *Ann Neurol*. 1999;46:22–35.
29. Lozano AM, Kumar R, Gross RE, et al. Globus pallidus internus pallidotomy for generalized dystonia. *Mov Disord*. 1997;12:865–870. https://doi.org/10.1002/mds.870120606.
30. Lozano A, Hutchison W, Kiss Z, Tasker R, Davis K, Dostrovsky J. Methods for microelectrode-guided posteroventral pallidotomy. *J Neurosurg*. 1996;84:194–202. https://doi.org/10.3171/jns.1996.84.2.0194.
31. Hassler R. Architectonic organization of the thalamic nuclei. In: Schaltenbrand G, Walker AE, eds. *Stereotaxy of the Human Brain*. Stuttgart: Thieme; 1982:140–180.
32. Garonzik IM, Hua SE, Ohara S, Lenz FA. Intraoperative microelectrode and semi-microelectrode recording during the physiological localization of the thalamic nucleus ventral intermediate. *Mov Disord*. 2002;17(suppl 3): S135–S144.
33. Narabayashi H, Ohye C. Nucleus ventralis intermedius of human thalamus. *Trans Am Neurol Assoc*. 1974;99: 232–233.
34. Crowell RM, Perret E, Siegfried J, Villoz JP. 'Movement units' and 'tremor phasic units' in the human thalamus. *Brain Res*. 1968;11:481–488.
35. Ohye C, Shibazaki T, Hirai T, Wada H, Hirato M, Kawashima Y. Further physiological observations on the ventralis intermedius neurons in the human thalamus. *J Neurophysiol*. 1989;61:488–500.
36. Tasker RR, Kiss ZH. The role of the thalamus in functional neurosurgery. *Neurosurg Clin N Am*. 1995;6:73–104.
37. Ohye C, Fukamachi A, Miyazaki M, Isobe I, Nakajima H, Shibazaki T. Physiologically controlled selective thalamotomy for the treatment of abnormal movement by Leksell's open system. *Acta Neurochir*. 1977;37:93–104.
38. Hassler R, Schmidt K, Riechert T, Mundinger F. Stereotactic treatment of action myoclonus in a case of combined status marmoratus and multiple sclerosis. A contribution to the pathophysiology of basal ganglia with multiple lesions in both the striatum and the substantia nigra. *Confin Neurol*. 1975;37:329–356.
39. Lenz FA, Dostrovsky JO, Tasker RR, Yamashiro K, Kwan HC, Murphy JT. Single-unit analysis of the human ventral thalamic nuclear group: somatosensory responses. *J Neurophysiol*. 1988;59:299–316.
40. Lenz FA, Tasker RR, Kwan HC, et al. Single unit analysis of the human ventral thalamic nuclear group: correlation of thalamic "tremor cells" with the 3–6 Hz component of parkinsonian tremor. *J Neurosci*. 1988;8:754–764.
41. McClean MD, Dostrovsky JO, Lee L, Tasker RR. Somatosensory neurons in human thalamus respond to speech-induced orofacial movements. *Brain Res*. 1990;513: 343–347.
42. Lenz FA, Kwan HC, Dostrovsky JO, Tasker RR, Murphy JT, Lenz YE. Single unit analysis of the human ventral thalamic nuclear group. Activity correlated with movement. *Brain*. 1990;113(Pt 6):1795–1821.
43. Raeva SN, Vainberg NA, Dubynin VA, Tsetlin IM, Tikhonov YN, Lashin AP. Changes in the spike activity of neurons in the ventrolateral nucleus of the thalamus in humans during performance of a voluntary movement. *Neurosci Behav Physiol*. 1999;29:505–513.
44. DeLong MR. Primate models of movement disorders of basal ganglia origin. *Trends Neurosci*. 1990;13: 281–285.
45. Smith Y, Bevan MD, Shink E, Bolam JP. Microcircuitry of the direct and indirect pathways of the basal ganglia. *Neuroscience*. 1998;86:353–387.
46. Carpenter MB, Whittier JR, Mettler FA. Analysis of choreoid hyperkinesia in the Rhesus monkey; surgical and pharmacological analysis of hyperkinesia resulting from lesions in the subthalamic nucleus of Luys. *J Comp Neurol*. 1950;92:293–331.
47. Aziz TZ, Peggs D, Sambrook MA, Crossman AR. Lesion of the subthalamic nucleus for the alleviation of 1-methyl-4-phenyl-1,2,3,6-tetrahydropyridine (MPTP)-induced parkinsonism in the primate. *Mov Disord*. 1991; 6:288–292. https://doi.org/10.1002/mds.870060404.
48. Benazzouz A, Boraud T, Feger J, Burbaud P, Bioulac B, Gross C. Alleviation of experimental hemiparkinsonism by high-frequency stimulation of the subthalamic nucleus in primates: a comparison with L-Dopa treatment. *Mov Disord*. 1996;11:627–632. https://doi.org/10.1002/mds.870110606.
49. Gao DM, Benazzouz A, Piallat B, et al. High-frequency stimulation of the subthalamic nucleus suppresses experimental resting tremor in the monkey. *Neuroscience*. 1999; 88:201–212.
50. Limousin P, Pollak P, Benazzouz A, et al. Effect of parkinsonian signs and symptoms of bilateral subthalamic nucleus stimulation. *Lancet*. 1995;345:91–95.
51. Parent A, Hazrati LN. Functional anatomy of the basal ganglia. II. The place of subthalamic nucleus and external pallidum in basal ganglia circuitry. *Brain Res Brain Res Rev*. 1995;20:128–154.
52. Monakow KH, Akert K, Kunzle H. Projections of the precentral motor cortex and other cortical areas of the frontal lobe to the subthalamic nucleus in the monkey. *Exp Brain Res*. 1978;33:395–403.
53. Bergman H, Wichmann T, Karmon B, DeLong MR. The primate subthalamic nucleus. II. Neuronal activity in the MPTP model of parkinsonism. *J Neurophysiol*. 1994; 72:507–520.
54. Bezard E, Boraud T, Bioulac B, Gross CE. Involvement of the subthalamic nucleus in glutamatergic compensatory mechanisms. *Eur J Neurosci*. 1999;11:2167–2170.

55. Wichmann T, Bergman H, DeLong MR. The primate subthalamic nucleus. I. Functional properties in intact animals. *J Neurophysiol*. 1994;72:494–506.
56. Levy R, Hutchison WD, Lozano AM, Dostrovsky JO. High-frequency synchronization of neuronal activity in the subthalamic nucleus of parkinsonian patients with limb tremor. *J Neurosci*. 2000;20:7766–7775.
57. Hutchison WD, Allan RJ, Opitz H, et al. Neurophysiological identification of the subthalamic nucleus in surgery for Parkinson's disease. *Ann Neurol*. 1998;44:622–628. https://doi.org/10.1002/ana.410440407.
58. Benazzouz A, Breit S, Koudsie A, Pollak P, Krack P, Benabid AL. Intraoperative microrecordings of the subthalamic nucleus in Parkinson's disease. *Mov Disord*. 2002;17(suppl 3):S145–S149.
59. Starr PA, Christine CW, Theodosopoulos PV, et al. Implantation of deep brain stimulators into the subthalamic nucleus: technical approach and magnetic resonance imaging-verified lead locations. *J Neurosurg*. 2002;97:370–387. https://doi.org/10.3171/jns.2002.97.2.0370.
60. Kondziolka D, Dempsey PK, Lunsford LD, et al. A comparison between magnetic resonance imaging and computed tomography for stereotactic coordinate determination. *Neurosurgery*. 1992;30:402–406; discussion 406–407.
61. Sumanaweera TS, Adler Jr JR, Napel S, Glover GH. Characterization of spatial distortion in magnetic resonance imaging and its implications for stereotactic surgery. *Neurosurgery*. 1994;35:696–703; discussion 703–694.
62. Kelly PJ, Derome P, Guiot G. Thalamic spatial variability and the surgical results of lesions placed with neurophysiologic control. *Surg Neurol*. 1978;9:307–315.
63. Brierley JB, Beck E. The significance in human stereotactic brain surgery of individual variation in the diencephalon and globus pallidus. *J Neurol Neurosurg Psychiatry*. 1959; 22:287–298.
64. Bejjani BP, Dormont D, Pidoux B, et al. Bilateral subthalamic stimulation for Parkinson's disease by using three-dimensional stereotactic magnetic resonance imaging and electrophysiological guidance. *J Neurosurg*. 2000;92:615–625. https://doi.org/10.3171/jns.2000.92.4.0615.
65. Lozano AM, Hutchison WD, Tasker RR, Lang AE, Junn F, Dostrovsky JO. Microelectrode recordings define the ventral posteromedial pallidotomy target. *Stereotact Funct Neurosurg*. 1998;71:153–163. https://doi.org/29659.
66. Giller CA, Dewey RB, Ginsburg MI, Mendelsohn DB, Berk AM. Stereotactic pallidotomy and thalamotomy using individual variations of anatomic landmarks for localization. *Neurosurgery*. 1998;42:56–62; discussion 62–55.
67. Reck C, Maarouf M, Wojtecki L, et al. Clinical outcome of subthalamic stimulation in Parkinson's disease is improved by intraoperative multiple trajectories microelectrode recording. *J Neurol Surg A, Cent Eur Neurosurg*. 2012; 73:377–386. https://doi.org/10.1055/s-0032-1326957.
68. Stefani A, Lozano AM, Peppe A, et al. Bilateral deep brain stimulation of the pedunculopontine and subthalamic nuclei in severe Parkinson's disease. *Brain*. 2007;130: 1596–1607. https://doi.org/10.1093/brain/awl346.
69. Morita H, Hass CJ, Moro E, Sudhyadhom A, Kumar R, Okun MS. Pedunculopontine nucleus stimulation: where are we now and what needs to be done to move the field forward? *Front Neurol*. 2014;5:243. https://doi.org/10.3389/fneur.2014.00243.
70. Mottonen T, Katisko J, Haapasalo J, et al. Defining the anterior nucleus of the thalamus (ANT) as a deep brain stimulation target in refractory epilepsy: delineation using 3 T MRI and intraoperative microelectrode recording. *NeuroImage Clin*. 2015;7:823–829. https://doi.org/10.1016/j.nicl.2015.03.001.
71. Laitinen LV. Brain targets in surgery for Parkinson's disease. Results of a survey of neurosurgeons. *J Neurosurg*. 1985;62:349–351. https://doi.org/10.3171/jns.1985.62.3.0349.
72. Hariz MI. Is MER necessary in movement disorder surgery? The case against. In: Israel Z, Burchiel KJ, eds. *Microelectrode Recording in Movement Disorder Surgery*. New York: Thieme; 2004:197–207.
73. Dogali M, Fazzini E, Kolodny E, et al. Stereotactic ventral pallidotomy for Parkinson's disease. *Neurology*. 1995;45: 753–761.
74. Samuel M, Caputo E, Brooks DJ, et al. A study of medial pallidotomy for Parkinson's disease: clinical outcome, MRI location and complications. *Brain*. 1998;121(Pt 1): 59–75.
75. Kirschman DL, Milligan B, Wilkinson S, et al. Pallidotomy microelectrode targeting: neurophysiology-based target refinement. *Neurosurgery*. 2000;46:613–622; discussion 622–614.
76. Koller W, Pahwa R, Busenbark K, et al. High-frequency unilateral thalamic stimulation in the treatment of essential and parkinsonian tremor. *Ann Neurol*. 1997;42: 292–299. https://doi.org/10.1002/ana.410420304.
77. Levesque MF, Taylor S, Rogers R, Le MT, Swope D. Subthalamic stimulation in Parkinson's disease. Preliminary results. *Stereotact Funct Neurosurg*. 1999;72:170–173. https://doi.org/29721.
78. Svennilson E, Torvik A, Lowe R, Leksell L. Treatment of parkinsonism by stereotatic thermolesions in the pallidal region. A clinical evaluation of 81 cases. *Acta Psychiatr Scand*. 1960;35:358–377.
79. Laitinen LV. Pallidotomy for Parkinson's disease. *Neurosurg Clin N Am*. 1995;6:105–112.
80. Maiti TK, Konar S, Bir S, Kalakoti P, Nanda A. Intraoperative micro-electrode recording in functional neurosurgery: past, present, future. *J Clin Neurosci*. 2016;32: 166–172. https://doi.org/10.1016/j.jocn.2016.03.028.
81. Larson PS, Starr PA, Bates G, Tansey L, Richardson RM, Martin AJ. An optimized system for interventional magnetic resonance imaging-guided stereotactic surgery: preliminary evaluation of targeting accuracy. *Neurosurgery*. 2012;70:95–103; discussion 103. doi:10.1227/NEU.0b013e31822f4a91.
82. Burchiel KJ, McCartney S, Lee A, Raslan AM. Accuracy of deep brain stimulation electrode placement using intraoperative computed tomography without microelectrode recording. *J Neurosurg*. 2013;119:301–306. https://doi.org/10.3171/2013.4.JNS122324.

83. Starr PA, Markun LC, Larson PS, Volz MM, Martin AJ, Ostrem JL. Interventional MRI-guided deep brain stimulation in pediatric dystonia: first experience with the ClearPoint system. *J Neurosurg Pediatr.* 2014;14: 400–408. https://doi.org/10.3171/2014.6.PEDS13605.
84. Mirzadeh Z, Chapple K, Lambert M, et al. Parkinson's disease outcomes after intraoperative CT-guided "asleep" deep brain stimulation in the globus pallidus internus. *J Neurosurg.* 2016;124:902–907. https://doi.org/10.3171/2015.4.JNS1550.
85. Starr PA, Martin AJ, Ostrem JL, Talke P, Levesque N, Larson PS. Subthalamic nucleus deep brain stimulator placement using high-field interventional magnetic resonance imaging and a skull-mounted aiming device: technique and application accuracy. *J Neurosurg.* 2010;112: 479–490. https://doi.org/10.3171/2009.6.JNS081161.
86. Ostrem JL, Galifianakis NB, Markun LC, et al. Clinical outcomes of PD patients having bilateral STN DBS using high-field interventional MR-imaging for lead placement. *Clin Neurol Neurosurg.* 2013;115:708–712. https://doi.org/10.1016/j.clineuro.2012.08.019.
87. Ostrem JL, Ziman N, Galifianakis NB, et al. Clinical outcomes using ClearPoint interventional MRI for deep brain stimulation lead placement in Parkinson's disease. *J Neurosurg.* 2016;124:908–916. https://doi.org/10.3171/2015.4.JNS15173.
88. Saleh S, Swanson KI, Lake WB, Sillay KA. Awake neurophysiologically guided versus asleep MRI-guided STN DBS for Parkinson disease: a comparison of outcomes using levodopa equivalents. *Stereotact Funct Neurosurg.* 2015;93:419–426. https://doi.org/10.1159/000442425.
89. Jimenez-Shahed J, York M, Smith-Gloyd EM, Jankovic J, Viswanathan A. MER vs. MRI guidance in placement of DBS electrodes for Parkinson's disease. *Mov Disord.* 2014;29(suppl 1):S1–S687. https://doi.org/10.1002/mds.25914.
90. Chen T, Mirzadeh Z, Chapple K, Lambert M, Dhall R, Ponce FA. "Asleep" deep brain stimulation for essential tremor. *J Neurosurg.* 2016;124:1842–1849. https://doi.org/10.3171/2015.6.JNS15526.
91. Jacob RL, Geddes J, McCartney S, Burchiel KJ. Cost analysis of awake versus asleep deep brain stimulation: a single academic health center experience. *J Neurosurg.* 2016;124: 1517–1523. https://doi.org/10.3171/2015.5.JNS15433.
92. Hertel F, Zuchner M, Weimar I, et al. Implantation of electrodes for deep brain stimulation of the subthalamic nucleus in advanced Parkinson's disease with the aid of intraoperative microrecording under general anesthesia. *Neurosurgery.* 2006;59:E1138; discussion E1138. https://doi.org/10.1227/01.NEU.0000245603.77075.55
93. Harries AM, Kausar J, Roberts SA, et al. Deep brain stimulation of the subthalamic nucleus for advanced Parkinson disease using general anesthesia: long-term results. *J Neurosurg.* 2012;116:107–113. https://doi.org/10.3171/2011.7.JNS11319.
94. Mathews L, Camalier CR, Kla KM, et al. The effects of dexmedetomidine on microelectrode recordings of the subthalamic nucleus during deep brain stimulation surgery: a retrospective analysis. *Stereotact Funct Neurosurg.* 2017;95:40–48. https://doi.org/10.1159/000453326.
95. Alkhani A, Lozano AM. Pallidotomy for Parkinson disease: a review of contemporary literature. *J Neurosurg.* 2001;94: 43–49. https://doi.org/10.3171/jns.2001.94.1.0043.
96. Palur RS, Berk C, Schulzer M, Honey CR. A metaanalysis comparing the results of pallidotomy performed using microelectrode recording or macroelectrode stimulation. *J Neurosurg.* 2002;96:1058–1062. https://doi.org/10.3171/jns.2002.96.6.1058.
97. de Bie RM, de Haan RJ, Schuurman PR, Esselink RA, Bosch DA, Speelman JD. Morbidity and mortality following pallidotomy in Parkinson's disease: a systematic review. *Neurology.* 2002;58:1008–1012.
98. Higuchi Y, Iacono RP. Surgical complications in patients with Parkinson's disease after posteroventral pallidotomy. *Neurosurgery.* 2003;52:558–571; discussion 568–571.
99. Zrinzo L, Foltynie T, Limousin P, Hariz MI. Reducing hemorrhagic complications in functional neurosurgery: a large case series and systematic literature review. *J Neurosurg.* 2012;116:84–94. https://doi.org/10.3171/2011.8.JNS101407.
100. Gorgulho A, De Salles AA, Frighetto L, Behnke E. Incidence of hemorrhage associated with electrophysiological studies performed using macroelectrodes and microelectrodes in functional neurosurgery. *J Neurosurg.* 2005;102:888–896. https://doi.org/10.3171/jns.2005.102.5.0888.
101. Deep-Brain Stimulation for Parkinson's Disease Study Group, Obeso JA, Olanow CW. Deep-brain stimulation of the subthalamic nucleus or the pars interna of the globus pallidus in Parkinson's disease. *N Engl J Med.* 2001;345: 956–963. https://doi.org/10.1056/NEJMoa000827.
102. Binder DK, Rau GM, Starr PA. Risk factors for hemorrhage during microelectrode-guided deep brain stimulator implantation for movement disorders. *Neurosurgery.* 2005; 56:722–732; discussion 722–732.
103. Hariz MI. Safety and risk of microelectrode recording in surgery for movement disorders. *Stereotact Funct Neurosurg.* 2002;78:146–157. https://doi.org/68960.
104. McClelland 3rd S. A cost analysis of intraoperative microelectrode recording during subthalamic stimulation for Parkinson's disease. *Mov Disord.* 2011;26:1422–1427. https://doi.org/10.1002/mds.23787.

CHAPTER 23

CT-Guided Asleep DBS

KIM J. BURCHIEL, MD, FACS

INTRODUCTION

Deep brain stimulation (DBS) for Parkinson disease (PD), essential tremor (ET), and dystonia has become an established therapy for patients with medically intractable movement disorders.[1] Indications for DBS for PD include frequent or unpredictable on/off motor fluctuations, disabling dyskinesia, or disabling tremor that is refractory to dopamine replacement medications. The indications for DBS for ET are less clear, but generally, DBS is reserved for patients with severe disabling, intentional or postural tremor. In the past 25 years, DBS has typically been performed with the patient awake in the operating room to allow for microelectrode recording (MER) to identify the targets for placement of the stimulating electrodes.[2] This procedure involves placement of recording microelectrodes into the brain to identify the location and borders of the subthalamic nucleus (STN) and globus pallidus pars interna globus pallidus internus (GPi) for patients with PD or dystonia, and the ventralis intermedius (Vim) for patients with ET. MER often necessitates multiple passes into brain tissue to achieve a satisfactory result,[3] a requirement that has been shown to be directly correlated with an increased incidence of intracerebral hemorrhage (ICH).[4]

The prospect of having an elective awake brain surgery is a barrier for many who are otherwise good candidates for this treatment, and there is no Class I or II evidence that MER improves the outcome of a DBS implant procedure. Often the MER procedure is accompanied by test stimulation with the patient awake to further verify target accuracy, further prolonging the duration of the procedure that might take up to 4 to 8 h.[5,6] With the advent of advanced magnetic resonance and computed tomography imaging, particularly intraoperative imaging, the argument for the continued use of MER during DBS implantation has been substantially weakened. Furthermore, although the risk of a serious adverse event related to MER, such as ICH, remains low, it is not zero. Metaanalyses of surgical risk for DBS have reported ICH rates of 3.2%–5%.[4,7,8] The risk of ICH is related to the use of MER, the number of MER penetrations, and sulcal or transventricular course of the electrode trajectory.[4] The bulk of the evidence indicates that multiple instrumented passes into the brain with the sharp tip of the recording microelectrode contributes to the risk of ICH, with the per-trajectory ICH rate estimated at 1.57%.[9]

ICH related to DBS may further be divided into asymptomatic, symptomatic, and that resulting in permanent deficit or death, at reported rates of 1.9%, 2.1%, and 1.1%, respectively.[4] The incidence of hemorrhage in studies adopting an image-guided and image-verified approach without MER was significantly lower than that reported with other operative techniques ($P < .001$ for total number of hemorrhages, $P < .001$ for asymptomatic hemorrhage, $P < .004$ for symptomatic hemorrhage, and $P = .001$ for hemorrhage leading to permanent deficit).[4]

Perhaps the most common argument for the use of MER is the sensitivity of this methodology in finding the precise target for implantation of DBS electrodes. Yet, a recent analysis of multiple databases between 2004 and 2013 revealed over 28,000 cases of DBS electrode placement, revision, and removal. Data from Medicare indicated that 15.2% of DBS procedures were for revision or removal. Similar analysis of the National Surgical Quality Improvement Program (NSQIP) dataset showed a 34.0% DBS removal or revision rate. The authors concluded that up to 48.5% of revisions may have been due to improper targeting or lack of therapeutic effect.[10] Combining the Medicare and NSQIP datasets, the proportion of these procedures performed for a first DBS electrode implant with MER was 73.9%, compared with 10.8% without MER. That is, the overwhelming majority of cases in the analysis were related to patients in whom MER had been used during the initial implant. This result suggests that the presumed location of DBS electrode implant using MER may not be as predictable as has been previously assumed.

Newer methods of performing DBS incorporate image guidance using intraoperative magnetic resonance image (iMRI) (Starr, 2010) or intraoperative computerized tomographic imaging (iCT)[11–13] without MER. When iCT is used, iCT images are coregistered with a preoperative 3-T MRI to plan the trajectory to avoid sulci and ventricles, which are known to cause adverse events, visualize the planned target, and confirm lead placement of the target electrode contact before the patient leaving the operating room.[11,13] This allows the patient to be asleep from the start to end of the entire procedure. Accuracy of lead placement using this method is excellent, with good outcomes.[11–13]

ASLEEP DEEP BRAIN STIMULATION PROCEDURE

Imaging

Before surgery, 3-T MRI is obtained for DBS targets in all patients using the following sequences: ventrointermediate nucleus (Vim; a standard 3D T1, TE: 4.61, TR: shortest, flip angle: 30, voxel size: 1.02, matrix 256 × 256), STN (a FLAIR sequence TE: 140, TR: 14,000, slice thickness 2.5 mm, voxel size: 1.02, matrix 256 × 256), and globus pallidus internus (GPi; an MPRAGE sequence TE: 80, TR: 8000, slice thickness: 2 mm, voxel size: 0.6, matrix 256 × 256).[14] These digital imaging and communications in medicine (DICOM) images are downloaded into a StealthStation (Medtronic Inc., Minneapolis, Minnesota, United States) via a network connection.

Surgical Technique

Implant procedures are carried out in two stages. The first stage is an inpatient procedure for implantation of the DBS electrodes, and the second stage is the implantation of the internal pulse generator (IPG), performed on an outpatient basis approximately 1 week later.

The implantation of the DBS electrode(s) uses the extraoperative MR images aforementioned, and surgical planning of electrode trajectories is carried out preoperatively on the StealthStation (Medtronic Inc.). GPi and STN targets are visualized directly, and the Vim target is derived from the Schaltenbrand and Wahren atlas, using the intercommissural plane and midcommissural point for reference.[15]

All procedures are performed under general anesthesia. After intubation, the patient's head is attached to the operating table using a Doro Halo Retractor System with carbon fiber extensions (Pro Med Instruments, Inc., Freiburg, Germany). After sterile preparation of the head, five skull-mounted fiducials (NexFrame, Medtronic Inc.) are placed. A stereotactic 1-mm thick, zero-gantry-angle CT image was then obtained using a CereTom CT scanner (NeuroLogica Corp., Danvers, MA).[16] Subsequently, these DICOM images are transferred to the StealthStation (Medtronic Inc.) surgical navigation system and merged with the preoperative MR images.

Using a passive planar blunt probe, a nonsterile registration of the skull fiducials is then performed to link image and surgical spaces. The burr hole entry point of the predetermined electrode trajectory is then marked on the skin, and a small pilot hole was drilled to mark that point on the skull.

After appropriate sterile preparation and draping, skin incisions are made and burr holes centered on the pilot hole are completed. The lead anchoring device (StimLoc, Medtronic, Inc.) and the NexFrame base are then attached to the skull, and a second sterile registration is performed using the implanted fiducials (target registration error <0.5 mm). The NexFrame tower is then attached and aligned to the corresponding target using FrameLink (Medtronic Inc.) software. Target depth is then calculated and set on the StarDrive (FHC Inc., Bowdoin, ME) positioning device. After opening the dura, a cannula is then placed to target, and fibrin glue is used to prevent egress of cerebrospinal fluid. A DBS lead (Medtronic lead model 3387) is then advanced through the cannula to the target position (Fig. 23.1). The cannula is then retracted, and the electrode is

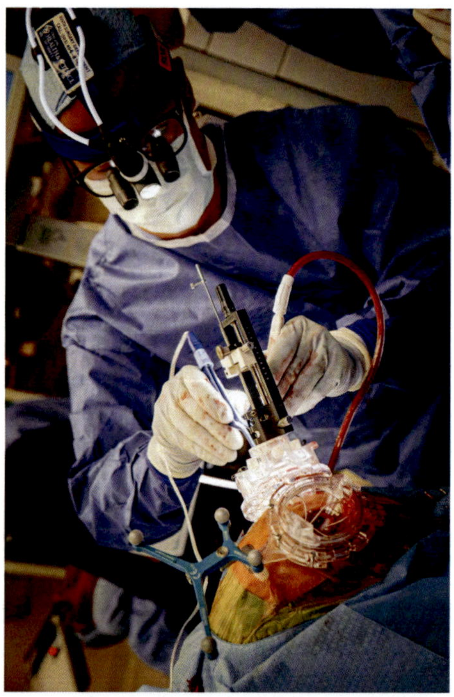

FIG. 23.1 Placement of DBS leads using the NexFrame and Stardrive. *DBS*, deep brain stimulation.

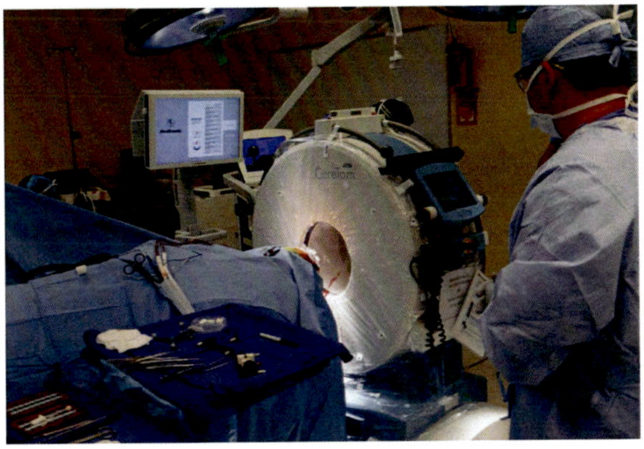

FIG. 23.2 An intraoperative CT scanner (Ceretom, NeuroLogica, Inc.) is used in conjunction with the StealthStation (Medronic, Inc.) to confirm accurate electrode location after the leads are placed and before completing the procedure. *CT*, computerized tomographic.

secured in the StimLoc system. The exposed electrode is then pulled back through the StarDrive, and in most cases, the process is repeated on the opposite side.

With the NexFrame towers in place, a second iCT scan is obtained to ensure satisfactory electrode placement (Fig. 23.2). This postplacement scan is then merged with the preoperative planning scans, and any off-target error is recorded. Vector error is calculated as the linear distance between the center of the intended target contact on the DBS electrode and the planned target. The electrode is repositioned if the vector error is >2.0 mm. Once the accuracy of the electrode placement is confirmed by intraoperative CT, no further imaging is carried out on these patients intra- or postoperatively (Fig. 23.3A and B).

After ensuring satisfactory electrode placement, the NexFrame towers are removed and the StimLoc caps are applied. The two leads are then capped and tunneled in the subgaleal plane to the side of the head just superior and posterior to the ear ipsilateral to the planned IPG subclavicular implant, after which the wounds are closed.

Within 4–7 days, an outpatient procedure is performed with the patient under general anesthesia during which the DBS leads are connected to extension leads and tunneled to a subclavicular pocket for the IPG implant.

OUTCOMES OF ASLEEP DEEP BRAIN STIMULATION

Electrode Accuracy

We have used two measures to assess electrode placement accuracy: (1) vector error, defined as the distance between the position of the center of the target DBS electrode contact ("1" for Vim and STN, and "0" for GPi) and the intended target location as determined by the Euclidean distance between these two points $[(x2 - x1)^2 + (y2 - y1)^2 + (z2 - z1)^2]^{1/2}$ and (2) deviation off trajectory, defined as the perpendicular distance from the target electrode to the planned trajectory, reflecting only the radial deviation from plan (Fig. 23.4). Both values are felt to be useful in determining the accuracy of placement because although vector error reflected the true accuracy of the procedure, off trajectory (radial) errors theoretically would be less easily correctable by assigning different active contacts during DBS therapy.

The accuracy of electrode placement has been compared among all three targets; GPi, STN, and Vim. The closest approach of the DBS lead trajectory to the lateral ventricle has also been measured and correlated with both the vector error and the deviation off trajectory. In all cases, the postimplantation CT scan is merged with the registration merged CT/MR used for planning the electrode trajectory and target to calculate both the vector error and the deviation off trajectory distances.

The initial 60 patients (33 PD, 26 ET, and 1 dystonia) who underwent DBS electrode placement by this method at Oregon Health and Science University (OHSU) were analyzed[11,13]. Over 18 months, 119 electrodes were placed (all bilateral, except one). Mean patient age was 64 ± 9.5 years, and electrode implant location was Vim (25 patients), GPi (23 patients), and STN (12 patients). Final intraoperative CT imaging showed no evidence of intracranial air or any other potential cause for brain shift in any case. The mean total operating room time (time in: time out), including anesthetic induction and recovery, was 190 ± 9.8 min.

In these cases, the closest approach of the electrode trajectories to the ventricle was 6.3 ± 3.4 mm (range, 1–13.9 mm), and there was no statistically significant difference between sides. Mean overall vector error was 1.59 ± 1.11 mm, and the trajectory deviation error was 1.24 ± 0.87 mm.

There was a significant correlation between (1) the distance from the ventricle and trajectory deviation error ($r2 = -0.325$, $P < .05$, $n = 77$) and (2) the distance from the ventricle and vector error ($r2 = -0.339$, $P < .05$, $n = 76$). Furthermore, when the distance from the electrode trajectory and the ventricular wall was <4 mm, the correlation of the ventricular distance to the deviation from the planned trajectory was stronger ($r2 = -0.419$, $P = .05$, $n = 19$; Fig. 23.5). Electrodes placed in the GPi were significantly more accurate than those placed in the Vim (mean vector error of 1.29 vs.

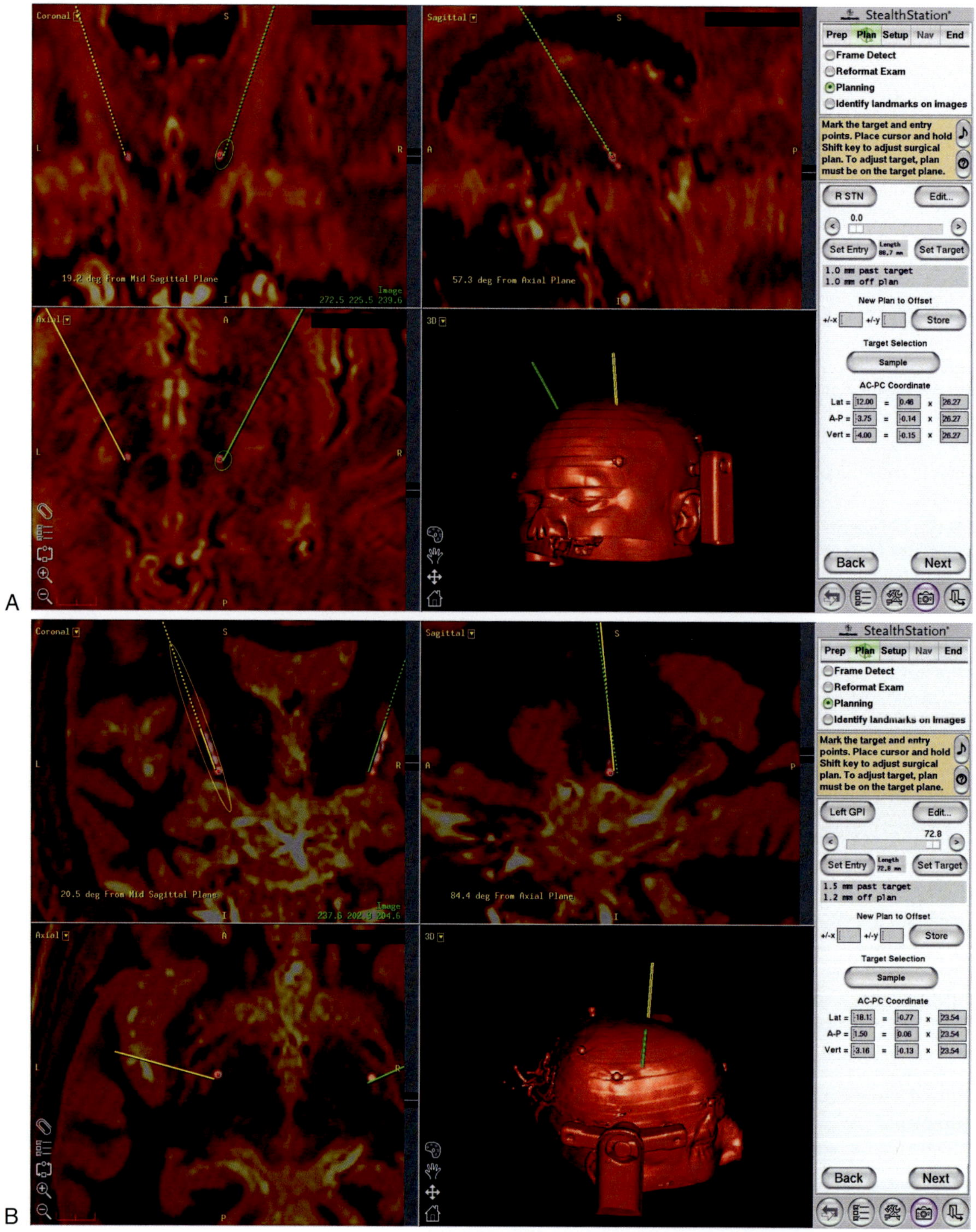

FIG. 23.3 Final postimplant CT scan merged with preoperative MRI scan to confirm accurate electrode placement. *Yellow* (left) and *green lines* represent the preoperative planned trajectory and target points for bilateral placements in the **(A)** subthalamic nucleus and **(B)** globus pallidus internus. *CT*, computerized tomographic; *MRI*, magnetic resonance image.

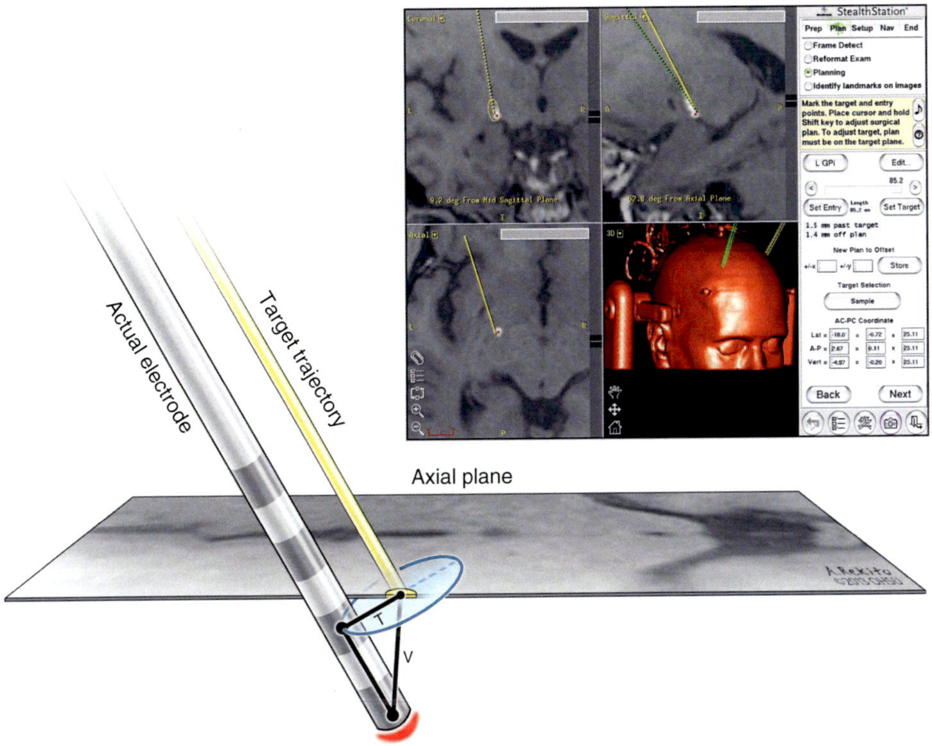

FIG. 23.4 Accuracy of electrode placement is measured by (1) vector error (V), defined as the distance between the position of the center of the target DBS electrode contact ("1" for Vim and STN, and "0" for GPi) and the intended target location as determined by the Euclidean distance between these two points: $[(x2 - x1)^2 + (y2 - y1)^2 + (z2 - z1)^2]^{1/2}$, and (2) deviation off trajectory (T), defined as the perpendicular distance from the target electrode to the planned trajectory, reflecting only the radial deviation from plan. *DBS*, deep brain stimulation; *GPi*, globus pallidus internus. (From the Burchiel KJ, McCartney S, Lee A, et al. Accuracy of deep brain stimulation electrode placement using intraoperative computed tomography without microelectrode recording. *J Neurosurg*. 2013;119(2):301–306 with permission.)

1.9 mm, $P = .01$). There was no statistically significant difference in accuracy comparing the GPi with STN, the STN with Vim, or the GPi with STN and Vim combined. Mean distance from the ventricle for GPi electrodes was 9 mm compared with 4.2 mm for the Vim and 5.15 mm for the STN, and these differences were significant ($P < .05$).

In this series, one implanted electrode had a vector error of >2 mm and was revised. There was one case of a late infection that required explant of the entire system. There were no hematomas, no new neurologic deficits, and there was no mortality.

Subsequent to this early experience, we have now analyzed 169 leads in 94 patients. Targets were GPi ($n = 86$), STN ($n = 31$), and Vim ($n = 52$); 85 leads were placed on the left and 84 on the right. Average Euclidean error was 1.63 mm (SD: 0.87). Error magnitude is higher for Vim (1.95 mm) than for GPi (1.44 mm), whereas STN (1.65 mm) did not differ from either Vim or GPi (ANOVA: $F = 6.15$, $P = 0.003$). Electrodes targeting Vim and STN were significantly more likely to deviate medially compared with GPi (ANOVA: $F = 9.13$, $P < 0.001$). Coronal approach angle affects error when targeting Vim ($\rho = 0.338$, $P = 0.01$). These findings were confirmed during multivariate analyses (Fig. 23.5).

Intracranial Air

The introduction of intracranial air may be a consequence of prolonged DBS implantation procedures under local anesthesia. In fact, it is the potential brain shift attendant upon cerebrospinal fluid drainage and brain

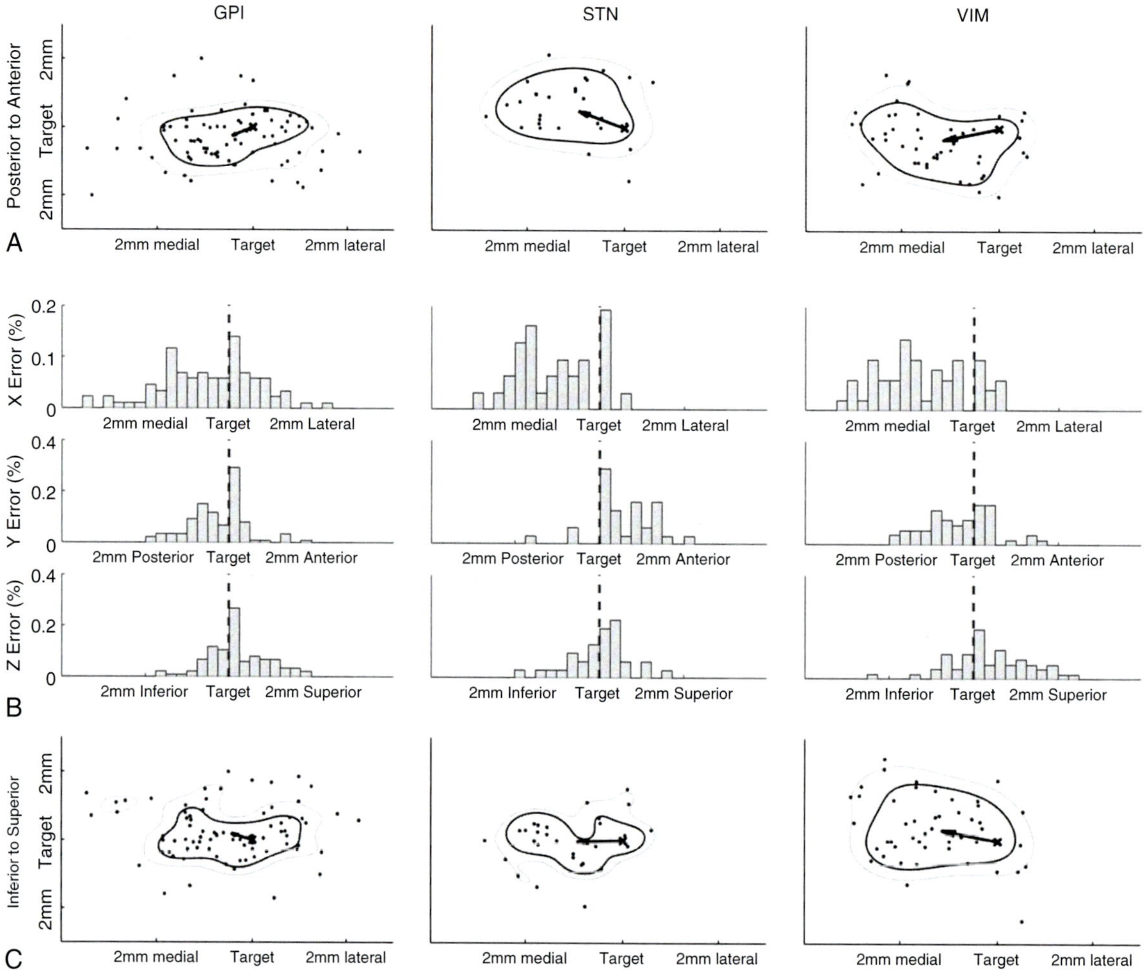

FIG. 23.5 Stereotactic error by target. **(A)** Distribution of electrode locations by target in the axial plane (average error in these directions is represented by the *back arrow*). Note that this error vector is greatest for Vim. *Contour lines* represent 50% (black) and 75% (gray) probability density estimates for electrode locations. **(B)** Histograms of error magnitudes in the X (*top*), Y (*middle*), and Z (*bottom*) directions for each target. No error (0 mm) is denoted with the *dotted line*. **(C)** Distribution of electrode locations in the coronal plane. Average error is again denoted with a black error, and probability density estimates for electrode locations are as above. *GPi*, globus pallidus internus; *STN*, subthalamic nucleus; *VIM*, ventralis intermedius.

"settling" that is often used as a rationale to perform procedures using iMRI as a means of accounting for this brain shift. To assess the incidence of intracranial air during iCT-guided DBS implantation procedures under general anesthesia, we conducted a retrospective review of our bilateral DBS cases performed from 2009 to 2013[17]; a time spanning 2 years before and 2 years after the implementation of asleep DBS at OHSU. Post- or intraoperative imaging was examined to determine the presence and volume of intracranial air during these procedures. A total of 163 electrode implantations in 156 patients were reviewed. Intracranial air was noted in 27% of cases, with an incidence of 10.1% and 61.1% during asleep and awake DBS, respectively. The incidence of intracranial air was significantly higher in our awake DBS cases ($P = .00$) (Fig. 23.6).

Clinical Outcomes

DBS candidates with PD referred to OHSU underwent asleep DBS with imaging guidance. Six-month outcomes were compared with patients who previously underwent awake DBS by the same surgeon and center.[18]

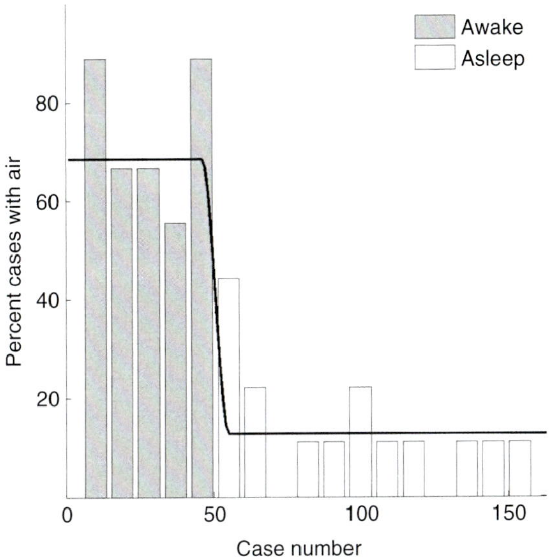

FIG. 23.6 Percentage of cases showing intracranial air after completion of the implant procedure. *Gray bars* reflect the incidence of intracranial air in 50 cases in which implants were performed with an awake patient, using MER. At case, 50 procedures were performed with the patient under general anesthesia without MER (*white bars*). *MER*, microelectrode recording.

Assessments included an off-levodopa Unified Parkinson's Disease Rating Scale (UPDRS) II and III, the PDQ-39 questionnaire, motor diaries, and speech fluency. Thirty patients underwent asleep DBS, and thirty-nine patients underwent awake DBS. No significant difference was observed in improvement of UPDRS III ($+14.8 \pm 8.9$ vs. $+17.6 \pm 12.3$ points, $P = .19$) or UPDRS II ($+9.3 \pm 2.7$ vs. $+7.4 \pm 5.8$ points, $P = .16$). Improvement in *on* time without dyskinesia was superior in asleep DBS ($+6.4 \pm 3.0$ h/day vs. $+1.7 \pm 1.2$ h/day, $P = .002$). Quality-of-life scores significantly improved in both groups ($+18.8 \pm 9.4$ in awake, $+8.9 \pm 11.5$ in asleep). Improvement in summary index ($P = .004$) and subscores for cognition ($P = .011$) and communication ($P < .001$) were superior in asleep DBS. Speech outcomes were superior in asleep DBS, both in category ($+2.77 \pm 4.3$ points vs. -6.31 ± 9.7 points, $P = .0012$) and phonemic fluency ($+1.0 \pm 8.2$ points vs. -5.5 ± 9.6 points, $P = .038$).[18]

Costs of Deep Brain Stimulation

We have compared the cost of DBS performed awake versus asleep at OHSU, and compared costs across the University Health System Consortium (UHC) Clinical Database.[19] Inpatient and outpatient demographics and hospital financial data for patients receiving a DBS lead implant (from the first quarter of 2009 to the second quarter of 2014) were collected and analyzed. Inpatient charges included those associated with International Classification of Diseases, Ninth Revision (ICD-9) procedure code 0293 (implantation or replacement of intracranial neurostimulator lead). Outpatient charges included all preoperative charges $\leq$30 days before implant and all postoperative charges $\leq$30 days after implant. The cost of care based on reported charges and a cost-to-charge ratio were estimated. The UHC database was queried (January 2011 to March 2014) with the same ICD-9 code. Procedure cost data across like hospitals (27 UHC hospitals) conducting similar DBS procedures were compared. 211 DBS procedures (53 awake and 158 asleep) were performed at OHSU during the study period. The average patient age ($\pm$SD) was 65 ± 9 years, and 39% of patients were female. The most common primary diagnosis was PD (61.1%) followed by essential and other forms of tremor (36%). Overall average DBS procedure cost was \$39,152 $\pm$ \$5340. The total asleep DBS cost was \$38,850 $\pm$ \$4830, which was not significantly different than the awake DBS cost of \$40,052 $\pm$ \$6604. The standard deviation for asleep DBS was significantly lower ($P \leq .05$). In 2013, the median cost for a neurostimulator implant lead (Ninth Revision [ICD-9] procedure code 0293 [implantation or replacement of intracranial neurostimulator lead]) was \$34,052 at UHC-affiliated hospitals that performed at least five procedures a year. At OHSU, the median cost was \$17,150, and the observed single academic health center cost for a neurostimulator lead implant was less than the expected cost ([ratio 0.97]) (Figs. 23.7 and 23.8).

DISCUSSION

Imaging technology has advanced to the degree that DBS electrode placement based entirely on imaging can be considered a feasible option. Several studies have demonstrated the reliability of image-defined STN and its dorsolateral subregion as location for movement-related cells during MER.[15] We capitalized on previous reports that combined the use of a skull-mounted frame (NexFrame), the use of intraoperative imaging, and general anesthesia.[6]

We have developed a method that uses an iCT scanner and a skull-mounted stereotactic system to place DBS electrodes. Our aim was to exploit the advantages of high-field extraoperative MRI, the availability of intraoperative CT scanning, and the capacity to merge images from both sources to provide the basis for target and trajectory planning for DBS surgery. Furthermore, this

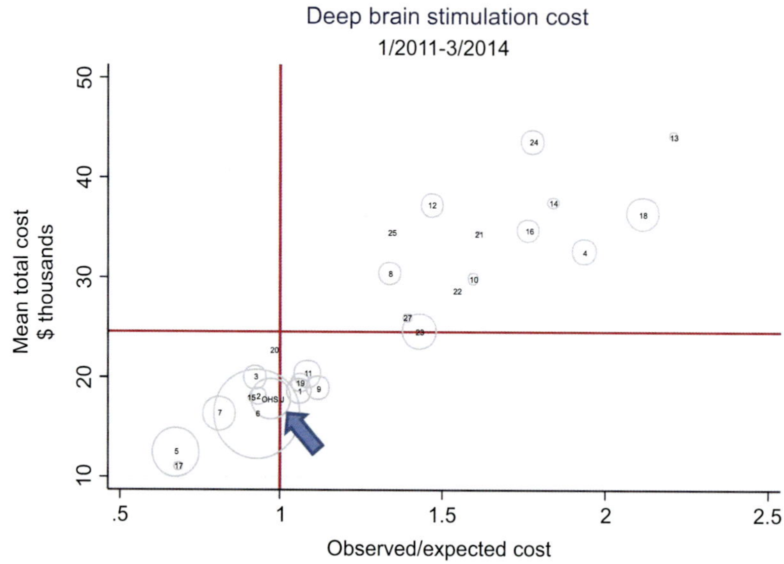

FIG. 23.7 Scatterplot of cost benchmarking of the ICD-9 code 0293 (neurostimulator implant lead) and adult inpatient cost data from 27 UHC hospitals from January 2011 to March 2014 compared with OHSU costs. *ICD-9*, International Classification of Diseases, Ninth Revision; *UHC*, University Health System Consortium. (Data source: UHC.)

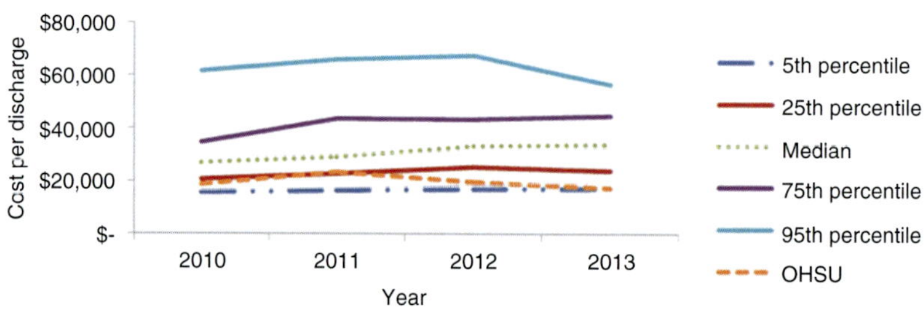

FIG. 23.8 Percentile average total cost per discharge for ICD-9 code 0293, using adult inpatient cost data from 27 UHC hospitals (2010–13). *ICD-9*, International Classification of Diseases, ninth revision; *UHC*, University Health System Consortium. (Data source: UHC.)

system could be used to confirm target acquisition and any operative complications (hematoma) before leaving the operating room. Because this method relies only on anatomic target determination, the use of MER was obviated, and therefore general anesthesia was feasible.

Electrode Accuracy

Using preoperative MRI, intraoperative CT, and a skull-mounted stereotactic system, we were able to achieve an unprecedented degree of accuracy for DBS electrode placement. Our results (1.59 mm vector error) compare favorably with previously reported vector errors for iMRI (2.18 mm),[13] intraoperative imaging (O-arm) combined with frame-stereotaxy (1.65 mm),[11] and conventional frame-based stereotaxy without intraoperative imaging (3 mm).[12] The mean trajectory deviation error in our series was 1.24 mm, indicating that displacement was mostly radial, and not along the planned trajectory (depth). Our data indicate that the electrode trajectory distance from the ventricle plays a major role in the radial deviation of the trajectory.

We attempted to correlate the vector error and trajectory deviation with factors that would impact location of the electrodes. The only significant correlation found was the distance of the electrode trajectory from the ventricle. Starr et al. previously reported on the correlation of the vector error and coronal approach angle, where the increased obliquity of the angle caused a higher positional error at the electrode tip.[20] A negative correlation was found between the distance of the electrode from the ventricle and both the vector error and trajectory deviation, i.e., both the vector error and the trajectory deviation were higher (less accuracy) when the electrode trajectory was closer to the ventricle. The strongest correlation was between the deviation error (radial displacement) and the distance from the ventricle in the range of 0–4 mm.

Our analysis also showed that electrode trajectories approaching the GPi are significantly ($P < .01$) more distant from the ventricle in comparison with other targets (GPi = 9 mm, STN = 4.5 mm, and Vim = 5.1 mm). Electrodes placed in the GPi were significantly more accurate than those placed in the Vim (mean vector error of 1.29 vs. 1.9 mm, $P = .01$) but not more accurate than those placed in the STN (mean vector error of 1.29 vs. 1.52, $P = .3$). Our data indicate that target trajectories that avoid a close approach to the ventricle are more likely to produce accurate placement. An alternative explanation is that traversing the internal capsule, e.g., approaching the Vim target from lateral to medial, may also cause distortion of the brain, with resultant electrode malposition. Trajectories that largely avoided the compact internal capsule, e.g., globus pallidus internus, were significantly more accurate. The reason behind this may well be the differential compliance of nuclei and white matter tracks to the penetrating cannula.

Intracranial Air

We have shown that asleep DBS significantly reduces the incidence of intracranial air, which is likely correlated to shift in brain structures and hence accuracy of electrode placement. Our experience now with over 800 electrode implantations indicates that the appearance of intracranial air is rare (<5%) during asleep DBS implantation. This finding would obviate the need for special imaging procedures, such as iMRI, where the rationale for the intraoperative imaging is to account for brain shift.

Outcomes of Asleep Deep Brain Stimulation

Asleep DBS for PD improved motor outcomes over 6 months on par with or better than awake DBS, was superior with regard to speech fluency and quality of life, and should be an option offered to all patients who are candidates for this treatment.

Cost

DBS performed asleep was associated with a lower cost variation relative to the awake procedure. Furthermore, costs compared very favorably to UHC-affiliated hospitals (50% of median UHC cost).

CONCLUSIONS

This method represents a clear departure from the use of MER and physiologic target confirmation during movement disorder surgery. It is our contention that MER has not been, nor will ever be, proven to add value to the implantation of DBS electrodes, or any other movement disorder procedure (Burchiel, 2004).[13] Furthermore, there is, in fact, new evidence that MER adds risk to these procedures by way of increased chances of ICH and the production of new neurologic deficits.[4] There is little question that MER requires additional expertise, added operative time, and the additional expense of the recording systems and electrodes. Effectively, MER also requires that procedures be performed under local anesthetic, a daunting prospect for most patients.

We have demonstrated the feasibility and accuracy of image-guided DBS electrode placement. If this procedure can be shown to produce clinical benefits that are equivalent to the more traditional methods using MER, and by historical comparison, proves to be a safer procedure, then the continuance of routine MER-based DBS electrode implantation should be questioned. MER may well then be relegated to the position of a research technique, potentially requiring additional informed consent by the patient.

As the demand for this procedure is expected to rise with the increasing prevalence of PD worldwide, the cost of this procedure is also an important issue. Prolonged duration of the DBS procedure and neurophysiologic assessments with MER may both add significantly to the cost of DBS. Costs associated with asleep DBS at our center were lower than comparable academic healthcare centers performing DBS[19] likely because of shorter operative time and elimination of the need for MER. iMRI is another method that has been used to target DBS electrode placement in the asleep patient; however, iMRI is a relatively more expensive and generally less available guidance system at surgical centers performing DBS compared with iCT. Image-guided asleep DBS procedures with iCT afford an accurate, cost-effective, and clinically effective alternative to traditional MER-guided approaches.

REFERENCES

1. Weaver F, Follett K, Stern M, et al. Bilateral deep brain stimulation vs best medical therapy for patients with advanced Parkinson disease. *JAMA*. 2009;301(1):63–73.
2. Israel Z, Burchiel K, eds. *Microelectrode Recording in Movement Disorder Surgery*. New York: Thieme Medical Publishers; 2005.

3. Starr PA, Christine CW, Theodosopoulos PV, et al. Implantation of deep brain stimulators into the subthalamic nucleus: technical approach and magnetic resonance imaging–verified lead locations. *J Neurosurg.* 2002;97:370–387.
4. Zrinzo L, Foltynie T, Limousin P, et al. Reducing hemorrhagic complications in functional neurosurgery: a large case series and systematic literature review. *J Neurosurg.* 2012;116:84–94.
5. Umemura A, Jaggi JL, Hurtig HI, et al. Deep brain stimulation for movement disorders: morbidity and mortality in 109 patients. *J Neurosurg.* 2003;98:779–784.
6. Oh MY, Abosch A, Kim SH, et al. Long-term hardware-related complications of deep brain stimulation. *Neurosurgery.* 2002;50:1268–1276.
7. Kleiner-Fisman G, Herzog J, Fisman DN, et al. Subthalamic nucleus deep brain stimulation: summary and meta-analysis of outcomes. *Mov Disord.* 2006;21(suppl 14):S290–S304.
8. Videnovic A, Metman LV. Deep brain stimulation for Parkinson's disease: prevalence of adverse events and need for standardized reporting. *Mov Disord.* 2008;23:343–349.
9. Kimmelman J, Duckworth K, Ramsay T, et al. Risk of surgical delivery to deep nuclei: a meta-analysis. *Mov Disord.* 2011;26(8):1415–1421.
10. Rolston JD, Englot DJ, Starr PA, et al. An unexpectedly high rate of revisions and removals in deep brain stimulation surgery: analysis of multiple databases. *Parkinsonism Relat Disord.* 2016;33:72–77.
11. Burchiel KJ, McCartney S, Lee A, et al. Accuracy of deep brain stimulation electrode placement using intraoperative computed tomography without microelectrode recording. *J Neurosurg.* 2013;119(2):301–306.
12. Mirzadeh Z, Chapple K, Lambert M, et al. Parkinson's disease outcomes after intraoperative CT-guided "asleep" deep brain stimulation in the globus pallidus internus. *J Neurosurg.* 2016;124:902–907.
13. Burchiel K. The future of microelectrode recording. In: Israel Z, Burchiel KJ, eds. *Microelectrode Recording in Movement Disorder Surgery.* New York: Thieme; 2004:209–210.
14. Sudhyadhom A, Haq IU, Foote KD, et al. A high resolution and high contrast MRI for differentiation of subcortical structures for DBS targeting: the fast gray matter acquisition T1 inversion recovery (FGATIR). *Neuroimage.* 2009;47(suppl 2):T44–T52.
15. Schaltenbrand G, Hassler RG, Wahren W. *Atlas for Stereotaxy of the Human Brain.* 2nd ed. Stuttgart: Thieme; 1977.
16. NeuroLogica Corporation. Available at: http://www.neurologica.com/ceretom.
17. Ko A, Ozpinar A, Hamzaoglu V, et al. Asleep DBS reduces incidence of intracranial air during electrode implantation. *J Funct Stereotact Neurosurg.* 2018. https://doi.org/10.1159/000488150.
18. Brodsky MA, Anderson S, Seier M, et al. Clinical outcomes of asleep versus awake deep brain stimulation for Parkinson's disease. *Neurology.* 2017;89:1–7.
19. Jacob RL, Geddes J, McCartney S, Burchiel K. Cost analysis of awake versus asleep deep brain stimulation: a single academic health center experience. *J Neurosurg.* 2016;124(5):1517–1523.
20. Starr PA, Martin AJ, Ostrem JL, et al. Subthalamic nucleus deep brain stimulator placement using high-field interventional magnetic resonance imaging and a skull-mounted aiming device: technique and application accuracy. *J Neurosurg.* 2010;112:479–490.

CHAPTER 24

Interventional MRI–Guided Deep Brain Stimulation

PAUL S. LARSON, MD

Traditional surgery for placement of deep brain stimulation (DBS) leads uses a combination of stereotactic and physiologic confirmation of proper lead placement. Both frame-based systems and frameless stereotaxy are widely used, and various forms of physiologic confirmation of the target can be used, including microelectrode recording (MER), local field potential recordings, and micro- or macrostimulation. Regardless of the technique used, DBS surgery has largely depended on an awake patient who is able to cooperate, communicate, and, in the case of Parkinson disease, do this off of their Parkinson medications during surgery. It also requires significant technical expertise and equipment to properly record and interpret physiologic data. In the case of MER, multiple brain penetrations are usually required.

Interventional MRI (iMRI)–guided DBS is an alternative to traditional awake surgery that uses direct visualization of the nucleus of interest on MRI as the only means of target localization. This obviates the need for physiologic mapping, which in turn eliminates the need for the patients to be awake. For this reason, iMRI DBS, along with intraoperative CT (iCT)–guided DBS, is often referred to as "asleep DBS." Unlike iCT, iMRI provides imaging that allows target visualization on properly optimized MR sequences, which eliminates dependence on image fusion with historical images (i.e., images that were acquired before surgery). A common misconception about iMRI DBS is that it requires a magnet that is located in a specially designed intraoperative MRI suite designed specifically for surgery. On the contrary, the technique was designed to be done on any standard, diagnostic 1.5- or 3-T MRI scanner located anywhere, whether it be in the radiology department or in surgery. Most centers performing iMRI DBS operate in scanners located in radiology.

At the time of this writing, the most commonly used system for performing iMRI DBS and the only one that takes full advantage of using MR as the imaging modality is the ClearPoint system (MRI Interventions, Irvine, CA). ClearPoint consists of disposable hardware components, primarily a skull-mounted aiming device with MR visible elements (the SmartFrame, Fig. 24.1) that works in conjunction with a sterile draping system and a software environment that runs on a laptop (ClearPoint software). MR images are streamed to the software, which in turn tells the MR technologist what

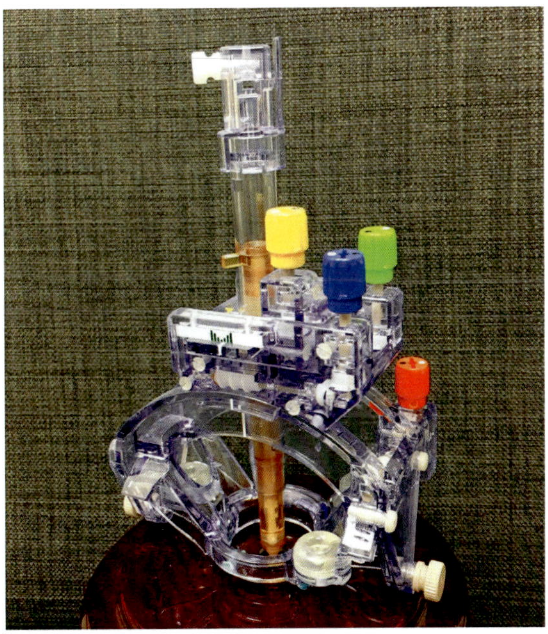

FIG. 24.1 SmartFrame. The fiducials can be seen in the SmartFrame base as yellow, doughnut-shaped objects; the targeting cannula occupies the center, vertical channel. The orange and blue knobs make pitch and roll movements, whereas the yellow and green knobs make parallel, offset adjustments.

sequences to acquire next and instructs the surgeon how to adjust the SmartFrame so that it is aligned with the chosen target. Each step in this process is based on MR images that were acquired just a few seconds before, which makes the workflow truly image-guided; there is no image fusion with image sets that were obtained before the time of surgery, and any brain shift or other changes in brain conformation are accounted for as the procedure progresses. The system was designed to work with any 1.5- or 3-T scanner from any of the major scanner manufacturers. In the United States, all MRI scanner rooms adhere to a minimum of air exchanges per hour. Although these minimums do not match the higher exchange rate seen in operating rooms (ORs), the infection rate in iMRI DBS is comparable with DBS performed in a standard OR.[1]

Patient selection for iMRI DBS is no different than selection for traditional surgery. The one exception is that patients must not have any contraindications to MR imaging, such as a noncompatible cardiac pacemaker. iMRI DBS does have the advantage of allowing DBS to be performed in patients who would otherwise not tolerate awake surgery because of anxiety, claustrophobia, or communication barriers. Despite changing Medtronic labeling over the years with regarding to MRI scanning guidelines of their hardware, we have been comfortable imaging patients with partially (lead only) or completely (lead and pulse generator) implanted systems at 1.5 T. We routinely perform staged lead implants using iMRI (i.e., second-sided implants in patients with an existing lead or complete system on the contralateral side). In these instances, we do use lower energy (low specific absorption rate, or SAR) sequences to reduce the potential for heating of the system components, but we have never experienced an adverse event related to imaging DBS hardware at 1.5 T since starting our iMRI program in 2004.

3-T scanners currently provide some challenges with regard to performing staged iMRI DBS implants, as the safety of imaging DBS components in a clinical setting has not been established at 3 T. As will be described below, the iMRI technique with ClearPoint differs from traditional micropositioner systems in that a flexible guide tube (a peel-away sheath) is delivered all the way to the target with a rigid, plastic-coated ceramic stylet within its lumen. Ceramic was selected as the material for the stylet because it leaves a small, discrete artifact on MR images as opposed to a nonferrous metal or the DBS lead itself. Therefore, when one obtains the scans to determine the accuracy of placement in ClearPoint, they are scanning a ceramic stylet, not the lead itself. All of the steps in the procedure are therefore safe to perform at 3 T, provided that the patient does not have any preexisiting DBS hardware. At 1.5 T, one can scan the DBS lead after it is passed down the peel-away sheath after removal of the stylet to double check the lead depth, but this step is not necessary and can be skipped if performing the procedure at 3 T.

The workflow for individual centers varies depending on factors such as the configuration of the MRI scanner room and adjacent spaces, anesthesia's preferred location for induction, and the preferences of the OR team. At our center, we have three distinct workflows for each of three different MRI scanners we operate in; the process described here is what is used at our main facility, where the majority of our cases are performed. The first step in preparation for the procedure is the so-called terminal cleaning of the MRI room, either in the evening before or the morning of the procedure. All surfaces are wiped down with disposable antiseptic cloths, and the floor is mopped. The flexible MR coils are wiped and wrapped in plastic to protect them from exposure to fluid. Once this cleaning is completed, the MRI room is treated as a standard OR; no one is allowed inside without fresh surgical scrub attire and hats. Once the sterile instruments are opened, masks must be worn as well. The MR technologist makes sure that the scanner is operating normally, usually by scanning a fluid or gel phantom. The SmartFrames contain MR-visible components, consisting of three fluid filled, doughnut-shaped fiducials on the SmartFrame base, and the targeting cannula or TC (Fig. 24.2). The TC is a fluid-filled hollow cannula with a sphere on its proximal end referred to as ball marker. The ball marker is the center of rotation of movement for the TC. During the procedure, the TC will be adjusted until it is aligned with the target; the stylet plus peel-away sheath assembly will ultimately be passed down the hollow TC to the target. The accuracy of the system is largely dependent on the ClearPoint software's ability to detect the position of these MR-visible components, particularly the ball marker. We therefore scan the nonsterile boxes containing the sterile SmartFrames before the procedure to make sure there has been no evaporation of fluid from these components. If they are not well visualized, the kits are rejected and new ones obtained from storage.

The cases are booked as if they are happening in a regular OR to secure an OR nursing team and anesthesia. We use two anesthesia machines: one MR-compatible unit in the MRI room and a regular machine in the adjacent MRI control room where the patient will be induced. The MR environment is unique and poses obvious safety issues, so early on we identified a small

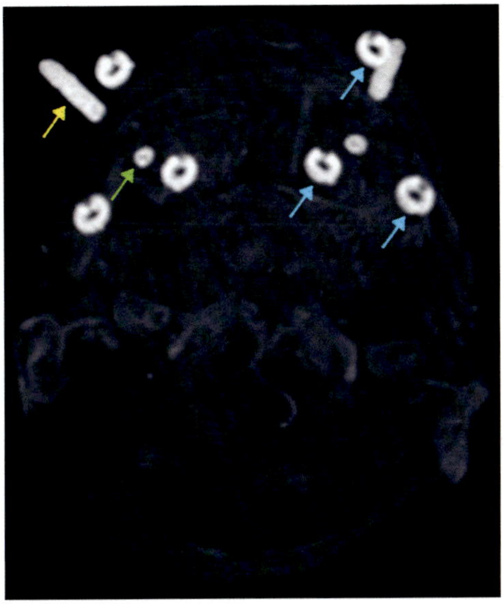

FIG. 24.2 A three-dimensional MR image reconstruction showing bilateral SmartFrames mounted in the frontal region. The targeting cannula (*yellow arrow*) and pivot point (*green arrow*) are seen on the left SmartFrame. The three fiducials in the SmartFrame base (*blue arrows*) are seen on the right.

collection of nurses and scrub technicians to perform these cases. Creating a culture of open questioning and double-checking is vital to maintain the safety of both the surgical team and the patient. Team members frequently ask each other if they are "clean" before entering the room during all phases of the case, which means are they free of metallic objects, cell phones, etc. Even highly experienced team members are asked these questions routinely, and many personnel will pause at the door and perform a physical "pat down" of themselves to ensure they are clean. Exhibiting such visible safety behavior is infectious and helps promote safe behavior in others. A particularly vulnerable time is at the end of the procedure, where many people start to relax or mistakenly believe that the scanner is not "on" if scanning is no longer being done.

The patient is checked in to the preoperative holding area and is transported on a regular gurney to the MRI control room adjacent to the MRI room. The patient is intubated and placed under anesthesia using the regular (non-MR compatible) anesthesia machine. MR-compatible EKG leads and pulse oximeter are placed. Our MRI gantry has a tabletop that can be rolled out of the MRI room on wheels; the tabletop is moved into the MRI control room, and the ClearPoint head holder is placed on the head end of the gantry. The patient is transferred to the tabletop, then slid up to place the head in the head holder. Care is taken to extend the head as much as possible to bring the anticipated frontal trajectory as close to horizontal as possible to avoid a bore collision (i.e., an inability to insert or remove the ceramic stylet due to contact with the walls of the bore when the patient's head is at isocenter, or the center of the bore). Downward pressure is placed on the forehead to help seat the occipital pins, whereas the temporal pins are tightened just above the pinna of the ear. The pressure points are padded appropriately, and a foley catheter is placed. If available, sequential compression devices are placed, but this usually requires waveguide (a tube that goes through the wall of the MRI scanner room) positioned such that the pump can be positioned outside the MRI room and the tubing can reach the patient's legs. We do not have a configuration that will accommodate this, so we do not use sequential compression devices during our DBS cases. Despite this, we have only had one DVT/PE event in our DBS program.

The patient is covered with blankets to maintain body temperature. The bore of the scanner is a warm environment, and we have not observed any issues with maintaining body temperature without a forced air warming blanket, but one can be used with a favorably position waveguide. We have occasionally used foley catheters with temperature probes, but in general, temperature probes are avoided as the wire loops contained within some of them can theoretically cause burns if they are in direct or close contact with tissue. Loops of conductive materials such as wires can focus electromagnetic energy during scanning and result in heating sufficient enough to cause burns.[2] The grounding pads for most monopolar cautery also contains loops, which is one of the reasons why only bipolar cautery is used. All MR-compatible EKG wires and any other wires or lines are inspected to ensure that they run down the body as close to each other as possible, as close to the center of the body as possible, and in a straight line without loops to avoid the potential for burns. These wires are also padded away from the skin as much as possible with thin foam padding. Finally, any medication patches that the patient might be wearing are removed, as many of them have a metallic backing that may cause burns. The hair in the frontal region is removed with electric clippers, the skin undergoes preliminary preparation with a surgical skin prep, and local anesthetic with epinephrine is infiltrated to cover the likely area of incision and aid in hemostasis. Although the exact location of the incision is not known at this point, it is usually at or just in front of the coronal suture. We infiltrate locally a row of 10 cc at the coronal suture, then two more rows of 10 cc each in front of coronal for a total of 30 cc.

All team members gather around the patient for a final MRI safety time-out. This involves all team members patting themselves down for any metallic objects, particularly pagers, cell phones, stethoscopes, scissors, ID badges with magnetic strips, and non-LCD watches. The patient and tabletop are also inspected for items that are not MR safe, including laryngoscope blades or handles, needles from IVs that may have been started after leaving the preoperative area and the electric clipper that was used to shave the head. Finally, the surgical plan is confirmed with the MRI technologist, including renal function test and planned dose of IV gadolinium, MR sequences planned to visualize the target and clarifying whether lower energy (lower SAR) sequences should be used if the patient already has implanted DBS hardware. The leader of the time-out asks if anyone has any questions regarding MR safety, and after verbal confirmation that everyone is ready to proceed, the patient is moved into the MRI scanner room.

The patient is placed in the scanner bore and connected to the MR-compatible anesthesia machine. IV pumps are kept outside the room, and extension tubing is used to accommodate the increased distance to the patient. The patient is then "landmarked" at the top of the head at the approximate level of the burr holes. This maneuver, performed by the MRI technologist, will ensure that when the head is at isocenter, the target below the skull and the SmartFrame above the skull will all be in the imaging "sweet spot" of the scanner (a spherical volume of space that straddles isocenter). The patient is then carefully moved into the bore, making sure that the ventilator circuit and IV lines are long enough to allow the head to protrude out the far end of the bore. The head is then definitely prepped and draped using the specially designed drape that comes with the ClearPoint System (Fig. 24.3). The drape has a central accordion-like section that works in combination with elastic tensioners to allow a sterile field to be maintained while the patient's head is moved from the edge of the bore to isocenter. At the same time, the nursing team ensures that the MR-compatible drill and the bipolar forceps are connected and working, and all of the titanium MR-compatible instruments are ready. Many bipolar forceps are MR compatible and can be tested with a hand magnet ahead of time to determine this. Disposable bipolar forceps are almost always MR safe; in general, the cheaper something is, the more likely it will be made out of low-grade metals

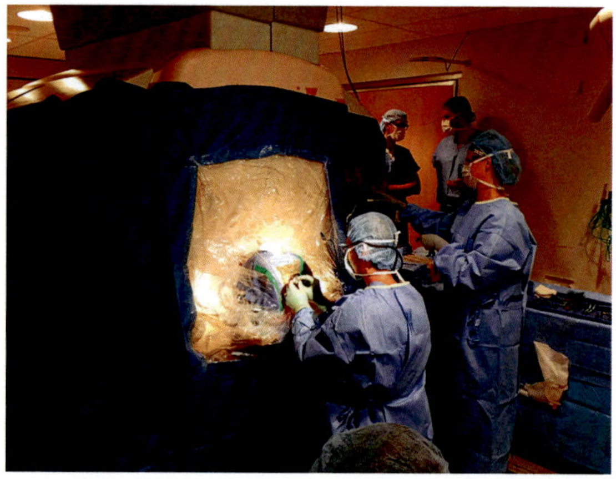

FIG. 24.3 Specially designed drape to allow surgical interventions to be performed in a standard, diagnostic scanner. This scanner is located in the radiology department.

that are MR compatible. Drills, on the other hand, must be specifically manufactured to be MR compatible. The nitrogen tank for the drill and console for the bipolar are kept outside the MRI room, with the associated hose and wires going through a waveguide. All surgical instruments are made of titanium and are commercially available. A spare MRI gantry top is used as a sterile back table. An MRI-compatible in-room monitor is positioned in the room such that the surgeon can see the ClearPoint software. The surgeon may choose to scrub out for certain tasks, particularly trajectory planning and targeting, but most other tasks can be accomplished by a nonsterile person on the ClearPoint laptop in the MRI control room with the surgeon supervising on the in-room monitor.

Dual-layer MR-visible marking grid(s), which have rows and columns of MR-visible cells, are placed over the anticipated entry site (or sites if a bilateral case). The patient is moved to isocenter, and IV gadolinium is administered. A volumetric T1 scan is obtained and transferred to the ClearPoint software. The surgeon then sets a preliminary target based purely on AC-PC (anterior commissure-posterior commissure)-based coordinates. We use $X = 12$, $Y = -3$, and $Z = -4$ for subthalamic nucleus (STN), $X = 21.5$, $Y = +2$, and $Z = 0$ for the globus pallidus internus (GPi). One could, if desired, obtain a high-resolution scan to directly visualize the target, but this is time-consuming and not necessary at this step for two reasons. First, we have discovered that the final target (selected later in the procedure) can change by as much as 5 mm without substantially changing the structures traversed during insertion; indeed, improper placement of the burr hole or poor SmartFrame placement are far more likely to result in an undesirable trajectory. Second, when one selects a point in the ClearPoint software, what they are really doing is selecting a three-dimensional point in MR space (the physical space within the bore of the scanner). It is therefore useful to think about the scanner as if it were a stereotactic frame; every time the patient is moved relative to the scanner, it is analogous to moving a frame on patient's head. Because the patient will need to be moved back to the edge of the bore for opening, we do not waste time getting a high-resolution scan that visualizes the target at this point.

The software detects the center of the marking grid and uses this as a preliminary entry point and trajectory. The trajectory is adjusted to avoid enhancing blood vessels, sulci, and the ventricles. Once the trajectory is finalized, the software shows the surgeon the proper location for centering the burr hole and mounting the SmartFrame base. The outer layer of the marking grid is removed to reveal an inner layer with printed rows and cells; a sharp trocar (the marking tool) is used to pierce the skin and make a divot in the underlying bone at the specified location. Gentle pressure should be used during this maneuver to not move the scalp, and the surgeon should approximate the anticipated trajectory to the target (much like drilling a hole to place a ventricular drain). The inner layer of the grid is then removed and an incision is planned. We use a linear incision that goes right through the puncture mark in the skin and parallels the coronal suture. This does place the incision directly over the dome of the Stimloc anchoring device (Medtronic, Minneapolis, MN). We have historically avoided incisions that go directly over the Stimloc in our awake, frame-based surgeries, but such an incision is extremely convenient for subsequent mounting of the SmartFrame and we have not had any wound healing issues related to this practice. The skin is opened with a disposable scalpel with a retractable blade; this is not MR compatible, but the blade is light and made of low-grade stainless, so the pull is minimal. Even so, the scrub should not let go of the blade when handing it to the surgeon until he or she has a firm grip on it, and vice versa. The blade should also be retracted before it is transferred between personnel.

The MR-compatible drill is used to make a burr hole about 15 mm in diameter. It is extremely important to center the burr hole precisely on the divot made in the bone by the marking tool. The burr hole must be as wide at the bottom as it is at the top; the SmartFrame will not be aligned with the target until after the head is back at isocenter, so it is imperative that there be a wide enough exposure at the bottom of the burr hole to avoid a collision with the bone edge. The trajectory is almost always close to the lateral edge of the burr hole, so we frequently undercut the lateral wall of the burr hole. The Stimloc is mounted in standard fashion, and the SmartFrame base is then mounted. The base is medialized slightly when mounted; this is another maneuver to avoid a collision with the lateral edge of the burr hole. The dura is traditionally opened widely, although we are currently studying a closed dura technique wherein the dura is pierced using a metal lancet after alignment of the SmartFrame is accomplished. Dural opening is performed as early as possible to allow any cerebrospinal fluid loss to occur early in the procedure. Brain shift is unpredictable, but when it occurs it can be upward of 2 mm or more in deep brain structures and is associated with the formation of pneumocephalus.[3,4] One of the advantages of the iMRI technique is that targeting is performed on an MR sequence that is obtained after opening, so any brain shift that occurs will be accounted for. Moreover, the images subsequently used to determine accuracy of stylet placement are also obtained in real-time and do not need to be fused back to a preoperative study. Image fusion, which is necessary with other forms of intraoperative imaging, can be problematic if there is pneumocephalus and shift present on the intraoperative image set and no shift on the preoperative, "historical" image set. This can be mitigated by using a closed dura technique, which minimizes or even eliminates brain shift.

The top of the SmartFrame is then mounted on the base, and the hand controller is connected. The hand controller allows the surgeon to easily adjust the SmartFrame orientation when the head is at isocenter. The SmartFrame is capable of making two types of movements that are used to align the TC with the target. Angular movements, referred to as pitch (forward-backward) and roll (side-to-side) adjustments, result in the TC pivoting above the ball marker, which remains in a fixed position just above the burr hole. Alternatively, parallel offset movements, referred to as X (medial-lateral) and Y (anterior-posterior) adjustments, result in the TC moving as a unit. This is similar to using an offset channel or an X-Y stage on a traditional stereotactic micropositioner. X-Y adjustments therefore do result in the ball marker changing position above the burr hole. We adjust the pitch and roll knobs on the SmartFrame to grossly align the TC with the target based on visualization of the TC relative to the head, then temporarily pass a bare stylet down the TC to see where the likely cortical entry point will be within the burr hole. If the likely trajectory is already very close to a burr hole edge, we will adjust either the X or Y knob (or both) up to 2 mm to stay away from the edge of the bone.

The patient is then moved to isocenter. Our 1.5-T Philips scanner does not have very reliable table movement, meaning that when the gantry tabletop is moved, it does not reliably go back to precisely the same position. For this reason, the gantry is not moved from this point forward until the DBS electrode is placed. On our 3-T Siemens scanner at another hospital, the table motion is quite precise and the gantry position is reproducible and reliable, so small table movements are allowed on that scanner to optimize imaging. A T1 volumetric scan is repeated and the field of view is large enough for the software to see and detect the position of the MR-visible fiducials in the SmartFrame and TC with the ball marker. The software can subsequently determine the position and angle of the TC relative to the fiducials and use this information to inform the alignment process. A high-resolution slab acquisition is obtained through the basal ganglia to directly visualize the target. Our current preferred scans for targeting are an interleaved T2 sequence for STN and either standard inversion recovery or Fast Gray Matter Acquisition T1 Inversion Recovery (FGATIR) for the GPi.

Targeting is performed using direct visualization of the nucleus. For the STN, we target on an axial plane 4 mm below AC-PC. If the structures are not well visualized on this plane, we may vary the axial depth but no more than ±1 mm. If one continues looking deeper than 5 mm below the AC-PC plane, the STN will eventually blend into the substantia nigra, and this can negatively impact target selection. The red nucleus is visible medially, and the medial border of the STN is always clearly visible even at 1.5 T. The lateral border of the STN, on the other hand, is often not distinct at 1.5 T or 3 T. To target the STN, we draw a horizontal line from the midline along the anterior border of the red nucleus and out to the STN. If the lateral border of the STN is visible, the target is centered in the nucleus along this line. If the STN is narrow in a particular subject or on a particular side, we make sure that the target is at least 2 mm away from the lateral border, but this is exceedingly rare. If the lateral border is not visible, we place the target 2 mm tangentially away from the medial border of the STN (Fig. 24.4).

For GPi, we target at the AC-PC plane. We draw a line along the border between the internal capsule and the GPi (the pallidocapsular line). This distance is usually 18–21 mm in most patients. This line is divided into thirds. A line is then drawn tangentially away from the medial border of the GPi at the junction of the anterior 2/3 and posterior 1/3 of the pallidocapsular line to a distance of 3–4 mm. The target is placed here (Fig. 24.5). Note that the target will be quite close to the GPi/GPe border. When selecting either target, one should keep in mind that targets will vary quite a bit from patient to patient, and significant asymmetries can exist within patients from one side to the other. This is particularly true in the anterior-posterior position of targets in GPi, which can vary significantly

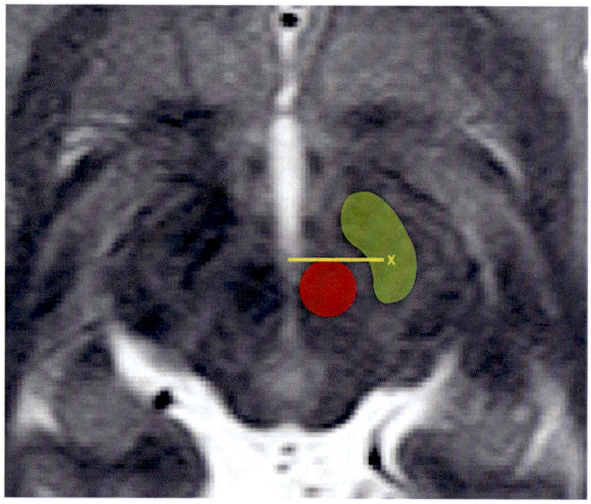

FIG. 24.4 Targeting the subthalamic nucleus, 4 mm below the AC-PC plane. T2 sequence at 1.5 T. *AC-PC*, anterior commissure-posterior commissure.

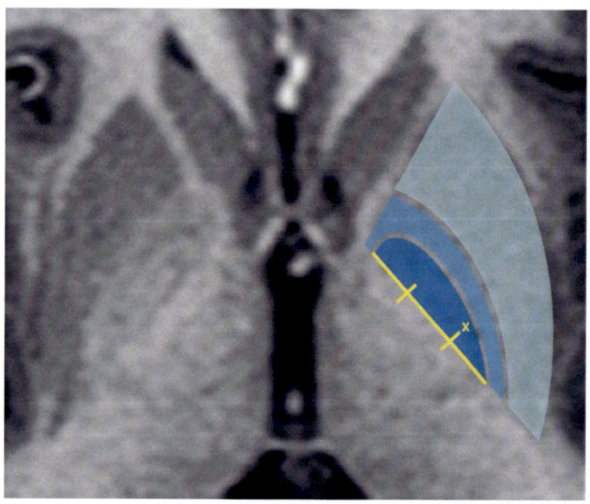

FIG. 24.5 Targeting the globus pallidus internus, at the AC-PC plane. Inversion recovery sequence at 1.5 T. *AC-PC*, anterior commissure-posterior commissure.

when one looks at the AC-PC coordinates of the final direct target. This is a demonstration of the power of direct targeting, which accounts for these variations up front unlike older methods which started with indirect, purely AC-PC-based targets and then depended on refinement with based on physiologic mapping.

Once the target is selected, the process of aligning the SmartFrame (or more specifically the TC) begins. First, the software instructs the MR technologist to obtain a single-slice acquisition through the TC and quickly (1) calculates the position of the TC in space, (2) determines the location of the lumen of the TC, and (3) predicts where a stylet inserted through the TC at that moment would cross the plane in which the target was selected. This process, including the scan, takes about 10–20 s. The software graphically depicts where the TC is currently aimed relative to the target and how much (and in which direction) the surgeon should turn the pitch and roll knobs to bring the TC in closer alignment to the target (Fig. 24.6). Another rapid, single-slice acquisition is obtained, and the process is repeated until the predicted overall error (that is, the vector difference between the target and predicted alignment of the TC) is below 1 mm. This process is fast but not that accurate, as it is a mathematically derived extrapolation of where the TC is aimed based on limited information. The purpose of this step is to get the TC grossly aligned to the target region.

In the next step, the software tells the MR technologist how to acquire thin slab scans that are obtained along the intended trajectory and include both the TC and the target. Two of these slabs are acquired, one an oblique coronal and the other an oblique sagittal. After both are transferred to ClearPoint, the software segments the entire TC and its lumen and predicts where the TC is aimed relative to the target based on an average of the prediction from both oblique scans (Fig. 24.7). Although this process is longer, with each oblique scan taking somewhere between 60 and 90 s, it is much more accurate. Options are given for the surgeon to make either another angular pitch-roll adjustment (recommended if the error is well over 1 mm or if the trajectory is already close to the bone edge) or a linear X-Y offset adjustment (recommended for smaller errors or if the direction of movement happens to be away from the bone edge if the trajectory is close to it). The process is again repeated until the overall predicted error is less than 0.4 mm. This "cutoff" for acceptable error may vary from scanner to scanner depending on the individual magnetic field inhomogeneity and/or biases of that particular machine. Such biases can only truly be learned over time and tracking predicted errors versus actual placement from case to case.

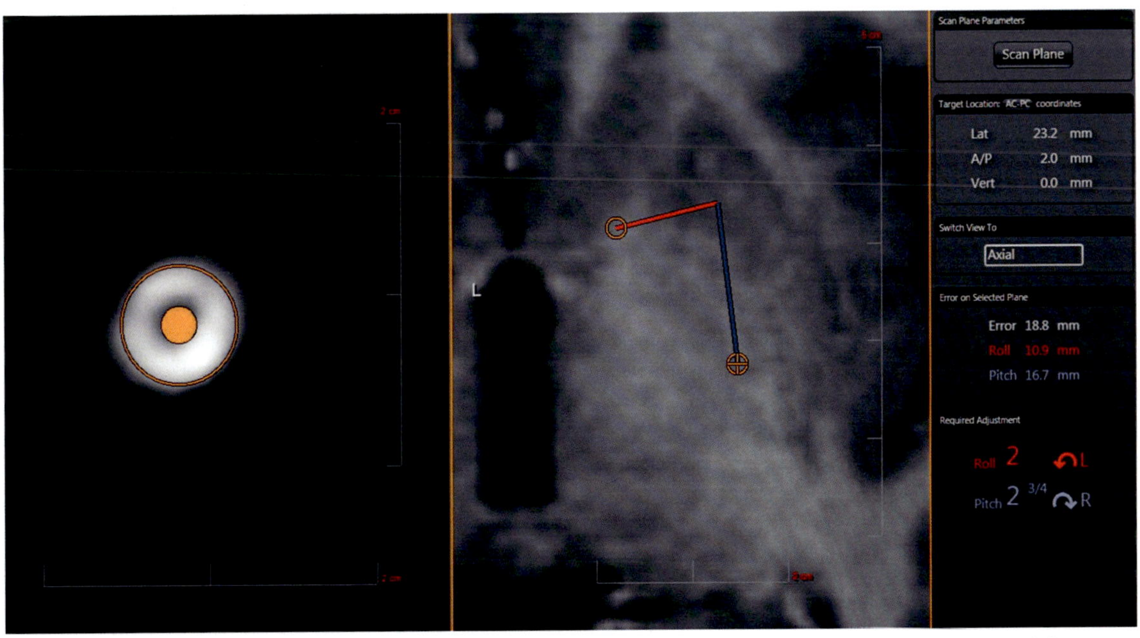

FIG. 24.6 Initial alignment of the SmartFrame. The single-slice acquisition through the TC is on the left; current alignment of the SmartFrame (*open circle*) and position of target (*crosshairs*) are on the right. Instructions for adjusting the pitch and roll knobs are in the lower right corner. *TC*, targeting cannula.

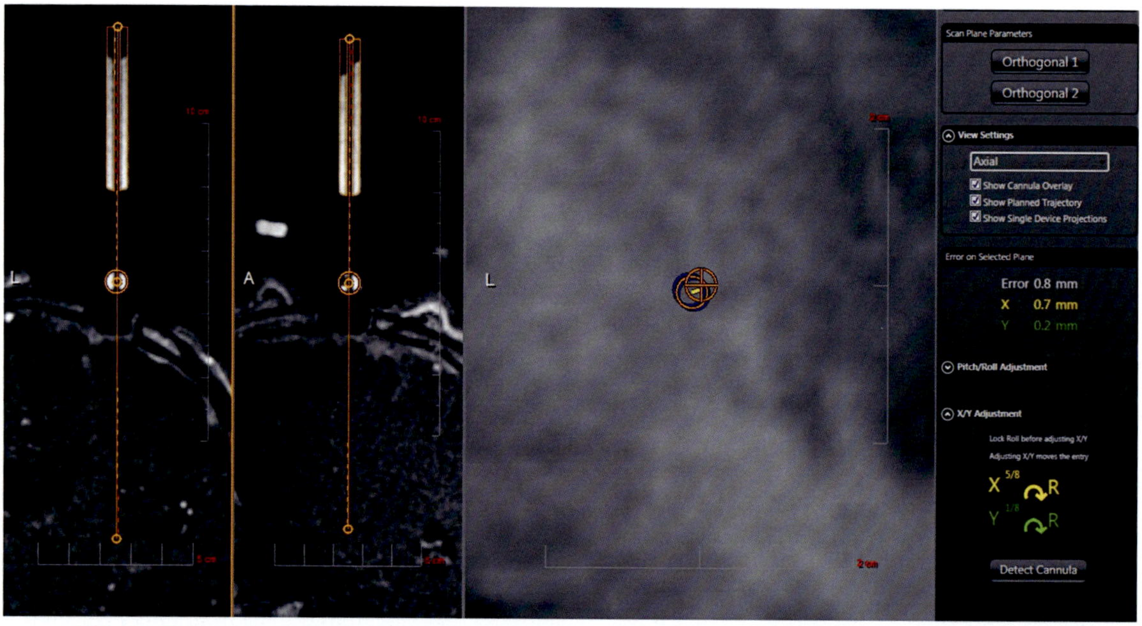

FIG. 24.7 Final alignment of the SmartFrame. Coronal and sagittal oblique scans are on the left; current alignment of the SmartFrame (*open circle*) and position of target (*crosshairs*) are on the right. Instructions for adjusting the X and Y knobs are in the lower right corner.

Once satisfactory alignment is achieved, the software measures the correct insertion depth for the ceramic stylet and presents that information to the surgeon. A depth stop is placed at the appropriate depth on a ceramic stylet, and a flexible peel-away sheath (which will act as the guide tube) is shortened to the appropriate length so the tip of the stylet is just protruding from beyond the end of the peel-away. The stylet and peel-away sheath assembly is then passed to the target by hand, with the patient remaining at isocenter and the surgeon reaching into the bore. Even when using the open dura technique, we usually use the sharp ceramic stylet provided in the ClearPoint kit (called a lancet) to make the initial pial entry into the cortex, then replace it with the blunt stylet to make the final pass all the way to the target. We typically stop when the blunt stylet is partially inserted and obtain images in at least one oblique plane along the insertion trajectory to make sure that the stylet is "on track" and there is no bleeding. When the stylet and peel-away are at target depth, coronal and sagittal oblique scans as well as a high-resolution T2 slab are obtained to determine if the placement is acceptable. In our experience, the initial placement is acceptable approximately 98%–99% of the time. The ceramic stylet is then withdrawn from the peel-away, and a depth stop is placed on a Medtronic DBS lead at the same insertion depth. As mentioned previously, if the procedure is being done at 1.5 T, we get one final scan to confirm the depth, but this is not absolutely necessary.

The patient is then moved back to the far end of the bore. The peel-away is removed, leaving the DBS lead in position. The Stimloc clip is applied, and the DBS lead stylet is removed. The SmartFrame is then disassembled, the Stimloc cap is placed, and the end of the DBS lead is capped. A blind pouch is created under the galea, and the end of the lead is tucked underneath the scalp. We use 3–0 Vicryl pop-off sutures (Ethicon, Somerville, NJ) that have standard needles that are not MR compatible. They will not be pulled toward the magnet unless they are within 3 or 4 ft of the bore because of their low mass, but it is important that the scrub technician or nurse load the needles on the needle drivers far away from the bore. When the surgeon pops the needle off the suture, he or she must be certain that the needle is clamped firmly with the needle driver and it is locked in the closed position. If a needle gets loose, it may fly toward the bore and be caught by the drape, but it is also possible that the needle may fly around and become stuck on the side of the scanner. It can be difficult if not impossible to find a needle that becomes free within the magnetic field, so care must be exercised. We close with staples and have found that most staplers are MR safe.

Clinical outcomes of iMRI DBS, mostly using the ClearPoint system, have been reported by individual centers in a number of small studies.[5–10] Improvements in UPDRS are comparable with awake surgery, which is not surprising; a properly positioned electrode that is optimally programmed will produce benefit (in a properly selected patient). iMRI does not place electrodes in a different location than awake surgery, it merely places them in a different manner. Our center maintains an ongoing database of statistics on our iMRI cases for quality assurance and research purposes, and our average placement error (the vector difference between intended placement and actual placement) in over 300 cases is 0.6 mm $\pm$ 0.4 mm. This is consistent with other centers using ClearPoint, who have reported average errors in the 0.7–1.2 mm range.[8,10] There is clearly a learning curve when switching from awake surgery to iMRI-guided procedures, and this may or may not be reflected in procedure time, accuracy, or simply getting used to a particular MRI scanner's individual biases and imaging characteristics.[11,12] Clinical outcomes of asleep DBS with iCT are also being published, and they too are comparable with awake surgery.[13,14] This lends more support to the argument that the need for physiologic confirmation in well-characterized DBS targets such as the STN and GPi is not necessary when direct, real-time intraoperative visualization of the target is available.[12,15]

REFERENCES

1. Martin AJ, Larson PS, Ziman N, et al. Deep brain stimulator implantation in a diagnostic MRI suite: infection history over a 10-year period. *J Neurosurg*. 2017;126(1):108–113.
2. Dempsey MF, Condon B. Thermal injuries associated with MRI. *Clin Radiol*. 2001;56(6):457–465.
3. Ivan ME, Yarlagadda J, Saxena AP, et al. Brain shift during bur hole-based procedures using interventional MRI. *J Neurosurg*. 2014;121(1):149–160.
4. Khan MF, Mewes K, Gross RE, Skrinjar O. Assessment of brain shift related to deep brain stimulation surgery. *Stereotact Funct Neurosurg*. 2008;86(1):44–53.
5. Starr PA, Martin AJ, Ostrem JL, Talke P, Levesque N, Larson PS. Subthalamic nucleus deep brain stimulator placement using high-field interventional magnetic resonance imaging and a skull-mounted aiming device: technique and application accuracy. *J Neurosurg*. 2010; 112(3):479–490.
6. Ostrem JL, Galifianakis NB, Markun LC, et al. Clinical outcomes of PD patients having bilateral STN DBS using high-field interventional MR-imaging for lead placement. *Clin Neurol Neurosurg*. 2013;115(6):708–712.
7. Ostrem JL, Ziman N, Galifianakis NB, et al. Clinical outcomes using ClearPoint interventional MRI for deep brain stimulation lead placement in Parkinson's disease. *J Neurosurg*. 2016;124(4):908–916.
8. Sidiropoulos C, Rammo R, Merker B, et al. Intraoperative MRI for deep brain stimulation lead placement in Parkinson's disease: 1 year motor and neuropsychological outcomes. *J Neurol*. 2016;263(6):1226–1231.
9. Sillay KA, Rusy D, Buyan-Dent L, Ninman NL, Vigen KK. Wide-bore 1.5 T MRI-guided deep brain stimulation surgery: initial experience and technique comparison. *Clin Neurol Neurosurg*. 2014;127:79–85.
10. Chansakul T, Chen Jr PN, Lee TC, Tierney T. Interventional MR imaging for deep-brain stimulation electrode placement. *Radiology*. 2016;281(3):940–946.
11. Southwell DG, Narvid JA, Martin AJ, Qasim SE, Starr PA, Larson PS. Comparison of deep brain stimulation lead targeting accuracy and procedure duration between 1.5- and 3-tesla interventional magnetic resonance imaging systems: an initial 12-month experience. *Stereotact Funct Neurosurg*. 2016;94(2):102–107.
12. Saleh S, Swanson KI, Lake WB, Sillay KA. Awake neurophysiologically guided versus asleep MRI-guided STN DBS for Parkinson disease: a comparison of outcomes using levodopa equivalents. *Stereotact Funct Neurosurg*. 2015; 93(6):419–426.
13. Burchiel KJ, McCartney S, Lee A, Raslan AM. Accuracy of deep brain stimulation electrode placement using intraoperative computed tomography without microelectrode recording. *J Neurosurg*. 2013;119(2):301–306.
14. Mirzadeh Z, Chapple K, Lambert M, et al. Parkinson's disease outcomes after intraoperative CT-guided "asleep" deep brain stimulation in the globus pallidus internus. *J Neurosurg*. 2016;124(4):902–907.
15. Chen T, Mirzadeh Z, Ponce FA. "Asleep" deep brain stimulation surgery: a critical review of the literature. *World Neurosurg*. 2017;105:191–198.

CHAPTER 25

Surgical Treatment of Psychiatric Disorders

HEATHER N. PINCKARD-DOVER, MD • ERIKA A. PETERSEN, MD, FAANS, FACS

HISTORY

Many historical clues point to the use of surgical techniques for the treatment of psychiatric disorders in very early times. Archeologists have found Neolithic skulls with trephinations, evidence supporting ancient writings describing treatment of "possessed" or sick people, scenes depicted in classic artworks such as the late 15th-century work attributed to Hieronymous Bosch, The Cure of Folly (The Extraction of the Stone of Madness).[1] Surgical treatments have evolved over time in conjunction with the increasing understanding of brain connections and their roll in psychiatric disorders.

In 1848, John Martyn Harlow was the first scientist to report on the relationship between frontal lobe function and behavior. He describes the infamous case of Phineas Cage who went from "a reliable altruistic individual to an immature, aggressive, and childishly selfish" individual after a metal rod was blown through his frontal lobes in a railroad construction accident.[1] Understanding of frontal lobe function in psychiatric disorders increased with study of other individuals with injuries to specific regions and their sequela, allowing surgical treatments to begin to develop.

Gottlieb Burckhardt was one of the first to attempt surgical treatment for psychosis after studying the effects of frontal topectomies on dogs. In 1891, he published his results on the use of bilateral topectomies on six institutionalized psychotic patients. He found that incisions to multiple foci in frontal, parietal, and temporal lobes showed some improvement in psychotic symptoms; however, there was a high incidence of adverse events which led to criticism of the procedure.[1,2] Working in Russia, neurologist Vladimir Bektherev's research centered on the anatomic connections within the brain underpinning behavior, including psychiatric disease. Between 1906 and 1910, Bektherev's protege Ludvig Puusepp performed three surgeries in which he severed the connections of the frontal lobe to treat psychiatric agitation. Puusepp's results were not widely reported, and several decades of inactivity and disinterest in surgical treatment of psychiatric disease followed.[3] Egas Moniz and Almeida Lima revived the interest in surgical treatment approaches to psychiatric disorders. They initially injected alcohol into subcortical white matter tracts in the prefrontal region. They then devised a leucotome that could be inserted through multiple burr holes to create similar lesions. After performing 20 cases, they found that patients with significant deterioration before surgery had little benefit but those without significant deterioration preoperatively showed only minor and temporary disturbances with prominent recovery from psychiatric disturbances. Moniz won the Nobel Prize for his work in 1949.[1,2]

Walther Freeman and James Watts performed similar operations and were the first to introduce surgical treatment for psychosis in the United States in the late 1930s. They developed a round blade with a lever arm that allowed coronal lesioning through multiple burr holes. The extent of lesioning was dependent on the severity of the patient's psychiatric symptoms. In 1946, Freeman revised his surgical technique to the transorbital lobotomy. With this technique, he would first use electric shock to induce unconsciousness, then pass a steel leucotome through the supraorbital rim and move it in the coronal plane. Freeman developed this approach until the technique took only 15–20 min and was increased in use to the point that it no longer required neurosurgeons, anesthetists, surgical settings, or sterile technique and could be performed from his "lobotomobile." By 1951, over 5000 lobotomies were performed per year. Several factors ultimately resulted in the decline in these procedures. The depiction of the procedure affected public sentiment. Inconsistently applied sterile technique led to rising morbidity and mortality, causing it to lose public favor.[1]

Around this same time, new nonsurgical treatments such as lithium, antipsychotic drugs, and electroconvulsive therapy (ECT) emerged, shifting interest away from the invasive surgical approach.[1]

Along with the development of medications and ECT, the 1930s and 1940s brought the development of Horsely's stereotactic apparatus and pneumoencephalography, allowing stereotactic targeting for lesioning. With Papez's introduction of the limbic circuit for emotion in 1937 came rationale for more specific anatomic targeting of lesions.[3] Ernest A. Spiegel and Henry T. Wycis targeted the dorsomedian nucleus of the thalamus for treatment of agitation and psychosis.[4] Hugh Cairns targeted the cingulate gyrus through open severing of the cingulum bundle, a procedure that became known as anterior cingulotomy. H.T. Ballantine converted this to a stereotactic ablative lesioning technique in 1967, and it has become the most reported psychosurgery in the United States and Canada. It has been used to treat chronic pain, major depressive disorder (MDD), and obsessive compulsive disorder (OCD) with 40%–60% reported improvement.[1,4]

Talairach's stereotactic lesioning to the anterior and middle third of the anterior limb of internal capsule (ALIC) at the level of the foramen of Monroe became known as the anterior capsulotomy (AC). Similar lesions were created by Lars Leksell using Gamma Knife radiosurgery. Effectiveness in treating OCD ranges between 48% and 78%.[1] Similar rates of effectiveness (40%–70%) have been found with Geoffrey Knight's subcaudate tractotomy (SCT). Initially performed by placing 1 × 7 mm yttrium rods into the anterior and inferior head of caudate to create 20 × 20 × 5 mm lesions, it evolved into a stereotactic radiofrequency (RF) lesioning procedure for the treatment of affective disorders, OCD, and anxiety.[1] Desmond Kelly and Alan Richardson created lesions similar to this SCT and combined them with lesions in the anterior cingulum for the treatment of resistant depression and OCD with response rates of 36%–50%.[1] These lesions remain an option for surgical treatment for refractory psychiatric disease (Fig. 25.1).

After stereotactic placement of the lesioning electrode but before lesioning these targets, many surgeons used low electric stimulation to confirm target placement. In 1952, José Delgado demonstrated that electric stimulation could be provided through implanted electrodes in deep structures. This stimulation could be used for both diagnostic and therapeutic purposes. Viktor Bektherev's daughter, Natalia Petrovna Bekthereva, was the first to use chronic depth stimulation, but her work did not reach world recognition because it was published in Russian. Carl Wilhelm Sem-Jacobsen placed depth electrodes for epilepsy and psychiatric disorder recording and stimulating in patients over the course of several months with minimal side effects, providing support for long-term implantation of electrodes. Irving S. Cooper performed chronic stimulation of the cerebellum and deep thalamic nuclei for cerebral palsy, spasticity, and epilepsy in 1977. Unfortunately, further studies did not show real efficacy. In 1991, Alim Benabid and colleagues reported on chronic stimulation of the ventral intermediate nucleus for tremor control, and their subsequent studies showed it was safer than thalamotomy and could be performed bilaterally. These results significantly increased the interest in neuromodulation for treatment of movement disorders, pain, and psychiatric disorders.[5]

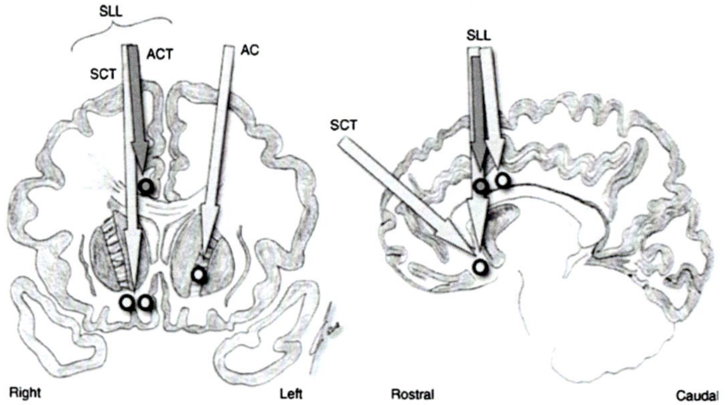

FIG. 25.1 Four stereotactic ablative procedures for refractory depression (schematic). Left, coronal; right, sagittal. *AC*, anterior capsulotomy; *ACT*, anterior cingulotomy; *SCT*, subcaudate tractotomy; *SLL*, stereotactic limbic leucotomy (essentially a combination of ACT and SCT). (From Lozano AM, Gildenberg PL, Tasker RR, eds. *Textbook of Stereotactic and Functional Neurosurgery*. Berlin: Springer, Figure 175.1.)

NEUROPHYSIOLOGY AND CONNECTIVITY

In 1937, J.W. Papez published a theory on an anatomic network integral in the processing of emotion. He recognized that emotion has two major parts: emotional expression and emotional experience, which he attributed to the medial and lateral regions of the hemisphere, respectively. He believed that primitive receptive organs relay their information to the thalamus, which then leaves the thalamus through one of the three streams. The first is the "stream of movement" from dorsal thalamus through internal capsule to the corpus striatum. The second is the "stream of thought" from thalamus through internal capsule to lateral cerebral cortex. The third is the "stream of feeling" from the ventral thalamus to the hypothalamus via the mammillary body and anterior thalamic nuclei to gyrus cinguli. In the hypothalamus, he denoted three specific regions: pars optica, tuber cinereum, and mammillary body. Researchers at the time found that damage to the pars optica and tuber cinereum caused severe autonomic symptoms but few emotional symptoms. When there was damage to the mammillary body, however, patients lacked emotive dynamics. Papez denoted the mammillary body as the ultimate recipient of afferent excitations because of its input from the fornix, mammillary peduncle, and the medial bundle of the forebrain. The fornix relays information from the hippocampal formation, which is thought also to be a part of the central olfactory apparatus. Its role in emotion, memory, and olfaction explains the significant importance olfaction can play with memory recall. The hippocampal formation receives input from prefrontal cortex via the angular bundle and subcallosal bundle.[6]

Information from the hippocampal formation passes through the fornix to the mammillary body and then to the anterior and anterodorsal nuclei of the thalamus via the mammillothalamic tract. Connections extend from the mammillothalamic tract to the region of the nucleus of campi foreli of the Vogts in which damage has been shown to cause significant drowsiness, somnolence, and emotional inactivity. The majority of afferent mammillothalamic projections terminate in the anterior and anterodorsal nuclei of the thalamus. Damage to these nuclei shows emotional disturbances including spontaneous laughing and crying.[4,6] Efferent projections from the anterior and anterodorsal nuclei of the thalamus pass through the anterior limb of the internal capsule to the gyrus cinguli. This structure lies just above the corpus callosum and becomes the precuneus, circling around to enter the hippocampal region completing the limbic loop of Papez. Damage to the gyrus cinguli has been shown to affect memory, personality, arousal, and emotion. Papez called it the "seat of dynamic vigilance by which environmental experiences are endowed with an emotional consciousness." La Peyronie called it the "seat of the soul."[4,6,7]

Papez knew the amygdala was connected to these areas through the stria terminalis, but he was unsure of its function at the time. Its role was further delineated by Walle Nauta, when he reported on the hippocampal projections in the cat. It has now been shown to play a major role in fear, learning, and memory. Other areas that are now appreciated as having a role in emotion, motor control of emotion, and psychiatric disorders include the prefrontal cortex, orbitofrontal cortex (OFC), subgenual cingulate cortex (SCC), and nucleus accumbens (NAc).[2,4,6,7]

As further understanding of cortical and subcortical structures and their connectivity increased, Alexander proposed that they were organized in cortico-striato-thalamo-cortical (CSTC) loops. Studying these loops, Modell et al. proposed in 1989 that a CSTC loop involving the OFC, basal ganglia, limbic striatum, and thalamus was responsible for OCD. He proposed that the frontothalamic portion of the loop was overactive and the limbic striatum was unable to inhibit the activity. He also believed there are structural changes within the OFC, prefrontal cortex, cingulate, and caudate that lead to this dysfunctional activity. Other studies have linked glutamate to the orbitofrontal-thalamic loop and glutamate, dopamine, serotonin, and GABA to the orbitofrontal-striatal-thalamic loop.[4,7]

Two major models of MDD have been proposed. The first designates three compartments: dorsal, ventral, and rostral. The dorsal compartment is responsible for attention and cognition and consists of the dorsal anterior cingulate cortex, dorsolateral prefrontal cortex (DLPFC), inferior parietal cortex, and striatum. The ventral compartment is responsible for arousal and somatic control and consists of the hypothalamus, insula, SCC, and brainstem. The third compartment is the rostral cingulate and is responsible for keeping the other two compartments in balance. The second model divided into the more dorsal exteroceptive region, dealing with cognitive function, and the more ventral interoceptive region, dealing with visceral-motor function. They also proposed a mood-monitoring region comprising the dorsomedial thalamus, amygdala, and basal ganglia and a mood-regulation region consisting of medial frontal cortex including the rostral anterior cingulate cortex (ACC). They theorized that MDD is due to lack of coordination in exteroceptive and interoceptive regions.[4]

Developments in neuroimaging and dissection techniques have helped support these theories. Anatomic white matter dissections and advanced diffusion tensor imaging (DTI) have confirmed Papez's and Nauta's proposed circuitry of the SCC to cingulate, hippocampus, amygdala, OFC, NAc, frontopolar cortex, and ventral striatum (VS).[8] Positron emission tomography (PET) studies have supported the theory of Modell. They have shown abnormalities in the caudate, OFC, and cingulate in patients with OCD. They showed increased metabolism in orbital gyri, caudate, and thalamus that significantly decreased in patients who had good response to treatment. PET also shows promise in predicting response to certain medications. One study found that increased metabolism in orbital gyri predicted poorer response to fluoxetine, whereas decreased orbital gyri metabolism predicted better response to behavioral therapy.[4,7]

PET has also been used to study MDD. Studies showed decreased glucose metabolism in lateral frontal cortex and lateral prefrontal cortex (PFC), whereas there was an increase in metabolism in medial PFC, ACC, and SCC. The degree of hypermetabolism in the SCC correlated well with the severity of depression and normalized in patients who responded well to treatment. The SCC even showed increased metabolism in controls with induced sadness. The degree of hypermetabolism in the left SCC and left thalamus also correlated with the increased response on the Beck Depression Inventory (BDI) at 12 months. Mayberg found similar results with the rostral ACC. Patients demonstrating hypermetabolism eventually became drug responders, whereas those with hypometabolism tended not to respond to medications.[4,7]

Significant advances have been made in magnetic resonance imaging (MRI) including the development of functional MRI (fMRI) and DTI. These studies have shown that patients with OCD have increased activity in lateral PFC, medial OFC, ACC, temporal and insular cortex, caudate, amygdala, and lenticulate nuclei. They tend to have reduced PFC, ACC, and caudate volumes and changes in white matter microstructure with asymmetric connections between the thalamus and PFC. The amygdala and hippocampal formations also seem to have abnormalities in structure.[4]

Similar studies in MDD showed increased activity in the cingulate cortex, PFC, amygdala, hippocampus, hypothalamus, and NAc. DTI may also be useful for patient-specific connectivity targeting in deep brain stimulation (DBS) for MDD. One study showed that patients who responded to DBS of the SCC for MDD had activation volumes within pathways connecting medial frontal cortex, rostral and dorsal cingulate cortex, and subcortical nuclei bilaterally. Nonresponders did not consistently show activation within these regions.[4]

INDICATIONS

Obsessive Compulsive Disorder

OCD is composed of intrusive thoughts and/or repetitive behaviors despite the patient's efforts to stop them. It affects approximately 2% of the population and comes with severe anxiety and inability to function socially. It is the 10th most common cause for disability in the world with 10%–27% attempted suicide rate. Studies show that 60%–90% of patients also have codiagnosis of MDD (67%), or an Axis II disorder. OCD is often seen in patients with Sydenham's chorea and Tourette's syndrome (TS), and 20% of OCD patients will also have motor tics, suggesting there may be similar mechanisms between OCD and movement disorders.[7,9–11]

The Yale-Brown Obsessive Compulsive Scale (YBOCS) is a common measure of symptoms severity. It consists of 10 questions and is scored 0–40 with higher score equivalent to worse severity. A clinically significant response is considered a reduction of 25%–35% of OCD symptoms. The remission rate is defined as YBOCS under 8.

As discussed earlier, Modell et al. proposed that OCD is due to overactivity in the frontothalamic portion of the CSTC loop, and the limbic striatum fails to inhibit the activity. This is accompanied by structural changes within the OFC, PFC, cingulate, and caudate. This has been supported by PET studies and fMRI and DTI studies.[4,7,10]

First-line therapy for OCD is serotonergic antidepressants. 40%–60% of patients will achieve clinically significant relief. Clomipramine, a tricyclic antidepressant, is second line because of its unfavorable side effect profile. If these are ineffective, then the regimen can be augmented with atypical antipsychotics. Cognitive-behavioral therapy (CBT) is also a significant contributor to patient response with as high as 76% response rate. Of those treated with above treatments, 7.1% will still fail to respond, and therefore surgical treatments have been considered.[10]

Before surgical intervention, it is recommended that patients be over 5 years out from initial diagnosis; have YBOCS score of 25–28; be refractory to CBT; have no or insufficient improvement after adequate administration for adequate time of three treatment attempts with selective serotonin reuptake inhibitors (SSRI) (one has to be clomipramine), augmentation with neuroleptic and benzodiazepine, and minimum of 16–20 CBT sessions.[9] Surgical options include lesioning techniques and neuromodulatory techniques. Lesioning techniques include capsulotomy, cingulotomy, limbic leucotomy (LL), and SCT. Lesions can be performed using glycerol infusion, RF, stereotactic radiosurgery, or laser interstitial thermal therapy. Cingulotomy is the most popular with burr holes placed just anterior to coronal suture and 1.5 cm from midline. Thermocoagulation electrodes are passed to a target 2–2.5 cm posterior to tip of frontal horn, 7 mm from midline, and 1–2 mm above corpus callosum. The 10-mm uninsulated tip is heated to 85° for 90 s giving a 1 cm × 8–10 mm lesion. More recent techniques place three lesions 7, 14, and 21 mm posterior to frontal horn. It can take 3–6 months before effects are appreciated. If no worthwhile improvement is noted after 6 months, more extensive lesioning can be considered. Close psychiatric follow-up is recommended.[7,10,11]

Neuromodulation through DBS has been studied in many targets including ALIC, ventral caudate, subthalamic nucleus (STN), NAc, and inferior thalamic peduncle (ITP). Target selection was based on effective lesioning targets with the most common target being the ALIC.[9,10,12] Reported complications include intracerebral hemorrhage and stimulation-induced side effects such as hypomania.[9]

Nuttin et al. were the first to study DBS for OCD in the 1990s. They performed a blinded crossover study in six patients targeting the ventral capsule/ventral striatum (VC/VS) and found four patients with >35% reduction in YBOCS score. Each arm was originally planned to be 3 months either on or off stimulation; however, each of the off phases were shortened due to worsening of symptoms.[9,12] Fayad et al. reported long-term results for the original six patients and found similar responder rates: four patients experienced more than 35% reduction in YBOCS, one patient had more than 25% reduction in YBOCS, and the other had his DBS off. They noted a significant increase in depressive symptoms over the study.[13] Gabriels et al. also studied DBS to the VC/VS. They defined the target as 3.5 mm anterior to posterior border of anterior commissure, 13 mm lateral on the right, and 14 mm lateral on the left at the level of the AC-PC plane. They studied 11 patients with mean YBOCS of 33.8 at baseline. Patients underwent double-blind assessments both on and off stimulation. The mean YBOCS was significantly lower on stimulation (17 vs. 33.8). They found 6 out of 11 patients were responders. Further study in five OCD DBS patients on the effects on frequency (FQ) and pulse width (PW) found combinations of high FQ (>10 Hz) and high PW (>60 mcs) decreased visual analog score (VAS) obsession scores, compulsion scores, and avoidance scores while increasing VAS self-confidence and well-being scores.[10] Greenberg also found that high-energy settings were required to reach optimal results, causing significant battery depletion. 26 patients were studied over 24 months with gradual adjustment of the VC/VS target more posterior during the trial, leading to three separate groups. With the anterior-most target, only a third of patients were responders, whereas three quarters of patients in the middle and posterior targets were responders.[9] Goodman studied a subset of these patients to determine whether a lesioning effect was responsible for the response rate. He performed a blinded staggered-onset study in which three patients were turned on 1 month after surgery and the remaining three turned on 2 months after surgery and found neither group displayed improvement until stimulation was turned on.[9] Abelson also studied DBS to internal capsule in four patients with 3-week periods of on or off stimulation with only modest differences.[9]

Only a few level 1 studies using DBS for treatment of OCD have been performed. Mallet et al. targeted the STN 2 mm anterior and 1 mm medial to common Parkinson disease (PD) target. He studied 16 patients at 10 academic centers. Patients received DBS, then experienced a 1 month washout period prior to be randomized to on or sham stimulation. The double-blind crossover study found significantly lower YBOCS scores at the end of the on phase compared with the sham phase (19 vs. 28, 32%, $P = .01$).[9,12] Tyagi et al. implanted six patients with both anteromedial STN and VC/VS electrodes. A double-blind crossover design was used to compare results after 12 weeks of continuous stimulation at each target, followed by a period where both targets were stimulated in combination. Five out of six patients were responders using VC/VS or combined stimulation, while only 3/6 responded to STN stimulation alone. Mean reduction in YBOCS scores was STN: 42%, VC/VS: 53%, and STN + VC/VS: 62%.[14]

Two level 2 studies have been performed, both targeting the NAc. Denys et al. designed a three-phase study: (1) open-label phase, (2) 2 week crossover blinded assessment on versus sham stimulation, (3) 12-month open-label maintenance period. Of 16 original participants, 14 agreed to the blinded phase. An 8.8 point reduction in YBOCS ($P = .003$) on stimulation was demonstrated. Huff et al. performed a three-phase trial studying the effects of right NAc stimulation. The first phase was in the operating room in which four 7-min blocks of test stimulation were used to determine optimal DBS settings. For the next 3 months, patients either received on or sham stimulation, they were then crossed over. Both the patients and the proctors of the test were blinded. Finally there was an open-label phase. There were no significant differences in YBOCS scores identified between the groups.[9,12]

A single level 3 study was performed by Jimenez-Ponce et al. targeting the ITP. Studying six patients, they found 100% of their patients had over 40% response ($P = .003$) with a mean 49% reduction in YBOCS at 12 months.[9,12] Pepper et al. compared 10 studies with 108 patients who underwent AC to 10 studies with 62 patients with VC/VS or NAc DBS. 62% of AC patients and 52% of DBS patients had significant response, a difference that was not clinically significant. AC had significantly greater remission rate than DBS (11% vs. 2%, $P = .02$). However, the DBS patients tended to have greater severity of disease and longer duration of symptoms than patients who had undergone AC. When adjusting for this difference, AC still had 50% greater chance of response than DBS in severe OCD patients. In extreme OCD patients, AC and DBS had similar response rates, but AC had 20% remission rate versus 2% for DBS ($P = .006$). Each technique carried a similar rate of adverse events.[11] These studies highlight how far we have come in the advancement of neuromodulatory treatments for OCD and the need for further level 1 studies to tease out more specific targets and allow better functional outcomes.

Major Depressive Disorder

MDD is defined as prolonged low mood with disinterest in normal activities and low energy lasting at least 2 weeks. It is the most common psychiatric disorder in North America. It has a lifetime prevalence of 9.5%, 14.6% across high-income countries. It is the third leading cause of disability in the world and has an estimated economic burden of $43.7 billion in the United States in 1990. Common measures of its severity include the Hamilton Depression Rating Scale-17 (HDRS-17) and the Montgomery-Asberg Depression Rating Scale (MADRS). First-line treatment includes antidepressants such as MAOIs, TCAs, SSRIs, and SNRIs combined with brief psychotherapies such as CBT and interpersonal psychotherapy. ECT, repetitive transcranial magnetic stimulation (rTMS), vagal nerve stimulation, and DBS have also emerged as potentially effective therapies for the treatment of MDD. Response to treatment is defined by 50% reduction on HDRS-17 or MADRS. Remission is defined by an HDRS-17 score <7 or MADRS score <10. Up to 30% of patients will fail to respond to four consecutive antidepressants, and 52% of these will fail to respond to ECT.[2,15–17]

Previous theories hypothesized that MDD was caused by a monoamine neurotransmitter deficit, whereas newer theories of MDD focus on the connectivity between CSTC loops. Imaging studies have shown abnormal activity within the limbic system and correction of this abnormality in patients who have responded to antidepressants, CBT, pharmacotherapy, sleep deprivation, and ablative techniques.[4,7,17] Genetic studies have shown patients with a short allele polymorphism of serotonin transporter gene are more likely to experience depression after adverse life events.[17]

Patients who have suffered for several years, have severe symptoms, and with MDD refractory to conventional therapies may be considered for surgical treatment. Patients with hysterical or sociopathic personalities, Axis II pathology, impaired cognitive function, organic brain lesions, advanced age, or serious medical illness should have considerable thought before surgical treatment. Historically, many lesioning techniques have been used with significant improvement in symptoms (Fig. 25.1). The most common technique in Great Britain was the SCT. Knight first described it as a stereotactic technique using yttrium seeds, but it has since been tailored to cryoprobes or diathermy. Reported response rates range from 34% to 68%. The AC may also be used, but is usually reserved for treatment of OCD or anxiety. Talairach first reported stereotactic lesioning of this area using cryoablation and Leksell performed his lesions using 110 Gy Gamma Knife. Leksell found a response rate of 48%. Kim et al. essentially combined the SCT and AC to create the LL. Response rates are reported as 61%–78%.[2,7]

Efforts to find an adaptable, possibly reversible treatment for MDD have led to the use of multiple DBS targets for the treatment of MDD refractory to medical treatments. Given the current three- and four-compartment models of MDD and the importance of the cingulate in these models, Johansen-Berg et al. studied the potential connectivity of the cingulate regions using diffusion MRI tractography. The common areas of connectivity included midcingulate cortex, frontal pole, hypothalamus, and NAc. Pregenual cingulate cortex connects with frontal pole, whereas subgenual cortex connects more strongly with OFC and medial temporal pole structures.[18] Each of these regions plays a strong role in MDD; therefore, it is no surprise the SCC has become a popular target for DBS treatment of MDD. The Toronto group performed PET scans in patients with severe MDD refractory to medical treatment. They found increased activity in Broadman area 25 (BA25) and decreased activity in prefrontal and premotor cortices, dorsal anterior cingulate gyrus, and anterior insula. Subsequently, Lozano and Mayberg performed DBS to the SCC for 8 weeks at 130 Hz, 60 ms, and 3–4 V. At 6 months, 4 of 6 (66%) of implanted patients were responders, and at 12 months 11 of 20 (55%)

patients were responders.[19] There was a 35% remission rate with most responders showing significant improvement at 1 month. Responders also showed a reversal in PET activity on repeat imaging. Comparison of pre- and posttreatment PET studies showed increased activity in SCC and decreased activity in dorsolateral prefrontal lobe, ventrolateral prefrontal and anterior cingulate at 3 months and was maintained at 6 months. Further publication of a 20-patient follow-up from this study shows sustained response, although a broader multicenter trial was less fruitful.[17,20,21]

Some studies report on stimulation to the anterior limb of the internal capsule, whereas others will label this as a ventral capsule/ventral striatum (VC/VS) target. Electrodes placed in this location are thought to affect the same area as stimulation, in part because high amplitude of stimulation likely creates a larger volume of tissue activation to exert its clinical effect. Greenberg's study of VC/VS stimulation discussed in the OCD section included eight patients who had concomitant MDD. He found that the depressive symptoms in these eight patients improved, but Fayad's long-term follow-up showed increased rates of depression in these individuals over time. Dougherty et al. completed the first multicenter, randomized double-blind sham-controlled trial of stimulation for MDD in this region. A 16-week blinded-treatment phase in which medications were not allowed to be adjusted was followed with an open-label continuation phase. They studied 30 patients and found 3 of 15 (20%) of active treatment patients responded with mean MADRS score change of 8 ± 13.7, whereas 2 of 14 (14.3%) control group responded with mean MADRS score change of 9 ± 10.6. In the 12-month follow-up open-label phase, they had 6/30 (20%) respond and 4/30 (13%) go into remission. At 24 months long-term follow-up, 23.3% were responders, 20% remission but no subjected maintained responder status throughout the study. However, 26/30 patients elected to continue DBS stimulation after the trial. There was significant cognitive decline in the active DBS group on tasks requiring mental flexibility in the context of response inhibition.[15,17,20]

Observation of antidepressant effects in patients whose electrodes were implanted slightly deeper than initially targeted resulted in further exploration of targets in the VS and NAc. So far there is a case study, a pilot study with three patients, and an open-label optimization phase study followed by a randomized, double-blind crossover active-sham phase study using this target. The patient in the case study did well with remission of depression sustained at 15 months; however, only one of the three patients in the pilot study was a responder at 23 weeks after implantation. The other study performed by Bergfeld et al. within two hospitals in the Netherlands showed mean time to first response in responders was 53.6 days, with decrease in mean HAM-D-17 scores from 22.2 to 15.9 ($P = .001$) and mean MADRS from 34 to 23.8 ($P < .001$) after open-label optimization phase. There was a 40% responder rate and 20% remission rate. After the randomized, double-blind crossover active-sham phase, they found significantly lower HAM-D-17 scores ($P < .001$) and MADRS scores ($P = .001$) in patients with active stimulation.[16,17,20]

Fenoy et al. released an interim report on a study of DBS to the medial forebrain bundle (MFB). Rationale for their study comes from the report by Schlaepfer et al. demonstrating significant improvements in MDD after 1 week of stimulation to the MFB. Fenoy reported on early results of the first four patients enrolled in his study. He used DTI imaging to select a target just lateral and anterior to the ventral tegmental area (VTA) based on its connectivity to the prefrontal cortex. After a 4-week blinded washout period, there was no significant reduction in MADRS scores at 4 weeks compared with baseline. However, 1 week after open-label stimulation, there was a significant reduction in MADRS (7 points, $P = .03$) from end of 4 week off period and from baseline (18 points, $P = .026$). Response rate was 75% at 1 week. Of note, the single nonresponder was found to have significantly lower connectivity through the area of proposed stimulation based on stimulation models. These findings support individualized targeting based on connectivity and the use of connectivity mapping in target selection.[22]

In 1979, a study of 36 psychiatric patients showed that stimulation to the rostral vermis caused significantly improved depressive symptoms in five of the six patients with MDD. They were all off medications at 30-month follow-up. Rationale for this study came from findings that stimulation to this area caused increased firing in anterior septal region and inhibition in hippocampal activity.[17] Similar stimulation studies showed that stimulation to the white matter bundle known as the ITP caused inhibitory effects on the OFC leading to the case study of a 49-year-old female with a 23-year history of MDD, bulimia, and comorbid borderline personality disorder. After bilateral implantation at the ITP, she experience significant reduction in depressive symptoms before stimulation. With 8 months of stimulation, she had HDRS-17 scores between 2 and 8. During the double-blind protocol, she had dramatic fluctuations in depression score, so stimulation was turned back on.[17,20] This case study is

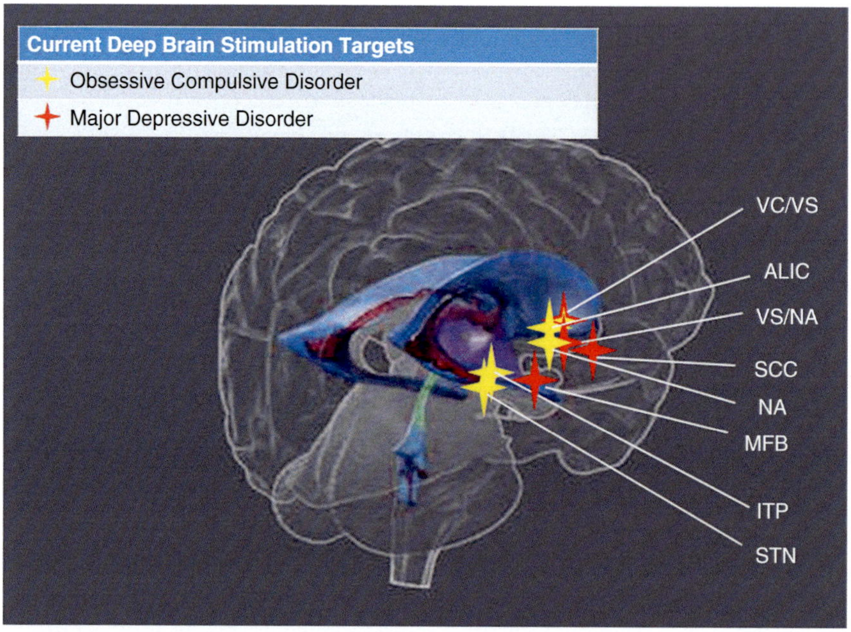

FIG. 25.2 Obsessive Compulsive Disorder targets include the ventral capsule/ventral striatum (VC/VS), anterior limb of the internal capsule (*ALIC*), nucleus accumbens (*NA*), subthalamic nucleus (STN), and the inferior thalamic peduncle (ITP). Major Depressive Disorder targets include the ventral capsule/ventral striatum (VC/VS), ventral striatum/nucleus accumbens (VS/NA), subgenual cingulate cortex (SCC), and medial forebrain bundle (MFB).

fraught with confounding factors highlighting the importance of excluding patients with Axis II pathology, recent suicide attempts, substance abuse, or diagnosis other then primary MDD.

Multiple targets have been advanced for treatment of both MDD and OCD (Fig. 25.2). Until successful targets can be isolated, studies should focus on individuals with minimal confounding factors. They must be educated that DBS is the beginning of a treatment process that will require psychiatric rehabilitation and chronic maintenance therapy. As there are no set parameters for stimulation in MDD, it is recommended that changes be made at least 4 weeks apart and that there be no concomitant changes in pharmacotherapy. If patients suddenly experience mania or psychosis or dramatic worsening of depressive symptoms such as suicidal ideations, it is recommended first to revert parameters to the last tolerated setting and observe for several hours. If no improvement is noted, then alteration of medications is recommended. [15,17,21]

TOURETTE'S SYNDROME

In 1885, Georges Gilles de la Tourette described "a neurological condition characterized by motor incoordination accompanied by echolalia and coprolalia."[23,24] Charcot later defined this disorder, Tourette's Syndrome. The DSM-IV now characterizes it as multiple motor tics and one or more vocal tics, not necessarily simultaneously. The disorder should develop before 18 years and occur multiple times per day, nearly every day or intermittently for at least 1 year with no more than three consecutive tic-free months. TS is often associated with other psychiatric disorders such as attention-deficit/hyperactivity disorder (ADHD) (21%–90%), OCD (11%–80%), MDD, anxiety, and personality disorders. Up to a third of patients will express self-injurious behavior. The reported prevalence of TS is 0.77%, and it is four times more prevalent in males. Mean age of onset is 7, with a peak around 10 and a subsequent improvement during adolescence. 59%–85% of patients will experience decline in tics during adulthood. Tics tend to be more frequent during periods of stress or fatigue and improve with relaxation and selective attention. The most recognizable symptom, coprolalia or uncontrollable use of obscene words, is only seen in 10% of patients. The Yale Global Tic Severity Scale (YGTSS) and modified Rush Video-Based Rating Scale (mRVRS) are the most common scales used to rate the severity of symptoms.

Current theories of underlying physiology causing TS suggest there is a dysfunction of basal ganglia and parallel striatal-thalamic-cortical circuits. Studies have shown that dopamine (DA) potentiates striatal neurons leading to excess inhibition of the globus pallidus internus (GPi) and substantia nigra pars reticulata (SNpr) thereby releasing thalamocortical transmission. This theory has been supported by fMRI studies showing that during tic suppression, there is decreased activity in the putamen, ventral pallidum, and thalamus bilaterally and increased activity in the head of the right caudate and frontal and temporal cortices.[23–27]

The treatment for TS is individualized by severity of disorder. In patients with mild TS, psychobehavioral therapies such as relaxation training, CBT, habit reversal training, and comprehensive behavioral intervention for tics are first-line therapies. In patients with more severe TS, pharmacologic treatment with α2-adrenergic agonists, typical or atypical neuroleptics, benzodiazepines, or botulinum toxin injection are used. Surgical treatment emerged in 1962 when E. F. Baker reported a case where bimedial leucotomy resulted in significant reduction in tic severity and panic attacks.[28] Other lesioning techniques have included prefrontal lobotomy, LL, ACT, thalamotomy, lesions to the zona incerta, red nucleus, and dentate. Adverse side effects included hemiplegia and dystonia. Veerle Visser-Vandewalle was the first to introduce DBS for the treatment of TS in 1999. He targeted the medial thalamus at the cross-point of the centromedian nucleus and the ventral oral internal nucleus.[23–27]

The patient selection criteria for DBS for TS have not been well determined, although usually it is reserved for patients with severe TS refractory to three medication regimens and trial of at least 10 sessions of behavioral therapy. The natural history of the disease is such that many individuals experience significant reduction of tics once reaching adulthood; therefore, treatment is usually reserved for those above 25 years who still have significant symptoms. Patients with severe psychiatric comorbidities, mental deficiency, suicidal ideation, structural abnormalities, or significant medical contraindication for surgery should not undergo DBS. There are multiple targets being explored currently. The most investigated target is the medial thalamus. Most reports are of case studies with some small open-label and blinded studies. These studies have found a 37%–90% reduction in tics and mixed results regarding improvement in depression, anxiety, and OCD symptoms. Similar studies have been performed targeting the globus pallidus (GP). There has been reported 15%–96% reduction in tic severity with most noting improvements in depression, anxiety, self-injurious behaviors, and quality of life. Early experience with GP DBS for TS suggests that there may be a need for increased stimulation amplitude over time to maintain effect, suggesting a tolerance to stimulation. Less studied targets include the anterior limb of the internal capsule reaching into the NAc with 20%–57% reduction in tic severity and the STN with 97% reduction in tic frequency. In studies that compared thalamic versus GP targets, in some patients, thalamic stimulation led to better tic control, whereas in others, GP showed greater control. This suggests that there may be subsets of patients who would benefit from different targets. More studies are needed to further delineate which patients would benefit from which target.[23–27]

OTHER PSYCHIATRIC DISORDERS

Like OCD, MDD, and TS, many psychiatric disorders are refractory to current therapies and therefore surgical options are being explored. Current human research includes addiction, aggression, anorexia, and anxiety disorders such as post-traumatic stress disorder (PTSD). Animal studies also suggest there may be a role for DBS in schizophrenia. The data available on the use of DBS for these disorders are limited to case reports, case studies, and small cohort studies. A brief summary of these studies can be found in Table 25.1.[29–36]

ETHICS

Ethical considerations for the use of DBS for psychiatric disorders are related to the scientific uncertainty of the benefit for specific patients and disorders and to the ability to obtain true informed consent. As has been reviewed, there is limited evidence available, primarily in the form of small case series with few placebo-controlled trials to support the use of DBS for psychiatric disease. When possible, DBS should be offered within a structured clinical trial. In some psychiatric disorders, the patient population that qualifies for treatment may be very small, making it difficult to arrange a clinical trial. In these cases, after internal review board approval, individual case studies may be performed. The use of national databases could help consolidate these findings and standardize treatment and follow-up paradigms. Patient selection, targets, and observation of outcomes are best done within a multidisciplinary team with open communication among collaborators. The use of prospective, randomized control trials is difficult in both psychiatric conditions and surgical treatments. Study designs should focus on controlling as

TABLE 25.1
Brief Summary of Studies for Deep Brain Stimulation for Other Psychiatric Disorders

Author	Study Design	Target	Number of Patients	Results
ADDICTION				
Kuhn et al.	Retrospective cohort	NAc	10	3/10 stopped smoking
Kuhn et al.	Case report	NAc	1	Reduced intake of alcohol
Muller et al.	Prospective open-label	NAc	5	All had disappearance of cravings, two remained abstinent
Mantoine et al.	Case report	NAc	1	Quit smoking
Zhou et al.	Case report	NAc	1	Abstinent from heroin and decreased cigarette consumption, sustained after removal of system
Ardouin et al., Bandini et al., Knobel et al., Witjas et al.	Four case studies	STN	12	Resolution of addictive behaviors
Smeding et al.	Case study	STN	1	PD patient developed pathologic gambling
Lim et al.	Retrospective cohort study	STN	19	PD with DA dysregulation syndrome or impulse control disorder with majority having no improvement in behavior and some worsened
AGGRESSION				
Broggi et al.	Case series	pHyp	6	Four patients had prompt improvement in aggressive behavior, one had no improvement at 2V and DBS turned off, one patient only at 1V 6 months postop with no improvement
Park et al.	Case report	NAc	1	40% decrease in SIB
ANOREXIA				
Lipsman et al.	Phase 1 pilot study	SCC	6	At 9 months: three had BMI > baseline, other three unchanged from baseline
Wu et al.	Prospective open-label study	NA	4	65% increase in body weight and significant reduction in YBOCS and HAM-A scores
Israel et al.	Case report	SCC	1	Maintenance of BMI 2 years postop
ANXIETY/PTSD				
Langevin et al.	Case report	BLA	1	37.8% reduction in CAPS scores

Author	Study Design	Target	Number of Patients	Results
SCHIZOPHRENIA				
Klein et al., Ewing et al., Mikell et al.	Animal studies	mPFC, GPe, MDN, hippocampus, NA, medial septum		Normalization of deficits in mice with mPFC, GPe, and MDN
				MDN stimulation induces long-term potentiation and synaptic plasticity in frontal cortex
				Inhibition of hippocampus and NA dampens DA systems alleviating psychotic symptoms
				vCA1 of hippocampus stimulation decreases output to PFC mitigating symptomatology.
				NA and medial septum stimulation normalizes psychotic behavior in mice.

BLA, basolateral amygdala; BMI, body-mass index; DA, dopamine; GPe, globus pallidus externa; HAM-A, Hamilton anxiety rating scale; MDN, mediodorsal nucleus of thalamus; mPFC, medial prefrontal cortex; NAc, nucleus accumbens; PD, Parkinson disease; pHyp, posterior hypothalamus; SCC, subcallosal cingulate cortex; SIB, self-injurious behavior; STN, subthalamic nucleus; YBOCS, yale-brown obsessive-compulsive scale.

many confounding variables while still allowing the results to be generalized to the general population. Oftentimes, psychiatric patients have questionable ability to give informed consent. Patients' families should be involved in the consenting process whenever possible. The consent process should emphasize the state of current evidence and suggested benefit and risks of the procedure. Some risks can be deduced from published DBS studies and the complications observed in DBS for movement disorders.[37,38]

OTHER TREATMENTS

Although DBS does offer a less invasive, potentially reversible treatment for psychiatric disorders, it is still invasive and comes with risks including bleeding, infection, and damage to important neural structures that might cause unintended alterations in neurologic function, stroke, coma, and even death. These risks are low, but there is still a desire for treatments that are noninvasive with reduced risks. Other treatment methods currently under investigation include rTMS, transcranial direct current stimulation (tDCS), and ketamine infusion. In rTMS, an electric current is passed through coils to create a magnetic field that can alter the axonal firing of certain brain structures. Current targets include the supplemental motor area (SMA) for TS and OCD; DLPFC for depression, PTSD, panic disorders, OCD, schizophrenia, and addiction; temporoparietal cortex for panic disorders and schizophrenia; and OFC for OCD. For tDCS, sponges with either a cathode or anode are placed over areas of the head and stimulation is applied. Currently, tDCS is being studied in the treatment of depression, OCD, and schizophrenia. Ketamine infusion has long been approved for use in anesthesia, but subanesthetic doses have also been used for treatment of pain. Because it was noted that ketamine-treated patients also experienced significant reduction in depressive symptoms, the infusion has also been used as a treatment for depression. Dosing is typically 0.5 mg/kg for 40 min as an IV infusion. The possibility of significant cardiovascular and psychiatric acute effects necessitates careful patient observation at time of administration. Each of these noninvasive methods shows significant promise and warrants further scientific investigation.[39–41]

FUTURE DIRECTIONS

Several variables in DBS stimulation can influence therapeutic efficacy beyond anatomic position of the electrode. Investigation of electric field changes and changes in molecular concentrations near the target may inform improved targeting. Imaging studies are useful in evaluating changes in metabolic activity and connectivity between these targets. This information is being combined to further our understanding of neuroconnectivity, to understand the mechanism of and impact on neurologic function, and to identify new targets for treatment. New technology includes closed-loop systems in which afferent information can be used to adapt stimulation provided at a given target. Micro and macro electrodes are being used to record activity of single and multicell units that can provide afferent feedback to these systems. Chemodes are microdialysis-like probes that can measure biomarkers and neurotransmitters and can use either microinjection or inverse dialysis to effect local changes. Chemodes may also be used to deliver drugs, gene therapy, neural grafts, and stem cells. Amperometry and voltammetry can offer local feedback closed-loop manipulation of targets. Optogenetics is another emerging therapy in which red to infrared light is used to arrest neuronal death.[42] The future of neuromodulation for psychiatric disorders will involve a coordinated multimodal approach that incorporates psychotherapy and behavioral modifications with medications and neurostimulation. As research progresses, it will be important for different specialties to come together and discuss their findings and develop multimodal treatment approaches for diseases.

REFERENCES

1. Bjarkam CR, Sørensen JC. Psychosurgery — a historical perspective. In: Lozano AM, Gildenberg PL, Tasker RR, eds. *Textbook of Stereotactic and Functional Neurosurgery*. Berlin: Springer; 2009:2067—2886.
2. Coenen VA, Honey CR. Ablative procedures for depression. In: Lozano AM, Gildenberg PL, Tasker RR, eds. *Textbook of Stereotactic and Functional Neurosurgery*. Berlin: Springer; 2009:2943—2952.
3. Lichterman BL. On the history of psychosurgery in Russia. *Acta Neurochir*. 1993;125(1—4):1—4. https://doi.org/10.1007/BF01401819.
4. Dyster TG, Mikell CB, Sheth SA. The co-evolution of neuroimaging and psychiatric neurosurgery. *Front Neuroanat*. 2016;10:68. https://doi.org/10.3389/fnana.2016.00068.
5. Sironi VA. Origin and evolution of deep brain stimulation. *Front Integr Neurosci*. 2011;5:42. https://doi.org/10.3389/fnint.2011.00042.
6. Papez JW. A proposed mechanism of emotion. *Arch Neurol Psychiatry*. 1937;38(4):725—743.
7. Cosgrove GR. Cingulotomy for depression and OCD. In: Lozano AM, Gildenberg PL, Tasker RR, eds. *Textbook of Stereotactic and Functional Neurosurgery*. Berlin: Springer; 2009:2887—2896.
8. Vergani F, Martino J, Morris C, et al. Anatomic connections of the subgenual cingulate region. *Neurosurgery*. 2016; 79(3):465—472. https://doi.org/10.1227/NEU.0000000000001315.
9. Blomstedt P, Sjöberg RL, Hansson M, Bodlund O, Hariz MI. Deep brain stimulation in the treatment of obsessive-compulsive disorder. *World Neurosurg*. 2013; 80(6):e245—e253. https://doi.org/10.1016/j.wneu.2012.10.006.
10. Gabriels L, Cosyn P, van Kuyck K, Nuttin B. DBS for OCD. In: Lozano AM, Gildenberg PL, Tasker RR, eds. *Textbook of Stereotactic and Functional Neurosurgery*. Berlin: Springer; 2009:2897—2924.
11. Pepper J, Hariz M, Zrinzo L. Deep brain stimulation versus anterior capsulotomy for obsessive-compulsive disorder. A review of the literature. *J Neurosurg*. 2015;122(5): 1028—1037. https://doi.org/10.3171/2014.11.JNS132618.
12. Hamani C, Pilitsis J, Rughani AI, et al. Deep brain stimulation for obsessive-compulsive disorder. Systematic review and evidence-based guideline sponsored by the American Society for Stereotactic and Functional Neurosurgery and the Congress of Neurological Surgeons (CNS) and endorsed by the CNS and American Association of Neurological Surgeons. *Neurosurgery*. 2014;75(4):327—333. https://doi.org/10.1227/NEU.0000000000000499. quiz 333.
13. Fayad Sarah M, Guzick Andrew G, Reid Adam M, et al. Six-nine year follow-up of deep brain stimulation for obsessive-compulsive disorder. *PLoS One*. 2016;11(12): e0167875. https://doi.org/10.1371/journal.pone.0167875.
14. Tyagi H, Zrinzo L, Akram H, et al. A randomised controlled trial of deep brain stimulation in obsessive compulsive disorder: a comparison of ventral capsule/ventral striatum and subthalamic nucleus targets. *J Neurol Neurosurg Psychiatry*. 2017;88(8). A8.2—A9.
15. Dougherty Darin D, Rezai Ali R, Carpenter Linda L, et al. A randomized sham-controlled trial of deep brain stimulation of the ventral capsule/ventral striatum for chronic treatment-resistant depression. *Biol Psychiatry*. 2015;78(4): 240—248. https://doi.org/10.1016/j.biopsych.2014.11.023.
16. Bergfeld Isidoor O, Mantione Mariska, Hoogendoorn Mechteld LC, et al. Deep brain stimulation of the ventral anterior limb of the internal capsule for treatment-resistant depression. A randomized clinical trial. *JAMA Psychiatry*. 2016;73(5):456—464. https://doi.org/10.1001/jamapsychiatry.2016.0152.
17. Giacobbe P, Kennedy S. Medical management and indications for surgery in depression. In: Lozano AM, Gildenberg PL, Tasker RR, eds. *Textbook of Stereotactic and Functional Neurosurgery*. Berlin: Springer; 2009: 2925—2942.

18. Johansen-Berg H, Gutman DA, Behrens TEJ, et al. Anatomical connectivity of the subgenual cingulate region targeted with deep brain stimulation for treatment-resistant depression. *Cereb Cortex*. 2007;18(6):1374–1383.
19. Lozano AM, Mayberg HS, Giacobbe P, et al. Subcallosal cingulate gyrus deep brain stimulation for treatment-resistant depression. *Biol Psychiatry*. 2008;64(6):461–467.
20. Hamani C, Snyder B, Laxton A. DBS for depression. In: Lozano AM, Gildenberg PL, Tasker RR, eds. *Textbook of Stereotactic and Functional Neurosurgery*. Berlin: Springer; 2009: 2953–2962.
21. Riva-Posse P, Holtzheimer PE, Garlow SJ, Mayberg HS. Practical considerations in the development and refinement of subcallosal cingulate white matter deep brain stimulation for treatment-resistant depression. *World Neurosurg*. 2013;80(3–4):S27. https://doi.org/10.1016/j.wneu.2012.11.074. e25-34.
22. Fenoy AK, Schulz P, Selvaraj S, et al. Deep brain stimulation of the medial forebrain bundle: distinctive responses in resistant depression. *J Affect Disord*. 2016;203:143–151.
23. Rotsides J, Mammis A. The use of deep brain stimulation in Tourette's syndrome. *Neurosurg Focus*. 2013;35(5):E4. https://doi.org/10.3171/2013.8.FOCUS13292.
24. Visser-Vandewalle V. Surgical procedures for Tourette's syndrome. In: Lozano AM, Gildenberg PL, Tasker RR, eds. *Textbook of Stereotactic and Functional Neurosurgery*. Berlin: Springer; 2009:2963–2970.
25. Huys D, Bartsch C, Koester P, et al. Motor improvement and emotional stabilization in patients with tourette syndrome after deep brain stimulation of the ventral anterior and ventrolateral motor part of the thalamus. *Biol Psychiatry*. 2016;79(5):392–401. https://doi.org/10.1016/j.biopsych.2014.05.014.
26. Zhang J, Ge Y, Stead M, et al. Long-term outcome of globus pallidus internus deep brain stimulation in patients with Tourette syndrome. *Mayo Clin Proc*. 2014;89(11): 1506–1514. https://doi.org/10.1016/j.mayocp.2014.05.019.
27. Kefalopoulou Z, Zrinzo L, Jahanshahi M, et al. Bilateral globus pallidus stimulation for severe Tourette's syndrome. A double-blind, randomised crossover trial. *Lancet Neurol*. 2015;14(6):595–605. https://doi.org/10.1016/S1474-4422(15)00008-3.
28. Baker EFW. Gilles de la Tourette syndrome treated by bimedial frontal leucotomy. *Can Med Assoc J*. 1962; 86(16):746–747.
29. Luigjes J, van den Brink W, Feenstra M, et al. Deep brain stimulation in addiction. A review of potential brain targets. *Mol Psychiatry*. 2012;17(6):572–583. https://doi.org/10.1038/mp.2011.114.
30. Müller Ulf J, Voges Jürgen, Steiner Johann, et al. Deep brain stimulation of the nucleus accumbens for the treatment of addiction. *Ann N Y Acad Sci*. 2013;1282:119–128. https://doi.org/10.1111/j.1749-6632.2012.06834.x.
31. Broggi G, Franzini A. Treatment of aggressive behavior. In: Lozano AM, Gildenberg PL, Tasker RR, eds. *Textbook of Stereotactic and Functional Neurosurgery*. Berlin: Springer; 2009:2971–2977. https://doi.org/10.1007/978-3-540-69960-6_178.
32. Park HR, Kim IH, Kang H, et al. Nucleus accumbens deep brain stimulation for a patient with self-injurious behavior and autism spectrum disorder. Functional and structural changes of the brain: report of a case and review of literature. *Acta Neurochir*. 2017;159(1):137–143. https://doi.org/10.1007/s00701-016-3002-2.
33. Lipsman N, Woodside DB, Giacobbe P, et al. Subcallosal cingulate deep brain stimulation for treatment-refractory anorexia nervosa. A phase 1 pilot trial. *Lancet*. 2013; 381(9875):1361–1370. https://doi.org/10.1016/S0140-6736(12)62188-6.
34. Wu H, van Dyck-Lippens PJ, Santegoeds R, et al. Deep-brain stimulation for anorexia nervosa. *World Neurosurg*. 2013;80(3–4):S29. https://doi.org/10.1016/j.wneu.2012.06.039. e1-10.
35. Reznikov R, Hamani C. Posttraumatic stress disorder. Perspectives for the use of deep brain stimulation. *Neuromodulation*. 2017;20(1):7–14. https://doi.org/10.1111/ner.12551.
36. Agarwal P, Sarris CE, Herschman Y, Agarwal N, Mammis Antonios. Schizophrenia and neurosurgery. A dark past with hope of a brighter future. *J Clin Neurosci*. 2016;34:53–58. https://doi.org/10.1016/j.jocn.2016.08.009.
37. Bell E, Leger P, Sankar T, Racine E. Deep brain stimulation as clinical innovation. An ethical and organizational framework to sustain deliberations about psychiatric deep brain stimulation. *Neurosurgery*. 2016;79(1):3–10. https://doi.org/10.1227/NEU.0000000000001207.
38. Appleby BS, Ravins PB. Ethical considerations. In: Lozano AM, Gildenberg PL, Tasker RR, eds. *Textbook of Stereotactic and Functional Neurosurgery*. Berlin: Springer; 2009: 2855–2864.
39. Lefaucheur JP, André-Obadia N, Antal A, et al. Evidence-based guidelines on the therapeutic use of repetitive transcranial magnetic stimulation (rTMS). *Clin Neurophysiol*. 2014; 125(11):2150–2206. https://doi.org/10.1016/j.clinph.2014.05.021.
40. D'Urso G, Brunoni AR, Mazzaferro MP, Anastasia A, Bartolomeis A de, Mantovani A. Transcranial direct current stimulation for obsessive-compulsive disorder. A randomized, controlled, partial crossover trial. *Depress Anxiety*. 2016;33(12):1132–1140. https://doi.org/10.1002/da.22578.
41. Sanacora G, Frye MA, McDonald W, et al. A consensus statement on the use of ketamine in the treatment of mood disorders. *JAMA Psychiatry*. 2017;74(4): 399–405. https://doi.org/10.1001/jamapsychiatry.2017.0080.
42. Nicolaidis S. Neurosurgery of the future. Deep brain stimulations and manipulations. *Metabolism*. 2017;69S:S16–S20. https://doi.org/10.1016/j.metabol.2017.01.013.

CHAPTER 26

Closed-Loop and Responsive Neurostimulation

KEVIN MANSFIELD, MD • AHMED M. RASLAN, MD, FAANS

INTRODUCTION

The goal of neurostimulation is to restore function to a malfunctioning nervous system. Ideally, neurostimulation should allow a patient to function in a manner that it is indistinguishable from "normal" both to an outside observer and to the patient himself. In other words, an ideal neurostimulation system should remove the awareness of both the pathology and the stimulator from the experience of the patient and those around him.

Because the nervous system is by its nature a dynamic and complex system, capable of shifting rapidly between many different operating states, the manifestation of pathology, as well as stimulation effects, can vary significantly with time and other treatment effects. Parkinson disease (PD) is a familiar example: external symptoms vary from bradykinesia to dyskinesia multiple times throughout the day with medication "on" and "off" times; longer-term, a change from appendicular to axial bradykinesia is often noted with progression of disease.[1] A simple, static, "always on" stimulation paradigm will not provide consistent, high-quality therapy in this setting.

With current technology, this requires repeated, ongoing adjustment of the stimulation parameters by medical personnel. During these sessions, adjustments are made empirically, using immediately observable or reportable changes in the patient's experience to guide program changes. Side effects such as mood alteration, compulsions, speech, or cognition may not be immediately evident and may only be revealed after weeks or months of stimulation; correction of these effects requires a return to the clinic and another empiric adjustment, using a protracted trial and error approach. Meanwhile, the underlying disease continues to progress, with concurrent changes in medication doses and schedules, evolution of new symptoms, and worsening of existing symptoms further confounding the challenge of programming the stimulator in a way that is intelligent, safe, and effective.

The development of responsive neurostimulation systems aims to integrate the decision-making and program adjustment tasks currently accomplished by human expertise into the control systems of the stimulators themselves. This should have the effect of increasing the efficiency of the optimization process (for the patient and provider) and minimizing the time that late-emerging side effects must be tolerated between system adjustments. Other benefits of this automation may become evident over time.

This chapter is intended to familiarize the reader with the concepts and basic principles of controlled systems and their applications to the problems of functional neurosurgery. We will begin with an explanation of control systems and their variations and conclude by exploring some of the many applications of these systems to neurosurgical problems.

CONTROL SYSTEMS

A control system is commonly defined as a system that "manages, commands, directs, or regulates the behavior of other devices or systems."[2] Examples range from the simple light switch in your home to the complex systems regulating automated fly-by-wire aircraft. In general, these systems are classified by how their various elements relate to one another. We will cover four broad types of control systems, each of which can be applied to neurostimulation: open-loop systems, closed-loop systems, adaptive systems, and responsive systems.

Open-Loop Systems

Open-loop systems are the simplest control systems, conceptually. They are useful for many applications and serve as a good starting place from which to build the other more complicated systems. Open-loop systems consist of an input signal (or simply, an input), a process that converts that input to another form (with or without some predefined parameters), and an output signal (Fig. 26.1).

An example of open-loop system is a gasoline engine. The operator changes the input signal by changing the throttle control position. The system then changes the amount of fuel fed into the combustion chamber (the "process"), and the result (or "output") is a change in engine speed. Open-loop systems have an advantage in that they are conceptually easy to understand and tend to be very stable, that is, the output does not vary significantly for a given input. Disadvantages of an open-loop system include the requirement for adjustment from outside the system to change the behavior of the system; put another way, they cannot adjust to changes in the operating context. Additionally, this static relationship of input to output is rarely the most efficient way to generate the desired output.

Despite the simple design, and its attendant limitations, open-loop designs are very useful. Current deep brain stimulators uses this design with very good results for a variety of indications; peripheral nerve stimulators and epidural spinal stimulators also use an open-loop design, as do intrathecal medication pumps. This type of control system is well suited for situations where (1) a stable system output is desired and (2) that output can be relatively independent from its effect on the global operating context or the effect of the output develops on a timescale that allows reasonable opportunity for human intervention to adjust the process.

Closed-Loop Systems

Closed-loop systems introduce an element of feedback which affects the operation of the system. This feedback generally takes the form of a comparison between the expected or desired output and the actual output; the result of the comparison is then used to adjust the process to minimize this difference, or error (Fig. 26.2).

To extend the example of the gasoline engine, consider a car with a simple cruise control mechanism: the throttle position signal drives the process of fuel delivery to produce engine speed (a surrogate for actual road speed), but now the actual road speed is compared with the desired road speed (the setpoint); the error in speed is used to increase or decrease the amount of fuel delivered to the engine so that the actual output is brought closer to the desired output.

The simple closed-loop system provides the principal advantages of increased system stability at the cost of increased complexity; it will tend to produce outputs within a specified range despite changing external conditions that could affect the process. An ideal closed-loop system will maintain the output at exactly the desired value (zero error) by instantaneously adjusting the input modulation function (often this is equivalent to the gain of the system) so that all possible combinations of the input signal and the environmental effects on the system produce exactly the correct output. In real systems, the rate of change of the actual output toward the desired output and threshold for output correction are design elements that will affect the performance of the system; the degree of output oscillation around the setpoint will be a function of these elements.

The simple closed-loop system introduces the elements of error and input modulation/gain into the control mechanism. Response time, thresholds, and system oscillation are properties of the system, which must be accounted for when the system is adjusted. More importantly, the selection of the measured output signal, which generally is built into the design of the system, is critical to the success of the control system. In neurologic disease, there are many potential choices for output signal that can be selected, each with their own advantages and disadvantages (see Biomarkers). Each will in some way serve as a surrogate for the ultimate goal of "normal function."

Simple closed-loop systems begin to allow for more intelligent design of neurostimulators. Their added complexity and the requirement of an appropriate output/feedback signal demand that a deeper understanding of the normal and pathologic physiology be applied in their design. This begins to allow for systems that respond more appropriately to the real-world dynamic changes that underlie the function of the nervous system. This was incorporated first outside the nervous system in the design of cardiac pacemakers that sense the heart rate and fire only when it falls below a set threshold. Currently, the vagus nerve stimulation

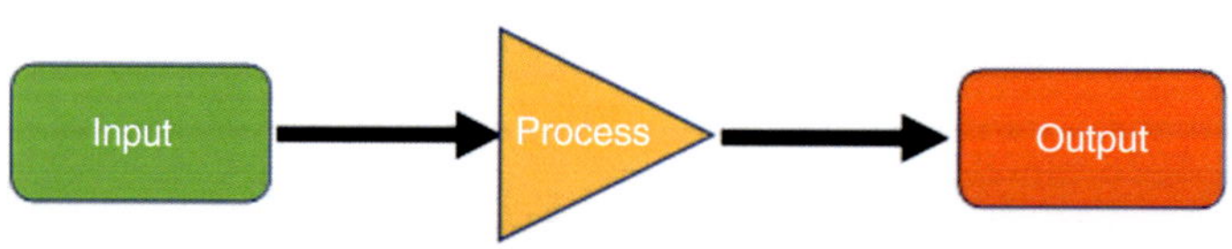

FIG. 26.1 A simple open-loop system.

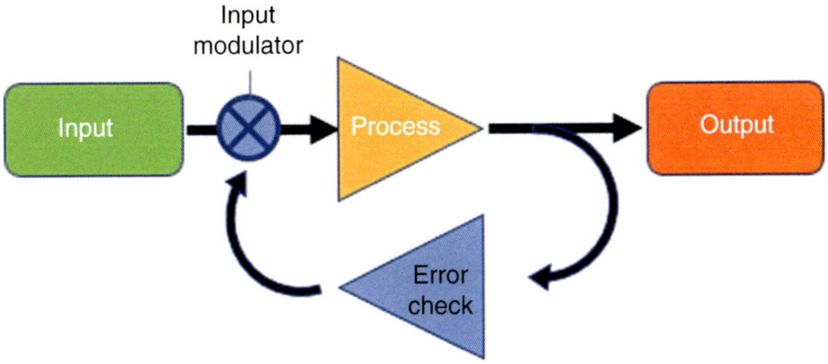

FIG. 26.2 A simple closed-loop feedback system.

(VNS) system (LivaNova) can use real-time tracking of a patient's heart rate, which frequently increases sharply at seizure onset, to trigger an increase in stimulation which lasts until the seizure is aborted.

Adaptive Systems

Adaptive control systems are a class of systems that use various methods of training to optimize a generic system to recognize and respond to a complex set of input signals. Using machine learning techniques, adaptive control systems can be "taught" to classify a set of signals by examining their relationships to each other and any other reference signal sets and evolving a model that predicts the classification of a novel signal set. This model can then be used in a control system to perform the same complex classification/prediction task repeatedly, either in a closed- or open-loop system. The training phase generally uses a closed-loop system design to iteratively adjust the various weights, biases, and other parameters that process the input data until an acceptably high prediction accuracy is achieved. These parameters are "frozen," and this system configuration is then used to process all future inputs as the system is implemented (Fig. 26.3).

Adaptive control systems increase the power of open- and closed-loop control systems, replacing generic, usually simple process control functions (on/off, more/less, or static combinations of several input signals), with more sophisticated control functions that are customized to the specific features of a given system. Furthermore, they can incorporate multiple input signals or multiple features of a single complex input signal on a scale that would be highly impractical to perform with traditional, explicit methods. For example, our cruise control system could be trained in the factory to use inputs about not only the vehicle speed but also road incline, wind speed, distance from the vehicle ahead, velocity and acceleration of that vehicle, and activation of brake lights on that vehicle to predict the adjustment to the throttle position most likely to prevent a collision while staying as close as possible to the user-defined desired speed. Creation of an explicit control function that appropriately incorporated all of those variables would be very difficult; by using machine learning techniques to allow the system to optimize itself using a training dataset, a control function can be efficiently derived that appropriately controls the throttle in an acceptable majority of real-world cases. The vehicles can then be distributed with that optimized control function in place.

Adaptive control systems used in neurostimulation require many of the same elements as closed-loop systems listed above for their training phase: an understanding of the normal and abnormal physiology of the system, one or more input signals, and intelligent selection of appropriate output signals used to compare the expected and actual results of the control function. The signals, particularly the input signals, should be detail-rich either alone or in combination, to justify the added complexity of the adaptive control system. The advantage of the adaptive system is that the designer no longer needs to know precisely the relative importance of the various input signals, the system will determine that. The trade-off is that the designer must choose inputs with an adequate signal-to-noise ratio and design a machine learning algorithm appropriate to the desired task. Once trained, the system should be able to reliably identify the desired triggering input conditions embedded within a complicated system. The ability to handle these complicated sets of variables makes adaptive systems well suited to advanced biomedical applications.

Currently, adaptive control systems are being used in the responsive neurostimulation system (RNS, NeuroPace). After implantation, the system records electrophysiologic data over the course of the subsequent weeks. These data are then downloaded and labeled with information about when a seizure occurred. The system is trained (aka optimized) to recognize novel instances of seizure that are similar to those recorded in

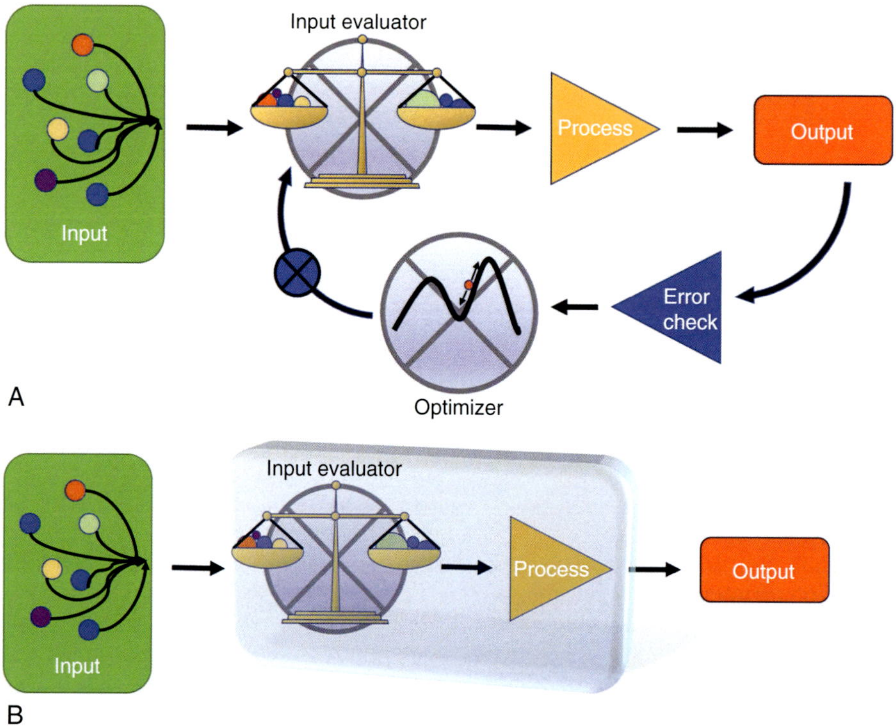

FIG. 26.3 **(A)** An adaptive control system takes a set of features, and via an iterative optimization process adapts a "generic" process into a process that very accurately produces the desired outputs for the specific inputs of the training environment. **(B)** A trained system is now optimized for the specific system it controls and is "frozen" in this configuration to produce a consistently accurate output as new input data are received in the implementation phase.

the dataset. It is important to note that during training, the system is not told why a given portion of the recorded data is a seizure, only that it is. The machine learning algorithms in the system automatically extract and key in on features of the training signals that yield accurate prediction results.

Responsive Systems

The most complicated control system is the responsive system. As in the adaptive system, a complex set of input variables is analyzed by the system and processed to produce the desired output in a highly consistent manner, despite the presence of extraneous signals. The responsive system adds an extra step to the algorithm by using a closed-loop design in the implementation phase (Fig. 26.4).

The value of using the closed-loop design lies in the system's ability to modulate and adapt its behavior to a dynamically changing situation. Our adaptive cruise control in the previous section, which could adjust the cruise control setting to account for traffic conditions, is now transformed into an active driver assist system that can learn and incorporate the driving patterns and response time of the driver to provide warnings, or even override certain actions to prevent an imminent collision. In biologic terms, it is the difference between the programmed stimulus-response loop of the biceps reflex and the feedback-controlled action of juggling. The RNS system includes this design element to a small degree, in that a feature of a successful output signal is the absence of continued seizure because the triggering input to the system includes the electrocorticography (ECoG) signals of a seizure, and the system is sampling at a high frequency for new input, a negative feedback control is intrinsic to the design of the system. However, more sophisticated input-output loops are possible and are the subject of ongoing research. We know, for example, that plastic changes within the central nervous system (CNS) occur with ongoing stimulation; a truly responsive system may be able to continuously monitor

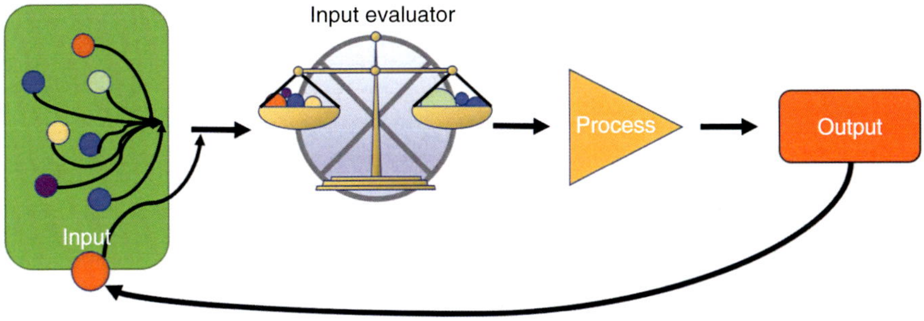

FIG. 26.4 A responsive system uses an adaptive control system with a closed-loop feedback signal.

the effectiveness of the trained system and retrain itself to account for these changes on an ongoing basis while continuing to provide effective therapy.

The limitations of adaptive and responsive systems are the limitations inherent to all machine learning applications; succinctly put, they are only as good as the training data provided to them and the base design of the underlying processing algorithm and optimizer. However, with thoughtful design and a solid understanding of the pathophysiology being addressed, these systems hold great potential for benefit in the complex and dynamic environment of the central nervous system.

BIOMARKERS

The Ideal Biomarker

Biomarkers are critical to the proper functioning of a neuromodulatory system. In this setting, a biomarker is any feature (or combination of features) that can be used to identify the state of the system being controlled. An ideal biomarker for use in a control system should exhibit the following characteristics:

- **Sensitivity**: The system should be able to detect the biomarker signal reliably despite reasonable extraneous signals and noise.
- **Specificity**: The biomarker should only vary with the condition being treated by the system.
- **Predictive utility**: The biomarker should be detectable on a timescale useful to allow intervention before the treated condition becomes symptomatic.
- **Temporal correlation**: The biomarker should fade rapidly as the condition resolves to allow detection of successful intervention.
- **Easy/Safe to obtain**: The biomarker should require minimal risk or discomfort to obtain. Its use should be practical on the timescale required for intervention.

As we use increasingly sophisticated control systems, biomarkers enter into the process at more and more points. They are not only use to decide if and which neuromodulatory systems should be used, but also become the triggers for open and closed loop systems, feedback signals in responsive systems, and responsive systems, and training patterns for adaptive systems. A wide variety of biomarkers is currently available and more are actively being researched. Some examples of biomarkers currently being applied to the problems of neuromodulation are explained below.

Physical Biomarkers

Sometimes a simple solution is best. Much of neuromodulation is focused on improving symptoms affecting physical movement. This is certainly the case with essential tremor, PD, and other movement disorders; however, physical movement is affected by many other neurologic pathologies and can therefore be used as elements in neuromodulation control systems. Seizures, for example, can generate excessive movement in the case of convulsions or movement arrest in certain types of partial epilepsy. Movement is easily trackable with wearable devices such as accelerometers. These biomarkers face challenges of sensitivity and specificity if raw movement data are used; however, with sophisticated detection algorithms, patterns of movement that are sensitive and specific for a given patient's condition can be used effectively as biomarkers. The benefit of physical biomarkers is that they can be obtained noninvasively and with minimal inconvenience to the patient (and the provider). They also have high temporal correlation with condition being treated, as they are a direct symptom of the pathologic state.

Subjective/Experiential Biomarkers

Ultimately, our neuromodulatory interventions are designed to improve our patients' quality of life. The subjective experience of our patients that impact this quality of life can be used as the control points for our systems. Consider the case of pain: tonic spinal cord stimulation (SCS) is accompanied by parasthesias in the covered dermatomes. The stimulator placement is frequently guided by the patient's subjective experience of these parasthesias, and the intensity of stimulation is often guided by these parasthesias in combination with the degree of pain experienced. This highlights the notion that people (either patients or clinicians) frequently function as vital control nodes in control systems. Systems that can be adjusted by the patient in real-time to optimally control their symptoms use experiential biomarkers to excellent effect. The risk of these biomarkers is somewhat higher than physical markers, in that the patient must be allowed to experience the undesired state (pain, dyskinesia, etc.) to adjust the system. The temporal variables are also potentially problematic, as the effect of adjusting the system may lag significantly behind the onset of the symptom. Conversely, the sensitivity and specificity of experiential biomarkers tends to be quite high.

Electric Biomarkers

Neuromodulation lends itself to conceptualizations of treatment centered around altering bioelectric processes. Electric signals are conceptually simple to measure and technically easy to process with current microcircuit technology. Because our control systems are built with electric machines, all biomarkers must eventually be converted into an electric signal before processing can occur; furthermore, because the vast majority of our neuromodulation is accomplished by electric stimulation, integration of electric biomarkers into these systems is an intuitive design choice. They have very high temporal fidelity to the conditions being treated. Their risk/ease of acquisition is very acceptable given that the acquisition of electric signals can often be done with the same devices used to administer the neuromodulatory stimulation; some systems, however, require recording from a site distant from the stimulation site, which requires a single episode of increased invasiveness and implantation risk to obtain the benefit of completely automated signal acquisition which does not intrude on the patient's perception. The exceptionally feature-rich electric signals acquired from the CNS offer the promise of highly sensitive and specific biomarkers. With increasing understanding of the electrophysiology of the CNS, electric biomarkers are very attractive choices for biomarkers.

Electric biomarkers are used heavily in epilepsy. The diagnosis of epilepsy itself depends on identification of characteristic electric signals generated in the brain. The RNS system is trained to identify specific features of a patient's unique seizure pattern on ECoG. Although seizure activity is detected, the system provides stimulation; when seizure is no longer detected, the system reverts to monitoring-only mode. There is the potential to apply similar techniques to deep brain stimulation (DBS) used for a multitude of other indications as our understanding of these conditions improves.

Chemical Biomarkers

The electric processes of the nervous system are predicated on the function of chemical processes ongoing at many points within and surrounding the cells that comprise the system. The inappropriate electric activity that is the hallmark of most neurologic diseases can usually be explained by alterations in the chemistry of the cells involved. This altered chemistry may therefore serve as a biomarker for these conditions and potentially even as a control signal that could be used as a trigger or as a feedback signal. Grahn et al. demonstrated that real-time measurement of dopamine levels in the medial forebrain bundle of rats could be used to modulate a feedback control signal during DBS.[3] However, integration of chemical biomarkers into routine clinical use is currently limited by available sensor technology. Measurement of chemical species in vivo currently requires consumptive/destructive reactions at the point of detection, severely limiting the useful lifespan of the detectors. However, if this barrier can be overcome, chemical biomarkers may provide a control system signal with similar flexibility and utility to electric biomarkers. Bennet et al. have shown the potential of novel materials such as boron-doped diamond to dramatically increase the longevity of in vivo detectors.[4]

Physiologic Biomarkers

Physiologic biomarkers for neuromodulation include other signals from within the body whose variance may correlate with the status of a neurologic pathology. For example, during a seizure, the heart rate often rapidly increases; the current version of VNS from LivaNova incorporates heart rate detection and increases stimulation when a rapid change in heart rate above a specified threshold is detected. Heart rate, body position, blood sugar levels, or any other measurement from body systems that may be affected by, or precipitate a change in, the disease condition being modulated may serve as a control signal.

Functional Biomarkers

The goal of neuromodulation is ultimately to alter the function of the nervous system and direct it toward a more "normal" state of function. The nervous system operates as a collection of complex neural networks working in series, parallel, or opposition to each other. Using the state of these networks as a biomarker in neuromodulation control systems can help directly tie the true desired outcome of the system to its function.

Anatomic network state

There are a number of known anatomic networks in the brain, which consist of "hardwired" connections between various structures in the brain. Anatomic networks such as the classically described direct and indirect pathways connecting the cortex, basal ganglia, and thalamus[5] or the circuit of Papez[6] are thought to play significant roles in different neuropathologic conditions. Measuring the patterns of activity at various points in these networks can potentially provide a rich source of information from which many potential biomarkers can be extracted and used to control advanced neuromodulation systems.

Functional network state

In the last decade, evidence has grown supporting the concept of nonanatomic, functionally connected networks within the brain whose purpose seems to be supporting the various higher cognitive and complex processing tasks that the brain handles on a daily basis.[7,8] These networks dynamically form and dissolve in a task-specific manner, using the hardwired connections and nodes within the brain to allow anatomically distant sites to work together on a complex task. This allows for a modular design within the brain that minimizes redundancy while maximizing task flexibility. Functional networks that are more active during introspection, executive function tasks, determining relevance of external stimuli to a situation, and several others have been identified.[8] These networks are also thought to be abnormally weak or strong in various disorders of consciousness or psychiatric disorders such as depression or schizophrenia.[7]

Anatomic or functional network states represent tantalizing targets for neuromodulatory feedback. Control systems that are able to stabilize a certain global network state or even switch between them have the potential to revolutionize the treatment of disorders of brain function. These potential biomarkers still require much study. Currently, they are best characterized through MRI techniques and thus are far from ideal in the metric of ease of acquisition. Like chemical biomarkers, however, technological and intellectual advances may soon remove the barrier of signal acquisition and allow use of these powerful biomarkers.

CURRENT AND FUTURE APPLICATIONS TO NEUROSURGERY

Current neuromodulation therapies, with a few notable exceptions mentioned previously in this chapter, continue to use a very simple open-loop design. The development of more intelligent, more efficient, and ultimately more effective therapies will depend mostly on identification of appropriate biomarkers to be used as positive or negative controls in the feedback loops of the systems. Recent advances in signal processing, machine learning, and pattern recognition software have largely removed this part of the process as an obstacle. Finding the best combination of signals and detectors to make use of that processing capability is the challenge facing the field of neuromodulation today.

Cranial Procedures

Cortical and DBS procedures are core techniques of functional and stereotactic neurosurgery. The relative complexity of the brain as compared with other parts of the nervous system, its involvement to some degree in almost all disorders of the nervous system, and its composition by anatomically distinct data processing and transmission elements make it an optimal target for closed-loop neuromodulation. The complexity of the brain, while daunting at first glance, provides feature-rich biomarkers that can be used in the various control points of advanced stimulation systems. Because central regulation of the peripheral nervous system and awareness of nervous system malfunction are generally the responsibility of brain structures, neuromodulation in the brain has the ability to dramatically impact the experience of neurologic disease, even in patients whose original pathology may exist in the periphery. Applying modulatory signals and measuring trigger/feedback signals in a highly targeted manner is predicated on measuring only the systems of interest and excluding noise from nearby, uninvolved systems; the ability to identify, stimulate or sample from discreet processing centers or pathways make subtle and precise neuromodulation applications possible in the brain.

Movement disorders

PD is perhaps the best-known example of successful neuromodulation. DBS has been shown repeatedly to improve the condition of Parkinson patients in multiple dimensions of analysis.[9–11] Essential tremor and dystonia also are commonly treated with DBS as well with similar dramatic results.[12–14] Despite more than 20 years of experience with DBS for movement disorders, the current standard of care is a simple, tonic, open-loop stimulation system, which has remained essentially unchanged since its introduction.[15] Current electrode designs available in the United States incorporate either four cylindrical platinum-iridium contacts (Medtronic) or two cylindrical contacts bracketing two segmented electrodes with three contacts covering 120 radial degrees each (total contacts = 8, Abbott). The electrodes can be configured such that any two contacts can be selected to serve as an anode-cathode pair, allowing 2^3 combinations (=8); alternatively, the casing of the generator in the chest may serve as an electrode, increasing the number of configurations to 12. Other variables that can be adjusted for each combination of electrodes are voltage/amplitude of the stimulation signal, frequency, and pulse width. This does not include more complex stimulation waveforms, which are currently under investigation. It is clear that even this relatively simple system has a very large space of stimulation variables that can be manipulated to provide the optimum stimulation paradigm for a given patient. The current method of identifying the "optimal" settings for a patient involves multiple visits to the clinic for evaluation and reprogramming. During these sessions, subjective reports from patient and family and clinical observations of symptoms, such as tremor over a time course of a few minutes, guide the adjustment of stimulation parameters. As many of the effects and side effects of DBS take days, weeks, or even months to become evident, this method of optimization lacks the sensitivity to take full advantage of the potential benefits offered by DBS. Even with experienced programming experts, the number of parameter combinations that can practically be trialed is only a small fraction of the available set. A more efficient method of parameter selection, using biomarkers that rapidly provide valuable feedback and trigger signals, is highly desirable. Additionally, incorporation of an adaptive/responsive, closed-loop system may help determine when stimulation is not necessary and reduce the net energy expenditure from the generator over time, thereby increasing the useful battery life of the device.

β-band oscillations (13–35 Hz) in the local field potential of the subthalamic nucleus (STN) and globus pallidus interna (GPi) have been shown to correlate with the severity of bradykinesia and rigidity in PD patients.[1] Phase amplitude coupling of the β-band in oscillations in the STN to cortical γ (50–200 Hz) signals and high-frequency oscillations in the upper γ band (200–400 Hz) of the STN local field potentials (LFPs) have also been shown to correlate with severity of motor symptoms in PD patients. Synchronization of corticocortical networks in the β-band has similarly been demonstrated to correlate with severity of PD symptoms.[16] Tremor, on the other hand, is highly associated with LFP frequencies around 5 and 10 Hz (θ- and α-band). Studies demonstrate that a typical 130-Hz stimulation decreases the β-band effects and that stimulation pulses timed to provide phase-interference to the tremor frequencies can disrupt that signal and reduce tremor.[1,16]

Little et al. demonstrated in 2013 that LFPs recorded from the unused contacts of the DBS electrode could be used as a feedback signal in an adaptive, closed-loop system.[17] They identified β-band frequencies with peak power in patients undergoing DBS and designed a closed-loop system that triggered a 100-ms burst of 130-Hz stimulation whenever the power in the predetermined subset of the β-band increased above a specified threshold. Little and Beudel showed in 2015 that this approach could be applied bilaterally and for a sustained period of time.[18] Both studies demonstrated that the adaptive (aDBS) produced improvements in movement equal to or surpassing traditional chronic DBS, with a reduction in power consumption by almost one half. There was suggestion in these studies that patients also had fewer side effects of stimulation with aDBS versus chronic DBS; however, the studies were not powered to make this determination. Beuter et al. proposed a similar method for closed-loop stimulation using cortical sensing and stimulation for PD that detects alterations in the behavior of an affected cortical network and applies stimulation to drive it back toward a nonpathologic state.[19] This sort of system would benefit greatly from the machine-learning techniques possible in adaptive and responsive closed-loop systems.

We should be careful to avoid the trap of confusing more complicated solutions with better solutions. As mentioned above, physical biomarkers work very well for conditions that generate altered patterns of movement. Many centers are currently investigating the use of wearable devices, usually incorporating accelerometers, to detect patterns of pathologic movement and adjust stimulation to return those patterns to a more normal state. Essential tremor is one condition where this seems easily applicable; however, dystonia and PD are also very reasonable applications of this process. In all the three conditions, the application of an adaptive algorithm will provide the greatest benefit in those patients with medication associated "on" and "off" times; in these patients, stimulation can be increased or decreased in real time to accommodate for the action of any medications by minimizing overtreatment effects (such as dyskinesia in PD) and accommodating undertreatment (such as when a medication dose is missed).

PD is certainly not the only movement disorder treated well by neuromodulation. Its multifaceted nature and the deep body of research related to the various symptoms of PD help develop our more global understanding of the control of movement within the brain. These developing insights can be applied to the development of more disease-specific neuromodulation therapies for isolated diseases of tremor, dystonia, and other abnormal movements.

Epilepsy

The responsive neurostimulation system from NeuroPace is perhaps the most well known of the closed-loop neuromodulation devices currently available. It is certainly the most fully developed and studied of the systems on the market today.[20–27] Its function is described previously in this chapter (sections Adaptive Systems and Electric Biomarkers) and highlights many of the advances that improved signal detection and data processing can bring to bear. The VNS (LivaNova) described above (sections Closed-Loop Systems and Physiologic Biomarkers) similarly uses personalized biomarker signals to provide a personalized neuromodulation system. Incorporation of feedback into other systems may help open more options for the treatment of medically refractory epilepsy. The SANTE trial evaluated chronic DBS similar to that used currently for traditional DBS for movement disorders applied to the anterior nucleus of the thalamus. The trial demonstrated positive results in terms of reduction of seizure frequency and several other secondary metrics, but the technology was ultimately not approved for general application by the US FDA, partially due to the risk of depression seen in some patients.[28] Use of an adaptive system such as the neural network–based system of the NeuroPace RNS or more specific features such as frequency band power as in the aDBS application to PD to provide a positive feedback signal may help fine-tune the system and target it better to interrupt seizure activity. Similarly, use of other biomarkers such as the functional network state to detect worsening depression states may provide a negative feedback signal useful for improving the safety profile of the system.

Psychiatric disorders

As suggested in the previous sections, closed-loop systems to modulate and treat psychiatric disorders are an attractive application of this developing technology. Currently, traditional chronic, open-loop DBS is being applied to obsessive compulsive disorder and has been investigated for obesity,[29,30] memory impairment in Alzheimer disease,[31] and depression.[32] These and other similar disorders share the common feature that no single anatomic or physiologic abnormality has been identified as the underlying mechanism responsible for the observed behavioral pathology. Rather, these disorders are likely the result of abnormalities in the function and control of more global functional networks. Identification of biomarkers to use as control signals will greatly aid the refinement of neuromodulation systems targeting these conditions. For some of them, simple subjective/experiential biomarkers may suffice: when the patient notes an increase in the severity of symptoms (i.e., a compulsion to perform a repetitive action), they might trigger their stimulator. This may have the added benefit of allowing the patient a sense of control over the disease and thereby (in a small way) helping to bootstrap the therapy in a successful direction. In other conditions, this patient-initiated feedback may be less appropriate. In these cases, more direct measurement of the functional network state may provide control signals that modulate the stimulus pattern to keep therapy effects and side effects in balance.

Central pain disorders

Medically refractory pain was one of the first indications to which DBS was applied.[33–36] Initial results were quite promising; many different areas were investigated, but thalamic targets and periaqueductal gray were the frequently selected sites in human trials.[37] Cortical stimulation, particularly motor cortex stimulation, has also been applied to patients with pain syndromes. In general, the chronic stimulation paradigms of open-loop systems tend to show good short-term results in conditions as varied as poststroke pain, headache/migraine syndromes, and deafferentation syndromes such as anesthesia dolorosa and brachial plexus avulsion.[37,38] The general trend, however, is for a large proportion of patients to have diminished efficacy (seen as a need for continually increasing stimulation voltage) or loss of effect after periods as short as 1 year, despite very positive stimulation trials. It is partly for this reason that DBS and other intracranial neurostimulator systems were not approved for use in treating chronic pain (although the techniques were approved in the United Kingdom). It is unclear why loss of effect occurs, but the possibility of plastic changes within the brain in the face of chronic stimulation is a leading theoretical explanation.[37] If that is true, then development of stimulation algorithms that activate only when needed may be the critical advancement that allows for durable and effective pain control in these conditions.

Here, as in the psychiatric disorders, identification of biomarkers to serve a control signals is key. Studies into the anatomic and functional networks of the brain may suggest novel targets for stimulation as well as sites to obtain feedback signals. Neurochemical signals may also feature prominently in the feedback loops directing these therapies. Ultimately, subjective control by patients themselves may prove to be a very powerful tool when combined with these advances.

Extracranial Procedures

Neuromodulation is not limited to electric stimulation of the brain. Epidural SCS and peripheral nerve stimulation are both established therapies with demonstrated efficacy in the treatment of various disorders. To date, the application of the technology, such as intracranial stimulation, has largely consisted of open-loop systems. These systems require manual adjustment in the clinic by empiric judgments, in the same fashion as intracranial stimulators.

Epidural spinal cord stimulation

- Pain: Stimulation for chronic pain, whether in the back or limbs, is the most common application of epidural SCS. Currently, there are systems available that sense patient position (horizontal or vertical) and can adjust where on the electrode stimulation is delivered to account for small changes in lead location. Otherwise, there is no ability to dynamically adjust the output of the system to maintain effectiveness. The challenge is in finding reliable and measurable biomarkers that can indicate the degree of pain being experienced by the patient. This is of course true generally in the treatment of pain, but in the case of SCS, there is the opportunity to take advantage of an implanted processor which is not available in other settings of pain management. Because pain is such a heterogeneous indication, it is likely that a variety of biomarkers may ultimately be needed to direct closed-loop therapy in a patient-specific manner. In the case of back pain associated with muscle spasms, electromyography may represent a source of signal indicating the relative severity of the patient's pain in real time. Alternatively, physical biomarkers such as a decrease in overall activity level may be useful in identifying states of increased pain. These may be combined with prompted patient input via a control device (to confirm that the activity level change is truly due to pain rather than simply changing activities) to form a customizable, responsive system.
- Angina and peripheral vascular disease: A special subset of pain conditions, medically refractory angina pectoris, and its related condition of peripheral ischemic pain are recognized indications for SCS, although this is more frequently used in Europe than the United States where it is not a separately approved indication. These conditions offer a broader range of potential biomarkers for use in control signals than simply the subjective experience of pain. In fact, biomarkers for these conditions already exist in the form of cardiac enzyme assays and other markers of ischemic tissue damage, as well as skin temperature/perfusion measurements. Incorporation of these elements via chemical analysis of blood, temperature sensors, or tissue oxygenation detectors may augment closed-loop designs.
- Bladder dystonia: Although pain can certainly be one aspect of bladder dystonia, there are many patients with this condition who cannot detect the pain consciously because of spinal cord or other injury but who nevertheless experience the effects of the dysfunction. This may take the form of urinary incontinence, frequency, or sympathetic dystrophy. These patients would potentially benefit from closed-loop SCS systems more than most, as they are much less able to assess the efficacy of the system until the symptoms become severely uncontrolled. Intelligent integration of data from sensors (moisture sensors, heart rate sensors) and patient input as appropriate could help to optimize these systems.
- Spinal cord injury: Spasticity or peri-injury pain is a common indication for placement of an SCS system in patients with spinal cord injury. New evidence is emerging; however, SCS may be beneficial in more directly treating the disability of spinal cord injury. Lumbosacral SCS has been demonstrated in a small number of patients with functionally complete spinal cord injury to allow voluntary movement of the lower limbs.[39,41] Animal studies have also recently demonstrated the potential for a closed-loop system using SCS and input signals from the premotor cortex to produce voluntary basic upper limb and hand motions in a model of injury to the primary motor cortex.[40] As our understanding of this new application of SCS grows, incorporation of increasingly advanced, adaptive and responsive control systems will potentially allow restoration of more sophisticated control of paralyzed limbs to patients. Many different biomarkers will likely need to be combined in the systems developed for this application, such as body position, speed and velocity, frequency of LFP oscillations within the spinal cord underlying the stimulator, activation

patterns of descending fiber tracts or cortical control areas, and many others.

- Dorsal root ganglion (DRG) stimulation: This technology has been available outside the United States for several years but was only FDA approved in January 2016. In a modified version of traditional epidural SCS, the electrodes are positioned in the epidural space just over the DRG, and microvolt stimulation is used to modulate the behavior of the DRG. Indicated for use in patients with neuropathic pain from peripheral nerve injury, this promises to be an effective therapy for patients with complex regional pain syndrome (CRPS) I and II. This is also an indication for traditional SCS; like SCS, DRG stimulation currently functions only with tonic, open-loop design. As with angina and peripheral ischemic pain, CRPS has objective findings such as temperature and color changes that may help to serve a biomarker for responsive control systems.

CONCLUSION

Adaptive neuromodulation is in its early stages of development. The goal is to convert comparatively simple open-loop systems to ones that provide optimized stimulation and symptom reduction in a patient-specific, customized fashion. In a sense, neurostimulation has always been responsive: clinicians have provided the sophisticated processing of information about the patient's symptoms to adjust the system's operating parameters and checking the results in a slow, manual, iterative process. Now, technology is allowing clinicians to replace more elements of the system with sensors and computers, making the systems more efficient and patient-specific.

Design of adaptive neuromodulation systems uses the following elements of an ideal closed-loop system:

- Well-defined biomarkers that are sensitive, specific, and appropriately temporally related to the pathology being addressed
- Well-designed sensors that can detect relevant biomarkers in a manner that are safe, convenient, and comfortable for patients and clinicians and that are durable under the conditions of typical clinical use
- Take advantage of sporadic (i.e., not constant) phenomenon to distinguish symptomatic states from normal states
- Produce an output that effectively modulates the system in a timeframe that is practical and relevant to the pathology
- Increased efficiency of energy delivery when the cost of signal detection is included (compared with simple open-loop stimulation)

Not all neuromodulation requires electric stimulation. Other modes, such as delivery of neuromodulatory pharmaceuticals to the CNS as in intrathecal baclofen pumps, can be optimized by application of these principles.

One of the principal challenges to advancing closed-loop neuromodulation to the problems of pain, behavior, epilepsy, and even movement disorders is the lack of robust clinical data to guide our next steps in developing these technologies. Designing ethical, safe, data-driven device studies is difficult, even when the underlying physiology is relatively well understood. In the complex systems of the nervous system, incorporation of the various basic science and clinical insights into a single, goal-directed effort will require an increasingly multidisciplinary approach.

REFERENCES

1. Beudel M, Brown P. Adaptive deep brain stimulation in Parkinson's disease. *Parkinsonism Relat Disord*. 2016;22: S123–S126.
2. Hambley AR. *Electrical Engineering, Principles and Applications: Engineering, Electronic Engineering*. CTI Reviews. 5th ed. Cram101 Textbook Reviews; 2016.
3. Grahn PJ, et al. A neurochemical closed-loop controller for deep brain stimulation: toward individualized smart neuromodulation therapies. *Front Neurosci*. 2014;8.
4. Bennet KE, et al. A diamond-based electrode for detection of neurochemicals in the human brain. *Front Hum Neurosci*. 2016;10.
5. Alexander GE, Crutcher MD. Functional architecture of basal ganglia circuits: neural substrates of parallel processing. *Trends Neurosci*. 1990;13(7):266–271.
6. Papez JW. A proposed mechanism of emotion. *Arch Neurol Psychiatry*. 1937;38(4):725–743.
7. Van Den Heuvel MP, Hulshoff Pol HE. Exploring the brain network: a review on resting-state fMRI functional connectivity. *Eur Neuropsychopharmacol*. 2010;20(8):519–534.
8. Heine L, et al. Resting state networks and consciousness: alterations of multiple resting state network connectivity in physiological, pharmacological, and pathological consciousness states. *Front Psychol*. 2012;3.
9. Weaver FM, et al. Bilateral deep brain stimulation vs best medical therapy for patients with advanced Parkinson disease: a randomized controlled trial. *JAMA*. 2009;301(1):63–73.
10. Williams A, et al. Deep brain stimulation plus best medical therapy versus best medical therapy alone for advanced Parkinson's disease (PD SURG trial): a randomised, open-label trial. *Lancet Neurol*. 2010;9(6):581–591.
11. Deuschl G, et al. A randomized trial of deep-brain stimulation for Parkinson's disease. *N Engl J Med*. 2006; 355(9):896–908.
12. Pahwa R, Lyons KE, Wilkinson SB, et al. Long-term evaluation of deep brain stimulation of the thalamus. *J Neurosurg*. 2006;104:506–512.

13. Kiss ZH, Doig-Beyaert K, Eliasziw M, et al. The Canadian multicentre study of deep brain stimulation for cervical dystonia. *Brain*. 2007;130:2879–2886.
14. Vidailhet M, Vercueil L, Houeto JL, et al. Bilateral, pallidal, deep-brain stimulation in primary generalized dystonia: a prospective 3 year follow-up study. *Lancet Neurol*. 2007;6: 223–229.
15. Arlotti M, et al. The adaptive deep brain stimulation challenge. *Parkinsonism Relat Disord*. 2016;28:12–17.
16. Silberstein P, et al. Cortico-cortical coupling in Parkinson's disease and its modulation by therapy. *Brain*. 2005; 128(6):1277–1291.
17. Little S, et al. Adaptive deep brain stimulation in advanced Parkinson disease. *Ann Neurol*. 2013;74(3):449–457.
18. Little S, et al. Bilateral adaptive deep brain stimulation is effective in Parkinson's disease. *J Neurol Neurosurg Psychiatry*. 2015. jnnp-2015.
19. Beuter A, Lefaucheur JP, Modolo J. Closed-loop cortical neuromodulation in Parkinson's disease: an alternative to deep brain stimulation? *Clin Neurophysiol*. 2014; 125(5):874–885.
20. Kossoff EH, et al. Effect of an external responsive neurostimulator on seizures and electrographic discharges during subdural electrode monitoring. *Epilepsia*. 2004;45(12): 1560–1567.
21. Fountas KN, et al. Implantation of a closed-loop stimulation in the management of medically refractory focal epilepsy. *Stereotact Funct Neurosurg*. 2005;83(4):153–158.
22. Morrell MJ. Responsive cortical stimulation for the treatment of medically intractable partial epilepsy. *Neurology*. 2011;77(13):1295–1304.
23. Heck CN, et al. Two-year seizure reduction in adults with medically intractable partial onset epilepsy treated with responsive neurostimulation: final results of the RNS System Pivotal trial. *Epilepsia*. 2014;55(3):432–441.
24. Bergey GK, et al. Long-term treatment with responsive brain stimulation in adults with refractory partial seizures. *Neurology*. 2015;84(8):810–817.
25. Loring DW, et al. Differential neuropsychological outcomes following targeted responsive neurostimulation for partial-onset epilepsy. *Epilepsia*. 2015;56(11):1836–1844.
26. King-Stephens D, et al. Lateralization of mesial temporal lobe epilepsy with chronic ambulatory electrocorticography. *Epilepsia*. 2015;56(6):959–967.
27. Meador KJ, et al. Quality of life and mood in patients with medically intractable epilepsy treated with targeted responsive neurostimulation. *Epilepsy Behav*. 2015;45:242–247.
28. Fisher R, et al. Electrical stimulation of the anterior nucleus of thalamus for treatment of refractory epilepsy. *Epilepsia*. 2010;51(5):899–908.
29. Halpern CH, et al. Amelioration of binge eating by nucleus accumbens shell deep brain stimulation in mice involves D2 receptor modulation. *J Neurosci*. 2013;33(17): 7122–7129.
30. Whiting DM, et al. Lateral hypothalamic area deep brain stimulation for refractory obesity: a pilot study with preliminary data on safety, body weight, and energy metabolism. *J Neurosurg*. 2013;119(1):56–63.
31. Laxton AW, et al. A phase I trial of deep brain stimulation of memory circuits in Alzheimer's disease. *Ann Neurol*. 2010;68(4):521–534.
32. Lozano AM, et al. Subcallosal cingulate gyrus deep brain stimulation for treatment-resistant depression. *Biol Psychiatry*. 2008;64(6):461–467.
33. Richardson DE, Akil H. Long term results of periventricular gray self-stimulation. *Neurosurgery*. 1977;1(2):199–202.
34. Hosobuchi Y, Adams JE, Linchitz R. Pain relief by electrical stimulation of the central gray matter in humans and its reversal by naloxone. *Science*. 1977;197(4299):183–186.
35. Thoden U, Doerr M, Dieckmann G, Krainick JU. Medial thalamic permanent electrodes for pain control in man: an electrophysiological and clinical study. *Electroencephalogr Clin Neurophysiol*. 1979;47(5):582–591.
36. Coffey RJ. Deep brain stimulation for chronic pain: results of two multicenter trials and a structured review. *Pain Med*. 2001;2(3):183–192.
37. Boccard SGJ, et al. Long-term outcomes of deep brain stimulation for neuropathic pain. *Neurosurgery*. 2013;72(2): 221.
38. Franzini A, et al. Stimulation of the posterior hypothalamus for treatment of chronic intractable cluster headaches: first reported series. *Neurosurgery*. 2003;52(5): 1095–1101.
39. Rejc E, Angeli C, Harkema S. Effects of lumbosacral spinal cord epidural stimulation for standing after chronic complete paralysis in humans. *PLoS One*. 2015;10(7): e0133998.
40. Zimmermann JB, Jackson A. Closed-loop control of spinal cord stimulation to restore hand function after paralysis. *Front Neurosci*. 2014;8.
41. Sayenko DG, et al. Neuromodulation of evoked muscle potentials induced by epidural spinal-cord stimulation in paralyzed individuals. *J Neurophysiol*. 2014;111(5): 1088–1099.

CHAPTER 27

Robotics in Stereotactic Neurosurgery

GEOFFREY STRICSEK, MD • OMADITYA KHANNA, MD • CHENGYUAN WU, MD, MSBmE

INTRODUCTION

The earliest use of stereotaxy for the localization of an intracranial target was conducted by Zernov, an anatomy professor at Moscow University. It consisted of three parts: a basal ring passing through the nasion and inion was fixed to the skull in the horizontal plane, an equator attached perpendicularly to the basal ring with the 0 point directly above the sagittal suture, and a meridian located in the sagittal plane that could translate along the equator.[1] Using an encephalometric map previously constructed by Zernov, spatial localization of a structure could be plotted using the frame; in 1889, it was successfully used to locate the Rolandic sulcus at which point an intracerebral abscess was drained.[2,3] Apparently unaware of the work in Russia, another report describing the methodology of stereotaxy emerged in 1897. A group based in Paris described an "operating compass" constructed of two Crookes tubes and two photographic film supports mounted orthogonally, which was then attached to a patient's skull. The contraption was then used to localize radio-opaque foreign bodies within the patient's cranium.[4] Sir Victor Horsley and Robert Clarke expanded on the work by the Parisian group through the pairing of an orthogonal coordinate system with relevant anatomic skull landmarks in animals.[5] In 1906, they commissioned a machinist to construct their machine using brass and subsequently patented the device and its application in humans in 1914.

These early forays into stereotaxy were severely constrained by the wide variability between bony landmarks and intracranial targets. Today's frame-based stereotaxy was first introduced by Ernest A. Spiegel and Henry T. Wycis in 1947; they paired the stereotactic work of Horsley and Clarke with pneumoencephalograms and Walter E. Dandy's work on ventriculography to improve the localization of intracranial targets in humans.[6] The earliest intracranial reference points were the foramen of Monro and the pineal gland, which could be easily characterized with pneumoencephalography; in addition, the anterior and posterior commissures (AC and PC) could be identified using contrast ventriculography. From these intracranial landmarks, Spiegel and Wycis were able to construct a stereotactic map of intracranial structures using the line that connects the PC with the bulbopontine sulcus as the primary reference by which they were defined.[7,8] Although they had also described the intercommissural line connecting the AC with the PC, targets were defined by distance in millimeters from a standardized reference, neglecting natural variation that exists from individual to individual.[8] Seeking to maintain accuracy across a population, Jean Talairach developed a three-dimensional, proportional coordinate system based on AC and PC as pivotal landmarks.[8,9] Using this space described by Talairach, Georges Schaltenbrand and Waldemar Wahren created a comprehensive stereotactic atlas of deep brain structures based on the analysis of more than 100 sectioned postmortem brain specimens.[10,11] The fundamentals of stereotaxy introduced by these pioneers remain in use today, as we have seen that improvements in frame-based technology (Fig. 27.1) lead to frameless methods of stereotaxy and more recently to automation with the incorporation of surgical robots.

ROBOTIC SURGERY

Broadly speaking, robots may be integrated into a surgical workflow as either a passive or active system.[12] A *passive system* functions as a platform to hold a surgical tool in a fixed position. It is set by the surgeon and does not move until redirected to do so. The earliest example of a passive robotic system was the one used for a stereotactic biopsy of an intracranial lesion.[13] In contrast, an *active system* is the one in which the robot can interact with the patient throughout the course of an operation while being monitored by the surgeon.[12] Active surgical

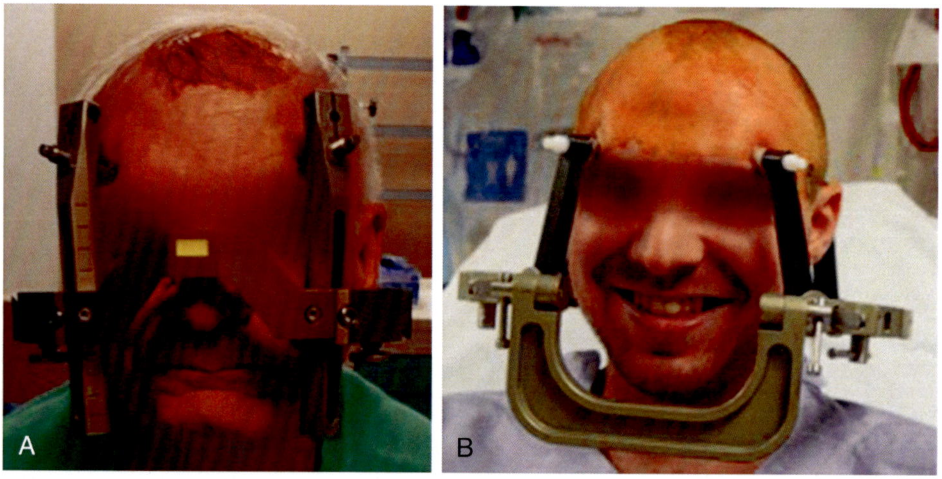

FIG. 27.1 Examples of different stereotactic headframes: **(A)** Leksell frame and **(B)** CRW frame.

systems come in three different forms: supervisory-controlled, robotic telesurgical, and shared-control systems.[12]

A *supervisory-controlled system* is dependent on preoperative planning of each action and position necessary during the course of a procedure; a formulated routine is transferred to the robot in preparation for surgery and then executed under observation of the surgeon.[12] The da Vinci Surgical System, made by Intuitive Surgical, Inc. (Sunnyvale, CA), is perhaps the most widely recognized surgical robot currently in practice and an example of a *robotic telesurgical system*. Specifically, it consists of a patient-side cart with multiple haptic-feedback robotic arms, which are under the direct control of a surgeon who is positioned at a remote three-dimensional viewing terminal. Lastly, in a *shared-control system* the surgeon and robot jointly control an instrument with the surgeon providing the action and direction, whereas the robot steadies the instrument and scales the motion for precision technique.[14]

ROBOTICS IN NEUROSURGERY

The Robotic Institute of America defines a robot as "a reprogrammable, multifunctional manipulator designed to move materials, parts, tools, or other specialized devices through various programmed motions for the performance of a variety of tasks."[15] Robots are particularly useful in assisting with complicated, often repetitive tasks. It is for this reason that robotic applications have found a home in stereotactic neurosurgery. With frame-based stereotaxy, neurosurgeons are accustomed to generating a surgical plan preoperatively and then executing that plan with the assistance of a frame-arc system. This workflow suits robotic systems, which also require a preoperative plan as described in the previous section with *supervisory-controlled systems*. Once formulated, the stereotactic plan can be programmed into the robot and then executed during the course of surgery. Furthermore, the absolute need for a high degree of accuracy in stereotaxy is well addressed by robotic solutions. Accordingly, the role of robots in stereotactic neurosurgery has continued to grow since its inception in the 1980s.

The first reported use of a robotic system used in surgery occurred in a neurosurgical setting in 1985 with the Programmable Universal Machine for Assembly (PUMA) device (Fig. 27.2). A patient with an intracranial lesion was placed in a stereotactic headframe and subsequently underwent target localization using CT imaging. The coordinates obtained from the CT were transferred to the PUMA robot, which then devised a trajectory to the target. The surgeon could adjust the entry point as necessary to avoid any critical structures, but the robot ensured that the target point remained constant; the first biopsy sample sent to the laboratory was positive.[13] The MINERVA system, introduced in the early 1990s, was the first robot designed specifically for neurosurgical application and offered integration of a robotic system with CT guidance to allow a surgeon to monitor instrument position and progress in real time.[16] At the time of this writing, current FDA-approved robots with applications in stereotactic neurosurgery include the Renaissance Guidance System by Mazor Robotics (Caesarea, Israel), the ROSA from Zimmer Biomet (Warsaw, IN), and the Neuromate by Renishaw (Wotton-under-Edge, UK).

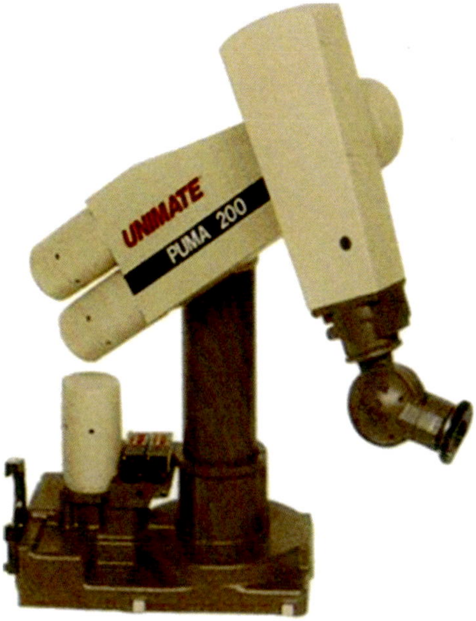

FIG. 27.2 Unimate PUMA robot used by Dr. Kwoh in the first robotic neurosurgical procedure. (Permission of Unimate.)

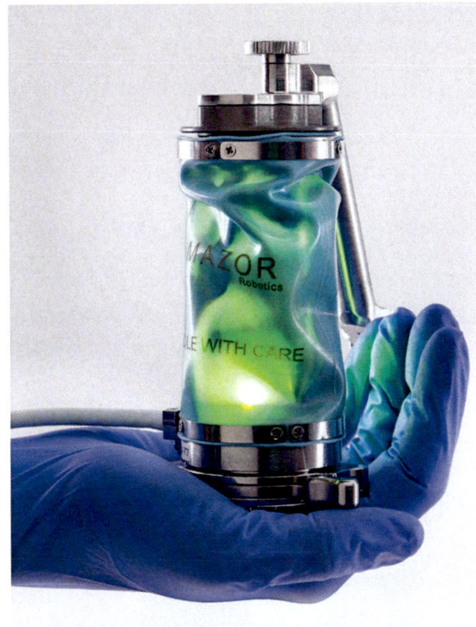

FIG. 27.3 MAZOR Renaissance—can be used for spinal or intracranial applications. (With permission from Mazor Robotics Ltd.)

NEUROSURGICAL ROBOTIC SYSTEMS

Mazor Robotics Renaissance Guidance System

The system from Mazor has six degrees of freedom and was initially designed to assist with pedicle screw placement (Fig. 27.3), gaining FDA approval for this application on 2004. It is approximately the size of a 12-ounce beverage can and has an arm attachment for purposes of trajectory guidance. For spine applications, a preoperative CT scan is obtained and screw entry points and trajectories are planned using proprietary software. Following induction of anesthesia and adequate patient positioning, a mounting platform is attached to the patient's spine and a series of fluoroscopic images are obtained to coregister the patient with the preoperative imaging and the robot. Once all equipment and registration is verified, the surgeon identifies a vertebra and the robot adjusts its position, bringing the cannulated drill guide to the prespecified entry point in the prespecified trajectory. Initially tested in cadavers, screw deviation from planned trajectory was only slightly greater than 1 mm.[17] Data from surgeon-reported in vivo robotic use suggest an accuracy of almost 99%; malpositioned screws were attributed to skiving of the drill bit at the cortex before cannulation.[18] Roughly 10% of planned screws were unable to be placed robotically, most often a result of poor registration.[18] Objective data from either intraoperative fluoroscopy[19] or postoperative CT[20–22] following robot-assisted pedicle screw placement largely support the surgeon observations, suggesting an accuracy of 90%–99%.

More recently, the Mazor platform was expanded to allow for intracranial stereotactic applications, with FDA approval in 2012. As with frame-based stereotaxy, the target, entry point, and trajectory are identified on a preoperative MRI. To begin the procedure, a low-profile reference platform is attached to the skull under local anesthesia. With an associated marker attachment secured to the reference platform, a CT scan is obtained and coregistered with the MRI. Once the coregistration is complete, the software is able to interpret the trajectories planned on the preoperative MRI by understanding its relationship relative to the reference platform. In the operating room, the robot can then be attached to the low-profile reference platform and manipulated into position to identify the preplanned entry point and trajectory.[23] In a retrospective case series of 20 deep brain stimulation (DBS) implants in a single center, the mean radial error was found to be 0.7 ± 0.36 mm with the Mazor Robotics Renaissance Guidance System.[24]

Neurosurgical Robotic Systems

ROSA® technology

The ROSA® Brain robot from Zimmer-Biomet (**Fig. 27.4**) also affords the surgeon with six degrees of freedom and exists as a free-standing system. It gained FDA clearance for neurosurgical applications in 2010 with the first generation of the robot: ROSA. More recently, in 2016, the latest generation of the robot, ROSA One, gained CE Mark in Europe, which integrates a spine application as well. This technology relies on the surgeon planning target trajectories using preoperative imaging. This preoperative planning is correlated to the patient at the time of surgery via several options: skin-based fiducials, bone fiducials, frame-based registration, or non-invasive laser registration. The laser registration system automatically captures several thousand individual points along the face and forehead.[25] In the operating room, the robot is secured in place near the head of the patient. After registration has occurred, the robot is locked in this position throughout the duration of the stereotactic procedure to preserve the registration and maintain accuracy. During the stereotactic procedure, the robot functions in a manner analogous to a stereotactic arc – providing guidance to trajectories planned on preoperative imaging.

A key feature of this system is the haptic feedback provided by a force sensor at the end of the robotic arm. Specifically, once providing the appropriate command, the surgeon can move the arm simply by directly manipulating the arm in the desired direction. Such movement can occur either along the designated trajectory of interest, or freely without restriction. When the movement has been completed, the arm locks into this new position.

ROSA technology can be utilized for a variety of surgical procedures where stereotactic positioning is appropriate. One such use is for the planning and guidance of stereoelectroencephalography (SEEG) electrodes with a high degree of accuracy. In this application, entry point error has been shown to be less than 2mm in more than 90% of cases and targeting error is less than 2mm in 83% of cases.[26] Similar to the Mazor Renaissance® Guidance System, spine applications of ROSA® have also been explored with pedicle screw placement accuracy cited at 90-97%.[27,28] Additionally, the haptic capabilities may be valuable in non-stereotactic procedures such as endoscopic transnasal surgery and ventricular endoscopic procedures – serving as a reliable endoscope holder.

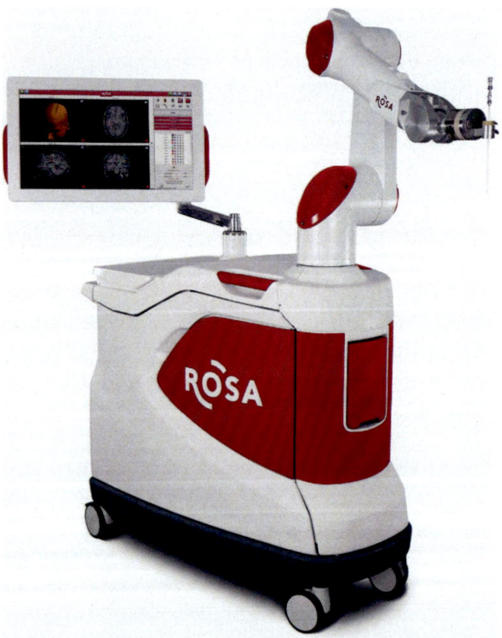

FIG. 27.4 ROSA robot by Zimmer Biomet. (With permission from Zimmer Biomet.)

Neuromate Robot

The Neuromate robot (Fig. 27.5) by Renishaw provides surgeons with five degrees of freedom in stereotactic applications. It gained FDA approval for intracranial procedures in 2014 and currently is not approved for use in spine surgeries. Before surgery, the surgeon plans the intended trajectories on preoperative images, which usually consists of a gadolinium-enhanced MRI and may also include other forms of vascular imaging or functional imaging. Registration can then be performed with either frame-based or frameless methods. In both

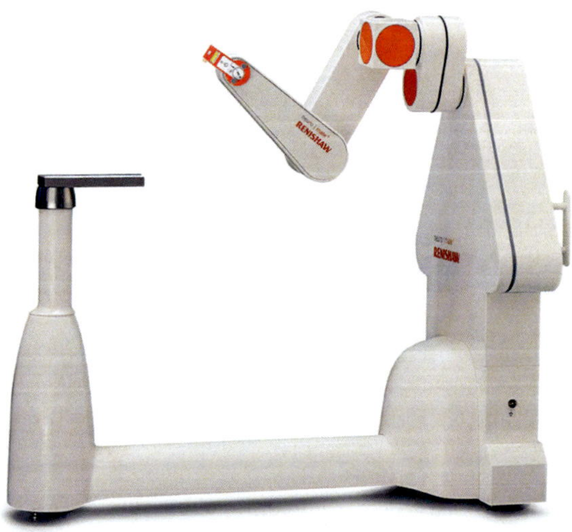

FIG. 27.5 Neuromate robot by Renishaw. (With permission from Renishaw.)

scenarios, once in the operating room, the patient's head is directly fixed to the robot base, which ensures that the robotic arm is at a standard and consistent distance from the patient's head. The head may be fixed within a Leksell frame or Cosman-Roberts-Wells (CRW) frame for frame-based registration or the Neuromate head holder in the case of frameless registration. Rather than laser registration of facial anatomy, the frameless registration of the Neuromate robot relies on ultrasound registration of the patient's head via a base plate fixed to the skull. Fidelity has been demonstrated in multiple studies: registration error averages 0.44–0.86 mm for frame-based and 1.6–1.95 mm for frameless setup; both have an average error of less than 2 mm, but the frame-based method is significantly more accurate than frameless.[30,31] Entry point error for frame-based application is 2 mm or less in 91%–96% of patients[26,32]; at the time of writing, there are no available published data regarding entry point accuracy with the frameless application. Target point error for frame-based averages has been cited as 0.86 mm in one study[33] with two other studies reporting median targeting error of 1.7 mm[26,32]; average targeting error for frameless application has been cited at 1.7 mm.[30]

ADVANTAGES OF ROBOTICS

Integration of robots into the neurosurgical operating room offers many benefits for both the patient and the surgeon. In this section, we will discuss the advantages of stereotactic robotic systems as compared with traditional frame and arc systems.

Reproducibility and Efficiency

In a stereotactic procedure, each trajectory requires adjusting and confirming multiple settings and an error at any one step could lead to a misplaced trajectory, which in turn could result in a poor patient outcome. Furthermore, although submillimeter precision for target coordinates in frame and arc systems is possible as well, their existing design in which the entry point of a trajectory is determined by the less precise arc and ring coordinates serves as a major limitation. Unfortunately, there exists no literature regarding the magnitude of entry point errors with frame and arc systems—yet less than 2 mm entry point error seen with robotic applications helps to demonstrate their ability to reliably reproduce the entire trajectory as initially planned.

As the number of trajectories increases, so does the opportunity for error. A robot is specifically designed to repetitively perform these precise tasks with submillimeter accuracy[34]; eliminating the human manipulation, transposition, and interpretation of frame coordinates can reduce targeting errors. Automation of these repetitive movements has the additional benefit of decreasing operative time in cases where multiple trajectories are used, such as with sEEG implants.[26] The value of decreased OR time cannot be overstated; one study cited an average decrease in OR time of 222 min when compared with traditional stereotactic frames.[26] If OR time is valued at $100 per minute,[35] the savings for a single robot case may exceed $22,000. All of these factors also help to reduce surgeon fatigue and ultimately to minimize the risk for associated adverse events.

Flexibility in Trajectory Planning

Current frame and arc systems limit the surgeon to entry points that are generally over the convexity of the patient's head. Such a limitation does not significantly affect DBS implantation or stereotactic biopsies; however, with sEEG implantation procedures, in which trajectories are oriented in a lateral to medial direction and orthogonal to the midsagittal plane, there is a need to be able to access trajectories that start from a more caudal position. Although the Leksell frame offers entry points within an arc of 170°, the CRW frame is limited to an arc of 120°. Even if the arc of either frame is positioned in a sagittal configuration, which is better suited for lateral trajectories, collisions between the platform or arc and the frame base limit such trajectories to a greater extent than robotic applications.

Marketability

An additional advantage to robotic surgery is the ability of robots to boost the commercial appeal of the hospital and perception of the procedure itself. It is logical that the term "robot" leads patients to perceive that the procedure itself is cutting-edge and to the belief that the hospital must be on the forefront of innovation and technology. A recent study quantified the effect of marketing robotic surgery as "innovative" or "state-of-the-art" and found that greater than 30% of patients would choose to undergo a novel procedure over a conventional alternative if it was framed in this manner.[36] As such, if the safety and efficacy of both conventional and novel techniques are at least equal, providing the "state-of-the-art robotic" alternative may provide not only a marketing advantage but also greater confidence in the surgeon by the patient.

DISADVANTAGES OF ROBOTICS

Although certainly a potential asset, it is important to also acknowledge some of the current disadvantages of robotic stereotactic neurosurgery.

Verification of Accuracy

In the prior section, we were careful to note that stereotactic robots confer greater surgical precision—but we did not claim that they provided greater accuracy. The literature to date has demonstrated that stereotactic robots provide accuracy that is comparable with existing frame-based, skull fiducial–based, and intraoperative MRI-based stereotactic systems.[31,37] As delineated above, a major benefit of a stereotactic robot is the advantage of greater reproducibility and efficiency when compared with frame and arc systems—particularly when several electrodes must be implanted, as with sEEG procedures. At the same time, there is no efficient intraoperative way to confirm that each implant is at the intended target, as one may do with the crosshair rings for the Leksell and CRW frames. If the Leksell frame is used in the robotic procedure, the X or Y as well as Z coordinates could be set on the frame to provide this confirmation; but doing so negates any efficiency gained with use of the robot. Therefore, the balance between surgical time and efficiency must be weighed with the potential reservations regarding accuracy.

Currently, most workflows for robotic stereotaxy have incorporated the execution of one or more test trajectories to surface landmarks as described earlier in this chapter. Although it still does not provide direct confirmation regarding the implant trajectories, it does inform the surgeon to the accuracy of the registration and test trajectories. Such information allows one to understand the overall accuracy of the planned trajectories, which the robot can place with a high degree of precision. If the accuracy of the initial test trajectories is not satisfactory, the surgeon may choose to abort the procedure or to fall back to traditional frame-based stereotaxy if the patient was initially placed in a stereotactic headframe.

Long-Term Reliability

As is the case with any piece of machinery, a robot is at risk for mechanical failure either preoperatively or during a case. It is also possible for its calibration to drift over time and, as a result, sacrifice accuracy. It is therefore necessary to have the system serviced and, if necessary, recalibrated on a routine basis to minimize the risk of intraoperative failure and loss of stereotactic accuracy.

Operating Room Space

Although the Mazor Renaissance Guidance System takes up little space, it needs to be mounted on the patient's skull and its short arm limits its use to DBS surgery and intracranial biopsies. In the case of the larger ROSA or Neuromate robots, which can be used for these procedures as well as sEEG implantations, the robot footprint requires an operating room that can accommodate it and its workstation as well as additional equipment that is often needed to supplement the robot's functionality, such as a C-arm or an O-arm (Fig. 27.6). Furthermore, its fixed position near the head of the patient can limit space around the surgical field (Fig. 27.7) and affect the overall surgical workflow.

As a new technology, there is the anticipated learning curve; but it is the one that includes not only the surgeon but also the support staff in the operating room. Both the surgeon and the support staff must be familiar with the nuances of incorporating the robot into the surgical procedure, which may include sterile draping of the robot, understanding when and where the robotic arm should and should not move, and how to preserve efficient instrument passing between the operator and assistant within the constraints of the robot position.

Cost

Stereotactic robotic systems can carry a steep financial price. At the time of this writing, initial capital investment can be up to six times greater than a traditional stereotactic headframe. In addition to this capital cost and as previously mentioned, there is also the need for an increased frequency of regular maintenance, which may increase the long-term cost of the device.

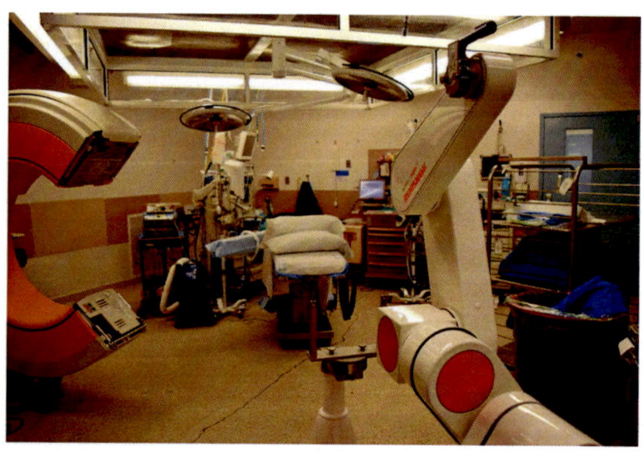

FIG. 27.6 Operating suite with Neuromate, O-arm, operating table, anesthesia machine, and additional ancillary equipment.

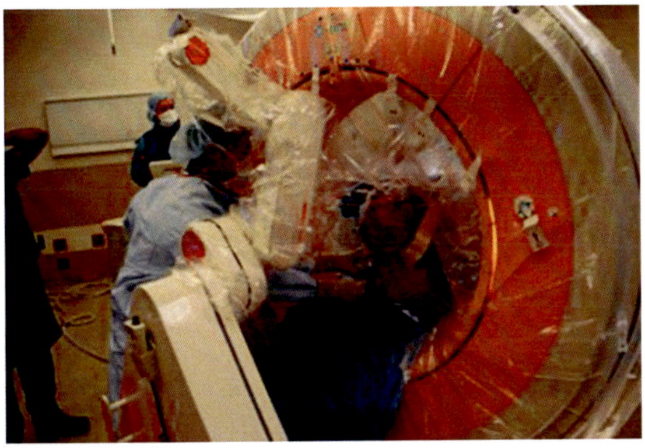

FIG. 27.7 Multiple pieces of equipment decrease available workspace around the patient.

FUTURE DIRECTIONS

Although robots have seen surgical applications in the past, it is only recently that they have reached early acceptance into clinical applications in neurosurgery, where there is certainly room for improvement. As we have seen with computer hardware in other industries, advancements in technology will allow for miniaturization of components, which will lead to a decreased robotic footprint and increased portability and, in turn, minimize the concerns of operating room space. Such advancements may also improve the reliability and longevity of these robots. In that same vein, improved production capabilities and expanded competition would help to lower overall costs.

As important are associated software advances, which have a broad scope, but in general can facilitate integration of the robotic system into the perioperative workflow by assisting the surgeon with preoperative trajectory planning,[38,39] intraoperative workflow, and postoperative assessments of the stereotactic procedure.

Beyond clinical applications, ongoing development may also push robots into a greater role in surgical education as robots with improved visual and haptic feedback can be used to create safe, but realistic, surgical simulators.[40] This scenario provides the tools necessary to objectively and reproducibly evaluate surgical trainees,[41] and as such, robots could potentially play a role in professional certification in the future.

SUMMARY

Robots have the ability to improve the execution of stereotactic procedures from DBS[30,33,34] and intracranial biopsies[13,23,42] to sEEG[32,43] and laser interstitial thermal therapy.[44] Their ability to rapidly and reproducibly execute precise movements can enhance patient safety, help optimize patient outcomes, and reduce operative times and potentially even operative costs. However, these benefits come at a cost: a monetary cost in terms of the initial investment and ongoing maintenance, a demand on infrastructure as a robot plus its ancillary equipment requires added operating room space, and the loss of the ability to intraoperatively confirm implant accuracy using the resources built into stereotactic headframes. Undoubtedly, robots will continue to develop and find themselves increasingly involved in surgery.

REFERENCES

1. Kandel E. *Functional and Stereotactic Neurosurgery*. New York, NY: Plenum Medical Book Company; 1989.
2. Willems P, Berkelbach van der Sprenkel J, Tulleken C, Viergever M, Taphoorn M. Neuronavigation and surgery of intracerebral tumours. *J Neurol*. 2006;253:1123–1136.
3. Altukhov N. *Encephalometric Investigations of the Brain Relative to the Sex, Age and Skull Indexes*. In: Moscow; 1891.
4. Benabid A, Chabardes S, Seigneuret E, History of stereotactic surgery in France. In: Lozano A, Gildenberg P, Tasker R, eds. *Textbook of Stereotactic and Functional Neurosurgery*. Berlin: Springer-Verlag.
5. Maryam R, Gregory J, Mocco J. Early history of stereotactic apparatus in neurosurgery. *Neurosurg Focus*. 2009;27(3):E12.
6. Gildenberg P. Spiegel and Wycis – the early years. *Stereotact Funct Neurosurg*. 2001;77(1–4):11–16.
7. Spiegel E, Wycis H, Marks M, Lee A. Stereotaxic apparatus for operations on the human brain. *Science*. 1947;106:349–350.
8. Lopes Alho EJ, Grinberg L, Heinsen H, Fonoff E. Review of printed and electronic stereotactic atlases of the human brain. In: Peres JFP, ed. *Neuroimaging for Clinicians – Combining Research and Practice*. InTech; 2011. https://doi.org/10.5772/24897. Available from: http://www.intechopen.com/books/neuroimaging-for-clinicians-combining-research-and-practice/review-of-printed-and-electronic-stereotactic-atlases-of-the-human-brain.
9. Talairach J, Tournoux P. *Co-planar Stereotaxic Atlas of the Human Brain: Three-Dimensional Proportional System: An Approach to Cerebral Imaging*. New York, NY: Thieme; 1988.
10. Schaltenbrand G, Bailey P. *Introduction to Stereotaxis with an Atlas of the Human Brain*. Stuttgart: Thieme; 1959.
11. Schaltenbrand G, Wahren W. *Atlas for Stereotaxy of the Human Brain with and Accompanying Guide*. Stuttgart: Thieme; 1977.
12. Nathoo N, Cavusoglu M, Vogelbaum M, Barnett G. In touch with robotics: neurosurgery for the future. *Neurosurgery*. 2005;56:421–433.
13. Kwoh Y, Hou J, Jonckheere E, Hayati S. A robot with improved absolute positioning accuracy for CT guided stereotactic brain surgery. *IEEE Trans Biomed Eng*. 1988;35(2):153–160.

14. Taylor R, Jensen P, Whitcomb L, et al. A steady-hand robotic system for microsurgical augmentation. *Int J Robot Res*. 1999;18:1201–1210.
15. Dowling K. Robotics FAQ. https://www.robotics.org/product-catalog-detail.cfm?productid=2953
16. Glauser D, Fankhauser H, Epitaux M, Hefti J-L, Jaccottet A. Neurosurgical robot Minerva: first results and current developments. *J Image Guid Surg*. 1995;1:266–272.
17. Lieberman I, Togawa D, Kayanja M, et al. Bone-mounted miniature robotic guidance for pedicle screw and translaminar facet screw placement: part I – technical development and test case results. *Neurosurgery*. 2006;59:641–650.
18. Hu X, Ohnmeiss D, Lieberman I. Robotic-assisted pedicle screw placement: lessons learned from the first 102 patients. *Eur Spine J*. 2013;22:661–666.
19. Kuo K, Su Y, Wu C, et al. Assessing the intraoperative accuracy of pedicle screw placement by using a bone-mounted miniature robot system through secondary registration. *PLoS One*. 2016;11(4):1–11.
20. Roser F, Tatagiba M, Maier G. Spinal robotics: current applications and future perspectives. *Neurosurgery*. 2013;72:A12–A18.
21. Kantelhardt S, Martinez R, Baerwinkel S, Burger R, Giese A, Rohde V. Perioperative course and accuracy of screw positioning in conventional, open robotic-guided and percutaneous robotic-guided, pedicle screw placement. *Eur Spine J*. 2011;20:860–868.
22. Devito D, Kaplan L, Dietl R, et al. Clinical acceptance and accuracy assessment of spinal implants guided with SpineAssist surgical robot. *Spine Phila Pa 1976*. 2010;35(24):2109–2115.
23. Grimm F, Naros G, Gutenberg A, Keric N, Griese A, Gharabaghi A. Blurring the boundaries between frame-based and frameless stereotaxy: feasibility study for brain biopsies performed with the use of a head-mounted robot. *J Neurosurg*. 2015;123:737–742.
24. VanSickle D. *Accuracy of Robotic Guided Subthalamic Nucleus Deep Brain Stimulation for Parkinson's Disease*. November 2014. http://cdn2.hubspot.net/hub/276703/file-2632119232-pdf/docs/RoboticDBSWhitePaper.pdf?__hssc=245777499.12.1432246476596&__hstc=245777499.6da3b5c-c931fc9e8e0fbe4303cef9c82.1398801594641.1432062359210.1432246476596.128&hsCtaTracking=7515dbde-0116-4cca-8d14-1c48129738e0%7C5900ad8d-fe55-4f82-aecd-22c598c7d06b&t=1487114006000.
25. Lefranc M, Capel C, Pruvot-Occean A, et al. Frameless robotic stereotactic biopsies: a consecutive series of 100 cases. *J Neurosurg*. 2015;122:342–352.
26. Gonzalez-Martinez J, Bulacio J, Thompson S, et al. Technique, results, and complications related to robot-assisted stereoelectroencephalography. *Neurosurgery*. 2016;78:169–180.
27. Lefranc M, Peltier J. Accuracy of thoracolumbar transpedicular and vertebral body percutaneous screw placement: coupling the ROSA Spine robot with intraoperative flat-panel CT guidance – a cadaver study. *J Robot Surg*. 2015;9:331–338.
28. Lonjon N, Chan-Seng E, Costalat V, Bonnafoux B, Vassal M, Boetto J. Robot-assisted spine surgery: feasibility study through a prospective case-matched analysis. *Eur Spine J*. 2016;25:947–955.
29. Hoshide R, Calayag M, Meltzer H, Levy M, Gonda D. Robot-assisted endoscopic third ventriculostomy. *Neurosurgery*. 2016;63(suppl 1).
30. Varma T, Eldridge P. Use of the NeuroMate stereotactic robot in a frameless mode for functional neurosurgery. *Int J Med Robot Comput Assist Surg*. 2006;2:107–113.
31. Li Q, Zamorano L, Pandya A, Perez R, Gong J, Diaz F. The application accuracy of the NeuroMate robot – a quantitative comparison with frameless and frame-based surgical localization systems. *Comput Aided Surg*. 2002;7:90–98.
32. Cardinale F, Massimo C, Castana L, et al. Stereoelectroencephalography: surgical methodology, safety, and stereotactic application accuracy in 500 patients. *Neurosurgery*. 2013;72(3):353–366.
33. von Langsdorff D, Paquis P, Fontaine D. In vivo measurement of the frame-based application accuracy of the NeuroMate neurosurgical robot. *J Neurosurg*. 2015;122:191–194.
34. Lefranc M, Capel C, Pruvot A, et al. The impact of the reference imaging modality, registration method and intraoperative flat-panel computed tomography on the accuracy of the ROSA stereotactic robot. *Stereotact Funct Neurosurg*. 2014;92:242–250.
35. Macario A. What does 1 min of operating room time cost? *J Clin Anesth*. 2010;22:233–236.
36. Dixon P, Grant R, Urbach D. The impact of marketing language on patient preference for robot-assisted surgery. *Surg Innov*. 2015;22(1):15–19.
37. Martin A, Larson P, Ostrem J, et al. Placement of deep brain stimulator electrodes using real-time high-field interventional magnetic resonance imaging. *Magn Reson Med*. 2005;54(5):1107–1114.
38. De Momi E, Caborni C, Cardinale F, et al. Multi-trajectories automatic planner for StereoElectroEncephaloGraphy (SEEG). *Int J Comput Assist Radiol Surg*. 2014;9(6):1087–1097.
39. Sparks R, Zombori G, Rodionov R, et al. Automated multiple trajectory planning algorithm for the placement of stereo-electroencephalography (SEEG) electrodes in epilepsy patients. *Int J Comput Assist Radiol Surg*. 2017;12(1):123–136.
40. McBeth P, Louw D, Rizun P, Sutherland G. Robotics in neurosurgery. *Am J Surg*. 2004;188:68S–75S.
41. Winckel C, Reznick R, Cohen R, Taylor B. Reliability and construct validity of a structured technical skills assessment form. *Am J Surg*. 1994;167:423–427.
42. Haegelen C, Touzet G, Reyns N, Maurage C, Ayachi M, Blond S. Stereotactic robot-guided biopsies of brain stem lesions: experience with 15 cases. *Neurochirurgie*. 2010;56(5):363–367.
43. Abhinav K, Prakash S, Sandeman D. Use of robot-guided stereotactic placement of intracerebral electrodes for investigation of focal epilepsy: initial experience in the UK. *Br J Neurosurg*. 2013;27(5):704–705.
44. Gonzalez-Martinez J, Vadera S, Mullin J, et al. Robot-assisted stereotactic laser ablation in medically intractable epilepsy: operative technique. *Oper Neurosurg*. 2014;10:167–173.

CHAPTER 28

Central and Peripheral Neurosurgical Ablative Techniques for Hypertonia

WALID AHMED ABDEL GHANY, MD, PHD •
MOHAMED ABDEL RAHMAN NADA, MD, PHD

KEY POINTS

- Neurosurgical ablative treatments have a very long history for hypertonic disorders starting in the late 19th century.
- Proper evaluation of hypertonia is crucial. Failure to distinguish between specific types of hypertonia may significantly affect the outcome of certain treatment modality.
- There are no worldwide accepted protocols for hypertonia. All existing treatment protocols are based on individual and\or institutional experience.

BACKGROUND AND DEFINITIONS

Hypertonia is the abnormal increase in muscle tone, which is a major component of chronic motor disorders and upper motor neuron syndrome (UMNS). This disorder results from damage to the motor pathways, which can be seen in many neurologic conditions (cerebral palsy, stroke, multiple sclerosis, posttraumatic brain or spinal cord injury, and many other central nervous system pathologies).[1]

Hypertonia involves abnormally increased resistance to externally imposed movement around a joint and is experienced by the examiner during attempts at passive movement of a joint. Examples of hypertonic disorders include spasticity, dystonia, and rigidity.

Spasticity is defined as a hypertonia that is associated with one or both of the following signs: (1) resistance to passive movement that increases with the increasing speed of stretch or (2) when the resistance to externally imposed movement rises rapidly above a threshold speed or joint angle.[2]

Dystonia is a movement disorder that is characterized by the involuntary intermittent or sustained muscular contractions that cause twisting and repetitive movements and\or abnormal postures. It is characterized by the simultaneous cocontraction of agonist and antagonist muscle groups.[2]

Rigidity is another hypertonic disorder that is characterized by isokinetic hypertonia that is present at very low speeds of movement that does not vary with the speed of movement and does not occur at a threshold.[3]

PATHOPHYSIOLOGY OF HYPERTONIA

The development of hypertonia is multifactorial; it can be summarized as a result of dysfunction of the motor control of the stretch reflexes and the local changes that occur in the muscle itself.

Abnormal Descending Control

The clinical patterns of the UMNS are largely determined by location of the lesion; the cortex, subcortical nuclei, the brainstem, and the spinal cord. These patterns are also dependent on the time after the lesion. Immediately after a lesion, there may be a period of shock, or depression of reflexes, which resolves and is replaced by hyperreflexia.

As a result of these defects, there is α and γ motor neuron hyperexcitability, decreased Ib inhibition, decreased recurrent (Renshaw cell) inhibition, and disordered reciprocal inhibition.[4,5]

Changes at the Spinal Level

These changes are a very good example for neuronal plasticity, in which a profound reorganization of spinal interneurons occurs in response to upper motor neuron (UMN) lesion. Collateral sprouting of afferents is shown to occur; this suggests that the Ia fibers may eventually constitute 10% of the synapses on motoneurons instead of the normal 1%, which may account for the exaggerated reflexes. Another well-known mechanism is denervation hypersensitivity of spinal neurons in response to diminished synaptic inputs. These changes are well established in patients with perinatal injury to the immature nervous system as cerebral palsy.[4]

Interestingly, complete transection of the spinal cord of cats at the midthoracic level leaves the hind limbs capable of generating coordinated walking movements. In general, circuits that give rise to rhythmic motor activity are called "central pattern generators." The simplest pattern generators, however, are single neurons whose membrane properties endow them with pacemaker properties. In an important series of experiments, Grillner showed that activation of *N*-methyl-D-aspartate (NMDA) receptors on spinal interneurons was sufficient to generate this locomotor activity.[6]

Changes in the Skeletal Muscles

Hyperactivity of the stretch reflex can also be due to contracture, and hypertonia can appear in some patients after contracture. With recent technical advances, it is becoming increasingly clear that there are dramatic changes within skeletal muscle as well as in the nervous system. One common finding in biopsy studies is that fiber size variability is increased in muscles from patients with spasticity.[7,8]

Recent studies demonstrated two sources that affect the passive elasticity in the muscle: first is the variation in the giant intramuscular cytoskeletal protein called "titin," and the second source is the extracellular matrix protein called collagen.[9]

There are many complex interactions between muscle cells and the extracellular matrix that may result from hypertonia. The UMNS seems to leave the muscle in a confused state in which the normal matching between the fiber size and type is lost.[8,9]

The normal control of movements is summarized in Fig. 28.1.[10]

EVALUATION OF HYPERTONIA AND MUSCULOSKELETAL CONSEQUENCES

Many of the features of the UMNS are actually more responsible for disability and consequent problems of participation than the more narrowly defined spasticity itself. The clinical features of the UMNS can be divided into two broad groups—negative phenomena and positive phenomena (Table 28.1).[11]

The clinical evaluation of hypertonia remains a complex problem. Observation of clonus or tendon hyperreflexia is easy, but it is not always easy to distinguish between resistance to stretching related to tonic spasticity or dystonic contractions and resistance related to increased intrinsic stiffness of the muscle.[12]

The clinical examination is then used to identify signs suggestive of hypertonia such as alteration of passive mobilization of the limb segment and abnormal deep tendon reflexes. The most important step consists of demonstrating that the hypertonia and\or its consequences interfere with the patient's natural movement and that treatment of this hypertonia will improve this movement.[7]

PHYSICAL ASSESSMENT

Physical examination of every patient should target the identification of type of hypertonia and its phenomenology. Physical assessment includes the assessment of the muscle tone, power, joints range of motion (ROM), and gait cycle assessment in ambulatory patients.

Many scales have been proposed for measurement of the muscle tone; the modified Ashworth scale[13] and the Tardieu scale[14] were the most validated scales.

ELECTROPHYSIOLOGIC ASSESSMENT

The technologic advances in gait laboratories, instrumented gait analysis, and dynamic surface electromyographic (EMG) measurement have developed very rapidly since the 1970s and have added much helpful data in the management of disabled patients.[15]

Electrophysiologic assessment can be useful to complete the clinical evaluation, especially to quantify the effect of treatments. Electromyographic measures of excitability of resting potentials, assessment of late responses in motor nerve conduction stimulation as H-reflex and Hmax/Mmax ratio, F-wave and F/M ratio, objective assessment of interference patterns, degree of impaired motor activity produced by paretic muscles, and timing of antagonist cocontraction using the dual channel EMG are considered in objective assessment and evaluation of these patients.[16–18]

The attribution of hypertonia to the disability should always be considered. Mobility and difficulty walking could be due to incoordination, combination of soft-tissue contractures, flexor or extensor spasms, and truncal spasticity or dystonia. Pain is another common associated problem that may be due to flexor or extensor spasms, osteoarthritic changes, joint subluxation, or dislocation.

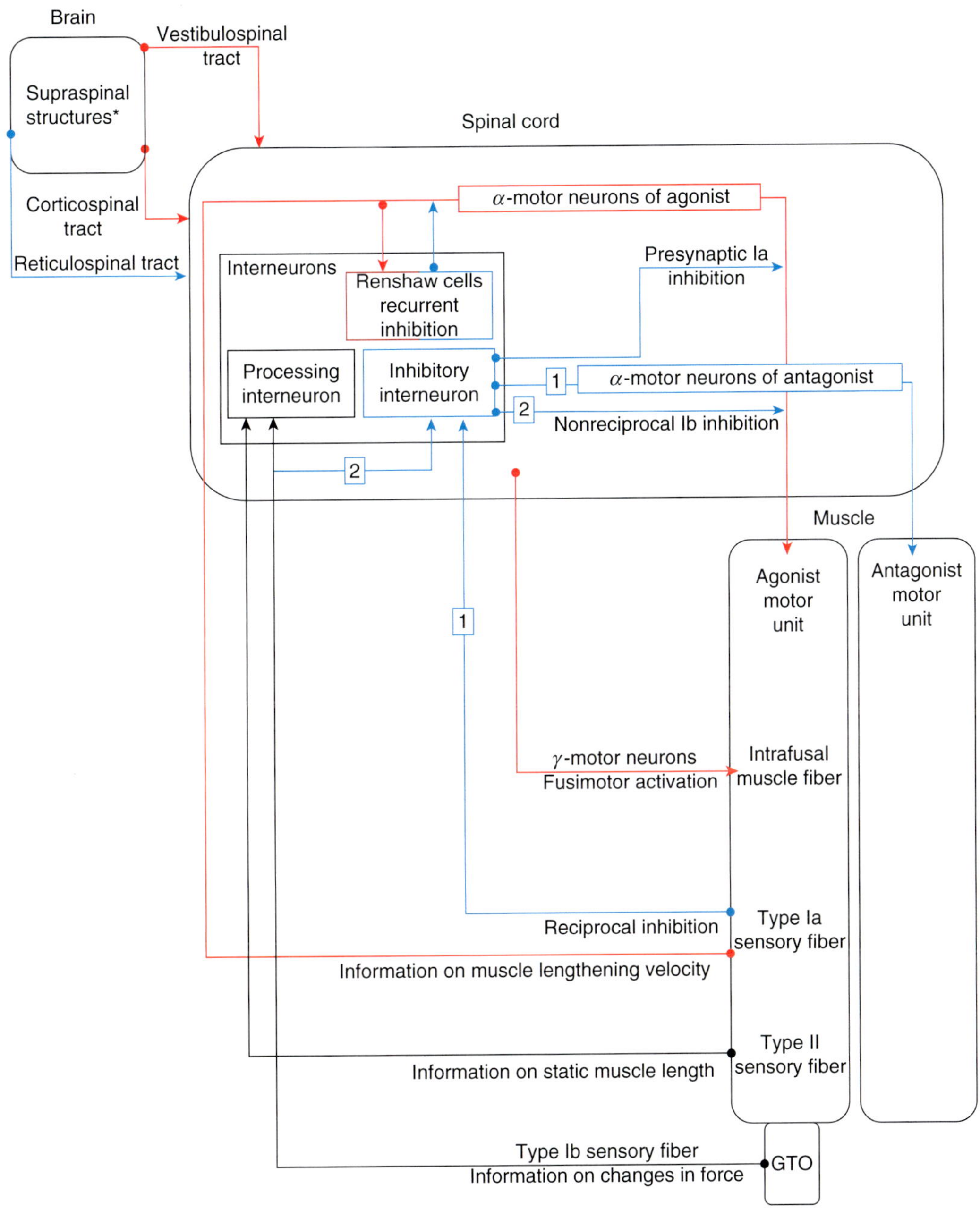

FIG. 28.1 Ascending and descending pathways controlling movement in humans: The major excitatory (red lines), inhibitory (*blue lines*), and processing (*black lines*) pathways involved in the reflex regulation contributing to normal trunk and limb muscle tone. Pathways numbered (1) and (2) travel first through interneurons before synapsing with alpha- (α-) motor neurons. *GTO*, golgi tendon organ. *Some extrapyramidal tracts (not shown in this figure) also contribute to the maintenance of normal muscle tone, and not all pathways shown are necessarily involved in increased stretch reflex due to spasticity. (Adapted from Lynn Bar-On, Molenaers G, Aertbelien E, Campenhout AV, Feys H, Nuttin B, Desloovere K. Spasticity and its contribution to hypertonia in cerebral palsy. Review article. *BioMed Res Int*. 2015.)

TABLE 28.1
Negative and Positive Signs of the Upper Motor Neuron Syndrome

Negative	Positive
Weakness	Increased tendon reflexes with radiation
Loss of dexterity	Clonus
Fatigability	Positive Babinski sign
	Hypertonia
	Extensor spasms
	Flexor spasms
	Mass reflex
	Dyssynergic patterns of cocontraction during movement
	Associated dyssynergic and stereotypical spastic dystonias

PREOPERATIVE DIAGNOSIS OF THE TYPE OF HYPERTONIA AND IMPACT ON OUTCOME MEASURES

The proper evaluation of each type of hypertonia is crucial for proper management. Spasticity is diagnosed by its length and velocity dependency, whereas the dystonic hypertonia is characterized by the cocontraction phenomenon and the overflow movement of one limb when moving the other. Dystonia may have a repetitive pattern or a specific posture, whereas rigidity is characterized by its isokinetic hypertonia, which is not related to velocity or stretch.

Failure to distinguish between specific types of hypertonia may significantly affect the outcome of certain treatment modality. For example, patients who are subjected to selective dorsal rhizotomy (SDR) may get a poor outcome or have a recurrence of hypertonia due to the presence of dystonia.

In addition, failure to distinguish between hypertonia and musculoskeletal changes (muscle contracture or joint deformity) can also lead to unfavorable outcome.[10]

HISTORY OF NEUROSURGICAL ABLATIVE TECHNIQUES

Neurosurgical treatments have a very long history for these different types of disorders. Lorenz did the first obturator neurotomy in 1887 to relieve focal adductor spasm,[19] and in 1889, Sherrington demonstrated that spasticity was associated with hyperexcitability of stretch reflex owing to loss of supraspinal inhibitory influence and that posterior rhizotomy led to reduction of spasticity in decerebrate animals. After this report, in 1908, Forester performed total dorsal rhizotomy to relieve spasticity in both lower limbs, but it was associated with loss of all types of sensation.[20]

In 1908, Horsley dramatically relieved spasmodic movements by resection of the precentral gyrus. Cortical resections for treatment of movement disorders, tremor, and spasticity followed through the 1930s. In 1939, Meyers examined the role of the basal ganglia in the production of movement disorders and the interruption of these structures as treatment. Putnam had opted for interruption of the descending motor fibers at the level of the cervical cord, and Walker had sectioned them to the level of the cerebral peduncles. These surgeons' efforts directed at the pyramidal motor system were effective in relieving involuntary movements but produced hemiparesis.[21]

In 1951, Bischof first described the longitudinal myelotomy. In 1960, Pourpre modified Bischof's technique to be less injurious. In 1972, surgery in the dorsal root entry zone (DREZ) of the spinal cord was introduced for the treatment of persistent pain. This technique also induced important hypotonia and was therefore used to treat severe focalized spasticity, not only of the lower limbs but also of the upper limbs.[22]

TREATMENT SELECTION AND MANAGEMENT ALGORITHMS

To the authors' knowledge, there is no worldwide accepted treatment protocol that set selection criteria for each treatment modality. All existing treatment protocols are based on individual and\or institutional experience and economic circumstances. For example, in model 1 (Fig. 28.2),[23] the author adopted a treatment protocol for muscle tone involving chemical neuromodulation techniques rather than ablative procedures.

Model 2 (Fig. 28.3), adopted by the author's institute, extensively involves multimodal evaluation hierarchy and multimodal treatment options (Ain Shams University Hospitals).

CENTRAL ABLATIVE TECHNIQUES

In Spinal Cord

Dorsal root entry zone ablation

The first trial of Marc Sindou in 1972, which was directed to control intractable pain, had resulted in marked hypotonia in the treated previously painful limbs. Since that observation, they suggested a new indication of dorsal root entry zone lesioning for treatment of intractable spasticity and the procedure was called microsurgical DREZotomy (MDT).[24]

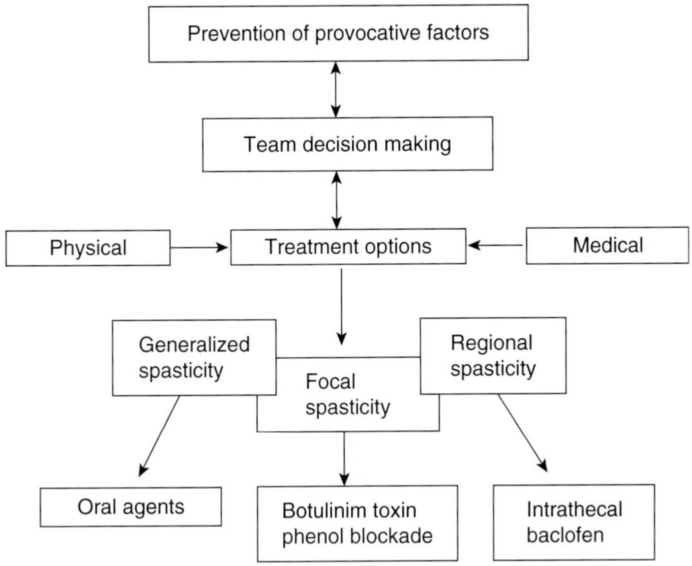

FIG. 28.2 Spasticity management strategy developed by Anthony B. Ward. (Adopted from Ward AB. Long-term modification of spasticity. *J Rehabil Med*. 2003;41(suppl.):60–65.)

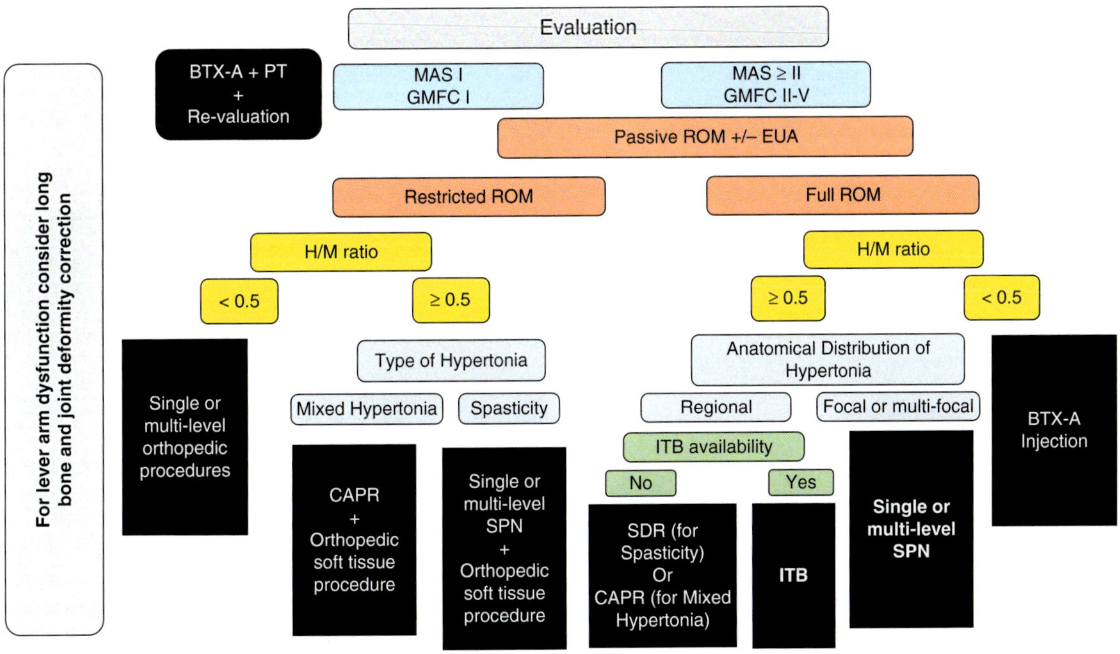

FIG. 28.3 Ain Shams University algorithm for management of hypertonia. *BTX-A*, Botulinum toxin type A; *CAPR*, combined anterior and posterior rhizotomy; *EUA*, examination under anesthesia; *GMFC*, gross motor function classification; *ITB*, intrathecal baclofen pump; *MAS*, modified Ashworth scale; *PT*, physical therapy; *SDR*, selective dorsal rhizotomy; *SPN*, selective peripheral neurotomy; *ROM*, range of motion.

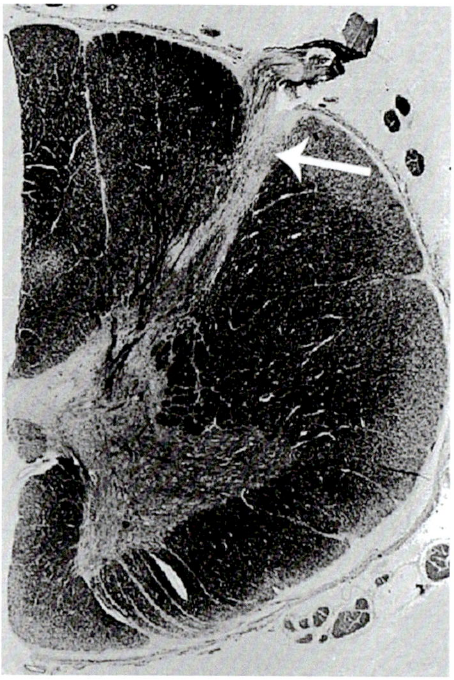

FIG. 28.4 Transverse hemisection of the spinal cord at the lower cervical level with myelin stained by Luxol-Fuchsin showing the dorsal root entry zone (*arrow*). (Adopted from Sindou M, Mertens P. Surgery in the dorsal root entry zone for pain. *Semin Neurosurg* 2004;15(2/3).)

The DREZ area includes the central segment of the dorsal rootlets, the tract of Lissauer, and the five dorsal-most layers of the dorsal horn where the primary afferents terminate (Fig. 28.4).

The purpose of the MDT is to preferentially interrupt both small (nociceptive) and large caliber (myotatic) tonigenic fibers of the dorsal roots, situated laterally and in the middle of the entry zone, respectively. The surgical lesion must partially, if not totally, preserve the medial large caliber fibers that project to the dorsal horn and must be located medially in the entry zone to preserve the sensory and inhibitory interneurons to the dorsal horn.[25]

Indications

1. The spastic hemiplegic upper limb can benefit from MDT, predominantly for shoulder and elbow functions, but much less at the level of the wrist and fingers, especially if there are irreducible deformities in flexion and no motor function in the extensors. So, MDT may be particularly indicated when there is an excess of spasticity in the proximal muscles.
2. For lower limbs, because MDT has generally a dramatic effect on tone, indications must be restricted to paraplegic patients with severe disability, unable to walk and uncomfortable in wheelchair and/or exposed to pressure sores in bed.

Surgical technique. MDT is performed under general anesthesia with short-acting muscle relaxant to allow for intraoperative stimulation of ventral roots for mapping of the spinal segments controlling the spastic muscles.

MDT consists of an incision and bipolar coagulations performed ventrolaterally at the entrance of the rootlets into the dorsolateral sulcus. This lesion should penetrate the lateral part of DREZ and the medial part of Lissauer tract extending downward to the apex of dorsal horn. The latter is recognized under the surgical microscope by its brown-gray color.[26]

The technical advances introduced other surgical techniques to produce the DREZ lesion. Radiofrequency thermocoagulation and laser beam lesioning were introduced in multiple articles aiming at producing less extensive lesions that do not encroach upon the neighboring corticospinal tract and dorsal column to minimize the side effects.[27]

Outcome. MDT was found to be very effective in reduction of spasticity and spasms. Sindou and his colleagues had the largest series of MDT; 94 patients had MDT in the cervical level for spastic upper limb, and 175 patients had MDT in the lumbosacral levels for spastic paraplegic lower limbs. For the paraplegic patients, 75% of patients had marked improvement in spasticity and 88% of patients had improved pain and spasms. For the hemiplegic patients, spasticity was abolished or reduced significantly in 87% of patients with better passive mobilization in 87% of patients.[28]

Complications. The main complication is the marked decrease in lemniscal sensitivity; nearly 70% of patients suffered this complication.[24] Permanent motor or sphincteric dysfunctions were also reported. Sepsis and death were reported in five patients with severe paraplegia due to multiple sclerosis. [27]

Other complications include cerebrospinal fluid (CSF) collection or leaks, spine deformities, or epidural hematoma.[29,30]

Myelotomy

Bischof was the first to describe the longitudinal myelotomy procedure. He aimed at interruption of the spinal reflex arc between the ventral and dorsal horns through a vertical coronal incision performed laterally from one side of the spinal cord to the other.[31]

Pourpre then modified the Bischof's technique to avoid interruption of the corticospinal tract fibers. Through a laminectomy from T9 to L1, the procedure consisted in making a posterior longitudinal sagittal incision before performing a cruciform myelotomy by transverse incision on either side with a stylet with a right-angled extremity. The purpose of this surgical lesion was to interrupt the spinal reflex arc between the ventral and dorsal horns without sectioning the fibers connecting the pyramidal tract to the motor neurons of the ventral horn.[32]

Laitinen and Singounas then designed a special surgical knife to perform less damaging myelotomies. Myelotomies are applied for the treatment of spasticity in bedridden paraplegic patients with triple flexion and severe sphincter disorders.[33,34]

Outcome. Laitinen and Singounas had favored the dorsal midline longitudinal myelotomies because of the suggested advantage of preservation of the connection between the pyramidal tracts and anterior horn cells. Sparing of these connections allows for the motor recovery after the myelotomy.[33] The effect of myelotomy was reported by many authors to be encouraging results.[33,35]

Brain Ablative Procedures

Stereotactic brain lesioning

Stereotactic neurosurgery was introduced by Spiegel and Wycis in 1950. Several targets for lesioning have been explored over time (different locations within the thalamus, dentate nucleus, globus pallidus internus, and subthalamic nucleus), and the results reported in the literature are miscellaneous. More recently, deep brain stimulation (DBS) has been implemented.[36]

Stereotactic functional procedures should be considered in individuals who are suffering from dystonic or rigid hypertonia that do not respond to conservative treatment options. We should consider the indications of each surgical option according to the etiology, the severity, the distribution, the presence of other neurologic symptoms, the patients' age, and the aimed goals to be achieved for each patient.

The principle of stereotactic approaches is the precise targeting of the basal ganglia in movement and hypertonic disorders. Many advances were developed recently in frameless stereotactic techniques and the older frame-based stereotaxy. Some neurosurgical centers recently favor the magnetic resonance–guided focused ultrasound lesioning or the use of the stereotactic radio surgery to induce a brain lesion.

Surgical technique. The stereotactic brain lesioning surgeries are preferably performed while patients are awake to allow for intraoperative assessment of motor, sensory, speech, and visual responses to macrostimulation (Fig. 28.5). If painful spasms or severe involuntary

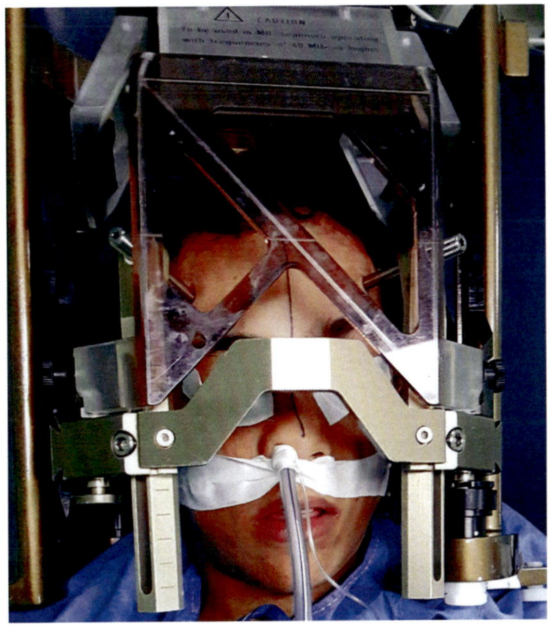

FIG. 28.5 Frame-based stereotactic targeting; the localizer is attached to the base ring and is ready for imaging.

movements make awake surgery difficult, conscious sedation with propofol or dexmedetomidine is used.

Thalamotomy. The thalamus was used as a target for decades before the posteroventral lateral GPi has been established as the first-line target for treatment of dystonia. Over the decades, it was considered to be advantageous in secondary dystonia. The thalamic target of choice for treatment of dystonia was variable among surgeons compared with the thalamic target for treatment of tremors. The targets included the ventralis oralis internus, the ventralis intermedius (Vim), the nucleus ventralis oralis anterior and posterior (Voa/Vop), the subthalamic region, the centrum medianum/nucleus parafascicularis complex (CM-Pf), and the pulvinar thalami. Nowadays, the thalamic Vim is used almost exclusively.[37]

Pallidotomy. The target for treatment of dystonia is located in the posteroventral lateral portion of the GPi (Fig. 28.6). Microelectrode recording is helpful in identifying the internal and the external borders of the GPi and the external segment of the globus pallidus (GPe). Usually, two lesions are placed with a distance of 2 mm along the trajectory of the radiofrequency probe. The effect of surgery on phasic movements may be apparent early postoperatively, whereas the tonic dystonic movements may be improved after a longer

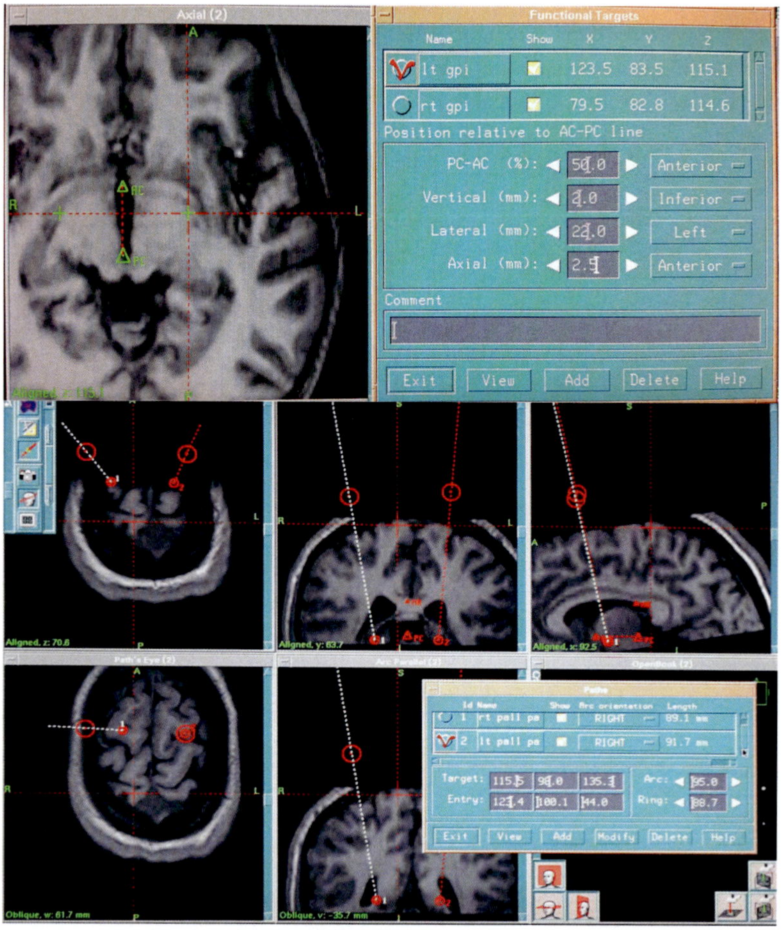

FIG. 28.6 Leksell SurgiPlan software showing the coordinates and path definition for bilateral GPi targeting.

period from weeks to months. Pallidotomy for dystonia has a risk of contralateral hemiparesis if the lesion is too close to the internal capsule in unilateral surgery, and for speech disturbance in bilateral surgery.[38]

Outcome. Many studies have reported that patients with atypical parkinsonian rigidity associated with some conditions such as progressive supranuclear palsy, multiple system atrophy, and dementia do not respond well to surgical lesioning.

In the mid-20th century, dystonia was treated with thalamotomy rather than pallidotomy. The success of pallidotomy to treat rigidity, dyskinesia, and dystonia in Parkinson disease led to the appearance of many striking articles recommending pallidotomy in primary generalized dystonia.[39]

A surge of reports followed this, reporting the success of pallidotomy in primary dystonia and more limited success in secondary dystonia. Coincidentally, the first publication on pallidotomy for dystonia by Iacono and colleagues[40] appeared in the same year of the paper on Vim DBS for tremors published by Benabid et al.[41] Rapidly the DBS began to replace pallidotomy for treatment of dystonia.

The advantages of the radiofrequency lesioning surgeries over DBS are the lower costs, no risk of hardware failure, the lower risk of infections, and there is no need for periodic battery replacements. However, DBS of the GPi and thalamus had replaced the lesioning procedures because of the lower risk of performing bilateral surgery in one session. Moreover, it avoids concern about the impact of lesioning on the developing brain in children.[42]

PERIPHERAL ABLATIVE TECHNIQUES

Selective Dorsal Rhizotomy

Dorsal rhizotomy is the oldest standard surgical technique for treating spasticity. Total dorsal rhizotomy was performed in 1908 by Forester, which was associated with loss of all types of sensation. In 1976, Gros and coworkers developed the SDR by sparing one-fifth of each root. In 1977, Fraioli and Guidetti reported a procedure by dividing the dorsal half of each rootlet in the selected dorsal root, which is known as partial dorsal rhizotomy. In 1979, Private and Frerebeau developed the sectorial dorsal rhizotomy, based on the preoperative topographic selection of the affected roots and confirmed by intraoperative localization by electrical stimulation. The more understanding of specially organized circuits of spasticity led Fasano and associates to propose the functional dorsal rhizotomy based on intraoperative stimulation and recording of EMG responses.[43–45]

Indications

SDR is designed mainly for children with nonprogressive disorders such as cerebral palsy, and the best results were seen in those with spastic diplegia where it is performed in the lumbosacral roots.

Contraindications

1. Mixed hypertonia with dystonia, rigidity, athetosis, or ataxia
2. Progressive neurologic disorders
3. Severe basal ganglia damage in children younger than 5 years
4. Severe thoracolumbar scoliosis and severe lumbar lordosis
5. Profound motor impairment with no head control
6. Lack of commitment to perform postoperative therapy

Surgical Techniques

Many technical variants for exposure of the cauda equina have been postulated. The most common technique was the Peacock technique.[46]

Patients are operated in prone position, under general anesthesia without or with short-acting muscle relaxant to allow for intraoperative stimulation and recordings. Then, laminotomy from L1 to S1 is performed, and the dura and arachnoid are opened longitudinally and then roots are identified at their exit foramina (Fig. 28.7).

Other limited exposure techniques were popularized by Park and colleagues in which they do a limited exposure below the conus level guided by intraoperative ultrasound. Then they perform a single-level laminectomy and make the dural and arachnoid opening to expose the cauda equine just below the conus medullaris.[47,48]

Recently, a minimally invasive interlaminar approach was developed by Sindou. The target roots are approached through a small laminotomy in the upper and lower laminae and excision of the ligamentum flavum, and then the dura is exposed at the target levels.[49]

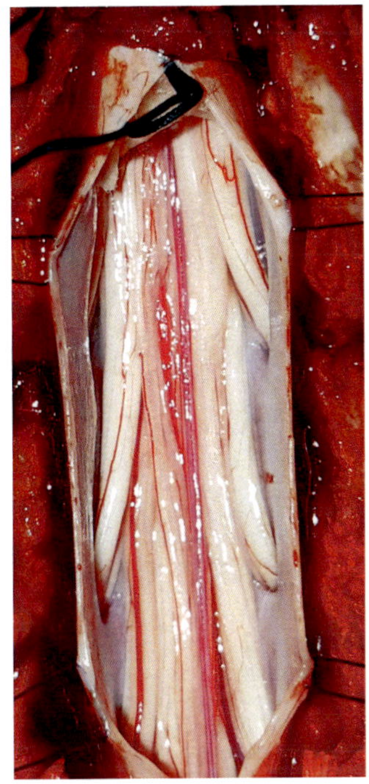

FIG. 28.7 After opening the dura and arachnoid, the roots are identified at their exit foramina. Intraoperative stimulation and recording is a very useful tool to help in identification of the segmental levels.

Sectioning of the roots is according to the intraoperative grading of the responses of each dorsal root to stimulation. First, the whole posterior root is tested with single stimuli, and then individual rootlets of the selected roots are dissected and tested separately. Single constant square-wave pulses of 0.1 ms duration are applied to the rootlet at a rate of 0.5 Hz. The stimulus intensity is increased stepwise until a reflex response appears from the ipsilateral muscles. After the reflex threshold is determined, a 50-Hz train of tetanic stimulation for 1 s is applied to the rootlet. The reflex response is then graded according to the criteria detailed in Table 28.2. The rootlets that produce a response of 0 are left intact. The rootlets producing 3+ and 4+ responses are cut, and those producing 1+ and 2+ responses are sometimes spared. If only 1+ and 2+ responses are detected, then rootlets with the most active responses are cut. Usually, no more than 75% of dorsal rootlets are sectioned, and monitoring of the pelvic floor muscles and sphincters is mandatory to avoid profound weakness or sphincteric dysfunctions (Fig. 28.8).[50]

Outcome

SDR has proven to be effective in tone reduction and has been validated in its long-term effect. Langerak

TABLE 28.2
Criteria for Grading of Electromyographic Responses for Dorsal Roots

Grade	Electromyographic Responses
0	Unsustained or single discharge to a train of stimuli
1+	Sustained discharges from muscles innervated through the segment stimulated in the ipsilateral lower extremity
2+	Sustained discharges from muscles innervated through the segment stimulated and immediately adjacent segments
3+	Sustained discharges segmentally innervated muscles as well as muscles innervated through segments distant to the segment stimulated
4+	Sustained discharges from contralateral muscles with or without sustained discharges from the ipsilateral muscles

and his colleagues have published a 20-year follow-up study that focused on the functional performance and gait. Patients with spastic diplegia showed functional improvements and prolonged reduction of spasticity.[51]

Complications

Complications could be classified according to the onset:

Intraoperative complications: The most common is aspiration pneumonia. Subdural hematoma and bronchospasm were experienced in Steinbok and Schrag series.[52]

Immediate postoperative complications: Bronchospasm is the most common in CP children, CSF leakage, sensory loss, ileus, meningitis, and wound infection.[53] In a series of 200 children, Abbott and his colleagues experienced serious complications in 35 children, urinary retention 7%, bronchospasm 5.5%, aspiration pneumonia 3.5%, minor dysesthesia 40%, and sensory loss 2%.[54]

Delayed complications: Sensory loss, dysesthesia, hypotonia, and spinal deformity due to extensive laminectomy; 20% of 99 patients developed isthmic spondylolysis or grade I spondylolisthesis following five-level laminectomy; and the majority of patients were ambulatory and active.[55]

Combined anterior and posterior rhizotomy

The mixed state of hypertonia is a common clinical problem especially in children with cerebral palsy; failure to detect this dystonic element may lead to failure of the treatment modalities used. Kim and his colleagues had tried to determine the preoperative clinical characteristics that might be predictive of poor outcomes after SDR surgery; the most important factors were the intellectual delay, truncal hypotonia, and mixed hypertonicity.[56]

Through this procedure, patients who suffer from mixed spastic dystonic diplegia—especially children with cerebral palsy (CP)—are subjected to intradural combined rhizotomy for both anterior and posterior roots. It is believed that rhizotomy of the anterior roots targets the dystonic element and sectioning of the posterior root affects the spastic element (Fig. 28.9).[57]

Recent reports demonstrated the efficacy of combined anterior and posterior rhizotomy in the control of hypertonia and involuntary dystonic movements.[57,58]

Best candidates who would benefit from this surgery are as follows:

1. Children with cerebral palsy due to a stationary pathology (e.g., perinatal hypoxic encephalopathy, postkernicterus encephalopathy, postencephalitic sequelae)
2. Age ranging from 4 to 18 years
3. Lower-extremity mixed hypertonia presented as a moderate to severe spasticity and dystonia with a predominance of the dystonia
4. Hypertonia intractable to other treatment modalities, such as tone-lowering medications, physical therapy, and\or botulinum toxin injections

Surgery is performed under general anesthesia without long-acting muscle relaxants. The fine adjustment of the depth of anesthesia and the use of drugs that do not interfere with neuromuscular transmission are important issues because of the extensive use of intraoperative electrophysiologic stimulation and recording (Fig. 28.10).

The cauda equine exposure is performed similar to the techniques of exposure in SDR.

- Lesioning of the dorsal roots: It is also performed according to Philips and Park's criteria (Table 28.2).
- The rationale of the anterior roots: Each individual anterior root from L1 to S1 is dissected into multiple rootlets (4–6 rootlets). Cutting of the anterior roots is performed according to the evaluation of the severity of preoperative dystonic elements. A maximum of 80% of the rootlets are cut in severe cases and 50% in moderate cases to avoid muscular atrophy (Fig. 28.11).[57]

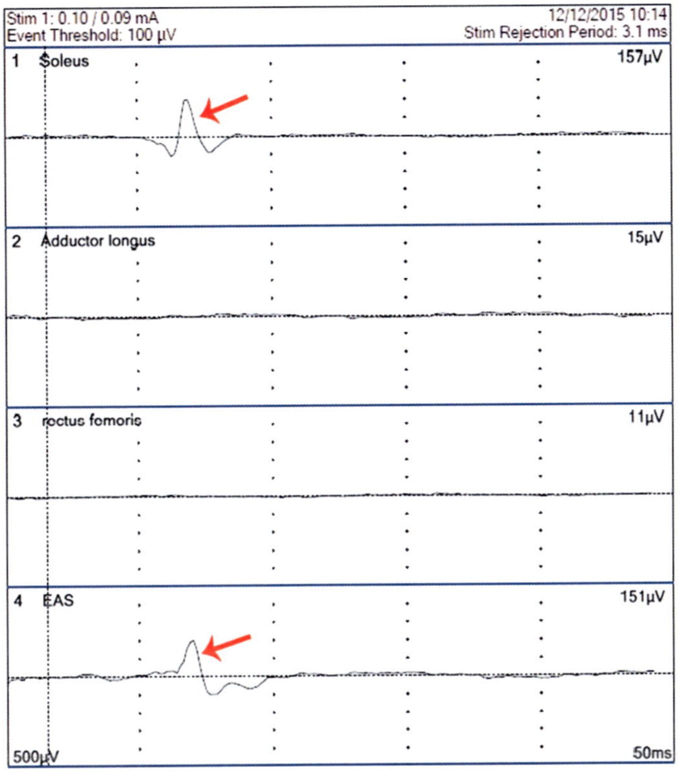

FIG. 28.8 Intraoperative screenshot of simultaneous EMG recording of the external anal sphincter (EAS) during stimulation of the S1 root.

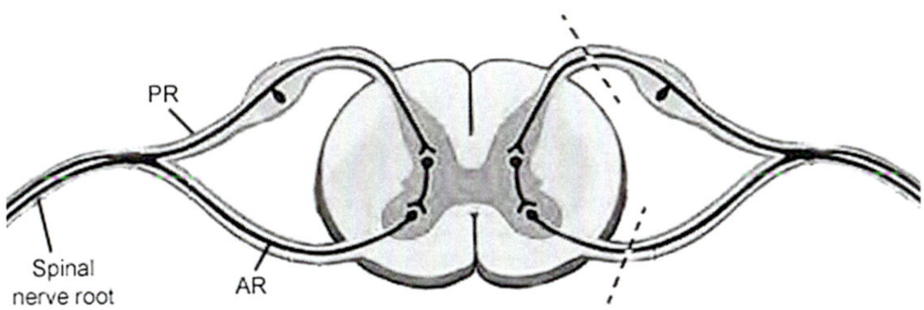

FIG. 28.9 Sectioning of the anterior (AR) and posterior (PR) rootlets in patients suffering from mixed dystonia and spasticity.

The postoperative improvement of the mixed state of spasticity and dystonia allows for the possibility of functional improvements as well as the improvement of the daily activities and care (Figs. 28.12 and 28.13).

Complications

In the authors' published series, four children (8%) developed postoperative complications. One boy developed subcutaneous CSF collection by the second postoperative day with no leakage through the suture line, which was managed conservatively. One girl had superficial wound dehiscence that required secondary sutures. One boy had abdominal distention due to ileus on the first postoperative day, and it was treated conservatively. One girl had urinary retention, which required urinary catheterization for 2 weeks postoperatively.[58]

Selective Peripheral Denervation (Bertrand procedure)

This procedure is an ablative surgery specific on peripheral motor nerves innervating dystonic neck muscles,

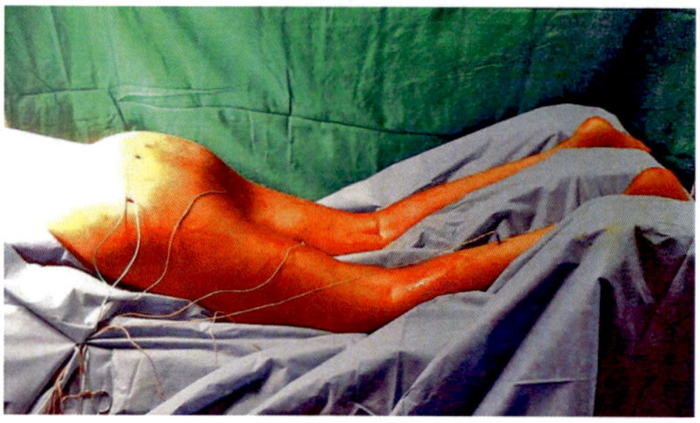

FIG. 28.10 A 16-year-old girl with mixed hypertonia of the lower limbs in prone position preparing for combined anterior and posterior rhizotomy (CAPR).

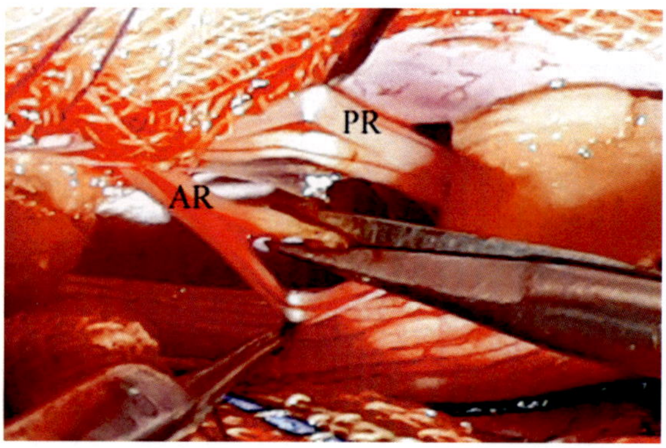

FIG. 28.11 Intraoperative picture demonstrating the sectioning of 50% of the anterior root (AR); the posterior root of the same level (PR) is suspended away from the AR.

whereas motor branches supplying normal muscles and sensory nerves are preserved.[59] Good to excellent outcome is often achieved by this procedure, so it has become a common surgical treatment for cervical dystonia.[60]

In Bertrand procedure, sectioning of the posterior rami of C3–C6 is performed, with either extraspinal C1–C2 rhizotomy or with posterior ramisectomy of C1–C2 to preserve anterior rami that are responsible for swallowing; this is followed by selective denervation of the contralateral sternocleidomastoid muscle (Fig. 28.14).[59]

Major sequela of Bertrand procedure is dysesthesia over the skin innervated by the C2 spinal nerve. The sensory disturbance of the C2 dermatome is inevitable in almost all patients who undergo this procedure. It always occurs in the early postoperative period as a result of resection of the proximal C2 dorsal ramus containing both motor and sensory nerve fibers.[61]

Additionally, there is a considerable risk of intraoperative bleeding from the paravertebral venous plexuses adjacent to the C1 and C2 posterior rami. Other potential complications include transient occipital neuralgia that usually disappears within 3 months, weakness of nondystonic muscles caused by excessive denervation, surgical site infection, and swallowing dysfunction.[62]

Taira has modified the classic procedure of Bertrand aiming to overcome these drawbacks. In his technique, he performed intradural anterior rhizotomy of C1–C2 and posterior ramisectomy of C3–C6 (Fig. 28.6).[62]

The cutting of peripheral branches supplying the sternocleidomastoid or levator scapulae endeavors to reduce their dystonia, resulting in improved neck posture and function.[59,61]

SELECTIVE PERIPHERAL NEUROTOMY

The first neurotomy was an obturator neurotomy for adductor spasm, which was performed in 1887 by Lorenz. In 1912, Stoffel proposed the first tibial neurotomy to treat spastic foot drop, and the first upper limb neurotomy was of the median nerve to treat forearm pronation spasticity. The first selective neurotomies in the nerve trunk were complicated by sensory disorders. Subsequently, the technique was modified following the studies by Gros in 1976. Only nerve branches innervating muscles identified by intraoperative electrical stimulation were sectioned. Peripheral neurotomies are designed to improve function or at least to improve comfort in maintenance of a deficient limb.[7]

THE PRINCIPLE OF ACTION

Partial Denervation and Differential Regeneration

The principle of peripheral neurotomy is based on the concept of differential regeneration. Neurotomy consists of partial section of the motor branches of the spastic muscle(s). This partial section involves afferent fibers to the spinal cord, especially large group I (Ia, Ib) and II myelinated fibers. Sectioning these fibers eliminates spasticity. In addition, sections of efferent motoneuron axons induce considerable denervation proportional to the number of sectioned fibers.[63]

Within several months, two types of regeneration occur, first is motor regeneration by sprouting of the remaining motor axons or enlargement of the already-existing endplates—about five times their original size to involve more muscle fibers. Second is sensory regeneration of the afferent proprioceptive fibers from the muscle spindle, which occur in disorganized pattern,

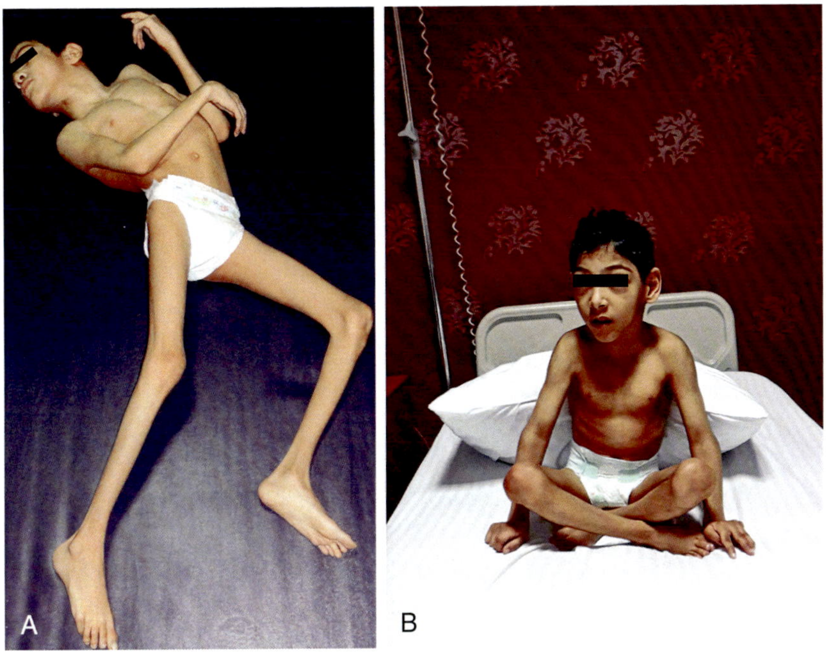

FIG. 28.12 A 6-year-old boy with CP and quadriplegia. **(A)** Preoperative dystonic posture. **(B)** The child can sit with self-support 1 year postoperatively.

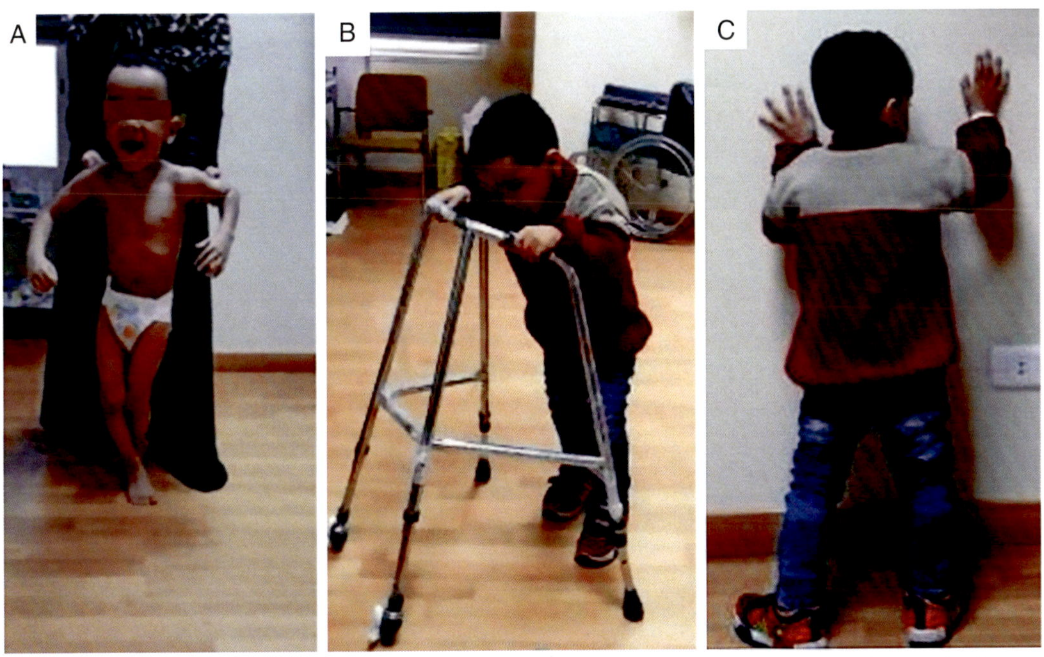

FIG. 28.13 A 5-year-old boy with CP diplegia. **(A)** Preoperative scissoring, knee flexion, and talipes equinovarus deformities. **(B** and **C)** 6 months postoperatively, the child can walk with a walker and can do side walking against the wall.

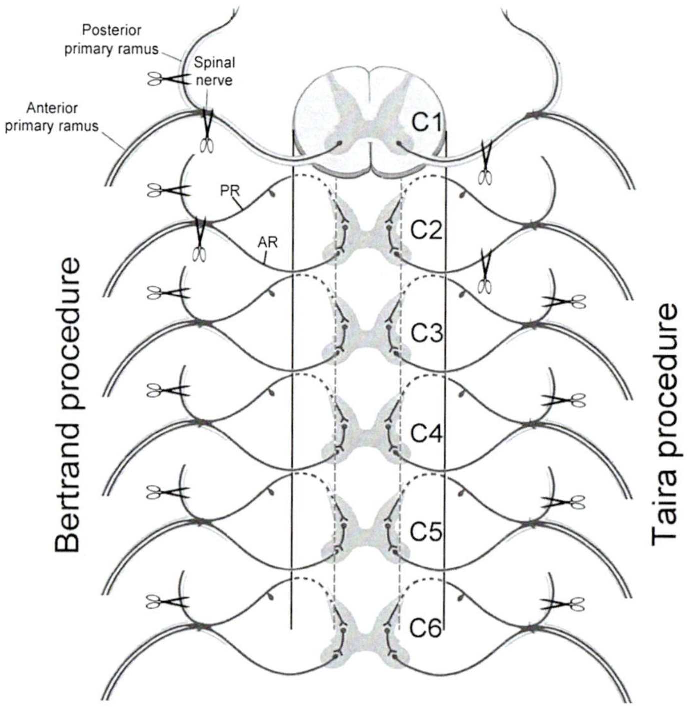

FIG. 28.14 Comparison between Bertrand procedure (left) and Taira's method (right). C1–C2 denervation in Bertrand procedure can be cut on either the spinal roots (extraspinal rhizotomy) or posterior ramisectomy. In Taira's method, intradural C1–C2 anterior rhizotomy is performed, while the C2 posterior root is preserved. C3–C6 posterior ramisectomy is identical in both procedures. The C1 posterior root and its dorsal root ganglion are usually absent in the majority of humans. *AR*, anterior root; *PR*, posterior root.

allowing long-term control of spasticity. This is proved either by histopathologic examination of spastic muscle biopsy after neurotomy or by the long-term absence of poor recovery of H-reflex and diminished Hmax/Mmax ratio.[64,65]

Indication

Selective peripheral neurotomy (SPN) is indicated in focal spastic disorder; however, a combination of several neurotomies can sometimes be considered in the case of multifocal and segmental disorders (multilevel neurotomies).

It is important to assure the presence of a good function of antagonists to help antagonize the residual spasticity. In the case of complete absence of antagonists, neurotomy can be indicated in combination with secondary tendon transfer surgery, when possible, to restore the deficient antagonists.

In case of coexistence of excessive contracture and marked spasticity, an isolated neurosurgical procedure in this context provides no benefit for the patient. An orthopedic procedure on contracture does not really treat spasticity and is associated with a high risk of recurrence. In these patients, orthopedic correction of these deformities is usually considered either in the same time or in another surgical session.[7]

Preoperative motor block

Clinical evaluation, especially by means of motor blocks, is crucial for defining the indications for these techniques and helps both the surgeon and patient to predict results and to increase their selectivity further.[66]

Surgical Techniques

SPN is performed under general anesthesia without long-acting muscle relaxants. The use of intraoperative stimulation is very crucial to help in mapping the motor branches of the targeted nerve. In addition, microscopic and microsurgical techniques should always be used in dealing with the peripheral nerve fascicles.

Selective Neurotomies in Lower Limbs

Obturator neurotomy

It aims at reducing spasticity of the hip adductors; the incision can be performed along the body of the adductor longus in the proximal part of the thigh. The anterior division of the obturator nerve is found after medial retraction of the adductor longus muscle (Fig. 28.15).

Sciatic neurotomy

Sciatic neurotomy is indicated in hamstring spasticity and knee flexion deformity. A longitudinal incision can be made in the midline of the posterior thigh while the patient is in prone position. Incision starts just below the gluteal skin crease, extending for 2 inches in the thigh. Then the main trunk of the sciatic nerve is identified after dissection between both groups of hamstrings. The branches to the medial hamstrings are identified, as they emerge from the main trunk of the nerve (Fig. 28.16).

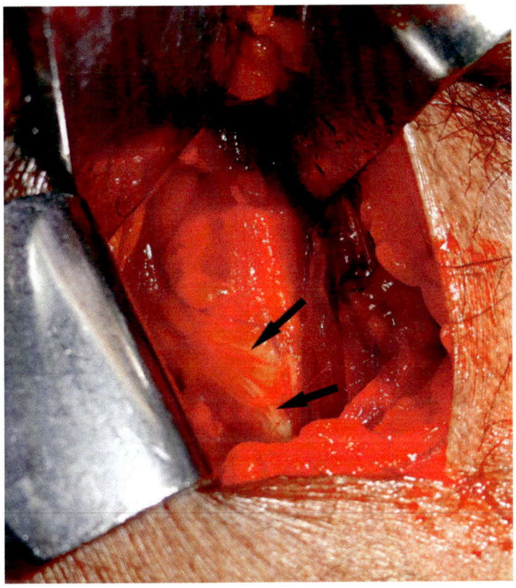

FIG. 28.15 Intraoperative view of the anterior division of the obturator nerve and its branches (*arrows*).

Tibial neurotomy

Tibial neurotomy is indicated in treatment of spastic foot; the nerve can be exposed in the popliteal fossa with either longitudinal or transverse incisions. The dissection is directed in the midline with caution not to injure the short saphenous vein or the sural nerve. The tibial nerve is found deeper to the two heads of the gastrocnemius muscle (Fig. 28.17).

Femoral neurotomy

Femoral neurotomy is indicated in patients with hypertonic quadriceps femoris, which may cause stiff knee gait and impair foot clearance during walking. The incision can be made vertically below the inguinal crease just lateral to the femoral pulsations; dissection is made medial to the sartorius muscle to expose the motor branches of the nerve (Fig. 28.18).

Common peroneal neurotomy

Common peroneal neurotomy is indicated in patients with spastic hitchhiker's toe or with peroneal spasticity; the nerve can be exposed at the lateral aspect of the leg

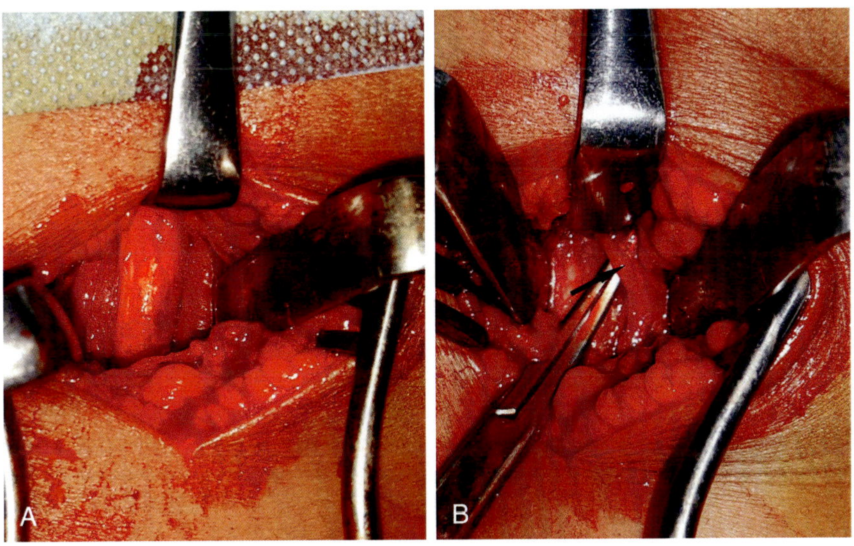

FIG. 28.16 Intraoperative picture showing exposure of **(A)** the left sciatic nerve main trunk and **(B)** the branch to the medial hamstrings (*black arrow*).

just above the palpable head of fibula, and the incision should extend obliquely toward the upper third of the leg to expose the branch to the extensor hallucis if needed (Fig. 28.19).

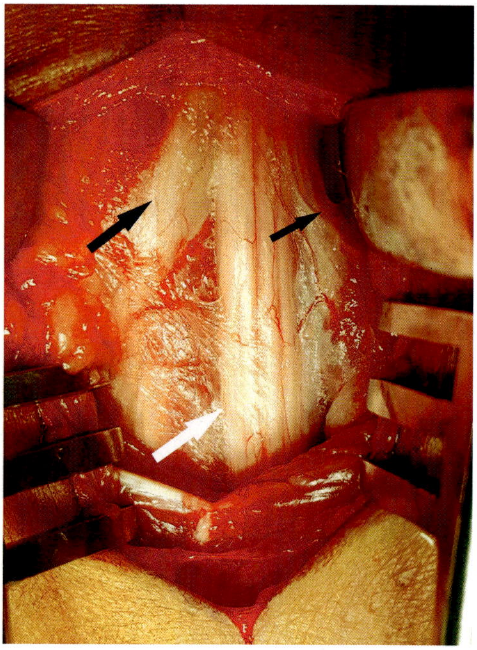

FIG. 28.17 Intraoperative view of the tibial nerve (*white arrow*); the branches to the medial and lateral heads of the gastrocnemius are viewed (*black arrows*).

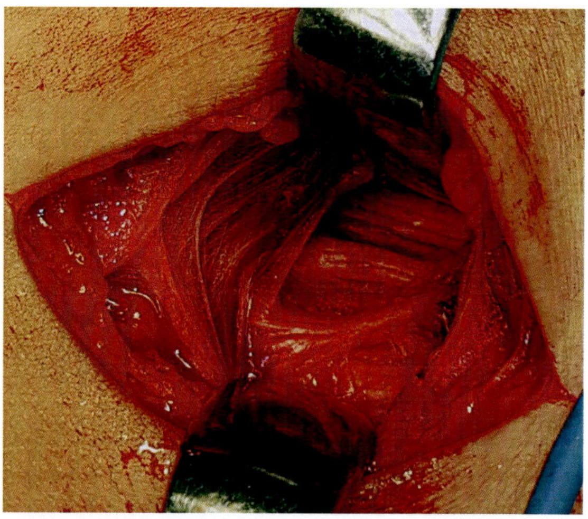

FIG. 28.18 Intraoperative exposure of the femoral nerve branches.

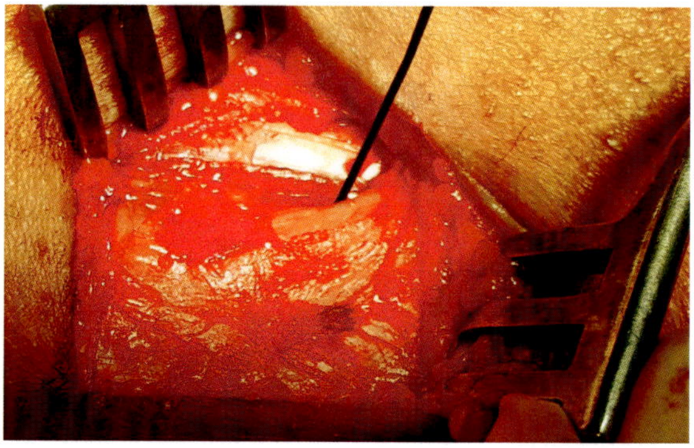

FIG. 28.19 Intraoperative picture of the right common peroneal nerve (*black arrow*); monopolar stimulation is performed for verification and mapping of the motor branches.

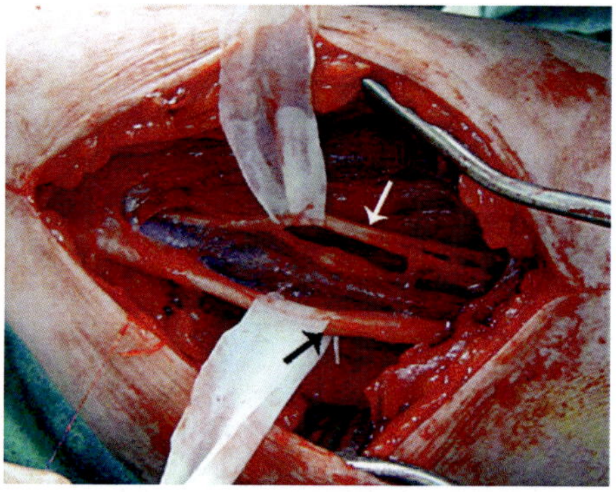

FIG. 28.20 Intraoperative picture of the left musculocutaneous (white arrow) and median nerve (black arrow) in the proximal arm.

Selective Peripheral Neurotomies in Upper Limbs

Brachial plexus neurotomy

This type of peripheral selective neurotomy involving the collateral branches of the brachial plexus has been used for treatment of the spastic shoulder. The target branches are the branches for the pectoralis major and teres major nerves, which are the main muscles attributed in shoulder spasticity.[67]

Musculocutaneous neurotomy

Musculocutaneous neurotomy is indicated in the spastic flexion of the elbow joint; the skin incision is performed longitudinally extending from the inferior edge of pectoralis major, medial to the biceps brachii, down to 5 cm dissecting through the plain between the biceps and brachialis proceeding in this space, where the musculocutaneous nerve lies anterior to the brachialis muscle (Fig. 28.20).

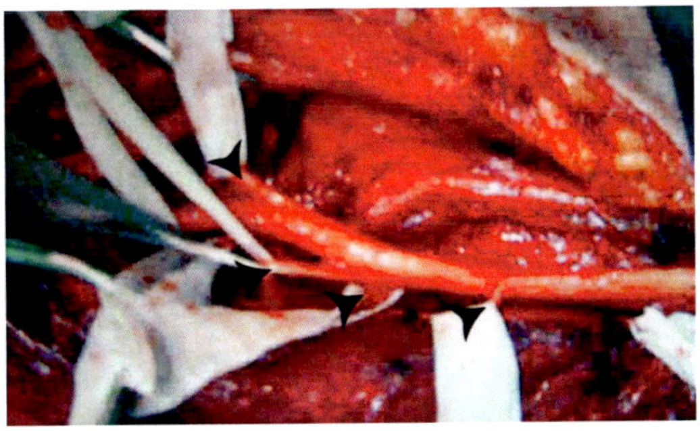

FIG. 28.21 Intraoperative picture of the right median nerve and its branches (black arrow heads) below the elbow.

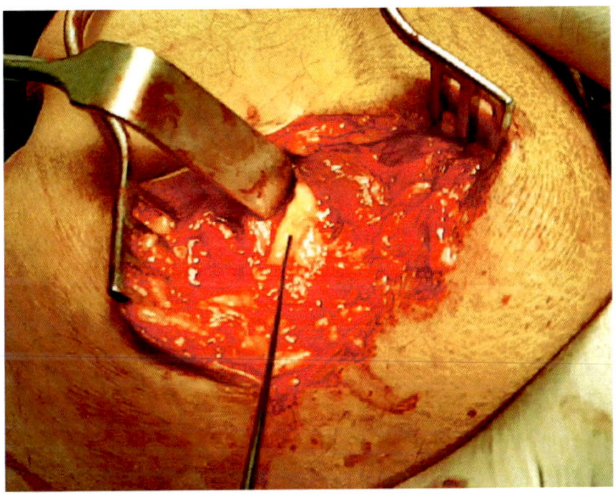

FIG. 28.22 Intraoperative picture of the left ulnar nerve behind the medial malleolus with elbow flexion for better view.

Median neurotomy

Median neurotomy is indicated in spastic flexed pronated hands; the skin incision begins 2–3 cm above the flexion line of the elbow, medial to the biceps brachii tendon, passes through the elbow, and curves toward the junction of the upper and middle thirds of the anterior forearm. Thereafter, the median nerve is searched medially to the brachial artery and recognized at the elbow, deeply under the lacertus fibrosus, which is cut. Sharp dissection is used to separate the branches of the median nerve (Fig. 28.21).

Ulnar neurotomy

Ulnar neurotomy is performed in patients with spastic wrist flexion especially in those with hyperactive flexor carpi ulnaris that leads to ulnar deviation of the wrist.

An arched skin incision is performed to expose the ulnar nerve at the medial part of the elbow. After subcutaneous dissection, the ulnar nerve is identified medially to the medial epicondyle, where it enters between the two heads of the flexor carpi ulnaris. There, the motor branches to this muscle are identified. More distally, the branches to the medial half of the flexor digitorum profundus can be found (Fig. 28.22).

Complications

Complications of neurotomies include hypothesia or paresthesia in the cutaneous distribution especially of the sural nerve in lower limbs and of the brachial cutaneous branches. Fortunately, most of these sensory complications are transient and show good response to antineuropathic medications.[68]

REFERENCES

1. Smania N, Picelli A, Munari D, et al. Rehabilitation procedures in the management of spasticity. *Eur J Phys Rehabil Med*. 2010;46:423–438.
2. Sanger TD, et al. Classification and definition of disorders causing hypertonia in childhood. *Pediatrics*. 2003;111(1):e89–97.
3. Delgado MR, Albright AL. Movement disorders in children: definitions, classification, and grading systems. *J Child Neurol*. 2003;18:S1–S8.
4. Penn RD, Corcos DM. Management of spasticity by central nervous system infusion techniques. In: Richard Winn H, ed. *Youmans Neurological Surgery*. 5th ed. Elsevier inc.; 2004:2875–2889. Part V, ch.177.
5. Smyth MD, Peacock WJ. The surgical treatment of spasticity. *Muscle Nerve*. 2000;23:153–163.
6. Bear MF, Connors BW, Paradiso MA. Spinal control of movement. In: Bear Mark F, Connors Barry W, Paradiso Micheal A, eds. *Neuroscience Exploring the Brain*. 2nd ed. USA: Lippincott Williams & Wilkins; 2001: 436–463. Ch 13.
7. Decq P, Filipetti P, Lefaucheur JP. Evaluation of spasticity in adults. *Oper Tech Neurosurg*. 2005;7:100–108.
8. Lieber RL, Stienman S, Barash IA, Chambers H. Structural and functional changes in spastic skeletal muscle. *Muscle Nerve*. 2004;29:615–627.
9. Friden J, Lieber RL. Spastic muscle cells are shorter and stiffer than normal cells. *Muscle Nerve*. 2003;27:157–164.
10. Bar-On Lynn, Molenaers G, Aertbelien E, et al. Spasticity and its contribution to hypertonia in cerebral palsy. Review article *BioMed Res Int*. 2015;2015.
11. Barnes MP. An overview of the clinical management of spasticity. In: *Upper Motor Neurone Syndrome and Spasticity*. 2nd ed. Cambridge University Press; 2008:1–2.
12. Gordon Laurie M, et al. Can spasticity and dystonia be independently measured in cerebral palsy? *Pediatr Neurol*. 2006;35(6):375–381.
13. Bohannon RW, Smith MB. Interrater reliability of a modified Ashworth scale of muscle spasticity. *Phys Ther*. 1987; 67(2):206–207.
14. Gracies JM. Evaluation de la spasticité. Apport de l'échelle de Tardieu. *Mot Cérébrale*. 2001;22:1–16.

15. Schwartz MH, Viehwege E, Stou J, Novacheck TF, Gage JR. Comprehensive treatment of ambulatory children with cerebral palsy: an outcome assessment. *J Pediatr Orthop.* 2004;24:45–53.
16. Lefaucheur JP. Evaluation electrophysiologique des boucles reflexes spinales potentiellement impliquées dans la spasticité. *Neurochirurgie.* 2003;49:205–214.
17. Daniel D. Special nerve conduction techniques. In: Daniel D, ed. *Electrodiagnostic Medicine.* Philadelphia: Hanley & Belfus, Inc; 1995.
18. Delwaide PJ. Human reflex studies for understanding the motor system. *Phys Med Rehabil Clin North Am.* 1993;4: 669–686.
19. Lorenz F. Über die chirurgische Behandlung der angeborenen spastischen Gliedstarre. *Wien Klin Rdsch.* 1887;21: 25–27.
20. Kennard MA, Fulton JF, de Gutiérrez-Mahoney CG. Otfrid Foerster 1873– 1941. An appreciation. *J Neurophysiol.* 1942;5:1–17.
21. Casey KF, Sekula R. Ablative surgery for spasticity. In: Richard Winn H, ed. *Youmans Neurological Surgery.* 5th ed. Elsevier Inc.; 2004:2863–2872. Part V, ch. 176.
22. Sindou MP. History of neurosurgical treatment of spasticity. *Oper Tech Neurosurg.* 2005;7:96–99. © Elsevier Inc.
23. Ward AB. Long-term modification of spasticity. *J Rehabil Med.* 2003;41(suppl):60–65.
24. Sindou M, Mertens P. Surgery in the dorsal root entry zone for spasticity in adults. *Oper Tech Neurosurg.* 2005;7: 157–162. © Elsevier Inc.
25. Sindou M, Mertens P. Surgery in the dorsal root entry zone for pain. *Semin Neurosurg.* 2004;15(2/3).
26. Sindou M. Microsurgical DREZotomy (MDT) for pain, spasticity and hyperactive bladder: a 20-years experience. *Acta Neurochir (Wien).* 1995;136:1–5.
27. Sindou M. Dorsal root entry zone lesions. In: Burchiel KJ, ed. *Surgical Management of Pain.* NY-USA: Thieme; 2002: 701–712. Part IV. Ch 56.
28. Sindou M. Microsurgical DREZotomy (MDT) for pain, spasticity and hyperactive bladder: a 20-year experience. *Acta Neurochir (Wien).* 1995;137:1–5.
29. Lazorthes Y, Sol JC, Sallerin B, Verdie JC. The surgical management of spasticity. *Eur J Neurol.* 2002;9(suppl 1):35–41.
30. Saris SC, Iacono RP, Nashold Jr BS. Dorsal root entry zone lesions for post-amputation pain. *J Neurosurg.* 1985;62(1): 72–76.
31. Bischof W. Die. Longitudinale myelotomie. *Zentralbl Neurochir.* 1951;11:79–88.
32. Pourpre H. Traitement neuro-chirurgical des contractures chez les paraplégiques posttraumatiques. *Neurochirurgie.* 1960;6:229–236.
33. Laitinen L, Singounas E. Longitudinal myelotomy in the treatment of spasticity of the legs. *J Neurosurg.* 1971;35: 536–540.
34. Laitinen LV. A myelotome for the treatment of spasticity. In: *Proceedings of the 25th Annual Meeting of the Nordisk Neurokirurgisk Förening (Scandinavian Neurosurgical Society), May 31–June 2, 1973, Turku/Abo, Compiled by P. Rasmussen*Acta Neurochir (Wien). Vol. 29. 1973:269.
35. Laha RK, Dujovny M, Osgood CP. Dorsal longitudinal myelotomy. *Paraplegia.* 1976;14:189–194. https://doi.org/10.1038/sc.1976.33.
36. Vasques XA, Cif L, Biolsi B, Coubes P. Central procedures for primary dystonia. In: Lozano AM, Gildenberg PL, Tasker RR, eds. *Textbook of Stereotactic and Functional Neurosurgery.* 2nd ed. Springer; 2009:1801–1834. ISBN 978-3-540-69959-0.
37. Krauss JK, Yianni J, Loher TJ, Aziz TZ. Deep brain stimulation for dystonia. *J Clin Neurophysiol.* 2004;21:18–30.
38. Ondo WG, Krauss JK. Surgical therapies for dystonia. In: Brin MF, Comella C, Jankovic J, eds. *Dystonia Monograph.* Philadelphia: Lippincott, Williams & Wilkins; 2003: 125–147.
39. Gross RE. What happened to posteroventral pallidotomy for Parkinson disease and dystonia? *Neurotherapeutics.* 2008;5:281–293.
40. Iacono RP, Kuniyoshi SM, Lonser RR, Maeda G, Inae AM, Ashwal S. Simultaneous bilateral pallidoansotomy for idiopathic dystonia musculorum deformans. *Pediatr Neurol.* 1996;14:145–148.
41. Benabid AL, Pollak P, Gao D, et al. Chronic electrical stimulation of the ventralis intermedius nucleus of the thalamus as a treatment of movement disorders. *J Neurosurg.* 1996;84:203–214.
42. Capelle H-H, Krauss JK. Functional stereotactic procedures for treatment of secondary dystonia. In: Lozano AM, Gildenberg PL, Tasker RR, eds. *Textbook of Stereotactic and Functional Neurosurgery.* 2nd ed. © Springer; 2009: 1835–1857. ISBN 978-3-540-69959-0.
43. Fasano VA, Barolat GR, Zeme S, Sguazzi A. Electrophysiological Assessment of Spinal Circuits in Spasticity) by direct dorsal root stimulation. *Neurosurgery.* 1979;4(2): 146–151.
44. Sindou M, Mertens P. Neurosurgical management of spasticity. In: Schmidek HH, ed. *Operative Neurosurgical Techniques. Indications, Methods and Results.* 4th ed. USA: W.B. Sounder; 2000:2460–2473; Vol. 188.
45. Farmer JP, McNeely PD. Surgery in the Dorsal Roots for Children with Cerebral Palsy. *Oper Tech Neurosurg.* 2005; 7:153–156. © Elsevier Inc.
46. Peacock WJ, Arens LJ. Selective posterior rhizotomy for the relief of spasticity in cerebral palsy. *S Afr Med J.* 1982;62: 119–124.
47. Park TS, Gaffney PE, Kaufman BA, Molleston MC. Selective lumbosacral dorsal rhizotomy immediately caudal to the conus medullaris for cerebral palsy spasticity. *Neurosurgery.* 1993;33(5):929–943.
48. Park TS, Johnston JM. Selective dorsal rhizotomy for spastic cerebral palsy. In: Goodrich JT, ed. *Pediatric Neurosurgery.* 2nd ed. New York: Thieme; 2008:177–183.
49. Sindou M. Radicotomies dorsales chez l'enfant. *Neurochirurgie.* 2003;49:312–323.
50. Abdel Ghany WA, Shalash AS, Desoky AE. Role of intraoperative electrophysiological monitoring during selective dorsal rhizotomy in children with spastic cerebral palsy regarding sparing of sphincter innervation. *Pan Arab J Neurosurg.* 2013;17(2).

51. Langerak NG, Lamberts RP, Fieggen AG, Peter JC, Peacock WJ, Vaughan CL. Functional status of patients with cerebral palsy according to the International Classification of Functioning, Disability and Health model: a 20-year follow-up study after selective dorsal rhizotomy. *Arch Phys Med Rehabil*. 2009;90(6):994–1003. https://doi.org/10.1016/j.apmr.2008.11.019.
52. Steinbok P, Schrag C. Complications after selective posterior rhizotomy for spasticity in children with cerebral palsy. *Pediatr Neurosurg*. 1998;28:300–313.
53. Park TS. Selective dorsal rhizotomy for spastic cerebral palsy. *J Neurosurg*. 2006;105(1 Suppl Pediatrics):8–15.
54. Abbott R, Murphy M, Maher T. Selective dorsal rhizotomy: outcome and complications in treating spastic cerebral palsy. *Neurosurgery*. 1993;33:851–857.
55. Peter JC, Hoffman EB, Arens LJ. Spondylolysis and spondylolisthesis after five-level lumbosacral laminectomy for selective posterior rhizotomy in cerebral palsy. *Childs Nerv Syst*. 1993;9:285–288.
56. Kim HS, Steinbok P, Wickenheiser D. Predictors of poor outcome after selective dorsal rhizotomy in treatment of spastic cerebral palsy. *Childs Nerv Syst*. 2005;22(1):60–66. https://doi.org/10.1007/s00381-005-1160-2.
57. Albright AL, Tyler-Kabara EC. Combined ventral and dorsal rhizotomy for dystonic and spastic extremities. *J Neurosurg*. 2007;107(4 Suppl Pediatrics):324–327.
58. Abdel Ghany WA, Nada M, Mahran MA, et al. Combined anterior and posterior lumbar rhizotomy for treatment of mixed dystonia and spasticity in children with cerebral palsy. *Neurosurgery*. 2016;79(3):336–344. https://doi.org/10.1227/NEU.0000000000001271.
59. Bertrand CM. Selective Peripheral Denervation for Spasmodic Torticollis. Surgical Technique, results, and observation in 260 cases. *Surg Neurol*. 1993;40(2):96–103. ISSN: 1879–3339.
60. Krauss JK. Surgical Treatment of Dystonia. *Eur J Neurol*. 2010;17(suppl 1):97–101. ISSN:1351–1501.
61. Sitthinamsuwan Bunpot, Nunta-Aree Sarun. Dystonia and Peripheral Nerve Surgery in the Cervical Area. In: Rosales Raymond, ed. *Dystonia - the Many Facets*. © InTech; 2012. ISBN 978-953-51-0329-5.
62. Taira T. Peripheral Procedures for Cervical Dystonia. In: Lozano AM, Gildenberg PL, Tasker RR, eds. *Textbook of Stereotactic and Functional Neurosurgery*. 2nd ed. © Springer; 2009:1885–1909. ISBN 978-3-540-69959-0.
63. Gordon T, Yang JF, Ayer K. Recovery potential of muscle after partial denervation: a comparison between rats and humans. *Brain Res Bull*. 1993;30:477–482.
64. Roujeau T, Lefaucheur JP, Slavov V, Gherardi R, Decq P. Long term course of the H reflex after selective tibial neurotomy. *J Neurol Neurosurg Psychiatry*. 2003;74:913–917.
65. Banks RW, Barker D. Specificities of afferents reinnervating cat muscle spindles after nerve section. *J Physiol*. 1989;408:345–372.
66. Mertens P, Sindou M. Surgical management of spasticity. In: Barnes MP, Johnson GR, eds. *Upper Motor Neurone Syndrome and Spasticity: Clinical Management of Spasticity*. Cambridge: Cambridge University Press; 2001:239–265.
67. Decq P, Filipetti P, Feve A, Djindjian M, Saraoui A, Kéravel Y. Peripheral selective neurotomy of the brachial plexus collateral branches for treatment of the spastic shoulder: anatomical study and clinical results in five patients. *J Neurosurg*. 1997;86(4):648–653.
68. Maarrawi J, Mertens P, Luaute J, et al. Longterm functional results of selective peripheral neurotomy for the treatment of spastic upper limb: prospective study in 31 patients. *J Neurosurg*. 2006;104:215–225.

IDDS for Spasticity, Dystonia, and Rigidity

JONATHAN WEYHENMEYER, MD, BSEE • ALBERT LEE, MD, MSECE, FACS

ORIGINS AND TREATMENT

Spasticity is defined as a hypertonic velocity-dependent state where antagonist muscle groups, i.e., knee flexors and extensors, are persistently activated resulting in increased rigidity on passive movement, hyperreflexia, poor coordination, and unwanted movements.[1] The increased spasticity is correlated with the velocity of the passive movement such that higher velocities result in greater spasticity. Spasticity arises secondary to a neurologic insult whereby upper motor neurons (UMNs) of the spinal cord, brainstem, or cerebrum are damaged, resulting in poor regulation of monosynaptic muscle stretch reflex pathways.[2] In a healthy individual, the spinal cord receives information regarding muscle length and rate of change of muscle length from Ia afferent fibers. Stretching or increasing the length of the muscle causes the Ia afferent neurons to fire an electrical impulse. Ia afferent neurons course to the spinal cord through the dorsal root ganglion and synapse directly on lower motor neurons (LMNs) that control the muscle in question. Specifically, when the Ia afferent neuron fires, it induces specific LMNs to fire, resulting in muscle contraction. Upon entering the spinal cord, the Ia neuron will also synapse on both inhibitory and excitatory interneurons. The excitatory neurons amplify the contraction response by synapsing on LMNs that innervate the muscle in question. The inhibitory neurons synapse on LMNs that innervate antagonist muscle groups, thereby inhibiting the stimulation of the antagonist muscles. The end result is that stretched muscles are contracted, whereas antagonist muscles are left unstimulated. The muscle stretch pathway is modulated by UMNs that upregulate or downregulate muscle stretch reflexes (MSRs) such that they are not continuously activated. The loss of UMN control results in poor tonic inhibition of the muscle stretch reflex arcs, leading to persistent activation of antagonist muscle, which manifests as clinical spasticity.

Many different insults may result in injury to UMNs contained in the cerebrum, brainstem, or spinal cord. As such, spasticity arises from many different injury mechanisms that may occur at varying points in a person's life. Spasticity of congenital origin is often found in patients who suffer from anoxic brain injury intrautero, myelomeningocele, or cerebral palsy. Spasticity may also be the end result of trauma to the cerebrum, e.g., stroke or traumatic brain injury. Untreated cerebral injury often leads to rigidity. Still, others suffer from chronic, progressive neurologic disease such as multiple sclerosis or other autoimmune diseases. The important point is that although the aforementioned diseases arise secondary to vastly different underlying pathologies, symptomatic spasticity is grounded in a consistent pathophysiologic mechanism that lends itself to a common targeted treatment pathway.

Clinically, spasticity is noted as a poor muscle control, posturing such as opisthotonus or scissoring of the legs, hyperreflexia on muscle stretch testing, and poor control of bowel and bladder. Patients are frequently confined to their bed or wheel chair. Contractures and rigidity often arise, which may be painful and/or require orthopedic release surgeries if not managed well.[3] Furthermore, the inability and lack of movement often results in the development of decubitus ulcers requiring hospitalization. The Ashworth scale is commonly used to grade a patient's spasticity ranging from normal tone to rigid in flexion and/or extension.[4] More recently, the modified Ashworth scale has gained acceptance as the method of choice in evaluating these patients.[5] The Ashworth scale is important for both initial grading and judging patient response to treatment.

Medical treatment for spasticity includes measures to avoid noxious stimuli, i.e., frequent repositioning, manual disimpaction, and bladder catheterization. Similarly, frequent physical therapy helps to keep the limbs loose and prevents contractures. Many patients have refractory spasticity and require oral medications, including benzodiazepines, α-2 agonists, and baclofen, all of which are dose-limited because of their side effect profile (see below). Finally, patients may also require intrathecal baclofen because of the inability to tolerate necessary oral doses of the medications, the main topic of this chapter.

BACLOFEN FOR SPASTICITY

As mentioned above, baclofen is frequently used to treat refractory spasticity. Baclofen acts at the $GABA_B$ receptor in the brain and spinal cord through the hyperpolarization of presynaptic neurons and inhibition of monosynaptic and polysynaptic reflexes.[6] It is through this mechanism that it inhibits the muscle stretch reflexes that underlie spasticity triggered by UMN disease. Originally, baclofen was administered via the oral route, but this was hampered by the fact that baclofen does not readily cross the blood-brain barrier.[7] High oral doses are often required to obtain clinical results, but more often than not, the side effects from oral medications are reached first before clinical benefits are achieved. Side effects often include gastrointestinal symptoms, cardiac symptoms such as bradycardia and orthostatic hypotension, and rarely, CNS depression, seizures, lethargy, dizziness, ataxia, and weakness.[6] Given these findings a new form of baclofen administration was attempted.

Intrathecal catheterization for intrathecal drug delivery (IDD) of baclofen has become the standard of care for patients with increased medically refractory spasticity, dystonia, and rigidity secondary to congenital or acquired neurologic abnormalities.[7–10] Intrathecal administration of baclofen allows for much higher therapeutic index, with a lower side effect profile compared with oral baclofen.[11] Intrathecal baclofen provides an automated, highly localized system for drug administration, decreasing the likelihood of missed or repeated doses. As such, intrathecal baclofen has decreased the incidence of baclofen withdrawal and overdose in spastic patients. Recent studies have shown that intrathecal baclofen delivery significantly decreases the lifetime cost of spasticity management because of the reduced incidence of baclofen overdose, withdrawal, and the need for hospitalization while improving the overall quality of life for these patients.[12]

ALTERNATIVE ORAL MEDICATIONS

As mentioned previously, baclofen is currently the first-line pharmaceutical for managing spasticity of cerebral and spinal origin. For patients who are unable to tolerate baclofen because of its side effect profile, there are a number of other oral options available. Previously, clonidine, an α-2 agonist, was widely used in the treatment of spasticity. It acts centrally by reducing afferent sensory transmission to the spinal cord, thereby toning down muscle stretch response.[13,14] Clonidine has fallen out of favor because of its side effect profile, which includes bradycardia and hypotension. Furthermore, titrating the dose within the therapeutic index can be challenging. Similarly, tizanidine, another α-2 agonist, works through presynaptic inhibition in the spinal cord and inhibits the firing of interneurons, suppressing the release of inhibitory amino acids.[15] This results in reduced LMN activation. Tizanidine tends to cause significant sedation and muscle weakness. Benzodiazepines work at the $GABA_A$ receptor, reducing CNS activity postsynaptically. These medications are quite sedating, and patients develop tolerance over time. Furthermore, withdrawal from benzodiazepines puts patients at high risk for epileptic activity. Dantrolene is unique in that it is the only antispasticity medication that works peripherally. Dantrolene works by inhibiting the release of calcium from the sarcoplasmic reticulum and subsequently inhibits muscle contraction.[16] Again, dantrolene tends to be limited by its side effect profile, which includes muscle weakness and liver failure. Although gabapentin has been identified as an agent that may be used to reduce spasticity, its lack of efficacy makes it a poor choice when compared with other available options.[13]

WORKUP BEFORE SURGERY

Intrathecal baclofen is indicated for patients with medically refractory spasticity or dystonia with or without rigidity who have failed oral baclofen because of either dose toxicity or poor dose-response. Typically, baclofen dosing of 40–80 mg per day divided in 3–4 daily doses is the range where side effects are observed. Some individuals can tolerate a much higher dose and, as such, do not require intrathecal therapy to help control their spasticity.

The workup for ITB (itchy, twitchy, bad behavior) includes making sure the patients' diagnosis is correct, i.e., if they have an undiagnosed genetic disorder instead of a standard cerebral palsy diagnosis, which should be identified, evaluated, and managed before instituting intrathecal therapy. Early initiation of physical and occupational therapy under the guide of a qualified physiatrist is an important step in management of the preoperative patient. A course of oral baclofen is attempted before considering a pump implant, as this will help to assess patient response to the medication. Botox is well tolerated and is often used as long as it achieves therapeutic goals. Once botox fails because of declining efficacy, it is reasonable to begin preoperative evaluation for ITB therapy.

During the preoperative evaluation, an intrathecal test dose of baclofen is administered through a lumbar puncture by a qualified provider with the documentation of Ashworth scores before and after administration. We recommend performing a lumbar puncture with a 50 μg baclofen test dose while patients are maintained on their standard oral regimen. The goal is to demonstrate that, despite maximum oral medications, intrathecal baclofen provides improved clinical results. If there is limited response to the 50 μg dose, it is reasonable to administer a 100 μg test dose and again evaluate the clinical response. We use the assistance of a physical therapist to assess before and after results. This provides an objective third-party evaluation and workup for ITB. If a lumbar puncture owing to spinal deformity correction has been performed, then intraventricular delivery of the drug through an Extraventricular Drain (EVD) is an alternative option but rarely used.

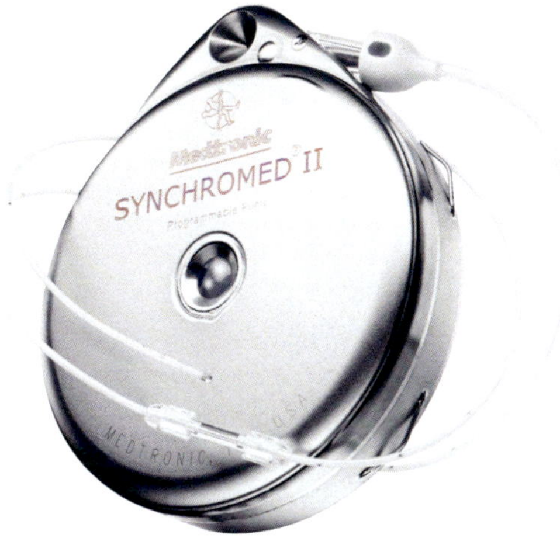

FIG. 29.1 Synchromed II intrathecal drug delivery pump by Medtronic. The pump is shown connected to an intrathecal catheter. The proximal catheter is connected to a distal catheter via a connector. (Reprinted with the permission of Medtronic, Inc. ©2018.)

HARDWARE OPTIONS

The Medtronic Synchromed II pump is now the standard of care for baclofen pump implantation along with the new Ascenda catheter released in 2013; see Figs. 29.1–29.3 that display the pump system and programmer. Codman Medstream was FDA-approved for intrathecal baclofen and morphine infusion but has been taken off the market owing to FDA recall. A rotatory motor system is far safer than any other system for intrathecal baclofen therapy because of the likelihood that patient may accidently receive an MRI in an emergency-type situation. If an uninformed care provider assumes the patient has a Synchromed II type of pump, the piezoelectric gating system will likely cause an overdose situation when the patient is placed in an MRI. This is why we recommend going only with a rotor-type drug delivery system for intrathecal baclofen.

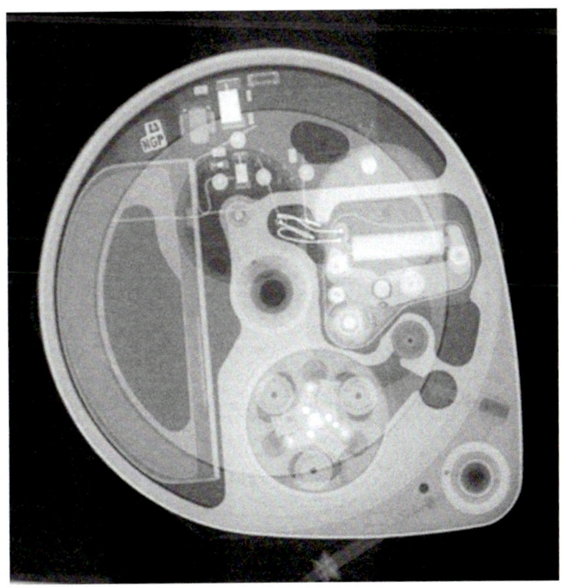
FIG. 29.2 Internal structure of Synchromed II pump by Medtronic, displaying the rotary system. (Reprinted with the permission of Medtronic, Inc. ©2018.)

SURGICAL TECHNIQUE

Before considering surgery, all routine surgical preoperative workup should be performed:

- The patient should be evaluated for low anesthesia risks.
- The patient should not have any active infections.
- The patient should not be on any blood thinning medications, e.g., aspirin, for at least 1 week before surgery.
- The patient should maintain their standard oral spasticity regimen and other appropriate medications.

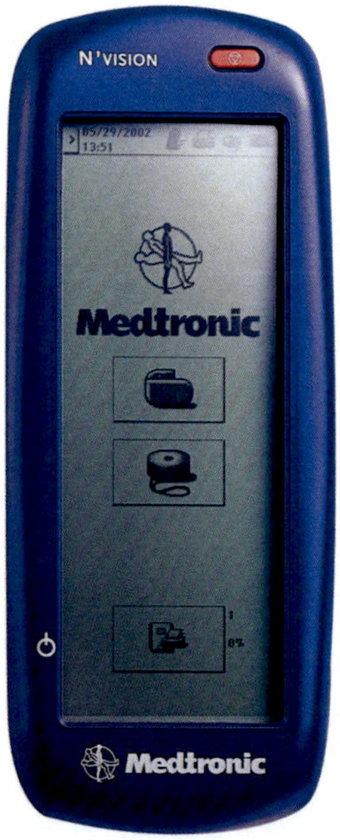

FIG. 29.3 Medtronic programmer for the Synchromed II intrathecal drug delivery pump system. (Reprinted with the permission of Medtronic, Inc. ©2018.)

Standard pre- and postoperative antibiotics should be given, and the patient should be monitored for cerebrospinal fluid (CSF) leak after surgery.

POSITIONING

The patient is positioned in the lateral decubitus position using sturdy tape directly placed on the hip, with the arms curled up toward the head. This provides increased positioning security such that the patient will not roll off of the bed. Some patients, e.g., patients with scoliotic spines, require a significant degree of bed rotation. The patients' arms are angled up, with the arm board parallel to the operative table. Angling the arms in this manner ensures that there is less tissue obstructing the fluoroscopy images that are required to image the catheter up to and including the C6 level. In addition, the posterior aspect of the patient should be placed at the edge of the bed, as this will assist with tunneling of the shunt passer to the anterior abdominal pocket. The shunt passer that is used for tunneling has a tendency to run into the side of the OR table if patients are not appropriately positioned with their back at the edge of the table.

SURGERY

A proper paramedian approach involves placing the Tuohy needle starting on the skin of the ipsilateral L3 pedicle; therefore fluoroscopy should be used in the placement of all intrathecal catheters. The needle is then walked up the lamina until it enters the intralaminar space and is advanced into the dura at the L1-2 interspace is desired and gives a good risk balance for avoiding spinal cord injury complications. The paramedian approach is preferable for a number of reasons; most importantly it helps to prevent catheter fracture at the time of insertion and postoperatively. Entering with a midline approach increases the risk of catheter fracture because the orientation of the spinous processes forces that catheter to exit the needle at approximately 90° within the dural sac. This makes it difficult to advance the catheter and may induce a catheter fracture. Second, placing the catheter within the interspinous ligament between spinous processes induces stress on the catheter with each flexion/extension of the spine, leading to increased risk of fracture over time.

For patients with upper- and lower-extremity spasticity and dystonia, we typically aim to place the catheter tip at C7. If there is a high amount of neck dystonia, a C6-7 level is achieved. We have found the higher cervical catheters require lower dosages compared with catheters placed at the upper thoracic levels. However, placement at the cervical levels may result in significant laxity of the neck. Increased neck laxity may be beneficial for patients suffering from neck dystonia. For spastic paraparesis and rigidity, we aim for the T5-7 level. This is due to the fact that catheters placed at the T10 level and below will occasionally become dislodged even after proper anchoring if there is a postoperative CSF leak.

The surgical technique for placement of the baclofen pump is as follows. First, the Tuohy needle infiltrates the thecal sac via that paramedian approach under fluoroscopy. Once the Tuohy needle infiltrates the intrathecal space, the intrathecal catheter is threaded into the intrathecal to the desired vertebral level under fluoroscopy. Next, a 4–5 cm incision is placed around the needle and the fascial plane is developed (Fig. 29.4), and the Tuohy needle is removed while securing the catheter so that it does not move from the space (Fig. 29.5). The incision should be made before removing the Tuohy needle to avoid inadvertently cutting the catheter. The catheter is then secured in place to the fascia using a securing device (Figs. 29.6–29.8). The surgeon's attention is next turned toward creating the pump pocket. A subdermal incision is made with

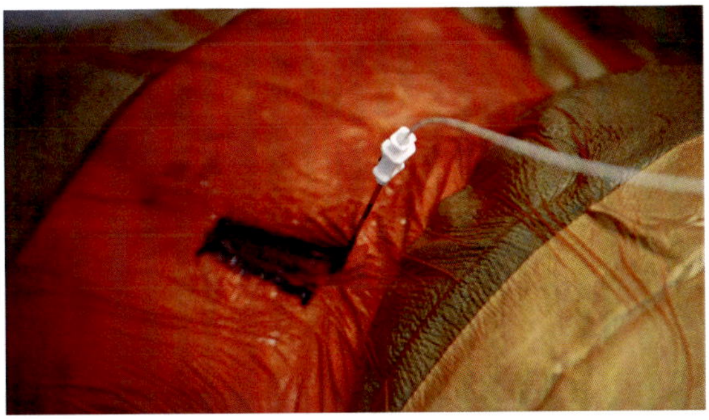

FIG. 29.4 After the Tuohy needle punctures the thecal sac, the intrathecal catheter is threaded up to the desired vertebral level and a 5 cm incision is made around the needle. (Reprinted with the permission of Medtronic, Inc. ©2018.)

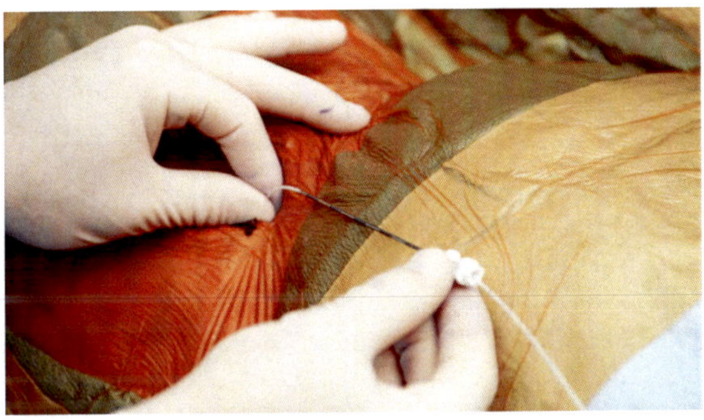

FIG. 29.5 The Tuohy needle is carefully removed while the catheter is held in place so that it is not displaced from the desired vertebral level within the intrathecal sac. If concerned that the catheter has changed position, additional X-rays should be obtained to confirm position. (Reprinted with the permission of Medtronic, Inc. ©2018.)

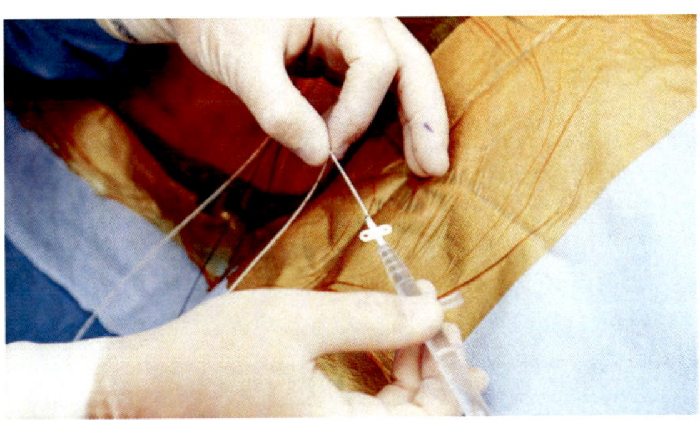

FIG. 29.6 The catheter securing device is threaded onto the catheter and advanced until it is at the level of fascia. (Reprinted with the permission of Medtronic, Inc. ©2018.)

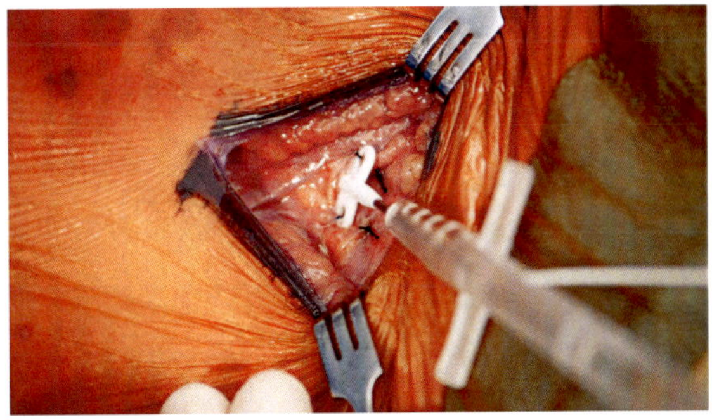

FIG. 29.7 Once the catheter is at the level of fascia, the butterfly securing device is fastened to the fascia with one or two sutures. A single suture involving both sides may be used. (Reprinted with the permission of Medtronic, Inc. ©2018.)

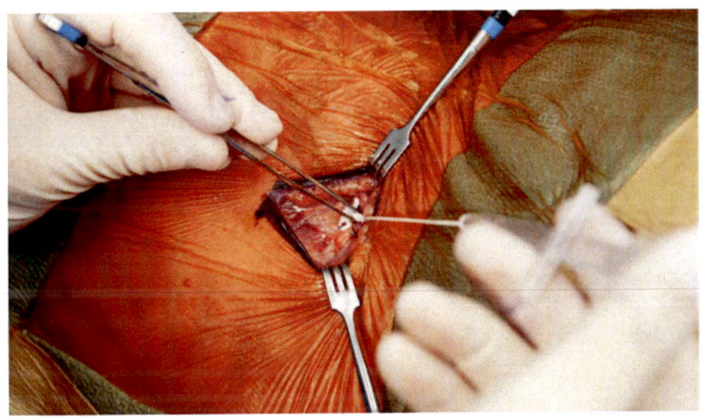

FIG. 29.8 When removing the applier and guidewire catheter, the securing device should be held with pickups to ensure that the catheter is not inadvertently pulled out. (Reprinted with the permission of Medtronic, Inc. ©2018.)

a #10 blade, and the Scarpa's fascia is exposed and undermined to create a pocket for the pump (Fig. 29.9). A shunt passer is then used to pass a new catheter from the pump pocket to the back (Figs. 29.10 and 29.11). This catheter will connect to the intrathecal catheter through a catheter connector that is compatible with the pump system being implanted (Fig. 29.12).

For younger and thinner patients, there is an increased risk of the baclofen pump eroding through the skin if it is placed too superficial. These patients have been noted to have a higher incidence of wound breakdown and postoperative pump-wound infections.[17] Many practitioners advocate for placing the pump subfascial in this subset of patients.[8,18] We agree that this method is very helpful but is often difficult in patients with larger body habitus. Indeed, the pump

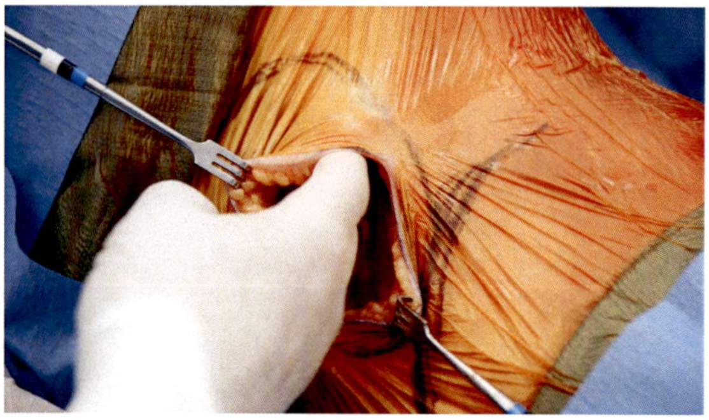

FIG. 29.9 An incision is made in the abdomen, and pump pocket is made with blunt dissection by undermining the fat and fascia of the abdominal wall. (Reprinted with the permission of Medtronic, Inc. ©2018.)

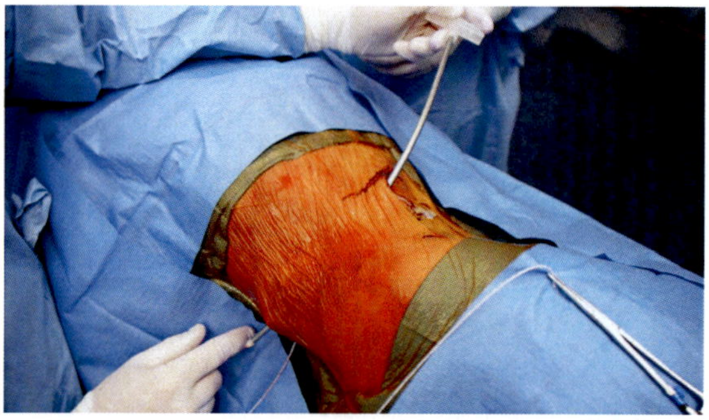

FIG. 29.10 A shunt passer is used to tunnel between the back and abdomen. Care should be taken to make sure that the tunnels are made between the lowest rib and the iliac crest. If the tunneler goes too high, there is a risk of injuring the lung. (Reprinted with the permission of Medtronic, Inc. ©2018.)

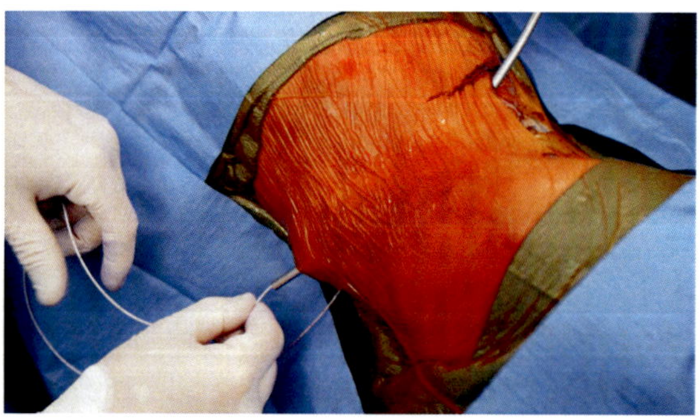

FIG. 29.11 The catheter tubing is pushed through the shunt passer. The shunt passer is then removed, and the catheter tubing is now visible through either incision. (Reprinted with the permission of Medtronic, Inc. ©2018.)

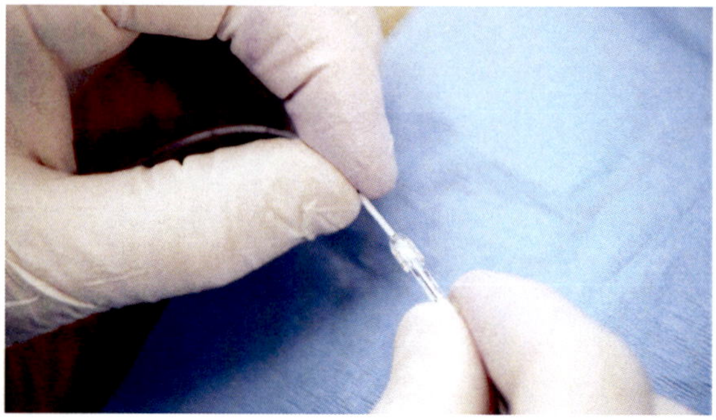

FIG. 29.12 The catheter is measured such that there is enough length of catheter on both the intrathecal and the pump segment side. Then the extra catheter is cut from both sides. The newly placed catheter is then connected to the intrathecal catheter via a catheter connector. (Reprinted with the permission of Medtronic, Inc. ©2018.)

should, ideally, not be placed more than 2–3 in. deeper than the skin, as this may lead to difficulty communicating with and filling the pump.

INFECTION CONTROL

Besides a CSF leak, infection is the second most frequent complication. Techniques that have been established in ventriculoperitoneal shunting should also be used for ITB implantation. Copiously scrubbing the surgical site with alcohol and chloraprep, sterile draping with ioban and a lap drape (we prefer the Turner lap drape for multiple reasons), and changing of outer gloves or overgloving are techniques that have reduced our incidence of infection. We also use Optifoam once skin incisions have been made to guard the skin edges from being exposed to the hardware. We believe that all of these methods have contributed a lower infection rate at our institution.

POSTOPERATIVE CONSIDERATIONS

The long-term data for the new Medtronic Ascenda catheter are not published to date. The primary advantages of the newer catheter are that it rarely kinks or suffers occlusions or fractures when compared with the older catheter, which is extremely beneficial to patients.[19] At our institution, we have attempted to institute multiple protocols to reduce postoperative complications. These protocols include keeping the head of the bed flat for 48 h postoperatively to prevent CSF leak and surgical techniques such as purse string suturing of the catheter at the fascia. Two discoveries we have found are that elevation of the head of bed immediately after surgery (often required if there is respiratory depression) and early mobilization with therapy and inpatient rehabilitation after surgery, leading to a higher frequency of resistant CSF leak. This likely occurs secondary to increased pressure at the catheter entry site with upright posture due to water column pressure that occurs in these positions.

We typically start patients with a standard dose of 50 μg/day especially with higher cervical catheters. The respiratory depression from intrathecal baclofen is a time-limited side effect. Regardless of a patient's preoperative oral medication dosing regimens, a high cervical catheter at an intrathecal level of C6-7 will cause significant respiratory depression if dosages are started at higher levels. We have not seen dose-related complications when starting patients at 50 μg/day. The dosage is increased slowly over time, helping to negate the onset of respiratory depression.

Routine end of service replacements should always be approached with the hypothesis that the catheter is nonfunctional unless a side port aspiration is performed in clinic during the preoperative visit. If a catheter malfunction is found at the time of pump replacement, it should be replaced unless there is a severe scoliotic deformity encountered at the time of surgery. We again recommend starting the patient at 50 μg/day if this situation is encountered. There is up to a 20% failure rate at 5 years with the older model catheter. This failure rate has decreased significantly with the newer catheter systems, i.e., Medtronic Ascenda catheter. For patients who require frequent catheter revisions such that they are at risk for arachnoiditis, intraventricular baclofen has been shown to be a well-tolerated option.[20] Although intraventricular catheter placement is beyond the scope of this chapter, it is an important option for patients who repeatedly fail intrathecal therapy.

WHERE IS THE DRUG?

When programming a new or existing pump, it is always important to know where the drug is or is not. When a side port aspiration is performed, it is important to know that the internal pump tubing is already primed in an existing pump. Improper programming can lead to fatal or near-fatal outcomes of baclofen overdose or withdrawal. When in doubt, always seek out more experienced help or call the manufacturer help line to speak to a clinical advisor. Please note in 2016 the FDA required Medtronic to change the bolus dosage time of the internal pump tubing; this may or may not affect the bolus programming that ITB patients receive, and patients should be warned of baclofen withdrawal symptoms.

BACLOFEN WITHDRAWAL

Baclofen withdrawal is the most concerning complication and can be rapidly fatal. Baclofen withdrawal is not typically seen in oral baclofen but can occur in a mild form. Baclofen withdrawal most commonly occurs in close proximity to the pump refill date as the pump reservoir empties.[21] There are two stages to baclofen withdrawal, an early and a late phase.

The early phase consists of symptoms that can be reversed if rapidly treated. Unfortunately, if patients, families, and care providers are not properly counseled, then the early phase can rapidly turn into a late-phase withdrawal, leading to death. We use the acronym "ITB—itchy, twitchy, bad behavior" to help remember the early symptoms: itchy being a rash or scratching episodes, twitch being increased spasticity, and bad behavior being mood or psychologic disturbances, which can progress into delirium or psychosis as the late phase is reached. These symptoms require a medical professional evaluation by a practitioner who has experience interrogating baclofen pumps.

Late-phase symptoms require an emergency department visit, usually intensive care unit (ICU) admission, and often intubation and or urgent/emergency surgery. Late-phase symptoms can include early-phase symptoms plus fever and tachycardia.[9] Neuropsychiatric manifestations are not uncommon and include delirium, hallucinations, delusions, and paranoia. Life-threatening manifestations of withdrawal are rhabdomyolysis, diffuse intravascular coagulopathy, and malignant hyperthermia.[21–23] Seizures are often reported as part of baclofen withdrawal symptoms, and quite often patients have a diagnosis of epilepsy and epilepsy medications. It is very important to know that baclofen withdrawal whether in its oral or intrathecal form does not cause seizures, but baclofen overdose may, as discussed below. The differential diagnosis of baclofen withdrawal includes syndromes with autonomic dysfunction, e.g., serotonin syndrome, malignant hyperthermia, and neuroleptic malignant syndrome.[22] Other common occurrences that can look like early-phase withdrawal include urinary tract infections, any type of inflammatory reaction from systemic illnesses, and constipation/GI issues. These should all be worked up routinely during evaluation of withdrawal.

Catheter-related issues, e.g., catheter fracture or obstruction, should always be assumed to be the etiology for withdrawal; however, pump malfunction, which is rare, should be worked up by interrogating the pump. Side port aspiration is the easiest way to work up catheter malfunction and often eliminates the need for consideration of surgical exploration if found to be adequate in flow.

The initial steps for managing baclofen withdrawal are evaluating and treating the patient's "ABC's" airway, breathing, and circulation followed by ICU admission. Given that a common reason for withdrawal is proximity to pump refill date, an experienced ITB physician should be consulted to interrogate the pump. Catheter X-ray series have been historically used to evaluate for catheter fracture; however, the new Ascenda catheter is radiolucent, so a CT scan of the abdomen and thoracic spine is often required. A "spiral CT" protocol, which is a CT myelogram using the side port to inject contrast, may also be performed to evaluate catheter function.[24]

There are multiple ways to treat baclofen withdrawal. For early-phase withdrawal with patients on less than 500 μg/day of intrathecal baclofen, starting with high-dose oral medications up to 20 mg QID is recommended. All intrathecal baclofen patients should have oral medications at home for rescue therapy. For late phase, a combination of oral baclofen 20 mg every 6 h (through an Nasogastric or Oralgastric (NG/OG) tube) and Valium 5−10 mg every 6 h is recommended. Oral Periactin 4 mg every 6 h should also be provided. On admission, the physician should adequately work up pump malfunction. Does the reservoir need a refill or does an intrathecal bolus dose help? Lumbar punctures may be performed to administer an injection of 50−100 μg of intrathecal baclofen but usually are not needed.[25] Clearly, the goal of any baclofen withdrawal situation is to reinstitute the patient's previous baclofen dose.

The first course of action is to secure the airway with an endotracheal tube; uncontrolled spasticity can cause laryngeal constriction, so laryngeal mask airways or bilevel positive airway pressure ventilation (BiPAP) is not recommended. An intravenous propofol infusion or a benzodiazepine infusion is administered and titrated to the patient's vital signs, e.g., tachycardia and hypertension, as this will be the guide on the dosing regimen. Both propofol and benzodiazepines work at the $GABA_A$ receptor, whereas Baclofen works at the $GABA_B$. The chronic administration of baclofen results in the downregulation of $GABA_B$ receptors on neuronal membranes. This downregulation will specifically occur at $GABA_B$ receptors, leaving $GABA_A$ receptors close to their natural levels. As such, benzodiazepines and low-dose propofol are highly efficacious in the management of baclofen withdrawal. Some studies have advocated for the use of dantrolene and cyproheptadine in acute withdrawal. Although dantrolene helps with muscle relaxation, it does little in the way of reversing the course of baclofen withdrawal. Cyproheptadine aids in the treatment of withdrawal by reducing symptoms of spasticity, fever, and pruritus. Regardless of how the acute phase of baclofen withdrawal is treated, the patient will eventually require reinstitution of intrathecal baclofen therapy. As stated above, the most efficacious method for treating baclofen withdrawal is the reinstitution of the patient's usual baclofen regimen. For some patients, refilling of the pump reservoir will be sufficient. For other patients, pump and/or catheter revisions may be necessary for the system to work appropriately again.

BACLOFEN OVERDOSE

The most common causes of overdose in intrathecal baclofen delivery are iatrogenic and are correlated with pump refilling and dose titration.[21] Baclofen overdose has become significantly less common since the advent of intrathecal drug delivery systems (IDDSs). This is largely due to the fact that intrathecal administration obtains an efficacious intrathecal concentration while keeping the intravascular concentration low. The intravascular concentration of baclofen with intrathecal administration is approximately 100-fold less than with oral dosing.[7] Furthermore, the automated process of drug administration either through scheduled boluses or continuous slow infusion rate helps to maintain a steady-state concentration that is difficult to achieve through oral administration. Unfortunately, baclofen toxicity may still occur with intrathecal administration because of high infusion rates. Less likely causes of baclofen overdose are pump malfunction, and/or catheter issues, as these situations typically cause baclofen withdrawal.

The clinical manifestations of baclofen overdose have been well established because of its long history as an antispasticity medication. Adverse effects of baclofen administration include headache, drowsiness, dizziness, orthostatic hypotension, and seizures.[26] These symptoms may occur with regular administration of the drug and do not necessarily imply overdose but should put the treating physician on alert. The clinical signs of baclofen overdose include profound central nervous system depression, respiratory depression, altered mental status, coma, rostral progression of hypotonia/flaccidity, decreased reflexes, bradycardia, miosis, mydriasis, and seizures.[21,26,27] Importantly, the cardiovascular and sympathetic systems may be either stimulated or depressed, so it is difficult to rely on these findings when making the diagnosis of overdose. Seizures typically occur in oral baclofen overdose and can happen in the setting of routine oral administration with patients with a known epilepsy history. ITB, even in an overdose state, does not typically cause seizures, and if seizures are found in a patient, intrathecal baclofen overdose should rank much lower on the differential diagnosis list. Some patients require both intrathecal and oral baclofen therapies, and in these situations, all oral baclofen therapies should be immediately discontinued.

The treatment of baclofen overdose begins with evaluation and management of the "ABC's" airway, breathing, circulation, and admission to the ICU. There should be a very low threshold for intubation, and central venous access is commonly required to administer intravenous medications for cardiovascular augmentation for hypotension and bradycardia. An experienced care provider should interrogate the pump and assess for the amount of baclofen delivered. The pump rate should be adjusted as needed. There are situations where the pump reservoir should be emptied and either refilled with baclofen at the same concentration or if necessary filled with saline, and a side port aspiration should be performed to remove baclofen in the tubing.

In the case of severe baclofen overdose, the CSF concentration is significantly increased and CSF aspiration in increments of 30 mL to reduce the total amount of baclofen may be indicated. As stated above, the catheter side port can be used instead of an Lumbar Puncture (LP) or ventricular tap.[21] Beyond therapeutic use of the catheter side port, aspiration of CSF allows for additional testing of baclofen concentration but is not typically needed as long as clinical improvement of the patient is seen. Following cessation of intrathecal baclofen delivery, supportive care is provided in the ICU setting throughout the critical overdose period. Supportive care includes intravenous fluids, intubation, and mechanical ventilation for management of the patient's inability to protect the airway and respiratory depression, and benzodiazepines for seizures.[25] The patient's response to baclofen cessation should be followed with serial clinical examinations of patient spasticity, deep tendon reflexes, and rigidity. Intrathecal baclofen should not be completely discontinued, as the pump rotor may lock up and cause frank baclofen withdrawal.[21] We do not recommend the use of activated charcoal and dialysis in the instance of oral overdose or end-stage renal disease, respectively, as has been reported in the literature.[28,29] Finally, there are no reversal agents for baclofen overdose. Physostigmine has been shown to have poor results when compared with therapies mentioned.[29a] The mainstay of treatment is supportive care and prevention of acute withdrawal following cessation of drug delivery.

MANAGING COMPLICATIONS

As with the implantation of any foreign device in the human, baclofen IDDSs have a high risk of infection. The postoperative infection is typically located in the pump pocket owing to the catheter site being surrounded by muscular tissue unless the patient also has a CSF leak. For a pump pocket infection, we have lovingly labeled the management technique as the "Dr. Michael S. Turner Switch Technique." This involves positioning the patient in the lateral decubitus position with the original pump side down, placing a new intrathecal catheter and pump on the contralateral side, and then closing the wounds. The original pump and catheter system is then removed by opening the original paramedian incision, removing the old intrathecal catheter while simultaneously fixing a CSF leak, and then flipping the patient supine to remove the rest of the infected catheter and pump system. A wound vacuum is placed after performing a deep abscess I&D of the wound over the old pump pocket. Next, long-term wound vacuum care and IV antibiotics are administered. This completely avoids the need to slowly wean down the pump over weeks to months, explanting the hardware and then treating for antibiotics for months followed by reimplantation. We have had zero reinfections after the "Dr. Michael S Turner Switch Technique" to date. Of note, it is often difficult if not impossible to reach under the same draping and perform the various maneuvers of this procedure, so the patient will need to be reprepped and draped multiple times during the procedure.

Catheter fracture/kinking is not seen with the new Medtronic Ascenda catheter except in cases of traumatic injury. If an older catheter (implanted before 2013) is being evaluated, it can occur. Catheter fracture may also occur during a routine pump replacement. If this does occur, it is recommended to place all new catheters from the intrathecal and tunneled side, as the catheter will fail later in life, and it will also eliminate the scenario where the wrong piece of catheter was repaired, thus requiring another surgery along with another episode of potential fatal baclofen withdrawal.

Despite case reports to the contrary, granulomas do not occur with intrathecal baclofen, single-drug therapy.[30] Intrathecal baclofen does not cause a histamine release, as intrathecal opioid medication does. We strongly believe that one patient reported in the literature at one time or concurrently had either intentionally or accidentally opioid pain medication delivered in the pump and that led to the granuloma.

CSF leak following intrathecal catheterization occurs at a much higher rate with the new catheter systems because of their low occlusion rate. Implantation of IDDSs requires penetration of the spinal dura. Dural infiltration results in a heightened risk of persistent CSF drainage from the dural defect.[31,32] CSF leak complications have been well established following dural puncture for spinal anesthesia, CSF collection, and chronic intrathecal catheterization.[8,33–37] Persistent CSF drainage creates a communicating tract between the intracranial or intrathecal space and the surrounding soft-tissue structures of the human body, resulting in subcutaneous seromas or persistent drainage through the surgical wound. CSF leaks may manifest with positional headaches secondary to intracranial hypotension, nausea, vomiting, pseudomeningoceles, meningitis, or cranial nerve deficits.[36] Postdural puncture headaches and persistent CSF leaks are overlapping pathologies that differ in time course. Approximately 90% of postdural puncture headaches occur within 48 h of dural puncture, whereas persistent CSF leaks may occur anywhere from a few days to many years after a procedure.[36]

Although CSF leak rates are well studied in relation to cranial and spinal surgery, leak rates range 0.8%–13%,[38] much remains unknown about CSF leaks following intrathecal catheterization for the chronic administration of intrathecal medication. A recent retrospective study found that postdural puncture headaches occur in 23% of chronic intrathecal catheterizations and 21% of these leaks require additional procedures, e.g., epidural blood patch or laminectomy for surgical identification and closure.[35] Unfortunately, there is a significant paucity of data regarding CSF leaks after intrathecal catheterization because most neurosurgical studies consider CSF leak complications to have occurred only if there is persistent CSF leakage from the surgical wound or palpable swelling in the lumbar region or along the catheter/pump tract while neglecting the incidence of symptomatic headache. As such, the true CSF leak rate following intrathecal catheterization for chronic administration of baclofen with the new Ascenda system is unpublished. Soon-to-be-published analysis of our institutional leak rate indicates that the true leak rate is likely closer to the upper end of the spectrum.

The previous standard of care for preventing CSF leaks after intrathecal catheterization includes an off-midline or paramedian approach for the Tuohy needle, using the smallest bore needle that is still adequate for catheter placement, minimizing the number of dural punctures, and placement of a purse string suture around the Tuohy needle before removal.[8] There is limited evidence that bevel position affects CSF leak rate. Rather, the incidence of CSF leaks after dural puncture is likely tied to the thickness of the dura at the infiltrated level and size of the puncture.[36] Unfortunately, a significant portion of the patient population receiving prolonged intrathecal catheterization demonstrates postdural puncture headache and persistent CSF leaks.[33,35]

CSF leaks from incidental and intentional dural puncture as well as prolonged intrathecal catheterization have been successfully treated with conservative measures, e.g., bed rest with the head of the bed kept flat, fluids, and caffeine.[36] For patients who remain symptomatic after conservative management, an invasive epidural blood patch is performed and is successful at a rate of 75% on the first attempt.[39] Subsequent blood patches improve overall efficacy.[36] A small proportion of patients have CSF leaks that are refractory to epidural blood patches and have traditionally been treated with open surgery, necessitating a laminectomy, direct visualization of the leak intraoperatively, and oversewing of the dural defect. Occasionally, intraoperative closure will also fail.[40] A number of case reports and small studies have demonstrated the efficacy of fibrin glue in the treatment of refractory CSF leak, following dural puncture and prolonged intrathecal catheterization.[33,40–45]

We are now using not only epidural blood patches but also intrathecal Tisseel to treat these leaks. The later seems to prevent the need for formal laminectomies and direct sew repairs of the CSF leaks. Later publications will likely show that this will be the standard of care for treatment of CSF leaks related to intrathecal catheterizations.

ORTHOPEDIC CONSIDERATIONS

As mentioned earlier in this chapter, IDD of baclofen has become the standard of care for patients suffering from spasticity of multiple origins.[7,9,10,46] Baclofen pumps are surgically placed in adults and children suffering from spinal and orthopedic deformities arising secondary to increased spasticity.[47] The administration of intrathecal baclofen has been shown to reduce the need for future orthopedic procedures in patients suffering from intractable spasticity. Furthermore, patients who were initially surgical candidates for orthopedic surgery, e.g., tendon release, have shown significant improvement after baclofen IDDS implantation such that orthopedic surgery was no longer warranted.[48] However, the implantation of the IDDS does not completely obviate that need for additional surgery, especially as it pertains to hip and spinal deformity. As such, it is frequently the case that the surgeon implanting the IDDS will either assist with the spinal or pelvic surgery or perform a concomitant operation.

BACLOFEN INTRATHECAL DRUG DELIVERY IN MAJOR DEFORMITY SURGERY FOR SCOLIOSIS

There is a high correlation between spasticity and scoliosis in the pediatric population. Although baclofen pumps are clearly efficacious for spasticity, the treatment of spasticity has not been shown to significantly alter the natural progression of scoliosis. At least one small case series postulated that intrathecal administration of baclofen increases the rate of progression of the scoliotic disease process.[49] Conversely, other studies have found a reduced rate of scoliotic progression following baclofen pump placement.[49] Regardless, given that long-segment deformity surgery involves significant spinal exposure and instrumentation, the complexity of the operation is increased in patients with IDDSs. As expected, there is an increased rate of complications following long-segment spinal deformity surgery in patients with baclofen IDDSs when compared with patients without (citation). Furthermore, there is also an increased risk of postoperative complications in patients undergoing concomitant placement of an intrathecal baclofen pump and spinal deformity surgery, including CSF leak.[49,50] A CSF leak following a long-segment deformity surgery with implanted graft material can be catastrophic and extremely difficult to manage. Finally, patients with baclofen pumps who require spinal surgery are at a much higher risk for the need for reoperation because of catheter malfunction, pump malfunction, infection, and persistent CSF leak.[50]

In some cases, the neurosurgeon performing the long-segment deformity operation may be the same surgeon who implanted the pump. In all other cases, it is imperative that the deformity surgeon coordinate with a surgeon familiar with IDDSs or with the surgeon who actually implanted the system. Careful attention should be paid to the spinal level at which the intrathecal catheter enters the spinal canal and the trajectory it takes to get there. Furthermore, the vertebral body at which the catheter tip is placed must be noted as moving the catheter tip cephalad or caudal may result in baclofen overdose or withdrawal, respectively. During the initial dissection to the spinal column, blunt dissection with Bovie electrocautery will permit visualization of the catheter with minimal risk of violation. If the catheter is fractured or accidentally removed from the intrathecal space, it will need to be replaced immediately or at the very latest within 24–48 h. Again, this is largely due to the high risk of baclofen withdrawal in patients who have become dependent on intrathecal baclofen.

When dissecting down to the spine, blunt dissection and Bovie electrocautery should be used. It is highly unlikely that a catheter fracture will occur with either of these dissection techniques. There should be no attempt to remove and/or replace the intrathecal catheter unless it is inadvertently removed from the thecal sac. The removal of the catheter will significantly increase the chances of a CSF leak and may lead to poor arthrodesis in the long-segment fusion.

CONCLUSION

Intrathecal baclofen can be an extremely effective treatment modality for a large population of patients suffering from medically refractory spasticity. The surgeon must be aware of proper techniques of implantation and must also have the tools to manage complications associated with the procedure to give patients the best outcome possible. Having knowledge of how to identify and treat patients in baclofen withdrawal and overdose adds the needed layer of safety that patients and families are looking for in the age of subspecialized care in medicine.

REFERENCES

1. Blumenfeld H. *Neuroanatomy Through Clinical Cases*. 2nd ed. 2010.
2. Francisco GE, Saulino MF, Yablon SA, Turner M. Intrathecal baclofen therapy: an update. *PM R*. 2009;1:852–858.
3. Lynn AK, Turner M, Chambers HG. Surgical management of spasticity in persons with cerebral palsy. *PM R*. 2009; 1:834–838.
4. Ashworth B. Preliminary trial of carisoprodol in multiple sclerosis. *Practitioner*. 1964;192:540–542.
5. Bohannon RW, Smith MB. Interrater reliability of a modified Ashworth scale of muscle spasticity. *Phys Ther*. 1987; 67:206–207.
6. Krach LE. Pharmacotherapy of spasticity: oral medications and intrathecal baclofen. *J Child Neurol*. 2001;16:31–36.
7. Penn RD, Kroin JS. Long-term intrathecal baclofen infusion for treatment of spasticity. *J Neurosurg*. 1987;66:181–185.
8. Albright AL, Turner M, Pattisapu JV. Best-practice surgical techniques for intrathecal baclofen therapy. *J Neurosurg*. 2006;104:233–239.
9. Coffey JR, Cahill D, Steers W, et al. Intrathecal baclofen for intractable spasticity of spinal origin: results of a long-term multicenter study. *J Neurosurg*. 1993;78:226–232.

10. Penn RD, Savoy SM, Corcos D, et al. Intrathecal baclofen for severe spinal spasticity. *N Engl J Med.* 1989;320: 1517–1521.
11. Lazorthes Y, Sallerin-Caute B, Verdie JC, Bastide R, Carillo JP. Chronic intrathecal baclofen administration for control of severe spasticity. *J Neurosurg.* 1990;72: 393–402.
12. Saulino M, Guillemette S, Leier J, Hinnenthal J. Medical cost impact of intrathecal baclofen therapy for severe spasticity. *Neuromodulation.* 2015;18:141–149; discussion 149.
13. Chang E, Ghosh N, Yanni D, Lee S, Alexandru D, Mozaffar T. A review of spasticity treatments: pharmacological and interventional approaches. *Crit Rev Phys Rehabil Med.* 2013;25:11–22.
14. Simon O, Yelnik AP. Managing spasticity with drugs. *Eur J Phys Rehabil Med.* 2010;46:401–410.
15. Nance PW, Shears AH, Nance DM. Clonidine in spinal cord injury. *Can Med Assoc J.* 1985;133:41–42.
16. Tilton A, Vargus-Adams J, Delgado MR. Pharmacologic treatment of spasticity in children. *Semin Pediatr Neurol.* 2010;17:261–267.
17. Albright AL, Awaad Y, Muhonen M, et al. Performance and complications associated with the synchromed 10-ml infusion pump for intrathecal baclofen administration in children. *J Neurosurg.* 2004;101:64–68.
18. Kopell BH, Sala D, Doyle WK, Feldman DS, Wisoff JH, Weiner HL. Subfascial implantation of intrathecal baclofen pumps in children: technical note. *Neurosurgery.* 2001;49:753–756; discussion 756–757.
19. Anderson VC, Burchiel KJ. A prospective study of long-term intrathecal morphine in the management of chronic nonmalignant pain. *Neurosurgery.* 1999;44:289–300. Discussion 300–281.
20. Turner M, Nguyen HS, Cohen-Gadol AA. Intraventricular baclofen as an alternative to intrathecal baclofen for intractable spasticity or dystonia: outcomes and technical considerations. *J Neurosurg Pediatr.* 2012;10:315–319.
21. Watve SV, Sivan M, Raza WA, Jamil FF. Management of acute overdose or withdrawal state in intrathecal baclofen therapy. *Spinal Cord.* 2012;50:107–111.
22. Coffey RJ, Edgar TS, Francisco GE, et al. Abrupt withdrawal from intrathecal baclofen: recognition and management of a potentially life-threatening syndrome. *Arch Phys Med Rehabil.* 2002;83:735–741.
23. Coffey RJ, Ridgely PM. Abrupt intrathecal baclofen withdrawal: management of potentially life-threatening sequelae. *Neuromodulation.* 2001;4:142–146.
24. Turner MS. Assessing syndromes of catheter malfunction with SynchroMed infusion systems: the value of spiral computed tomography with contrast injection. *PM R.* 2010;2:757–766.
25. Saulino M, Anderson DJ, Doble J, et al. Best practices for intrathecal baclofen therapy: troubleshooting. *Neuromodulation.* 2016;19:632–641.
26. Wall GC, Wasiak A, Hicklin GA. An initially unsuspected case of baclofen overdose. *Am J Crit Care.* 2006;15: 611–613.
27. Leung NY, Whyte IM, Isbister GK. Baclofen overdose: defining the spectrum of toxicity. *Emerg Med Australas.* 2006;18:77–82.
28. Dias LS, Vivek G, Manthappa M, Acharya RV. Role of hemodialysis in baclofen overdose with normal renal function. *Indian J Pharmacol.* 2011;43:722–723.
29. Perry HE, Wright RO, Shannon MW, Woolf AD. Baclofen overdose: drug experimentation in a group of adolescents. *Pediatrics.* 1998;101:1045–1048.
29a. Delhass EM, Brouwers JR. Intrathecal baclofen overdose: report of 7 events in 5 patients and review of the literature. *Int J Clin Pharmacol Ther Toxicol.* 1991;29(7): 274–280.
30. Murphy PM, Skouvaklis DE, Amadeo RJ, Haberman C, Brazier DH, Cousins MJ. Intrathecal catheter granuloma associated with isolated baclofen infusion. *Anesth Analg.* 2006;102:848–852.
31. Hutter G, von Felten S, Sailer MH, Schulz M, Mariani L. Risk factors for postoperative CSF leakage after elective craniotomy and the efficacy of fleece-bound tissue sealing against dural suturing alone: a randomized controlled trial. *J Neurosurg.* 2014;121:735–744.
32. Jankowitz BT, Atteberry DS, Gerszten PC, et al. Effect of fibrin glue on the prevention of persistent cerebral spinal fluid leakage after incidental durotomy during lumbar spinal surgery. *Eur Spine J.* 2009;18:1169–1174.
33. Crul BJ, Delhaas EM. Technical complications during long-term subarachnoid or epidural administration of morphine in terminally ill cancer patients: a review of 140 cases. *Reg Anesth.* 1991;16:209–213.
34. Motta F, Antonello CE. Analysis of complications in 430 consecutive pediatric patients treated with intrathecal baclofen therapy: 14-year experience. *J Neurosurg Pediatr.* 2014;13:301–306.
35. Neuman SA, Eldrige JS, Qu W, Freeman ED, Hoelzer BC. Post dural puncture headache following intrathecal drug delivery system placement. *Pain Physician.* 2013;16: 101–107.
36. Turnbull DK, Shepherd DB. Post-dural puncture headache: pathogenesis, prevention and treatment. *Br J Anaesth.* 2003;91:718–729.
37. Vender JR, Hester S, Waller JL, Rekito A, Lee MR. Identification and management of intrathecal baclofen pump complications: a comparison of pediatric and adult patients. *J Neurosurg.* 2006;104:9–15.
38. Esposito F, Angileri FF, Kruse P, et al. Fibrin sealants in dura sealing: a systematic literature review. *PLoS One.* 2016;11:e0151533.
39. Safa-Tisseront V, Thormann F, Malassine P, et al. Effectiveness of epidural blood patch in the management of post-dural puncture headache. *Anesthesiology.* 2001;95:334–339.
40. Freeman ED, Hoelzer BC, Eldrige JS, Moeschler SM. Fibrin glue to treat spinal fluid leaks associated with intrathecal drug systems. *Pain Pract.* 2014;14:570–576.
41. Crul BJ, Gerritse BM, van Dongen RT, Schoonderwaldt HC. Epidural fibrin glue injection stops persistent postdural puncture headache. *Anesthesiology.* 1999;91:576–577.

42. Gerritse BM, van Dongen RT, Crul BJ. Epidural fibrin glue injection stops persistent cerebrospinal fluid leak during long-term intrathecal catheterization. *Anesth Analg*. 1997; 84:1140–1141.
43. Mihlon F, Kranz PG, Gafton AR, Gray L. Computed tomography-guided epidural patching of postoperative cerebrospinal fluid leaks. *J Neurosurg Spine*. 2014;21: 805–810.
44. Patel MR, Caruso PA, Yousuf N, Rachlin J. CT-guided percutaneous fibrin glue therapy of cerebrospinal fluid leaks in the spine after surgery. *Am J Roentgenol*. 2000; 175:443–446.
45. Patel MR, Louie W, Rachlin J. Postoperative cerebrospinal fluid leaks of the lumbosacral spine: management with percutaneous fibrin glue. *Am J Neuroradiol*. 1996;17: 495–500.
46. Albright AL, Cervi A, Singletary J. Intrathecal baclofen for spasticity in cerebral palsy. *JAMA*. 1991;265:1418–1422.
47. Rawicki B. Treatment of cerebral origin spasticity with continuous intrathecal baclofen delivered via an implantable pump: long-term follow-up review of 18 patients. *J Neurosurg*. 1999;91:733–736.
48. Gerszten PC, Albright AL, Johnstone GF. Intrathecal baclofen infusion and subsequent orthopedic surgery in patients with spastic cerebral palsy. *J Neurosurg*. 1998;88:1009–1013.
49. Caird MS, Palanca AA, Garton H, et al. Outcomes of posterior spinal fusion and instrumentation in patients with continuous intrathecal baclofen infusion pumps. *Spine (Phila Pa 1976)*. 2008;33:E94–E99.
50. Segal LS, Wallach DM, Kanev PM. Potential complications of posterior spine fusion and instrumentation in patients with cerebral palsy treated with intrathecal baclofen infusion. *Spine (Phila Pa 1976)*. 2005;30:E219–E224.

Index

Note: Page numbers followed by "f" indicate figures, "t" indicate tables.

Q

R

T

U

V

FSC
www.fsc.org
MIX
Papier | Fördert
gute Waldnutzung
FSC® C083411

Kolibri 360 GmbH
Ferdinand-Jühlke-Straße 7
99095 Erfurt, Deutschland
produktsicherheit@kolibri360.de